The Clinical Chemistry
of Laboratory Animals

Pergamon Titles of Related Interest

Altman   PATHOLOGY OF LABORATORY MICE AND RATS

Chapman   PREDICTION OF TUMOR TREATMENT
RESPONSE

Kallman   RODENT TUMOR MODELS IN EXPERIMENTAL
CANCER THERAPY

Related Journal*

Current Advances in Clinical Chemistry

*Free sample copies available on request.

The Clinical Chemistry
of Laboratory Animals

Edited by

Walter F. Loeb, VMD, PhD
MetPath Inc., Rockville, Maryland

and

Fred W. Quimby, VMD, PhD
Cornell University, Ithaca, New York

PERGAMON PRESS

NEW YORK · OXFORD · BEIJING · FRANKFURT
SÃO PAULO · SYDNEY · TOKYO · TORONTO

U.S.A.	Pergamon Press, Inc., Maxwell House, Fairview Park, Elmsford, New York 10523, U.S.A.
U.K.	Pergamon Press plc, Headington Hill Hall, Oxford OX3 0BW, England
PEOPLE'S REPUBLIC OF CHINA	Pergamon Press, Room 4037, Qianmen Hotel, Beijing, People's Republic of China
FEDERAL REPUBLIC OF GERMANY	Pergamon Press GmbH, Hammerweg 6, D-6242 Kronberg, Federal Republic of Germany
BRAZIL	Pergamon Editora Ltda, Rua Eça de Queiros, 346, CEP 04011, Paraiso, São Paulo, Brazil
AUSTRALIA	Pergamon Press Australia Pty Ltd., P.O. Box 544, Potts Point, N.S.W. 2011, Australia
JAPAN	Pergamon Press, 5th Floor, Matsuoka Central Building, 1-7-1 Nishishinjuku, Shinjuku-ku, Tokyo 160, Japan
CANADA	Pergamon Press Canada Ltd., Suite No. 271, 253 College Street, Toronto, Ontario, Canada M5T 1R5

First edition 1989

Library of Congress Cataloging-in-Publication Data
The Clinical chemistry of laboratory animals/edited by
Walter F. Loeb, Fred W. Quimby.
p.   cm.
Includes bibliographies and index.
ISBN 0-08-035180-8
1. Laboratory animals—Metabolism—Tables. 2. Laboratory animals—Composition—Tables. 3. Chemistry, Clinical—Tables. I. Loeb, Walter F. II. Quimby, Fred W.
[DNLM: 1. Animals, Laboratory.   QY 50 C641]
SF772.635.C57 1988
619—dc19
DNLM/DLC
for Library of Congress 88-28944

British Library Cataloguing in Publication Data
The clinical chemistry of laboratory animals
1. Man. Diseases. Models: Diseases in
laboratory animals
I. Loeb, Walter F. II. Quimby, Fred W.
619
ISBN 0-08-035180-8

Printed in Great Britain by A. Wheaton & Co. Ltd., Exeter

Preface

Millions of individual clinical chemistry determinations are performed annually on specimens from rats, mice, and other laboratory animal species in the course of biomedical studies. The information obtained is used in a plethora of journal publications and reports to regulatory agencies, which, as a whole, tend to be inaccessible to and unread by much of the user community responsible for interpretation of the data so generated. No single text is available to guide the scientist in the selection and interpretation of clinical chemical analyses on laboratory animals. In compiling this book, our principal objective was to bring this information to the user. It is our hope and belief that this book will be a valuable resource to laboratory animal veterinarians, clinical pathologists and clinical chemists, experimental toxicologists, and the host of other biomedical researchers, technologists, and technicians responsible for the optimal interpretation of clinical laboratory data from animals in research.

Each contributing author of this book has knowledge of both laboratory animals and clinical chemical evaluation, a rarely found combination. Each is a well-informed authority in his or her discipline and was given free rein with respect to the content, organization, and style of his or her chapter. As a result there is considerable variation among the chapters, reflecting both the available body of information and the author's vantage point. This brings us to the second objective of this book: to familiarize the reader with areas that have been well studied and areas in which information is lacking, fruitful new areas for investigation.

Internationally, the biomedical professions have agreed to use a system of units termed *Système International* (SI) built upon molar concentrations and metric units. Although most of the world has adopted this system, the United States has been slow to do so. Consequently, most of the values in this book are in conventional units. An introduction to SI is given in Chapter 15.

This book represents the participation and unselfish contributions of innumerable persons. To each we express our gratitude.

To the reader go our thanks for your support and for sharing our interest in upgrading the study of laboratory animals by the tools of clinical chemistry. In the future, we or others will revise this book, or others will be able to write a better book because this beginning was made. We will be grateful for your feedback, for calling to our attention the errors and omissions of this book which surely exist, and for sharing with us the information that will improve subsequent editions.

Walter F. Loeb
Fred W. Quimby

Contents

List of Contributors

Richard B. Bankert, VMD, PhD
Department of Molecular Immunology
Roswell Park Memorial Institute
Buffalo, New York 14263

Richard Carroll, PhD
Department of Preventive Medicine and
Community Health
University of Texas Medical Branch
Galveston, Texas 77550

Larry M. Cornelius, DVM, PhD
Department of Small Animal Medicine
College of Veterinary Medicine
University of Georgia
Athens, Georgia 30602

Louis DePaolo, PhD
Department of Physiology
University of Texas Health Science Center
San Antonio, Texas 78284

Lloyd Dillingham, DVM
New York State College of Veterinary Medicine
VRT 221
Cornell University
Ithaca, New York 14853

Elaine Feldman, MD
Medical College of Georgia
Department of Medicine
Section of Nutrition BG-230
Augusta, Georgia 30912-3102

Richard Fox, PhD
The Jackson Laboratory
Bar Harbor, Maine 04609

Tracy French, DVM
Department of Pathology
New York State College of Veterinary Medicine
Cornell University
Ithaca, New York 14853

Walter E. Hoffman, DVM, PhD
College of Veterinary Medicine
Department of Veterinary Pathobiology
University of Illinois
Urbana, Illinois 61801

Charles Howard, PhD
Oregon Regional Primate Research Center
505 N.W. 185th Avenue
Beaverton, Oregon 97006

Jiro J. Kaneko, DVM, PhD, DVCSc(Hon)
Department of Clinical Pathology
School of Veterinary Medicine
University of California
Davis, California 95616

Randy Kidd, DVM, PhD
RT 1 Box 466
St. George, Kansas 66535

John W. Kramer, DVM, PhD
Clinical Pathology Section
Department of Veterinary Clinical Medicine
and Surgery
College of Veterinary Medicine
Washington State University
Pullman, Washington 99164-6610

Samuel Krukenberg, DVM, PhD
Department of Pathology
College of Veterinary Medicine
Manhattan, Kansas 66506

C. Max Lang, DVM
Department of Comparative Medicine
M. S. Hershey Medical Center
P.O. Box 850
Hershey, Pennsylvania 17033

Walter F. Loeb, VMD, PhD
Metpath Inc.
Rockville, Maryland 20850

A. Russell Main, PhD (Deceased)

Edward Masoro, PhD
Department of Physiology
University of Texas Health Science Center
7703 Floyd Curl Drive
San Antonio, Texas 78284

Paul K. Mazzaferro, PhD
Phillips Petroleum Co.
Biotechnology Division
Bartlesville, Oklahoma 74004

Robert G. Meeks, PhD
School of Public Health
University of Alabama at Birmingham
University Station
Birmington, Alabama 35294

Hai T. Nguyen, VMD, MS
Research Animal Resource Center
Cornell University Medical College
1300 York Avenue
New York, New York 10021

Fred W. Quimby, VMD, PhD
New York State College of Veterinary
Medicine
221 VRT
Cornell University
Ithaca, New York 14853-6401

Harvey A. Ragan, DVM
Battelle Pacific Northwest Laboratories
Richland, Washington 99352

Julia Riley, DVM, MS
Experimental Pathology Laboratories
P.O. Box 12766
Research Triangle Park, North Carolina 27709

Juan L. Torres, PhD
Department of Chemical Engineering
North Carolina State University
Raleigh, North Carolina 27650-7905

Gerald L. Van Hoosier, DVM
Division of Animal Medicine SB-42
University of Washington
Seattle, Washington 98195

K. Jane Wardrop, DVM, MS
Department of Veterinary and Comparative
Anatomy, Pharmacology and Physiology
College of Veterinary Medicine
Washington State University
Pullman, Washington 99146

William J. White, VMD, MS
Charles River Laboratories Inc.
251 Ballardvale Street
Wilmington, MA 01887

PART A

Clinical Chemical Studies
Applicable to Laboratory Animal
Species and Their Interpretation

1

The Mouse

FRED W. QUIMBY, VMD, PhD

In the United States, the mouse is the most widely used mammalian species in biomedical research, with 8,500,000 mice being used in 1983 (127). It is estimated that the use of mice exceeds twofold that of rats (next most popular mammal). Mice represented 61 per cent of all vertebrate mammals used in 1983. In addition, although the number of other commonly used research animals is declining, the number of mice used during the 1980s is increasing (127). Since 1901 when the first Nobel prize for physiology and medicine was awarded, 11 Nobel laureates have received this award based on work specifically involving mice (119). Many characteristics of mice, such as small body size, ease of care, availability in a disease-free state, inexpensiveness, and genetic purity, make this species well suited for biomedical research; however, perhaps the greatest advantage of this species over other animals used in research is its well-described genetic composition.

Often, in biomedical research, there is a need to understand if the observations recorded are due to genetically or nongenetically determined factors. This type of discrimination is possible using the mouse, because of development of inbred strains, congenic lines, and recombinant inbred strains. Inbreeding has been used successfully to produce strains of mice with genetic homogeneity. The most common method employs 20 successive generations of brother by sister matings, which leads to progeny with a theoretical inbreeding coefficient of 0.986 (4); this coefficient measures the probability that both alleles at a locus are identical by descent. Inbreeding gains tend to plateau before the inbreeding coefficient reaches 1 because of the countering effects of new mutations. However, the theoretical probability of reaching total homozygosity and genetic fixation takes place between inbred generations 35 to 40. Two practical implications arise from these observations: (1) following 20 inbred generations, each animal within the strain is essentially uniform in genotype, and (2) a strain maintained in isolation by inbreeding after 20 generations should be designated as an individual subline because continued mutations may allow this stock to become genetically divergent.

Once inbred strains are established, additional lines and strains can be generated through genetic manipulation. A congenic line may be developed when an inbred strain is bred to an individual bearing a distinctive gene, and the progeny bearing this gene are selectively backcrossed to the inbred strain. If backcrossing continues, eventually all genes except the distinctive gene are homozygous and identical to the original inbred strain. These congenic lines can then be used to evaluate the effect of a single locus (or closely linked loci) on a similar background. Inbred strains and congenic lines have allowed investigators to map the various murine chromosomes, recognize mutations, determine if isoenzymes are the result of multiple alleles or multiple loci, and explore such complex phenomena as immunoglobulin gene rearrangement, genetic control of immune responsiveness, and changes in the phenotypic expression of a single gene product associated with its interaction with other genes such as the expression of thymic alymphoplasia associated with the nude (nu) mutation in various inbred strains.

A third type of inbred animal, the recombinant inbred strain (RI), results from crossing two inbred strains and systematically inbreeding the first generation progeny by brother by sister matings for 20 generations. Each substrain, repeatedly inbred from a single brother by sister cross, will have a reassortment of loci with a fixed allele at each locus which is derived from one of the two original parental strains. The pattern of inheritance for the various genetic loci will be unique for each RI strain if no selection takes place during inbreeding. These RI strains have been particularly useful for assigning new traits to linkage groups (4).

Mutations at a single locus may have profound biochemical and physiologic effects on the host. Proper identification and characterization of mutations in the mouse have led to the development of a large number of murine models for some of man's most serious afflictions. In fact, the number of models for human disease available for study in the mouse is unparalleled by any other species. The Jackson Laboratory maintains 260 mutant genes in 400 different strains and stocks (68).

Because of the complexity of murine inbred strains, lines, and substrains, as well as the recognition of multiple alleles at single loci and mutant alleles, a standardized nomenclature has been developed. By following the rules of nomenclature, researchers can easily identify individually maintained sublines, indicate special procedures used in the maintenance of a strain, such as foster nursing, ova transfer, and ovary transplant, and give precise information relating to specific genes, such as allele, recessive or dominant mutation, and wild type (4). Lists of inbred strains (155), congenic lines, and segregation inbred strains and recombinant inbred strains (54,63) are also available.

Given the tremendous genetic complexity of the mouse, it is not surprising that mice that are not genetically pure occasionally make their way into the research laboratory (49). The reasons include residual heterozygosity, recent mutations (not fixed by inbreeding), and pedigree errors or contamination. To ensure the genetic purity of breeding colony mice, a system of genetic monitoring should be employed. Such programs have employed mandible shape analysis (172), biochemical and serologic markers (54,116), and DNA restriction enzyme analysis (85).

The amount of clinical chemistry information available on the mouse is tremendous, relates in large part to investigations of murine models of human disease, and is impossible to review completely in this chapter. However, in the discussion of specific tests, clinical chemistry data will be presented in several popular murine model systems.

SAMPLING TECHNIQUE

One problem that has prevented the mouse from being used more widely in the evaluation of serum chemistries is its small body size and the difficulty in obtaining an adequate blood sample. However, the recent development of micromethodology for many chemistry assays allows the mouse to be used for sequential small blood sampling. Three techniques used for blood collection in the mouse are retroorbital plexus sampling (69), tail vein sampling (31), and heart puncture (56,152). In each procedure, 0.5 to 0.7 ml of blood may be obtained from adult mice as a survival procedure that can be repeated. The orbital plexus may be used successfully to collect small volumes (30 to 80 μl) from mice 14 to 16 days old. Larger volumes may be obtained from the tail vein if a vacuum apparatus is used (124). General anesthesia is recommended for orbital plexus and heart puncture techniques (31). Lewis et al. (96) found that heparinization of the mouse before tail bleeding increases the yield. Prewarming the mouse under a lamp or by immersion in warm water facilitates the bleeding procedure.

Disadvantages associated with tail bleeding techniques include stimulation of the sympathetic nervous system, significant differences between samples and between tail vein blood and orbital plexus blood, and mixing of venous and arterial blood (147).

Loeb (99) found that when mice were bled via

the orbital plexus, there was an elevation of the enzymes alanine aminotransferase, aspartate aminotransferase, and lactic dehydrogenase on subsequent bleeding from the contralateral orbital sinus. The effect was observed on rebleeding within 1 minute or as long as 48 hours after the initial collection.

Patrick et al. (133) compared the values of several routine clinical chemistry measurements conducted on N:NIH(S) mice submitted to intracardiac or jugular vein collection. They found that the sample collection technique greatly affected two chemical parameters and that intracardiac collection was associated with a higher glucose and a lower creatine phosphokinase (CPK) level.

The anesthetic or physical restraint method used during blood collection may also lead to increased variation among certain analytes; this problem has been reviewed by Pfeiffer and Muller (136).

Four additional bleeding procedures that yield greater volumes of blood have been described, but each requires anesthesia and all are terminal. These are jugular vein (5), abdominal aorta (100), brachial artery (170), and exposed heart bleeding techniques (30,114). The technique of Young and Chambers (170) is reputed to be associated with minimal hemolysis.

The author has found that the use of heparized microhematocrit tubes, when combined with either tail vein or orbital plexus procedures, has the added advantage of immediately separating plasma from cellular components after centrifugation and breaking the capillary tube above the buffy coat line (140). This procedure maximizes the retrievable plasma volume and minimizes hemolysis.

A variety of inhalation and injectable anesthetics are available and safe for use in mice (31). Several anesthetics, such as ether, chloral hydrate, and tribromoethanol, have been associated with increased mortality in mice and rats caused by respiratory irritation, which may lead to airway obstruction (for ether), and the development of adynamic ileus after intraperitoneal injection of chloral hydrate and tribromoethanol (53,159). However, tribromoethanol is the anesthetic of choice at Jackson Laboratory (31). Halothane, methoxyflurane, and pentobarbital sodium have all been widely used and are safe; however, very little is known con-

cerning their effects on clinical chemistry values. Carbon dioxide narcosis provides sedation and analgesia for 1 to 2 minutes and is a good anesthetic for orbital bleeding (31). Fowler et al. (55) found no alterations in packed cell volume, urea, prothrombin, or alanine aminotransferase when rats anesthetized with CO_2 were compared with rats anesthetized with ether; however, CO_2 did alter plasma glucose levels. Naturally CO_2 anesthesia would be unsatisfactory when blood gases are being measured. Ether anesthesia in mice is not associated with hematologic changes (31).

Restraint devices allowing for collection of blood from the tail of a conscious mouse have been described (156), as have devices designed for collection of urine from mice for periods in excess of 24 hours (153,165).

Hemolysis is a continuing problem associated with serum collection in mice. Hemolyzed samples are associated with elevations in various enzymes. Everett and Harrison (42) have addressed this problem, providing advice on collection sites and animal numbers, and recommend heparinized plasma for routine chemical determinations.

REFERENCE RANGES

Variables

The usefulness of compiled control data will depend on controlling a large number of variables known to influence chemistry determinations. Included among those variables known to affect the host adversely are environmental factors, pathogens, and shipment. In addition, nutrition, time of sample collection, and storage techniques may all contribute to variability.

Everett and Harrison (42) illustrate the effect of strain, sex, and age differences on selected chemistry determinations. Finch and Foster (50), evaluating the effect of age on 16 hematologic and electrolyte values, found no alterations in electrolytes providing the aged population were free of gross pathologic lesions. However, significant age-associated changes in serum calcium determinations have been reported in certain strains of mice (9). Profound differences in chemistry determinations may be seen between strains of mice (173). Strain-associated changes appearing in healthy animals have been documented for complement components (61), cholesterol (37,111), testosterone (79), cortisol-binding protein (62), and serum protein (14). The sex of the mouse is known to exert an effect on many parameters (9), and the increased variability seen in certain analyte levels of female mice is thought to be the effect of estrus (42).

The degree of hydration, exposure to noise, degree of confinement, and environmental temperatures have all been shown to affect the metabolism and toxicity of drugs in mice (23); therefore, it is not surprising that similar environmental factors influence serum chemistry determinations (12,15,80,98,149).

Diet is known to influence the blood levels of many plasma (serum) analytes. Perhaps the best studied of these is the effect of atherogenic diets on serum cholesterol (117). Similarly, significant differences in both serum cholesterol and blood urea nitrogen are seen in mice maintained on a semipurified (AIN-76) diet (64). The mouse is unique among mammals because it carries neither carnosine nor anserine (18). Because carnosine probably serves as a resource for histidine when its intake is low, one may speculate that the mouse is more sensitive than other animals to dietary histamine (130).

The presence or absence (axenic) of intestinal microbial flora is associated with dramatic changes in immunoglobulin levels (163) and may be associated with changes in other analytes as well (161). Certainly, the presence of pathogens is associated with dramatic changes in various analytes (76,137), even when infection by those agents is subclinical (143).

These effects are particularly well known for lactic dehydrogenase-elevating virus in which infection is associated with major elevations in lactic dehydrogenase, isocitric dehydrogenase, malic dehydrogenase, aspartate aminotransferase, and glutathione reductase (142, 143,145).

Alterations in clinicopathologic parameters can be attributed to stress in mice. Landi et al. (91,92) found that plasma corticosterone concentrations in mice tested on arrival or 24 or 48 hours after arrival (by plane or truck transport) were significantly higher than those of control mice. Mice sensitized on arrival with sheep red cells as an antigen had significantly lower antibody titers, fewer plaque-forming cells, and a decreased delayed type of hypersensitivity reac-

tion when compared with normal mice allowed to acclimate to the facility for 48 hours.

The effect of serum storage at various temperatures and for varying periods has been reported in several domestic (84) and laboratory (114) species. Falk et al. (44) evaluated the effect of storage time (after freezing) on 20 serum analytes in 6 laboratory species. They found that in the mouse, only creatinine phosphokinase activity changed significantly with storage up to 28 days.

Quality Assurance

Everett and Harrison (42) stressed the importance of a clinical pathology quality assurance program that would include regular assays of pooled and commercially prepared preassayed sera. In addition, they encourage participation of the laboratory in a subscription quality assurance program. The within-day and day-to-day coefficient of variation should be known for each analyte being measured.

Because of the tremendous number of variables known to influence clinical chemistry values in mice, it is often prudent to test adequate numbers of control specimens along with the experimental samples. This technique is often impractical when tests are being conducted strictly for diagnostic purposes, and in those situations, compiled values controlled for as many variables as possible may be sufficient. Compilation of murine clinical chemistry data was accomplished by the Laboratory Animal Data Bank (National Technical Information Service).

Statistics

The normal values that define a reference range for a particular analyte in mice may be described using several methods. For values that fall into a Gaussian distribution, parametric methods, such as mean and standard deviation, are appropriate. Regardless of the distribution of data, it is generally useful to describe the limits that include 95 per cent of the test results in a disease-free population. For Gaussian distributed data, this is the range that includes 2 standard deviations above and 2 below the mean (167).

Certain murine analytes have non-Gaussian distributions and must be evaluated using non-parametric methods. A variety of methods are available and include the percentile method (42,105) and logarithm-transformed data analyzed using parametric methods (16).

The method of percentile estimates is more vulnerable to bias because of extreme values (outliers) than is the log-transformed parametric method. Boyd (16) asserts that a sample size of at least 120 is required to give 90 per cent confidence intervals using the percentile method, whereas a sample size of 50 may give reliable ranges if parametric analyses are used. Neither statistical method just described will replace raw data in certain situations.

SPECIFIC TESTS

Glucose

The concentration of blood glucose has been studied intensely in mice because of the availability of several murine models of diabetes mellitus (27,59,77,83). Glucose determinations generally are conducted on fresh serum; however, if some delay before analysis is anticipated, fluoride should be used as an anticoagulant and preservative because it inhibits glycolysis (114). Blood glucose in mice has been measured using a modification of Faulkner's method (59), the Somogyi-Nelson method (21), and the o-toluidine method (42). Each appears to give reliable results.

Glucose tolerance tests (GTT) have also been conducted in mice. A 1-hour GTT was performed by comparing preinjection serum to serum collected 1 hour following the administration of 2 mg/g (2 g/kg) of glucose intraperitoneally (128). A 4-hour GTT has also been described in which mice are given 10 ml/kg of 10 per cent glucose orally (59). This assay was very sensitive in measuring the differences in glucose tolerance following implantation of normal islet cells in New Zealand obese mice.

The hypoglycemic response to insulin also has been described in mice (21).

Serum Protein

Total serum proteins have been evaluated in mice using the Lowry (14,50) and Biuret (42,114) techniques. The Lowry method can accurately measure protein in a sample size of only 2 μl (50). Hyperproteinemia may be seen in mice during severe dehydration (42) and hypoproteinemia is associated with increased renal loss of protein as seen in glomerulonephritis (73).

Electrophoresis has been used to evaluate the major classes of serum (or plasma) protein. Cellulose acetate electrophoresis in barbital buffer is the most popular method used and gives excellent separation of α_1-, α_2-, β- and γ-globulins (50,114,150). This method has been used to demonstrate the murine myeloma monoclonal spike (95), alterations in serum proteins in mice afflicted with immune complex glomerulonephritis (157), and protein alterations in mice of the mottled locus with an intestinal copper transport defect (150).

The major serum protein, albumin, has been measured accurately in mice using the radial immunodiffusion technique with goat anti-mouse albumin antibody (14,73). This technique also has sufficient sensitivity to measure urinary albumin in mice with glomerulonephritis (73).

Zizkovsky (173) identified three specific murine fetal serum proteins using immunoelectrophoresis. These fetal proteins correspond to α_1-fetoprotein, lipoprotein esterase, and a counterpart to rat α_2-slow globulin. Alpha-1-fetoprotein was also found in the serum of mice receiving a transplantable hepatoma (1).

Three murine pregnancy-associated serum proteins, PAMP-1, PAMP-2, and PAMP-4, which correspond to human pregnancy zone protein, human pregnancy-specific β_1-glycoprotein, and α-fetoprotein, respectively, may be demonstrated using a sensitive line immunoelectrophoresis technique (66). The dependency of these serum proteins on pregnancy was demonstrated by Lin et al. (97).

Lipids

Total serum cholesterol in mice has been measured using the enzymatic oxidation method of Roschlay (111), the Lipid Research Clinics Program protocol (117), and the Abell technique (114). These methods have the necessary sensitivity to measure differences in serum cholesterol associated with H-2 haplotype (111) and diet (117,132). Dunnington et al. (37) also used serum cholesterol determinations as a factor for genetic selection to produce hypercholesterolemic, high activity mice. Mark et al. (103) measured changes in blood cholesterol in autoimmune disease-prone mice on various diets.

Serum triglycerides have been measured using

the Lipid Research Clinics Program protocols, and normal as well as abnormal triglyceride levels have been reported (19,103,117).

The distribution and characterization of murine serum lipoproteins and apoproteins have been reported (20). Using density gradient ultracentrifugation, nine subfractions of murine lipoproteins were identified and later characterized by electrophoretic, immunologic, chemical, and morphologic analyses. Similar methods were used to evaluate changes in serum lipoproteins during diet-induced atherosclerosis in mice (117).

Electrolytes

Sodium and potassium levels are easily measured in murine serum using flame photometry (lithium reference) (42,50). Serum sodium levels are slightly higher in mice than in most other mammalian species with reported values of 174 ± 23 (SD) mEq/l (50) and 147 ± 15 (SD) mEq/l (42). No differences in serum sodium were seen during aging (50). Serum chloride has been measured using mercuric thiocyanate (42) and the chloridometric (114) techniques, and inorganic phosphorus in mice has been measured using the phosphomolybdate technique (42, 114).

Calcium

Total serum calcium in mouse serum has been measured using the sodium alizarin sulfonate technique (42) or atomic absorption spectrometry (9,114). Two reports, using different techniques, list similar reference ranges of 9 ± 1 (SD) mg/dl (9,42), whereas a third report lists reference ranges of 5.6 ± 0.4 (SD) mg/dl for male and 7.4 ± 0.50 (SD) mg/dl for female albino mice (114). The latter values reported for male mice were significantly lower than those for six inbred strains of mice in two different age groups using the same technique (9). Likewise, no differences associated with sex were reported by Everett and Harrison (42) who also examined random bred albino mice. However, Bonella et al. (13) demonstrated a significantly higher level in female Swiss albino mice.

Total calcium levels reflect both ionized (active) calcium and protein-bound calcium; therefore, mice with decreased serum albumin levels are expected also to have decreased total calcium levels. Alcock and Shils (3) found that in mice fed magnesium-deficient diets hypocalcemia developed as it did in mice receiving intramuscular injections of heparin (13). Bonella et al. (13) demonstrated significantly elevated calcium levels when blood was collected by orbital puncture versus cardiac puncture.

Enzymes

Alkaline Phosphatase (AP)

This production enzyme (in which serum concentrations change as a result of synthesis) is found in the highest concentrations in the kidney and intestine in mice (25) with virtually no detectable activity in the liver when measured using the Hausamen technique (67). Kinnett and Wilcox (88) assayed murine AP by measuring the rate of hydrolysis of p-nitrophenyl phosphate in the presence of isoenzyme (52). They found evidence of two isoenzymes of AP in mouse liver, both cytosolic in location and each requiring different pH and manganese requirements for optimal measurement. Fassati et al. (45) measured AP fluorometrically using 2-naphthyl phosphate as a substrate and quantitated two liver isoenzymes of AP that changed in activity in the liver during the course of mouse hepatitis virus infection with the appearance of the anodic isoenzyme in the plasma after 48 hours. Intestinal AP activity was shown to vary fourfold between two strains of Swiss mice (123). This difference in activity was under polygenic control and was influenced by a strain-specific factor in milk (122). Whether these differences reflect changes in catalytic activity or tissue concentration is unknown. In most species, changes in the serum activity of AP do not occur in hepatocellular disease unless accompanied by cholestasis (42). Clampitt and Hart (25) stress that the method used to measure AP in mice may be important.

Alanine Aminotransferase (ALT, GPT)

Alanine aminotransferase is a leakage enzyme (reflects alterations in cell membrane function) found in highest concentration in the liver of mice; however, tissue activity can also be demonstrated in intestine, kidney, heart, muscle, brain (25), skin, pancreas, spleen, and erythrocytes (24). Activity in spleen and erythrocytes was not found by others (38). Ruscak et al. (146) demonstrated that most species have two proteins with ALT activity, one located in the cytosol and the other in mitochondria. Despite its widespread tissue distribution, ALT is a useful analyte to measure as an index of hepatocellular damage (42). An 11,000 per cent increase in serum ALT activity has been reported following infection with mouse hepatitis virus (33).

Aspartate Aminotransferase (AST, GOT)

Aspartate aminotransferase is a leakage enzyme associated with both cytosol and mitochondria in the mouse (36). Dooley (36) found that 59 per cent of the total activity of liver AST was mitochondria associated in the mouse. The tissue distribution of AST includes liver, blood vessels, brain, intestine, kidney, lung, testes, and cardiac and skeletal muscles (129); however, the activity in lung, kidney, intestine, and skeletal muscle was very low (25) as measured by the technique of Bergmeyer and Bernt (11). With histochemical techniques, AST was shown to be nonuniformly distributed in the liver, with periportal hepatocytes containing greater enzymatic activity (129). The highest specific activity of AST was found in mouse cardiac muscle, and skeletal muscle had the lowest activity of those tissues studied (70). Because of its widespread distribution, injury to several organs may be associated with serum elevations of AST in the mouse (42); however, the differential location of 2 isozymes in liver cytosol and mitochondria has been used to assess the degree of hepatic injury in mice infected with mouse hepatitis virus (45). Reference values for murine AST have been reported (19,42).

Lactic Dehydrogenase (LDH)

Lactic dehydrogenase is a leakage enzyme that in mouse and man is characterized by five isozymes identified as LDH-1 through LDH-5 (46). In tissues LDH is under control of 2 structural genes that determine the A and B polypeptides. The rate of synthesis of each in various tissues determines the specific isozyme distribution (82). The enzyme itself is composed of multiple subunits constructed of either A or B polypeptides. During early fetal development, all murine tissues contain LDH-5 (more A sub-

units) activity. As the embryo matures, tissues develop shifts in A or B subunit production so that during adulthood, each tissue contains a characteristic LDH profile (46). In adult mice, the heart contains LDH-1 and LDH-2, and most other tissues have intermediate LDH-3. Skeletal muscle and liver fail to exhibit this developmental shift and are composed predominantly of LDH-5 (104). Destruction of a particular tissue is characterized by the presence of the tissue-specific activity in the blood. Erythrocyte LDH-B subunits are under partial control of the Ldr regulatory gene located on chromosome 6. The Ldr-B$^-$ phenotype (negative isozyme phenotype) is present in the red cells of most mouse strains except SWR which contain LDH-4 (A^3B^1) in their red cells (46). The mouse has highest activity of LDH in skeletal muscle, with decreasing activity in the heart, liver, kidney and intestine, respectively (25). The sera and liver of normal mice contain each of the five isozymes with LDH-5 in highest concentration (42). LDH-5 rises in the blood within 72 hours after inoculation of mice with mouse hepatitis virus (45). Mice infected with the LDH virus (LDV) exhibit increased serum concentrations of LDH, isocitric dehydrogenase, malic dehydrogenase, phosphohexase isomerase, and AST (126). Notkins (126) showed that increased enzymatic activity was due to a decreased rate of endogenous clearance by infected mice. Decreased plasma protein turnover has also been associated with LDV in mice (142).

Ornithine Carbamoyltransferase (OCT)

Ornithine carbamoyltransferase is a mitochondrial enzyme found primarily in the liver of mice (115). Increases in the serum of mice reflect severe injury to hepatocytes, resulting in disruption of mitochondrial membranes (42). There is no simple method to assay for OCT; therefore, it is not frequently measured. An abnormal OCT has been described in mice having the sparse-fur mutation (32).

Creatine Phosphokinase (CPK)

Creatine phosphokinase participates in the production of creatine phosphate from adenosine triphosphate (ATP) and creatine. The reaction is reversible, and it is thought that high amounts of CPK in muscle and brain tissues may allow maintenance of a constant ATP level and ensure immediate rephosphorylation of adenosine diphosphate (ADP) (39). The CPKs are dimeric enzymes with M and B subunits, and three dimeric combinations are found in mouse serum (42). In the mouse, the greatest activity of CPK is found in skeletal muscle with much less activity found in the heart and brain (25). The skeletal muscle contains the MM isozyme, cardiac muscle contains MM, MB, and BB isozymes, and brain contains the BB enzyme (2). No CPK activity is found in kidney, spleen, and liver; therefore, it is a useful marker enzyme for muscle injury.

The MM isozyme of CPK found in skeletal muscle cytosol is also localized in the thick filaments and on sarcoplasmic reticulum. Mitochondrial CPK is bound to the exterior aspect of the inner mitochondrial membrane (107). There is some evidence now that normal myocardium in man actually contains very little MB isozyme, but that during ischemia (myocardial infarction) there is expression of the fetal form of CPK (B-subunit), resulting in a greater tissue and serum concentration of the MB isozyme (78). Similar findings for other mammals have not been documented.

Aldolase

Aldolase is a cytosolic enzyme that can alter its distribution between soluble and particulate forms according to the metabolic status of the tissue (107). In adult mice, nine aldolase isozymes are known to occur in tissues with significant activities in muscle, brain, liver, kidney, and spleen (2). Everett and Harrison (42) report no apparent advantages in the measurement of aldolase over other enzymes known to have specific liver or muscle activity.

Sorbitol Dehydrogenase (SDH)

Sorbitol dehydrogenase is located primarily in the cyotplasm and mitochondria of liver, kidney, and seminal vesicles (25,34). The activity of SDH is usually low in the serum and rises during hepatic injury (34). A mechanized method for centifugal analyzer determination of SDH in the serum of mice has been developed which is based on conversion of D-fructose to sorbitol with simultaneous oxidation of NADH

(34). Reference values in normal mice are 26.8 ± 2.1 (SD) U/L.

Amylase

Amylase is a gene product in mouse pancreas and salivary gland. Production is controlled by two distinct but closely linked loci in mice, designated Amy-1 (salivary) and Amy-2 (pancreatic) (112). The product of Amy-1 gene appears to be a single enzyme; however, mouse pancreatic amylase is complex with electrophoretic diversity. Recent evidence suggests that the Amy-2 gene region comprises multiple gene copies with some divergence of regulation (112). Based on electrophoretic patterns, pancreatic amylase isozymes of inbred strains may be assigned to four classes: A_1, A_2, B_1, and B_2.

Mackenzie and Messer (101) found that mouse serum predominantly contained amylase of salivary gland origin, and urine contained only pancreatic amylase. When pancreatic amylase was injected into the blood of mice, it rapidly cleared through the urine.

Ross et al. (144) reported two to threefold increases in serum amylase activity in mice infected with Coxsackie virus of salivary and pancreatic trophism. Alterations in the activity of specific pancreatic isozymes have been shown in streptozotocin-induced diabetes in mice (112).

Other Enzymes

Pancreatic lipase containing two isozymes has been measured in mice (17). The enzyme 5'-nucleotidase was measured in the serum of normal mice using a simple one-step kinetic method (35). A reference range of 10.9 ± 4.5 (SD) U/L has been recorded in 100 mice, and it is thought but not proven to be a good indicator of hepatic injury.

Glutamate dehydrogenase (GDH) has been measured in the tissues (25) and serum (19) of mice. The activity of GDH is fivefold greater in the liver than in the kidney and brain, and the authors speculated that its measurement would be a sensitive indicator of hepatic cell injury (25). Cranmer and Peoples (29) found that the substrate 3-dimethyl butyl acetate was not acceptable in the measurement of cholinesterase in mouse plasma in which high levels of non-specific esterase complicate interpretation. Much is known concerning the function and molecular genetics of other murine enzymes (74); however, few have proven useful as predictors of disease.

Kidney Function

Urea Nitrogen

The kidneys play a complex role in maintaining homeostasis in the body and are involved in such functions as water and electrolyte balance, nutrient conservation, maintenance of blood pH, and removal of the end products of nitrogen metabolism, such as urea, creatinine, and allantoin. In addition, the kidney produces and responds to a variety of hormones (84). However, assessment of renal function is often compromised by their large functional capacity reserve. For instance, increases in blood urea nitrogen (BUN) do not occur until 70 to 75 per cent of the organ's mass has become functionally compromised (42).

Causes for increased BUN levels (azotemia) include prerenal, renal, and postrenal syndromes. Renal causes include agents and processes known to cause tissue destruction and loss of functional nephrons (42). Three causes for loss of glomerular function in mice are amyloidosis (22), immune complex disease (103), and polycystic disease (162). Each is associated with elevations in BUN.

Creatinine

Creatinine is the end product of muscle metabolism, with serum levels directly related to muscular conditioning and total muscular mass (42). Because creatinine is not metabolically active, it is excreted in urine. Creatinine is known to increase in the serum for reasons similar to those that cause elevations of BUN and offers no interpretative advantage (42).

Urinalysis

Proteinuria is a common finding in normal mice and includes uromucoid, small quantities of alpha and beta globulins, and a family of prealbumins known as major urinary protein (MUP)(4). The MUP has three electrophoretic variants, designed as 1, 2, and 3, that are under both genetic and hormonal control. A regulatory locus designed Mup-1 with codominantly expressed alleles a and b (located on chromosome 4) controls the urinary levels of the three variants. The MUP is synthesized in the liver, secreted into the blood, and excreted into the urine (4). Males are more proteinuric than are females (51) with levels of 5 mg/ml, and age-related increases are seen in mice of both genders (73). Increases in other urinary proteins have been associated with a variety of renal diseases in mice (22, 89, 106).

Complement

The mouse has been widely used as a model for studies concerning the biosynthesis and molecular biology of individual complement components (120). Currently, seven individual components have been identified (60,125). Complement component 4(C4) exists in the mouse as an active (true) C4 as well as an inactive form. The locus for active C4 is designated Ss and for the inactive (hemolytically inactive) form Slp (48). Both loci are located close to each other on chromosome 17, are linked to the major histocompatibility locus, and appear to have arisen by gene duplication. Heterologous antisera raised by C4 often cross-react with the Slp product and must be absorbed by Slp to be monospecific; however, various strains differ in their ability to express the Slp product, and therefore a monospecific antibody may be raised by inoculating serum from an Slp$^+$ individual into an Slp$^-$ individual (121).

The fifth component of complement is the product of a structural gene found on the second chromosome (40). Many strains of mice do not express the product of this locus because of a posttranslational defect and are therefore deficient in their capability to form a membrane attack complex, C5-9 (40).

Specific antisera directed against murine C3, C4, and C5 are commercially available and may be used to quantitate these proteins using radial immunodiffusion or rocket electrophoresis (47,134). Complement levels vary greatly in several spontaneous autoimmune diseases of mice (6), as well as during certain viral infections (94), as a result of endotoxemia (93) and after injection with various foreign substances (26). Mice of certain H-2 haplotypes have lower levels of C4 than do most strains (151), and the expression of the Slp product is sex dependent (131).

Circulating Immune Complexes

Circulating immune complexes (CIC) are multimolecular substances composed of antigen, antibody, and activated complement components. They generally signal the recognition by an antibody of a foreign substance in the blood. In the mouse, all IgM and subclasses of IgG including IgG1, IgG2a, and IgG2b have a complement activation region (43). Assays to detect immune complexes in mice usually involve binding of C3b to the CR1 receptor or precipitation of C1q using polyethylene glycol (58). A commonly used method involves the binding of immune complexes to the C3b, C3d, and C1a (160) receptors present on the Raji cell line (a mouse lymphoblastic leukemia cell). Circulating immune complexes have been measured using a sensitive ELISA in which a C1q substrate and AP-conjugated rabbit anti-mouse IgG antibody are employed (81).

In addition to foreign substances producing CIC, complexes are frequently found in NZB, BWF1 hybrids, MRL/Lpr/Lpr, and BXSB strains, in all of which a lupus erythematosus-like syndrome develops (58,81). The CIC levels in serum are found to fluctuate with sex (6) and diet (103) in these strains. The CIC may also arise as a result of viral infection and are classically associated with the congenital acquired infection with lymphocytic choriomeningitis virus (94). The CIC are cleared from the circulation by phagocytic cells generally expressing Fc or CR1 receptors (87). During periods characterized by high serum levels of CIC, tissue deposition may be associated with vasculitis (103), glomerulonephritis (89), and inflammation of the choroid plexus (90).

Immunoglobulins

The immunoglobulins of mice have been well characterized and include members of the heavy chain classes IgM, IgG, IgA, IgE, and IgD (139). Commercially prepared antisera are readily available for the quantitation of each class and most subclasses. Several companies manufacture radial immunodiffusion kits capable of quantitation of IgA, IgM, and all IgG subclasses. The levels of various immunoglobulin classes generally fluctuate with the activation of the immune system by antigenic substances; however, certain murine strains appear deficient in their ability to produce particular subclasses. For example, CBA/N mice have deficiencies of IgM and IgG3 (72,135,148), and other strains (characterized by an inherited defect in the thymic derived lymphocyte system, i.e., nudes) have a poor IgM to IgG shift, resulting in a deficiency of most IgG subclasses in the serum (113). In addition, at least one mouse strain, Balb/c, has serum IgA of unusual disulfide structure (65), and most mouse strains have a predominance (95 per cent) of kappa light chains in their sera (75).

Immunoglobulin levels are also greatly reduced in germ-free mice (166), and the offspring of mice on zinc-deficient diets (10) and in mice on protein-deficient diets (28). In the neonatal mouse, intestinal transport of immunoglobulin from milk is restricted to the IgG subclasses, involves enterocyte Fc receptors, and stops abruptly at 16 days of age (102). Antibody-secreting plasmacytomas or myelomas are easily induced in Balb/c mice (138), and their presence is characterized by a monoclonal spike of a particular antibody molecule (idiotype) easily demonstrated using immunoelectrophoresis (138).

Acute Phase Reactants

Serum Amyloid A (SAA)

Certain strains of mice are prone to develop secondary amyloidosis as a result of chronic inflammation (41), infection (164), or injection with casein (86,110). Mice of the LLC (low leukocyte count) strain (22) and KK strain (prone to diabetes mellitus) (154) appear to be particularly susceptible to renal amyloidosis. Endotoxin is a potent inducer of SAA in most strains of mice (158). Normally SAA, which is secreted by hepatocytes, a mechanism regulated by lymphoid cells and macrophages, behaves as an acute phase reactant and is quickly cleaved into a small molecular weight product (57). It is believed that in human amyloidosis, there is a defect in the SAA degradation pathway (109); however, in the amyloid susceptible Balb/c mouse, it has been shown that a serum amyloid A isotype (SAAL) is the only SAA product deposited in the mouse amyloid tissues (168). The gene that controls expression of this isotype is defective in the amyloidosis-resistant SJL mouse (168). Serum Amyloid A may be quantitated using radioimmune or ELISA assays;

however, antisera specific to the murine protein must be used (110).

Certain strains of mice are also prone to primary amyloidosis, which may be associated with aging (108,174) and kidney disease (71), and have not involved the AA protein (or AL protein).

C-Reactive Protein (CRP) and Serum Amyloid P Component (SAP)

C-reactive protein and serum amyloid P component are plasma proteins known as pentraxins. They share a common electron microscopic appearance, have a similar subunit structure, extensive amino acid homology, and calcium-dependent binding specificity for appropriate ligands (8). In the mouse, both these plasma proteins behave as acute phase reactants.

The SAP levels are sustained and high in response to daily casein injections in the amyloid-susceptible strains, CBA, and C57B1/6 (141); however, the role of SAP in amyloid induction in mice is unknown. Using electroimmunoassay and radiolabeling techniques, Baltz et al. (8) found that the in vivo half-life of SAP in the mouse is 7.0 to 8.25 hours. This was constant in all strains including those with different genetically determined plasma concentrations, those undergoing acute phase responses, and mice with casein-induced amyloidosis. The authors concluded that the circulating levels of SAP in mice are independent of clearance and catabolism and are determined by the rate of synthesis.

Levels of CRP in the mouse differ greatly from those of most mammalian species in that during an acute phase reaction, they are elevated in the microgram per liter range as opposed to the 100 mg/l range in most other species (7). Although the function of murine CRP is unknown, passively infused human CRP protects mice against lethal pneumococcal infection (169). This has been attributed to the ability of CRP to bind the c-polysaccharide (CPS) of pneumococci (118). Baltz et al. (7,8) studied the plasma clearance of radiolabeled human CRP in several strains of mice and found the half-life to be 4 hours. The half-life was independent of circulating levels of murine CRP and was not affected by the presence of CPS in the plasma. These authors concluded that CRP did not provide a mechanism for extremely rapid clearance

of its ligands from the circulation. Details on the measurement of CRP in mice are given in the chapter on Specific Proteins.

REFERENCES

1. Abelev GI, Perova SD, Khramkova NI, Postnikova ZA, Irlin IS (1963) Production of embryonal alpha-globulin by transplantable mouse hepatomas. Transplation 1: 174–180
2. Adamson ED (1976) Isoenzyme transitions of creatine phosphokinase, aldolase and phosphoglycerate mutase in differentiating mouse cells. J Embryol Exp Morphol 35: 355–367
3. Alcock NW, Shils ME (1974) Comparison of magnesium deficiency in the rat and mouse. Proc Soc Exp Med 146: 137–141
4. Altman PL, Katz DD (1979) Inbred and genetically defined strains of laboratory animals, part 1. Mouse and rat. Federation of American Societies for Experimental Biology, Bethesda, MD
5. Ambrus JL, Ambrus CM, Harrison JWE, Leonard CA, Moser CE, Cravitz H (1951) Comparison of methods for obtaining blood for mice. Am J Pharmacol 123: 100–104
6. Andrews BS, Eisenberg RA, Theofilopoulos AN, Izui S, Wilson CB, McConahey PJ, Murphy ED, Roths JB, Dixon FJ (1978) Spontaneous murine lupus-like syndromes. Clinical and immunological manifestations in several strains. J Exp Med 148: 1198–1215
7. Baltz ML, Rowe IF, Pepys MB (1985) In vivo turnover studies of C-reactive protein. Clin Exp Immunol 59: 243–250
8. Baltz ML, Dyck RF, Pepys MB (1985) Studies of the in vivo synthesis and catabolism of serum amyloid P component in the mouse. Clin Exp Immunol 59: 235–242
9. Barrett CP, Donati EJ, Volz JE, Smith EB (1975) Variations in serum calcium between strains of inbred mice. Lab An Sci 25: 638–640
10. Beach RS, Gershwin ME, Hurley LS (1982) Gestational zinc deprivation in mice: Persistence of immunodeficiency for three generations. Science 218: 469–471
11. Bergmeyer HU, Bernt E (1974) In Bergmeyer HU (ed), Methods of Enzymatic Analysis, 2nd English edition, Vol 2, Section C. Academic Press, New York, p 727
12. Besch EL (1985) Definition of laboratory animal environmental conditions. In Moberg GP (ed), Animal Stress, American Physiological Society, Bethesda, MD, pp 297–315
13. Bonella CA, Stringham RM, Lytle IM (1968) Effects of heparin on serum calcium concentrations in mice. Nature 217: 1281–1282
14. Borovkov A, Svirdov SM (1981) Albumin content in blood of inbred mice strains. Genetika 17: 1690–1692
15. Boyd JW (1983) The mechanisms relating to increases in plasma enzymes and isoenzymes in diseases of animals. Vet Clin Pathol 12: 9–24

16. Boyd JW (1985) The interpretation of serum biochemistry test results in domestic animals. Vet Clin Pathol 13: 7–14

17. Bradshaw WS, Rutter WJ (1972) Multiple pancreatic lipases. Tissue distribution and pattern of accumulation during embryological development. Biochem 11: 1517–1528

18. Brewer NR (1986) A note about histadine. Synapse 19: 12

19. Caisey JD, King DJ (1980) Clinical chemical values for some common laboratory animals. Clin Chem 26: 1877–1879

20. Camus M-C, Chapman MJ, Forgez P, Laplaud PM (1983) Distribution and characterization of the serum lipoproteins and apoproteins in the mouse, *Mus musculus*. J Lipid Res 24: 1210–1229

21. Carpenter KJ, Mayer J (1958) Physiologic observations on yellow obesity in the mouse. Am J Physiol 193: 499–504

22. Chai CK (1978) Spontaneous amyloidosis in LLC mice. Am J Pathol 90: 381–398

23. Chance MRA (1947) Factors influencing the toxicity of sympathomimetic amines to solitary mice. J Pharmacol Exp Ther 89: 289–296

24. Chen SH, Donahue RP, Scott CR (1973) The genetics of glutamic-pyruvic transaminase in mice: Inheritance, electrophoretic phenotypes and post natal changes. Biochem Genet 10: 23–28

25. Clampitt RB, Hart RJ (1978) The tissue activities of some diagnostic enzymes in ten mammalian species. J Comp Pathol 88: 607–621

26. Cockrane CG, Muller-Eberhard HJ, Aikin BS (1970) Depletion of plasma complement *in vivo* by a protein of cobra venom: Its effect on various immunologic reactions. J Immunol 105: 55–69

27. Coleman D (1982) Diabetes-obesity syndromes. In Foster HL, Small JD, Fox JG (eds), The Mouse in Biomedical Research, Vol 4. Academic Press, New York, pp 126–132

28. Cooper WC, Good RA, Mariani T (1974) Effects of protein insufficiency on immune responsiveness. Am J Clin Nutr 27: 647–664

29. Cranmer MF, Peoples AJ (1973) Measurement of blood cholinesterase activity in laboratory animals utilizing dimethylbutyl acetate as a substrate. Lab An Sci 23: 881–884

30. Cubitt JGK, Barrett CP (1978) A comparison of serum calcium levels obtained by two methods of cardiac puncture in mice. Lab An Sci 28: 347

31. Cunliffe-Beamer TL (1983) Biomethodology and surgical techniques. In Foster HL, Small JD, Fox JG (eds), The Mouse in Biomedical Research, Vol 3. Academic Press, New York, pp 401–437

32. DeMars R, LeVan SL, Trend BL, Russell LB (1976) Abnormal ornithine carbamoyltransferase in mice having the sparse-fur mutation. Proc Natl Acad Sci (USA) 73: 1693–1697

33. deRitis F, Cacciatore L, Ruggiero G (1969) Glutamic oxaloacetic and glutamic pyruvic transaminase of bile in different conditions of experimental hepatic pathology. Enzymol Biol Clin 10: 281–292

34. Dooley JF, Turnquist LJ, Racich L (1979) Kinetic determination of serum sorbitol dehydrogenase activity with a centrifugal analyzer. Clin Chem 25: 2026–2029

35. Dooley JF, Racich L (1980) A new kinetic determination of serum 5'-nucleotidase activity, with modifications for a centrifugal analyzer. Clin Chem 26: 1291–1297

36. Dooley JF, Masullo KM, Tse PH (1981) Hepatocellular aspartate aminotransferase activity and isoenzyme distribution in several laboratory animals. Clin Chem 27: 1038 (abstr)

37. Dunnington EA, White JM, Vinson WE (1981) Selection for serum cholesterol, voluntary physical activity, 56-day body weight and feed intake in random bred mice. II. Correlated responses. Can J Genet Cytol 23: 545–555

38. Eicher EM, Womack JE (1977) Chromosomal location of soluble glutamic-pyruvic transaminase-1 (GPT-1) in the mouse. Biochem Genet 15: 1–8

39. Eppenberger HM, Perriard J-C, Willimann T (1983) Analysis of creatine kinase isozymes during muscle differentiation. Isozymes: Current Topics in Biological and Medical Research 7: 19–38

40. Erickson RP, Tachibana DK, Herzenberg LA, Rosenberg LT (1964) A single gene controlling hemolytic complement and a serum antigen in the mouse. J Immunol 92: 611–615

41. Erikin N, Ericsson LH, Pearsall N, Lagunoff D, Benditt EP (1976) Mouse amyloid protein AA: Homology with non-immunoglobulin protein of human and monkey amyloid substance. Proc Natl Acad Sci 73: 964–967

42. Everett RM, Harrison SD, Jr. (1983) Clinical Biochemistry. In Foster HL, Small JD, Fox JG (eds.), The Mouse in Biomedical Research, Vol 3. Academic Press, New York, pp 313–325

43. Ey PL, Russell-Jones GJ, Jenkin CR (1980) Isotypes of mouse IgG. I. Evidence for non-complement fixing IgG1 antibodies and characterization of their capacity to interfere with IgG2 sensitization of target red blood cells for lysis of complement. Mol Immunol 17: 699–710

44. Falk HB, Schroer RA, Novak JJ, Heft SM (1981) The effect of freezing on various serum chemistry parameters from common lab animals. Clin Chem 27: 1039

45. Fassati M, Stepan J, Schon E, Hacker J (1969) Alkaline phosphatase, lactate dehydrogenase and aspartate aminotransferase and their isoenzymes as indicators of the development of experimental hepatitis in mice. Clin Chim Acta 26: 497–504

46. Felder MR (1980) Biochemical and developmental genetics of isozymes in the mouse, *Mus musculus*. Isozymes: Current Topics in Biological and Medical Reseach 4: 1–68

47. Ferreira A, Nussenzweig V (1975) Genetic linkage between serum levels of the third component of complement and the H-2 complex. J Exp Med 141: 513–517

48. Ferreira A, Takahasho M, Nussenzweig V (1977) Purification and characterization of mouse serum protein with specific binding affinity for C4 (Ss protein). J Exp Med 146: 1001–1018

49. Festing MFW (1982) Genetic contamination of laboratory animal colonies. An increasingly serious problem. ILAR News 25: 6–10

50. Finch CE, Foster JR (1973) Hematologic and serum electrolyte values of the C57 Bl/6j male mouse in maturity and senescence. Lab An Sci 25: 339–349

51. Finlayson JS, Baumann CA (1958) Mouse proteinuria. Am J Physiol 192: 69–72

52. Fitt PS, Peterkin PI (1976) Isolation and properties of a small manganese-ion-stimulated bacterial alkaline phosphatase. Biochem J 157: 161–167

53. Fleischman RW, McCracken D, Forbes W (1977) Adynamic ileus in the rat induced by chloral hydrate. Lab An Sci 27: 238–243

54. Foster HL, Small JD, Fox JG (1981) (eds) The Mouse in Biomedical Research, Vol 1. Academic Press, New York

55. Fowler JSL, Brown JS, Flower EN (1980) Comparison between ether and carbon dioxide anesthesia for removal of small blood samples in rats. Lab An 14: 275–278

56. Frankenberg L (1979) Cardiac puncture in the mouse through the anterior thoracic aperture. Lab An 13: 311–312

57. Franklin EC (1982) The amyloid diseases. In Lachmann PJ, Peters DK (eds), Clinical Aspects of Immunology, 4th ed, Vol 2. Blackwell Scientific Publications, Oxford, pp 1231–1245

58. Fujiwara M, Kariyone AI, Shiraki M (1985) Studies on the role of the Lpr gene in the development of immunological abnormalities and lupus nephritis. Analysis in F_2 mice. Clin Exp Immunol 59: 161–168

59. Gates RJ, Hunt MI, Smith R, Lazarus NR (1972) Return to normal of blood-glucose, plasma-insulin and weight gain in New Zealand obese mice after implantation of islets of Langerhans. Lancet 2: 567–570

60. Gigli I, Austen KF (1971) Phylogeny and function of the complement system. Ann Rev Microb 25: 309–329

61. Goldman MB, Goldman JN (1976) Relationship of functional levels of early components of complement to the H-2 complex of mice. J Immunol 117: 1584–1588

62. Goldman AS, Katsumata M, Yaffe SJ, Gasser DL (1977) Palatal cytosol cortisol-binding protein associated with cleft palate susceptibility and H-2 genotype. Nature 265: 643–645

63. Green MC (1981) (ed) Genetic Variants and Strains of the Laboratory Mouse. Fischer, Stuttgart

64. Greenman DL, Fullerton F, Gough B, Suber R (1982) Clinical chemistry and hematology of mice: A comparison of cereal-based and semipurified diets (abstr). Lab An Sci 32: 414

65. Grey HM, Sher A, Shalit N (1970) The subunit structure of mouse IgA. J Immunol 105: 75–84

66. Hau J (1985) Immunological cross-reaction between pregnancy associated serum proteins in different species. In Archibald J, Ditchfield J, Rowsell HC (eds), The Contribution of Laboratory Animal Science to the Welfare of Man and Animals. Gustav Fischer Verlag, Stuttgart, pp 71–77

67. Hausamen TU, Helger R, Rick W, Gross W (1967) Optimal conditions for the determination of serum alkaline phosphatase by a new kinetic method. Clin Chim Acta 15: 241–245

68. Heiniger H-J, Dorey JL (1982) (eds) Handbook on Genetically Standardized Jax Mice, Jackson Laboratory, Bar Harbor, ME

69. Herbert WJ (1978) Laboratory animal techniques for immunology. In Weir DM (ed), Handbook of Experimental Immunology, 3rd ed. Blackwell Scientific Publications, Oxford, pp A4.1–A4.29

70. Herzfeld A, Knox WE (1971) The distribution of aspartate aminotransferases in normal and neoplastic rat and mouse tissues. Enzyme 12: 699–703

71. Heston WE, Deringer MK (1948) Hereditary renal disease and amyloidosis in mice. Arch Pathol 46: 49–59

72. Hiernaux JR, Jones JM, Rudbach JA, Rollwagen F, Baker PJ (1983) Antibody response of immunodeficient (xid) CBA/N mice to *Escherichia coli* 0113 lipopolysaccharide, a thymus-independent antigen. J Exp Med 157: 1197–1207

73. Hoffsten PE, Hill CL, Klahr S (1975) Studies of albuminuria and proteinuria in normal mice and mice with immune complex glomerulonephritis. J Lab Clin Med 86: 920–930

74. Homes RS, Duley JA, Burnell JN (1983) The alcohol dehydrogenase gene complex on chromosome 3 of the mouse. Isozymes: Current Topics in Biological and Medical Research 8: 155–174

75. Hood L, Grant JA, Sox HC (1969) In Steryl J, Riha I (eds), Developmental Aspects of Antibody Formation and Structure, Vol 1. Academic Press, New York, 283

76. Hsu CK, New AE, Mayo JG (1980) Quality assurance of rodent models. In: Seventh ICLAS Symposium. Gustav-Fischer Verlag, New York

77. Hummel KP, Dickie MM, Coleman DL (1966) Diabetes, a new mutation in the mouse. Science 153: 1127–1128

78. Ingwall JS, Kramer MF, Fifer MA, Lorell BH, Shemin R, Grossman W, Allen PD (1985) The creatine kinase system in normal and diseased human myocardium. N Engl J Med 313: 1050–1054

79. Ivanyi P, Hampl R, Starka L, Mickova M (1972) Genetic association between H-2 gene and testosterone metabolism in mice. Nature (New Biol) 238: 280–282

80. Jensen MM, Rasmussen AF (1963) Stress and susceptibility to viral infection. J Immunol 90: 17–20

81. Jones MG, Harris G (1985) Prolongation of life in female NZB/NZW (F_1) hybrid mice by cyclosporin A. Clin Exp Immunol 59: 1–9

82. Jungmann RA, Derda DF, Kelley DC, Miles MF, Milkowski D, Schweppe JS (1983) Regulation of lactate dehydrogenase gene expression. Isozymes: Current Topics in Biological and Medical Research 7: 161-174

83. Khan CR, Neville DM, Roth J (1973) Insulin-receptor interaction in the obese hyperglycemic mouse. J Biol Chem 248: 244–250

84. Kaneko JJ (ed) (1980) Clinical Biochemistry of Domestic Animals, 3rd ed. Academic Press, New York

85. Katoh H, Esaki K, Shoji Y, Nomura T, Moriwaki K, Yonekawa H (1985) Demonstration of genetic profiles in various lines of ARR and NZB by a genetic monitoring system. In Archibald J, Ditchfield J, Rowsell HC (eds), The Contribution of Lab-

oratory Animal Science to the Welfare of Man and Animals. Gustav Fischer Verlag, Stuttgart, pp 495–502

86. Kedar I, Ravid M, Sohar E, Gafni J (1974) Colchicine inhibition of casein-induced amyloidosis in mice. Israel J Med Sci 10: 787–791

87. Kimberly RP, Parris TM, Inman RD, McDougal JS (1983) Dynamics of mononuclear phagocyte system Fc receptor function in systemic lupus erythematosus. Relation to disease activity and circulating immune complexes. Clin Exp Immunol 51: 261–268

88. Kinnett DG, Wilcox FH (1982) Partial characterization of two mouse liver alkaline phosphatases that require manganese for activity. Int J Biochem 14: 977–981

89. Knight JG, Adams DD (1978) Three genes for lupus nephritis in NZB X NZW mice. J Exp Med 148: 1652–1660

90. Lampert PW, Oldstone MBS (1973) Host immunoglobulin and complement deposits in choroid plexus during spontaneous complex disease. Science 180: 408–410

91. Landi M, Kreider JW, Lang CM, Bullock LP (1982) Effect of shipping on the immune function of mice. Am J Vet Res 43: 1654–1657

92. Landi M, Kreider JW, Lang CM, Bullock LP (1985) Effect of shipping on the immune functions of mice. In Archibald J, Ditchfield J, Rowsell HC (eds), The Contribution of Laboratory Animal Science to the Welfare of Man and Animals. Gustav Fischer Verlag, Stuttgart, pp 11–18

93. Landy M, Pillemer L (1956) Elevation of properdin levels in mice following administration of bacterial lipopolysaccharides. J Exp Med 103: 823–833

94. Lehmann-Grube F (1982) Lymphocytic choriomeningitis virus. In Foster HL, Small JD, Fox JG (eds), The Mouse in Biomedical Research, Vol 2. Academic Press, New York, pp 231–266

95. Lewis RM, Andre-Schwartz J, Harris GS, Hirsh MS, Black PH, Schwartz RS (1973) Canine systemic lupus erythematosus: Transmission of serologic abnormalities by cell-free filtrates. J Clin Invest 52: 1893–1970

96. Lewis VJ, Thacker WL, Mitchell SH, Baer GM (1976) A new technique for obtaining blood from mice. Lab An Sci 26: 211–213

97. Lin TM, Halbert SP, Kiefer D (1974) Pregnancy associated serum antigens in the rat and mouse. Proc Soc Exp Biol (NY) 145: 62–64

98. Lindsey JR, Conner MW, Baker HJ (1978) Physical, chemical and microbial factors affecting biologic response. In: Laboratory Animal Housing, National Academy of Sciences, Washington, pp 31–43

99. Loeb W (1986) Personal communication

100. Lushbough CH, Moline SW (1961) Improved terminal bleeding method. Proc An Care Panel 11: 305–308

101. MacKenzie PI, Messer M (1976) Studies on the origin and excretion of serum alpha-amylase in the mouse. Comp Biochem Physiol 54B: 103–106

102. Mackenzie N (1984) Fc receptor-mediated transport of immunoglobulin across the intestinal epithelium of the neonatal rodent. Immunol Today 5: 364–366

103. Mark DA, Alonso DR, Quimby F, Thaler T, Kim YT, Fernandes G, Good, RA, Weksler ME (1984) Effects of nutrition on disease and life span. I. Immune responses, cardiovascular pathology, and life span in MRL mice. Am J Pathol 117: 110–124

104. Markert CL (1983) Isozymes: Conceptual history and biological significance. Isozymes: Current Topics in Biological and Medical Research 7: 1–17

105. Martin HF, Gudzinowicz BJ, Fanger H (1975) Normal Values in Clinical Chemistry. Marcel Dekker, New York

106. Maruyama N, Ohta K, Hirose S, Shirai T (1980) Genetic studies of autoimmunity in New Zealand mice. Immunol Letters 2: 1–5

107. Masters C (1983) Subcellular localization of isozymes—an overview. Isozymes: Current Topics in Biological and Medical Research 8: 1–21

108. Matsumura A, Higuchi K, Shimizu K, Hosokawa M, Hashimoto K, Yasuhira K, Takeda T (1982) A novel amyloid fibril protein isolated from senescence-accelerated mice. Lab Invest 47: 270–275

109. Maury CPJ, Teppo A-M, Salaspuro MP (1983) Amyloid A fibril degrading activity in serum and liver disease—relation to serum acute phase and other protein levels. Clin Chim Acta 131: 29–37

110. McAdam KPWJ, Sipe JD (1976) Murine model for human secondary amyloidosis: Genetic variability of the acute-phase serum protein SAA response to endotoxin and casein. J Exp Med 144: 1121–1127

111. Meade CJ, Gore VA (1982) An H-2–associated difference in murine serum cholesterol levels. Experientia 38: 1106–1107

112. Meisler M, Strahler J, Wiebauer K, Thomsen KK (1983) Multiple genes encode mouse pancreatic amylases. Isozymes: Current Topics in Biological and Medical Research 7: 38–57

113. Mink JG, Radl J, Van den Berg P, Haaijman JJ, Van Zwieten MJ, Benner R (1980) Serum immunoglobulins in nude mice and their heterozygous littermates during aging. Immunology 40: 539–545

114. Mitruka BM, Rawnsley HM (1977) Clinical Biochemical and Hematological Reference Values in Normal Experimental Animals. Masson Publishing Inc., New York

115. Mizutani A (1968) Cytochemical demonstration of ornithine carbomoyl transferase activity in liver mitochondria of rat and mouse. J Histochem Cytochem 16: 172–180

116. Moriwaki K, Miyashita N, Yonekawa H (1985) Genetic survey of the origin of laboratory mice and its implication in genetic monitoring. In Archibald J, Ditchfield J, Rowsell HC (eds), The Contribution of Laboratory Animal Science to the Welfare of Man and Animals. Gustav Fischer Verlag, Stuttgart, pp 239–247

117. Morrisett JD, Kim HS, Patsch JR, Datta SK, Trentin JJ (1982) Genetic susceptibility and resistance to diet-induced atheroschlerosis and hyperlipoproteinemia. Arteriosclerosis 2: 312–324

118. Nakayama S, Mold C, Gewurz H, DuClos TW (1982) Opsonic properties of c-reactive protein in vivo. J Immunol 128: 2435–2441

119. National Academy of Sciences, Models for Biomedical Research: A New Perspective. National Academy Press, Washington, DC, 1985

120. National Academy of Sciences, Immunodeficient rodents. National Academy Press, Washington DC, 1988

121. Natsuume-Sakai S, Kaidoh T, Nonako M, Takahashi M (1980) Structural polymorphism of murine C4 and its linkage to H-2. J Immunol 124: 2714-2720

122. Nayudu PRV, Moog F (1966) Intestinal alkaline phosphatase: Regulation by a strain specific factor in mouse milk. Science 152: 656-657

123. Nayudu PRV, Moog F (1967) The genetic control of alkaline phosphatase activity in the duodenum of the mouse. Biochem Genetics 1: 155-170

124. Nerenberg ST, Zedler P (1975) Sequential blood samples from the tail vein of rats and mice obtained with modified Liebig condenser jackets and vacuum. J Lab Clin Med 85: 523-526

125. Nillson UR, Muller-Eberhard HJ (1967) Deficiency of the fifth component of complement in mice with inherited complement defect. J Exp Med 124: 1-16

126. Notkins AL (1965) Lactic dehydrogenase virus. Bacterial Rev 29: 143-160

127. Office of Technology Assessment (1986) Alternatives to Animal Use in Research, Testing and Education. U.S. Government Accounting Office, Washington, DC

128. Oldstone MBA, Rodriguez M, Daughaday WH, Lampert PW (1984) Viral perturbation of endocrine function: Disordered cell function leads to disturbed homeostasis and disease. Nature 307: 278-280

129. Papadimitriou JM, Van Duijn P (1970) The ultrastructural localization of the isozymes of aspartate aminotransferase in murine tissues. J Cell Biol 47: 84-98

130. Parker CJ, Riess GT, Sardesai VM (1985) Essentiality of histamine in adult mice. J Nutr 115: 824-826

131. Passmore HC, Shreffler DC (1970) A sex-limited serum protein variant in the mouse: Inheritance and association with the H-2 region. Biochem Genetics 4: 351-365

132. Patel ST, Newman HAI, Mervis RF (1982) Effects of choline deficiency on mouse serum lipids and alpha-lipoproteins. Clin Chem 28: 1576

133. Patrick DH, Werner RM, Lewis LL (1983) Clinical chemistry values of the N:NIH(S) mice and parameter variations due to sampling techniques (abstr). Lab An Sci 33: 504

134. Pepys MB, Dash AC, Fielder AHL, Mirjah DD (1977) Isolation and study of murine C3. Immunology 33: 491-499

135. Perlmutter RM, Nahn M, Stein KE, Slack J, Zitron I, Paul WE, Davie JM (1979) Immunoglobulin subclass specific immunodeficiency in mice with an x-linked B-lymphocyte defect. J Exp Med 149: 993-998

136. Pfeiffer CJ, Muller PJ (1967) Physiologic correlates depending on the mode of death. Toxicol Appl Pharmacol 10: 253-260

137. Piazza M (1969) Experimental Viral Hepatitis. Charles C Thomas, Springfield, IL

138. Potter M (1972) Immunoglobulin-producing tumors and myeloma proteins of mice. Physiol Rev 52: 631-719

139. Potter M (1983) Immunoglobulins and immunoglobulin genes. In Foster HL, Small JD, Fox JG (eds), The Mouse in Biomedical Research, Vol 3. Academic Press, New York, pp 348-380

140. Quimby FW (1986) Personal communication

141. Ram JS, DeLellis RA, Glenner GG (1969) Amyloid. VIII. On strain variability in experimental murine amyloidosis. Proc Soc Exp Biol Med 130: 462-464

142. Riley V (1974) Persistence and other characteristics of the lactate dehydrogenase-elevating virus. Prog Med Virol 18: 198-213

143. Riley V, Spackman DH, Santisteban GA, Dalldorf G, Hellstrom I (1978) The LDH virus: An interfering biological contaminant. Science 200: 124-126

144. Ross ME, Hayashi K, Notkins AL (1974) Virus induced pancreatic disease: Alterations in concentrations of glucose and amylase in blood. J Infect Dis 129: 669-676

145. Rowson KED, Mahy BWJ (1975) Lactic dehydrogenase virus. In Goard S, Hallaver C (eds), Virology, monograph 13. Springer-Verlag, New York

146. Ruscak M, Orlicky J, Zubor V (1982) Isoelectric focusing of the alanine aminotransferase isoenzymes from the brain, liver and kidney. Comp Biochem Physiol 74B: 141-144

147. Sakaki K, Tanaka K, Hirasawa K (1961) Hematological comparison of the mouse blood taken from the eye and the tail. Exp An 10: 14-19

148. Scher I (1982) CBA/N immune defective mice: Evidence for the failure of a B-cell subpopulation to be expressed. Immunol Rev 64: 117-136

149. Serrano LJ (1971) Carbon dioxide and ammonia in mouse cages: Effects of cage covers, population and activity. Lab An Sci 21: 75-85

150. Sheedlo HJ, Beck ML (1982) Electrophoretic analysis of the plasma and urinary proteins and the ceruloplasmin oxidase activity of heterozygous tortoiseshell ($Mo^{to/+}$) female mice (*Mus musculus*). Comp Biochem Physiol 71B: 309-311

151. Shreffler DC, Owen RD (1963) A serologically detected variant in mouse serum: Inheritance and association with the histocompatibility-2 locus. Genetics 48: 9-25

152. Simmons ML, Brick JO (1970) The Laboratory Mouse—Selection and Management. Prentice-Hall, Englewood Cliffs, NJ

153. Smith CR, Felton JS, Taylor RT (1981) Description of a disposable individual-mouse urine collection apparatus. Lab An Sci 31: 80-82

154. Soret MG, Peterson T, Wyse B, Block EM, Dulin WE (1977) Renal amyloidosis in KK mice that may be misinterpreted as diabetic glomerulosclerosis. Arch Pathol Lab Med 101: 464-468

155. Staats J (1985) Standardized nomenclature for inbred strains of mice: 8th listing. Canc Res 45: 945-977

156. Stoltz DR, Bendall RD (1975) A simple technique for repeated collection of blood samples from mice. Lab An Sci 25: 353-354

157. Sugai S, Pillarisetty RJ, Talal N (1973) Monoclonal macroglobulinemia in NZB/NZW mice. J Exp Med 138: 989-993

158. Sztein MB, Vogel SN, Sipe JD, Murphy RA, Mizel

SB, Oppenhein JJ, Rosenstreich DL (1981) The role of macrophages in the acute-phase response: SAA inducer is closely related to lymphocyte activating factor and endogenous pyrogen. Cell Immunol 63: 164–176

159. Tarin D, Sturdee A (1972) Surgical anesthesia of mice: Evaluation of tribromoethanol, ether, halothane and methoxyflurane and development of reliable technique. Lab An 6: 79–84

160. Theofilopoulos AN, Wilson CG, Dixon FJ (1976) The Raji cell radioimmune assay for detecting immune complexes in human sera. J Clin Invest 57: 169–182

161. Tsuda M, Saheki T, Takado S, Kusumi T, Ohkubo T, Sase M, Katsunuma T (1981) Effect of intestinal flora on the metabolism of amino acids and proteins in the rat and mouse. In Sasaki et al. (eds), Recent Advances in Germ-free Research. Tokai University Press, Tokyo, pp 237–242

162. Ueyama Y, Kuwahara Y, Takahashi H, Maruo K, Hioki K, Saito M, Esaki K, Nomura T, Tamaoki N (1984) Usefulness of double-mutant athymic/renal failure mice in experimental therapy of nephrogenic anemia by an erythropoietin-producing human tumor. In Sordat B (ed), Immune-deficient Animals. Karger, Basel, pp 73–75

163. van der Waaij D (1980) The role of the microbial flora in the development, maintenance and modulation of host immune functions. Adv Physiol Sci 29: 443–477

164. Weisbroth S (1982) Arthropods. In Foster HL, Small JD, Fox JG (eds), The Mouse in Biomedical Research, Vol 2. Academic Press, New York, pp 385–402

165. West RW, Stanley JW, Newport GD (1978) Single mouse urine collection and pH monitoring system. Lab An Sci 28: 343–345

166. Wostman BS (1959) Serum proteins in germfree vertebrates. Ann NY Acad Sci 78: 255–268

167. Wulff HR (1976) Rational Diagnosis and Treatment. Blackwell Scientific Publications, Oxford

168. Yamamoto K, Shiroo M, Migita S (1986) Diverse gene expression for isotypes of murine serum amyloid A protein during acute phase reaction. Science 232: 227–229

169. Yother J, Volanakis JE, Briles DE (1982) Human c-reactive protein is protective against fatal *Streptococcus pneumoniae* infection in mice. J Immunol 128: 2374–2380

170. Young L, Chambers T (1973) A mouse bleeding technique yielding consistent volume with minimal hemolysis. Lab An Sci 23: 428–430

171. Yuhas JM, Angel CR, Mahin DT, Ferris RD, Woodward KT, Storer JB (1967) Plasma enzyme activities in inbred mice. Genetics 57: 613–624

172. Zborowska E, Zborowski M, Czarnomska A (1985) The use of mandible shape analysis for genetic quality control of inbred and congenic mice. In Archibald J, Ditchfield J, Rowsell HC (eds), The Contribution of Laboratory Animal Science to the Welfare of Man and Animals. Gustav Fischer Verlag, Stuttgart, pp 485–494

173. Zizkovsky V (1975) Specific fetal serum proteins of 13 mammalian species. Comp Biochem Physiol B 51B: 87–91

174. Zurcher C, van Zwieten MJ, Solleveld HA, Hollander CF (1982) Aging research. In Foster HL, Small JD, Fox JG (eds), The Mouse in Biomedical Research, Vol 4. Academic Press, New York, pp 11–35

2

The Rat

ROBERT G. MEEKS, PhD

Detailed guidelines have been developed in recent years for assessing the potential health risks associated with exposure to drugs and chemicals. In the United States most of these guidelines have been published by various regulatory agencies such as the Food and Drug Administration (52) and the Environmental Protection Agency (24), and elsewhere by international agencies such as the Organization for Economic Cooperation and Development (43). All contain recommendations for the measurement of biochemical parameters to detect possible organ injury. The laboratory rat (*Rattus norvegicus*) has generally become the animal species of choice for such use.

Analysis of various biochemical parameters in this species is not particularly difficult, especially with the recent development of many automated clinical chemistry analyzers. Most of these instruments require 1.5 to 50 μl of serum or plasma and are pre-programmed with as many as 20 different clinical chemistry tests. The primary challenge of the clinical pathology laboratory is to develop or adapt procedures designed for human use into reliable tests for the evaluation of organ function and toxicity in rats.

Under conditions of genetic, pathogenic, and environmental quality control (2,38), the laboratory rat provides the investigator with a powerful test system. All of the animals in a study are stabilized in normal health before

initiation of treatment with the test compound. An end point of the study then is to determine whether administration of the test compound produces a change, be it morphologic or functional. In an organ system, pathologic evaluation at the end of a study allows identification of changes at organ and tissue levels (ie, morphologic changes), whereas clinical chemistry measurements provide an assessment of functional changes. The ultimate goal of a study then should be to integrate the changes in function and morphology into an overall understanding of the mechanisms by which the chemical produces its effect(s). Repeated sampling during a study should provide information on the temporal relationship between onset of tissue damage and administration of the compound.

SOURCES OF VARIATION

One major difference between conducting biochemical determinations in rats versus human subjects is the seemingly infinite number of variables in rats that must be considered and controlled to the extent possible. Experimentalists must be aware of these variables and must address them when reporting their results.

Sources of variation can be divided into at least three general categories: (1) variation related to the physiologic status of the animal and its environmental condition, (2) variation related to sampling, and (3) variation related to analytic instrumentation and methodology.

Several reports address the effect of these variations on many of the common clinical chemistry procedures. Variations related to the physiologic status of the rat and its environment include disease status (11,14), age (35,55,58), sex (34,35,55,58), husbandry (9,34,56), and nutritional condition and degree of hydration (5,29,47,63). Variations related to sampling include (but are not limited to): method of collection (4,54), anesthetic used (30), sampling time, that is, time of day (46), restraint technique (4,30,54,59), anticoagulant used (33,36), hemolysis (28,50), sample processing and storage (3,5,8), and site of sampling. Blood samples may be collected from the retroorbital sinus, tail veins and arteries, or jugular veins as a survival procedure. Cardiac puncture on anesthetized rats is performed as a survival procedure but entails a greater risk. Terminally, samples may be drawn from the aorta or vena cava or by decapitation. The last of these is generally unsatisfactory because of gross contamination.

Jugular venipuncture is particularly recommended in the rat. It is performed by two persons and requires a simple restraining board. The rat is placed on its back on the board and its forelegs are gently separated and immobilized using leather thongs hooked to the board. A hood made of plastic, perforated to allow air access, is placed over the rat's head by the phlebotomist and the head is turned to one side. The result is a triangular configuration in the jugular furrow on the opposite side. The jugular vein lies superficially in this triangle. Venipuncture may be performed with a 5/8 of an inch, 23-gauge needle attached to a syringe or vacuum collection tube. Three milliliters of whole blood can readily be collected from an adult rat without undue risk or stress. Skilled teams consisting of a phlebotomist and an assistant can perform the entire procedure at a continuous rate of two animals per minute. Because of the brevity of the restraint, blood samples can be collected before stress-dependent alterations in analytes take place. The collection of specimens from an endothelial-lined channel with minimal trauma makes them suitable for coagulation studies and similar analyses that are invalidated by tissue trauma (23).

From 1.25 to 2 ml of blood can be collected monthly from young adult Fischer 344 rats with-

out any perceptible hematologic or biochemical effects. However, this volume slightly reduces the rat's weight gain (10,60). Volumes of blood as large as 5 ml have been drawn daily for 3 consecutive days by cardiac puncture from adult anesthetized Sprague-Dawley rats without fatality (39).

In the collection of serum for clinical chemical analysis in the rat as in other species, prompt separation of serum from cells is critical. Hemolyzed or visually clear serum that has remained in contact with erythrocytes has falsely elevated values for potassium and lactic dehydrogenase, less consistently and to a lesser degree for phosphorus, and sometimes for bilirubin. Prolonged contact of serum with erythrocytes reduces serum glucose. Hemolysis falsely elevates protein levels. The use of thixotropic gel, centrifugation no more than 30 minutes after collection, and prompt removal of the serum from the clot are essential in collecting serum that will yield reliable data.

The effect of the sampling site on clinical chemistry parameters was recently documented (16,17,26,42). Analysis of the blood sampling site coupled with various collection methods was performed on Fischer 344 rats. Sampling sites included the right ventricle, aorta, vena cava, retroorbital sinus, and tail. Collection methods included vacuum tube, syringe, capillary tube, and exsanguination. Nineteen frequently measured clinical chemistry parameters including serum enzyme, cholesterol, and triglyceride levels were determined. No collection method proved to be the most appropriate for all parameters measured. Nevertheless, samples collected into a vacuum tube from the right ventricle produced the most consistent results in most procedures when compared with the overall mean obtained by all methods. The most significant differences from the overall mean were seen in samples obtained from the tail and orbital sinus. Major differences for some parameters also were found in samples obtained by exsanguination. It was concluded that selection of a sampling site can be a major source of variation in clinical chemistry values and that in selecting an appropriate sampling method, consideration should be given to which clinical chemistry parameters are likely to be of greatest interest (42). Dunn and Scheuing (22) showed that when rats were housed in pairs, the first rat of the pair to be bled consistently had a significantly lower level of serum corticosterone than did its cagemate, demonstrating the need to randomize the sequence of bleeding among treated and control animals. Finally, analytic instrumentation and different methodologies will affect most clinical chemistry parameters (7,12,20,52); however, the extent of this variation can be determined and controlled by quality control programs that include the determination of intra- and interassay variability. Further control of variability arising from analytical instrumentation is assured by following rigid equipment maintenance and calibration by qualified field engineers.

ESTABLISHMENT OF REFERENCE RANGES

Because all of the variables just discussed cannot be controlled to the same extent in all laboratories, it becomes extremely important for each laboratory to establish its own normal range for each biochemical parameter based on the sex, age, and species used; however, the large number of inbred strains, outbred stocks, and other less defined laboratory subline strains, as well as the suppliers of rats, complicates the process of establishing baseline data (1). It is exceedingly difficult to compare a single value from an individual rat with a laboratory reference range that has been accumulated over months or years without regard to sex, age, strain or species, and husbandry conditions (25). Several attempts to document reference ranges for various strains and stocks of rats (40,56) have shown differences in various individual tests.

In general, however, studies are conducted in which there is a control population and a test population. The control population is untreated or is treated with the vehicle used to carry the test substance. The criteria used to assess the effects of the test compound on clinical chemistry parameters are based on a comparison of differences between the control and test populations and should not be based on differences between test populations and historical reference ranges.

INTERPRETATION OF RESULTS

Interpretation of results on samples obtained from rats requires a thorough understanding of the problems and variables just alluded to. For example, parameters sensitive to stress from restraining techniques used during sampling would be expected to show much greater fluctuation that would parameters less affected by stress (25). The great variability in the activities of particular enzymes, such as lactate dehydrogenase and alkaline phosphatase, limits the diagnostic significance of these tests unless isoenzyme patterns are determined concomitantly. Furthermore, consideration must be given to differences in the biochemistry of a particular test (6,18,19). For example, differences in enzyme substrate and/or pH optimum that have an effect on the maximal velocity (Vmax) of the reaction have been reported. The biochemistry of a test becomes extremely important when rat samples are assayed using diagnostic kits that are designed for human samples.

SPECIFIC TESTS

The choice of specific tests for assessing the effects of chemical agents on the functioning of various organ systems must be made judiciously. The selection of parameters for the various studies should be based on clinical usefuless; therefore, the tests chosen should be particularly sensitive to tissue damage. Conversely, some consideration must be given to the analysis of parameters that might be considered important in fulfilling the requirement set forth by the various regulatory agencies (24,43,52). Choice of appropriate tests should be aided by a consideration of the tissue distribution of the various biochemical entities and in particular enzyme activities. Boyd (7) has compiled the enzyme activities in the tissues and serum of various species including the rat. It is important to know not only the tissue distribution but also the subcellular localization of the various enzymes. This knowledge aids in determining the damage to specific subcellular organelles if an increase in a particular serum enzyme activity occurs. Furthermore, many enzymes such as asparate aminotransferase (AST, or serum glutamic oxalacetic transaminace), lactic dehydrogenase, and isocitrate dehydrogenase are nonspecific, that is they are distributed widely to many tissues; therefore, increases in serum or plasma activities of these enzymes should not be considered specific for damage to any particular organ or tissue.

Glucose

Glucose levels may vary with blood collection methods (4). Furthermore, handling, anesthesia, restraint techniques, method of collection, and fasting state contribute to the variation. Cells must be separated from serum as quickly as possible after collection because glycolysis can account for a rapid fall in levels; however, the effect of glycolysis can be diminished by the addition of fluoride as well as thymol. There are several analytic techniques for determining glucose levels, but true glucose levels are measured enzymatically. The plethora of analytic techniques plus differences in husbandry and sample collection probably accounts for the considerable variation in reported means (9,25,35,40).

Urea Nitrogen

The usefulness of blood urea nitrogen in determining the extent of kidney and/or renal tubular damage is questionable unless damage to the nephron is extensive (37,48,49). This is most likely related to the tremendous functional reserve capacity of the kidney resulting from the large number of nephrons (37). This lack of sensitivity has prompted several investigators to make extensive use of urinary enzyme activities for detecting renal tubular damage (15,44, 53,62). It is apparent from their results that this approach does offer greater sensitivity. Blood urea nitrogen in rats does not appear to vary with age or sex (25,35).

Creatinine

Creatine metabolism in muscle tissue results in the formation of creatinine which is filtered in the kidney. As for blood urea nitrogen, the usefulness of the test in assessing kidney damage is limited because extensive damage must occur for a gross change in creatinine levels to be seen (48,49). A number of endogenous and exogenous materials will interfere with the Jaffe reaction, which is the primary analytic method used to determine creatinine levels (13,51). Interfering substances include barbituates, ketones, ascorbic acid, and glucose (51). Bromsulfaphthalein has also been reported to interfere with creatinine measurements. Sex differences in serum levels (35) disappear as the rat ages.

Bilirubin

Bilirubin is formed from the breakdown of hemoglobin molecules by the reticuloendothelial system. Prehapatic bilirubin, loosely linked to albumin, is transported to hepatocytes where it is conjugated in part as glucuronide. Total serum bilirubin is elevated in hemolytic or hepatocellular disease or obstructive disease of the biliary tree. Measurement of conjugated and unconjugated fractions permits a differential diagnosis of these conditions (50). Selection of a method for determining direct and total bilirubin presents a dilemma because of the many methods available and the problems associated with them (13,28). This problem is further complicated by the lack of a reference method that prohibits assessment of accuracy (28). Thus, selection of a method is somewhat arbitrary.

Both direct and indirect bilirubin undergoes photooxidation and/or dehydrogenation on exposure to light. Therefore, measurement should be performed as soon as possible following sample collection. Samples can be stored up to 8 hours at room temperature or overnight at 4°C if they are protected from light (28,61). Hemolysis also interferes with bilirubin determination (28).

Serum Protein

Albumin and globulin, both free and in combination with other substances containing lipids and carbohydrates, make up the serum proteins in rats. Slightly higher total protein values are obtained in plasma than in serum because of the presence of fibrinogen. The major protein component, albumin, can be determined by several methods. The globulin fraction is generally considered as the difference between the measured total protein and albumin. It has been reported that the major globulin fractions in rat serum are α_1- or β-fraction followed by α_2- and γ-globulin (57). It has been noted that total protein values tend to fall following freezing, possibly the result of cryoprecipitation of some proteins. Serum protein mean values of the rat apparently are not affected by age, sex, and the like (35, 40,41).

Serum Enzyme Activity

The level of enzyme activity in the serum of rodents depends primarily on the rate of release of the enzyme from cells as well as the uptake of the enzyme from the circulation (7). Therefore, an increase in serum enzyme activity above control levels signals either (1) an increased release of enzyme, (2) overproduction of enzyme by the cells, or (3) a decrease in the clearance rate of enzyme from the circulation (7).

Furthermore, as noted earlier, some enzymes are found in numerous tissues; therefore, an increase in serum activity of an enzyme that has widespread distribution is not as powerful a diagnostic tool for assessing injury of a particular tissue as is an increase in enzyme activity that has limited tissue distribution (7,45).

The use of measurements of rat serum for specific enzymes has generally been directed toward the early and precise identification of organ damage.

Lactate Dehydrogenase (LDH)

Lactate dehydrogenase activity can be found in myocardial tissue, kidney, liver, and skeletal muscle (7). This enzyme can be separated by electrophoresis into five major bands corresponding to the five isoenzymes, and each tissue has its own unique isoenzyme pattern (45). Normal values for serum LDH are highly variable and depend on the method of analysis (27,28,35).

Alkaline Phosphatase (ALP)

The most significant levels of ALP are found in the osteoblasts, kidney, and intestine, with limited activity in a number of other tissues (7). Because of its diffuse distribution, an increase in serum ALP activity is not a definitive indication of tissue activities. Isoenzyme patterns may be used to differentiate various disease states (27,28). Male rats have significantly higher serum ALP activity than do female rats (41,50).

Aspartate Aminotransferase (AST)

The enzyme is widely distributed to several tissues in rats with the highest concentrations found in the liver, heart, skeletal muscle, and kidney (40). Because of this ubiquitous tissue distribution, increases in the activity of this enzyme in serum are of limited diagnostic utility. Normal values apparently do not differ significantly with repect to age or sex (35).

Alanine Aminotransferase (ALT)

Alanine aminotransferase is a liver-specific enzyme in rats (7). Because of this tissue specificity, increases in serum enzyme activity are indicative of hepatocellular damage. As with AST, ALT serum levels apparently do not vary significantly in rats with regard to sex or age (35).

Sorbitol Dehydrogenase (SDH) and Ornithine Carbamyltransferase (OCT)

These two enzymes are highly specific to the liver parenchyma in rats (7) and therefore are fairly specific indicators of hepatocellular damage.

A correlation between increases in OCT and ALT activities and morphologic changes has been reported in rats receiving experimental drugs (31). Ornithine carbamyltransferase is a mitochondrial enzyme and is only elevated when hepatocellular necrosis occurs, whereas SDH is a cytosol enzyme that would be released following early changes in membrane permeability. Therefore, the more sensitive indicator of induced minimal liver damage in the rat is SDH (21,32). Dooley and Racick (21) have shown no differences in normal values for rats based on the sex of the animal.

Gamma Glutamyltransferase (GGT)

Rat kidneys contain the highest activity of GGT, whereas levels are close to nondetectable in serum (7). When kidney damage occurs GGT levels increase more in urine than in plasma (55) Likewise, serum GGT levels are only slightly increased in hepatocellular necrosis. Therefore, measurement of this enzyme in the serum of rats may be of no real diagnostic use.

CONCLUSION

Performance of clinical chemistry determinations on plasma or serum samples obtained from rats is not difficult. Rats are an ideal species in that reasonably good volumes of samples can be obtained, they are easy to work with, and they are relatively inexpensive. As noted however, it is critical that the variables that affect the results are controlled and that each laboratory establish its own reference range for the strain used in its

studies. Lastly, the choice of tests to be performed must be judicious, that is, the selection
of parameters for the various kinds of studies
anticipated should be based on clinical usefulness. Therefore, tests that are particularly sensitive to tissue damage should be chosen.

REFERENCES

1. Animals for Research, A Directory of Sources (1979)
   National Academy of Sciences, Washington, DC
2. Baker HJ, Lindsey JR, Weisbroth SH (1979) In Baker
   HJ, Lindsey JR, Weisbroth SH (eds), The Laboratory Rat, Vol I. Academic Press, New York, pp
   169–191
3. Bayard SP (1974) Another look at the statistical
   analysis of changes during storage of serum specimens. Health Lab Sci 11: 45–49
4. Besch EL, Chou BJ (1971) Physiological responses
   to blood collection methods in rats. Proc Soc Exp
   Biol Med 138: 1019–1021
5. Bolter CP, Critz JB (1974) Plasma enzyme activities
   in rats with diet-induced alterations in liver enzyme
   activities. Experientia 30: 1241–1243
6. Boyd JW (1966) The extraction and purification of
   two isoenzymes of L-aspartate: 2-Oxoglutarate
   aminotransferase. Biochim Biophys Acta 113: 302
7. Boyd JW (1983) The mechanism relating to increases
   in plasma enzymes and isoenzymes in diseases of
   animals. Vet Clin Pathol 12: 9–24
8. Bramanti G, Ravina A, DeFina V (1972) Pre-
   servability of rat serum in delayed determinations of
   some hematochemical parameters. Boll Chim Farm
   111: 694–699
9. Burn KF, Terrimons EH, Portey SM (1971) Serum
   chemistry and hematological values for axenic (germ-
   free) and environmentally associated inbred rats. Lab
   An Sci 21: 415–419
10. Cardy RH, Warner JW (1979) Effects of sequential
    bleeding on body weight gain in rats. Lab An Sci 29:
    179–181
11. Cotchin E, Roe FJC (1967) Pathology of Laboratory
    Rats and Mice. Davis, Philadelphia
12. Cutter MG (1974) The sensitivity of the function
    tests in detecting liver damage in the rat. Toxicol
    Appl Pharmacol 28: 349–357
13. Davidson I, Henry JB (1983) Clinical Diagnosis by
    Laboratory Methods, 16th ed. Saunders, Phi-
    ladelphia
14. Deb C, Hart JS (1956) Hematological and body fluid
    adjustments during acclimation to cold environment.
    Can J Biochem Physiol 34: 959–966
15. Dieter MP, Powers MB, Riley JH, Thorstenson JH,
    Uriah LC (1984) Utilization of urinary enzyme assays
    to monitor renal toxicity in F344 rats after prolonged
    mercuric chloride treatment. The Toxicologist 4: 119
16. Dohler KD, Von Der Mulen A, Gartner K, Dohler
    U (1977) Effect of various blood sampling techniques
    on serum levels of pituitary and thyroid hormones in
    the rat. J Endocrinal 74: 341–342
17. Dohler KD, Wong CC, Gaudssuhn D, Von Zur
    Muhler A, Gartner K, Dohler U (1978) Site of blood

18. sampling in rats as a possible source of error in hor-
    mone determinations. J Endocrinal 79: 141–142
18. Dooley JF (1979) The role of clinical chemistry in
    chemical and drug safety evaluation by use of lab-
    oratory animals. Clin Chem 25: 345–347
19. Dooley JF (1981) Clinical chemistry in animal drug
    safety testing. Lab An 10: 32–35
20. Dooley JF (1983) The role of alanine amino-
    transferase for assessing hepatotoxicity in labora-
    tory animals. Lab An 13: 20–23
21. Dooley JF, Racick L (1976) The sensitivity of serum
    sorbital dehydrogenase in thioacetamide induced
    liver toxicity in rats. Laboratory animal Clinical
    Analyses Group Symposium, Houston, TX
22. Dunn J, Scheuing L (1971) Plasma corticosterone in
    rats killed sequentially at the "trough" or "peak" of
    the adrenocortical cycle. J Endocrinal 49: 347–348
23. Everett RM (1982) Personal communication
24. Federal Register, Tuesday, November 29, 1983,
    53922–53969
25. Fowler JSL (1982) Animal clinical chemistry and
    hematology for the toxicologist. Arch Toxicol Suppl
    5: 152–159
26. Friedel R, Trautschold I, Gartner K, Helle-Feldman
    M, Gaudssuhn D (1975) Einflus verschiedener
    Methoden zur Blutgewinnung auf Enzym-Akti-
    vitaten im Serum kleiner Laboratoriumstiere. Z Klin
    Chem Klin Biochem 13: 499–505
27. Garrick LM, Sharma VS, Ranney HM (1974) Struc-
    tural studies of rat hemoglobins. Ann NY Acad Sci
    241: 434–435
28. Henry RJ, Cannon DC, Winkelman JW (1974) Clini-
    cal Chemistry, Principles and Technics, 2nd ed.
    Harper, New York
29. Horowitz M, Borut A (1973) Blood volume regu-
    lation in dehydrated rodents: Plasma colloid osmotic
    pressure, total osmotic pressure and electrolytes.
    Comp Biochem Physical A44: 1261–1265
30. Irvine ROH, Dow J, Fong J (1966) Effect of anes-
    thesia on the collection of blood for acid-base stud-
    ies in the rat. Med Pharmacol Exp 14: 557–562
31. Kosrud GO, Grice HG, Goodman TK, Knipfel JE,
    McLaughlan JM (1973) Sensitivity of several serum
    enzymes for the detection of thioacetamide-, dime-
    thylnitrosamine-, and diethanolamine-induced liver
    damage in rats. Toxicol Appl Pharmacol 26: 299–313
32. Kosrud GO, Grice HC, McLaughlin JM (1972) Sen-
    sitivity of several enzymes in detecting carbon-tetra-
    chloride-induced liver damage. Toxicol Appl Phar-
    macol 22: 474–483
33. Kosrud GO, Trick KD (1973) Activities of several
    enzymes in serum and heparinized plasma from rats.
    Clin Chim Acta 48: 311–315
34. Kozma CK (1967) Electrophoretic determination of
    serum proteins of laboratory animals. J Am Vet Med
    Assoc 151: 865–869
35. Kozma CK, Weisbroth SH, Stratman SL, Conejeros
    M (1969) Normal biological values for Long-Evans
    rats. Lab An Care 19: 746–755
36. Ladenson JH, Tsai LB, Michael JM, Kessler G, Jorst
    JH (1974) Serum versus heparinized plasma for eigh-
    teen common chemistry tests. Is serum the appro-
    priate specimen? Am J Clin Pathol 62: 545–552
37. Lameire NH, Lifschitz MD, Stin JH (1977) Het-

erogeneity of nephron function. Annu Rev Physiol 39: 159–184

38. Lindsey JR, Conner MW, Baker HJ (1978) Physical, chemical, and microbial factors affecting biologic response. In Laboratory Animal Housing. National Academy of Sciences, Washington DC, pp 31–43

39. Loeb WF (1976) Personal communication

40. Mitruka BM, Rawnsley HM (1977) Clinical Biochemical and Hematological Reference Values in Normal Experimental Animals. Masson, New York

41. Nakave HS, Dost FN, Bukler DR (1973) Studies on the toxicity of hexachlorophene in the rat. Toxicol appl Pharmacol 24: 239–249

42. Neptun D, Smith CN, Irons R (1985) Effect of Sampling Site and Collection Method on Variations in Baseline clinical Pathology Parameters in Fischer 344 Rats. 1. Clinical Chemistry Fundamental and Applied Tox 5: 1180–1185

43. OECD Guidelines for Testing of Chemicals, Section 4, 75775 Paris, Cedex 16, France

44. Raab WR (1972) Diagnostic value of urinary enzyme determinations. Clin Chem 18: 5–25

45. Ringler DH, Dabich L (1979) In Baker HJ, Lindsey JR, Weisbroth SH (eds), The Laboratory Rat, Vol 1. Academic Press, New York, pp 105–121

46. Scheving LE, Pauley JE (1967) Daily rhythmic variations in blood coagulation times in rats. Anat Rec 157: 657–666

47. Schwartz E, Tornaben JA, Boxill GC (1973) The effects of food restriction on hematology, clinical chemistry, and pathology in the albino rat. Toxicol Appl Pharmacol 25: 515–524

48. Shanatt M, Frazer AC (1963) The sensitivity of function tests in detecting renal damage in the rats. Toxicol Appl Pharmacol 5: 36–48

49. Slunnil MS (1974) A review of the pathology and pathogenesis of acute renal failure due to acute tubular necrosis. J Clin Pathol 27: 2–13

50. Tietz NW (1976) Fundamentals of Clinical Chemistry. Saunders, Philadelphia

51. Toro G, Ackerman PG (1975) Practical Clinical Chemistry. Little, Brown, Boston

52. 21 Code of Federal Regulations: Part 58 (1978). Good Laboratory Practice for Nonclinical Laboratory Studies

53. Ulright PJ, Leathwood PD, Plummer DT (1972) Enzymes in rat urine: Alkaline phosphatase. Enzymology 42: 317–327

54. Upton PK, Morgan DJ (1975) The effect of sampling technique on some blood parameters in the rat. Lab An 9: 85–91

55. Vondruska JF, Greco RA (1973) Certain hematologic and blood chemical values in Charles River CD Albino rats. Bull Am Soc Vet Clin pathol 2: 3–17

56. Weil CS (1982) Statistical analyses and normality of selected hematologic and clinical chemistry measurements used in toxicologic studies. Arch Toxicol Suppl 5: 237–253

57. Weimer HE, Benjamin DC, Darcy DA (1965) Synthesis of the Alpha-glycoprotein (Darcy) of rat serum by the liver. Nature (London) 208: 1221 1222

58. Weisse VI, Knappen F, Frölke W, Guénard J, Kállmer H, Stótzer H (1974) Blutwerte der Rathe in Abhangigkeit van Alter und Geschlecht. Arzeim-Forsch 24: 1221–1225

59. Whelan G, Combes B (1975) Phenobarbital-enhanced biliary excretion of administered unconjugated and conjugated sulfo-bromophthalein (BSP) in the rat. Biochem Pharmacol 24: 1283–1286

60. Wiersma J, Kastelijn J (1986) Haematological, immunological and endocrinological aspects of chronic high frequency blood sampling in rats with replacement by fresh or preserved donor blood. Lab An 20: 57–65

61. Winsten S (1968) Collection and preservation of specimens. In Faulkner WR, King JW, Damm HC (eds), CRC Handbook of Clinical Laboratory Data, 2nd ed. Chem. Rubber Publ. Co., Cleveland

62. Wright PJ, Plummer DT (1974) The use of urinary enzyme measurements to detect renal damage caused by nephrotoxic compounds. Biochem Pharmacol 23: 65–73

63. Zbinden G (1963) Experimental and clinical aspects of drug toxicity. Adv Pharmacol 2: 1–112

3

The Guinea Pig

WILLIAM J. WHITE, VMD, MS and C. MAX LANG, DVM

The guinea pig (*Cavia porcellus*) is a hystricomorph mammal belonging to a family of burrowing rodents native to the western hemisphere. In the wild, guinea pigs live in small groups in open grasslands of Bolivia, Western Peru, Argentina, Uruguay, and Brazil (23). They have been domesticated and are used as food animals in several South American countries. Guinea pigs were first brought to Europe in the early 1600s where they were bred for food and as pets. In the early 1900s they were first used as laboratory animals, primarily in genetic research (24). Since then, they have proved to be useful laboratory animals for research in immunology, audiology, toxicology, and teratology.

The use of guinea pigs has remained relatively constant over the last decade at slightly more than 2 per cent of the laboratory rodents used in biomedical research (13). The popularity of guinea pigs in research has declined from a peak in the 1930s, but their use as pets has increased.

SAMPLING TECHNIQUE

Although the term "guinea pig" is commonly used synonymously with laboratory animal by lay people, data relating to the clinical chemistry of the guinea pig are rather sparse. This may be due to the relatively small number of these animals used in research and the difficulty in obtaining blood samples from their peripheral veins; their deep vessels are often covered with many layers of fat. Methods of obtaining repeated blood samples have been described (Table 3.1) in addition to single sample terminal methods such as decapitation or surgical intervention. With the exception of cardiac puncture, femoral puncture, and orbital sinus bleeding, sample volumes are usually low and often contaminated. Cardiac puncture, femoral puncture, and orbital sinus bleeding have a low degree of repeatability and may be stressful to the animal.

Blood and plasma volumes of guinea pigs average 6.96 and 3.88 ml per 100 g of body weight respectively. These figures vary considerably with age (19,9). They are highest at birth and decline steadily until 900 g of body weight is reached, at which point they level out.

When guinea pig serum is prepared in plastic rather than glass tubes, serum electrolyte changes occur. This finding is directly associated with the clotting mechanism and results in lower serum potassium levels (4). During clotting, blood cellular elements of the guinea pig release lactic dehydrogenase and gamma glutamyl transferase (GGT) into the serum. This is in sharp contrast to many other mammalian species in which no release of GGT occurs (4). Of the common laboratory animal species, only the guinea pig, rabbit, and nonhuman primate have detectable serum levels of GGT; cats, dogs, rats, and mice do not. Guinea pig serum levels of GGT are only one sixth of those reported for

Table 3.1. Methods for Obtaining Blood from Guinea Pigs

Method	Comments
Cutting nail bed	Small quantities of blood (<1 ml); may be contaminated
Marginal ear vein laceration	Small quantities of blood (<1 ml); may be contaminated
Dorsal metatarsal vein laceration	Small quantities of blood (<1 ml); may be contaminated
Orbital sinus	Moderate quantities of blood (>2 cc); little contamination; requires anesthesia
Lateral metatarsal vein laceration (vacuum assisted)	Moderate quantities of blood (>2 cc); may be contaminated
Femoral puncture	Moderate quantities of blood (>2 cc); not contaminated
Cardiac puncture	Large quantities of blood (>5 cc); not contaminated; cardiac or pulmonary laceration may cause death; best performed under anesthesia
Vena cava or other large internal vessels	Large quantities of blood (>5 cc); not contaminated; must be performed surgically under anesthesia; usually a terminal procedure
Decapitation	Large quantities of blood (>5 cc); usually contaminated; terminal procedure

nonhuman primates, and they may be associated with release during blood clotting (4).

ENZYMES

Serum alkaline phosphatase in the guinea pig has been shown to decrease with increasing body weight, comparable to the decrease with maturation observed in other species. A dramatic increase in the serum alkaline phosphatase activity is induced by zinc-deficient diets (under 20 ppm) or managanese-deficient diets (1,22). Although conflicting conclusions have been drawn concerning the effect of ascorbic acid on serum alkaline phosphatase, Degkwitz (7) demonstrated that ascorbic acid deficiency did not decrease this enzymatic activity when ascorbic acid-deficient guinea pigs were compared with appropriate control animals.

In the guinea pig, in sharp contrast to such species as the dog or rat, alanine aminotransferase is an extremely insensitive and nonspecific marker of hepatocellular injury. This is in part due to the low total activity of alanine aminotransferase in guinea pig hepatocytes and in part the low cytosol and high mitochondrial distribution of the enzyme (6).

DRUG METABOLISM

Methods for determining drug levels in guinea pig serum are similar to those used in humans and other mammalian species. Drug metabolism and hence plasma drug levels following similar dosing rates vary with the age of the guinea pig.

Newborn guinea pigs generally lack activity of many microsomal drug-metabolizing enzymes, especially those responsible for glucuronide formation, n-demethylation, and o-dealkylation (10). Activity is absent at 24 hours but appears within the first week of life at about one third the adult levels. Full drug-metabolizing activity in the liver and hence normal plasma half-lives are not reached until 8 weeks of age (10).

CHOLESTEROL AND LIPOPROTEINS

Mammals generally differ in the way they react to dietary cholesterol. Feeding diets high in cholesterol (1 to 2 per cent) to species such as rats, dogs, nonhuman primates, and man does not cause extensive or rapid expansion of body cholesterol pools (5,25). Hypercholesterolemia is uncommon in these species in contrast to the guinea pig, rabbit, and prairie dog in which it is common (9,16,24). In the guinea pig, hypercholesterolemia is often accompanied by fatty infiltration of many tissues including the liver.

In the guinea pig as in man, the intestine is the principal site of cholesterol synthesis, whereas in most species the liver is the principal site of cholesterologenesis. Swann et al. (21) showed in the guinea pig that the liver to ileum ratio of acetate incorporation into cholesterol is 0.061, whereas in the rat it is 1.57. All cholesterologenic tissues in the guinea pig are subject to feedback inhibition (21,26).

High dietary cholesterol induces hemolytic anemia in the guinea pig. This anemia is accompanied by splenic enlargement and bone marrow hyperplasia, and may lead to death before the formation of atherogenic plaques (14,27,28).

Guinea pigs on a normal diet have little if any high density lipoprotein (HDL) until they are fed cholesterol. Cholesterol bound to this HDL is predominantly nonesterified (26).

Because dietary cholesterol as low as 0.1 per cent may induce biochemical changes and lesions in the guinea pig, dietary considerations should always be taken into account in interpreting serum levels of lipids and lipoproteins in the guinea pig (14,27).

HORMONES

Most plasma steroid radioimmunoassay methods used for other mammalian species are applicable to the guinea pig. Cortisol is the principal adrenoglucocorticoid produced by the guinea pig in contrast to the rat and mouse which produce predominantly corticosterone. The guinea pig has a high rate of interconversion between cortisol and cortisone (12). Sexual dimorphism in plasma cortisol levels of the guinea pig occurs after 30 days of age, with males having higher levels than females. These differences are related to differences in metabolism and binding of cortisol by transcortin (8). In guinea pigs between 90 and 120 days of age, basal and stress plasma cortisol levels are the same for both sexes, but sexual dimorphism in plasma cortisol levels reappears in adult guinea pigs. These changes seem to correspond to changes in testosterone levels. In addition to corticosteroid-binding globulin (transcortin) identified in many species, which binds either cortisol or progesterone, the pregnant guinea pig has a second steroid-binding protein, progesterone-binding globulin, which specifically binds progesterone but not cortisol. Guinea pig transcortin has a much higher affinity for cortisol than for progesterone in contrast to human transcortin which has a similar affinity for both steroids. Progesterone-binding globulin appears to be unique to hystricomorph rodents (26).

Insulin

Insulin from most species is remarkably similar. Cyclostomes, boney fishes, mammals, and birds all possess insulin whose molecules are closely related structurally (11,20). The guinea pig

and several other hystricomorph rodents represent exceptions to this orderly relationship (3). Guinea pig insulin differs from other mammalian insulins in one third of its amino acids (11,20) as reflected in a reduction in the biologic activity of the molecule to a level that is only 1 to 5 per cent of that of other mammalian insulins (29). The guinea pig compensates for this by producing a high circulating level of insulin and higher tissue concentrations of insulin receptors (29). Circulating guinea pig insulin is poorly reactive with standard antiinsulin antibodies, does not dimerize at high concentrations, does not form crystals, and does not bind zinc (29,30).

Guinea pigs produce insulin in small quantities in extrapancreatic tissues (17,18). This insulin is immunologically similar to that of other mammalian tissues, and reacts well with standard anti-beef– or anti-pork–insulin antibodies (17), and seems to be confined to the cells in which it is produced, with none being detected in the plasma. It is metabolically as active as other mammalian insulins, but it does not appear to be responsible for controlling variations in plasma glucose levels (18). This apparently is done by the biologically less active guinea pig pancreatic insulin.

Commercially available insulin radioimmunoassay kits are not valid for measuring plasma insulin levels in guinea pigs, but they can be used to measure tissue levels of nonpancreatic guinea pig insulin. Some commercial plasma insulin kits utilize antiinsulin antibodies produced in guinea pigs, which further limits their use in this species.

Unlike in many other species, little if any chromuim ion is required for binding insulin to cell receptors; hence, guinea pig chromium requirements are low when compared to those of other species (15).

ACID-BASE BALANCE

Bar-Ilan and Marder (2) studied the acid-base status of unanesthetized, unrestrained guinea pigs implanted with chronic cannulas and observed values similar to those in rats under similar conditions. Because the core body temperature of unrestrained and unanesthetized guinea pigs is between 38.6° and 40.4°C, it is essential that all determinations of acid-base status be appropriately temperature corrected. This is particularly important when such determinations are made on anesthetized animals, which is often the case because of the relative inaccessibility of peripheral arteries in the guinea pig which limits percutaneous sampling (2).

In summary, relatively little information is available on the clinical chemistry of the guinea pig. This tractable and easily maintained laboratory animal requires much more study if its clinical chemistry and idiosyncracies are to be documented and understood.

REFERENCES

1. Alberts J, Lang L, Reyes P, Briggs G (1977) Zinc requirements of the young guinea pig. J Nutr 107: 1517–1527
2. Bar-Ilan A, Marder J (1980) Acid base status in unanesthetized, unrestrained guinea pigs. Pflügers Arch 384: 93–97
3. Blundell J, Wood S (1975) Is the evolution of insulin darwinian or due to selectively neutral mutation? Nature 257: 198–203
4. Caisey J, Kling D (1980) Clinical chemical values for some common laboratory animals. Clin Chem 26: 1877–1879
5. Chantuin A, Ludewig S (1933) The effects of cholesterol ingestion on the tissue lipids of rats. J Biol Chem 102: 57–65
6. Clampitt RB, Hart RJ (1978) The tissue activities of some diagnostic enzymes in ten mammalian species. J Comp Pathol 88: 607–621
7. Degkwitz E (1982) Activity of alkaline phosphatase in the serum of normal and ascorbic acid-deficient guinea pigs. Z Ernahrungswiss 21: 51–56
8. El Hani A, Dalle M, DeLost P (1980) Sexual dimorphism in binding and metabolism of cortisol during puberty in guinea pigs. J Physiol (Paris) 76: 25–28
9. Green M, Crim M, Traber M, Ostwald R (1976) Cholesterol turnover and tissue distribution in the guinea pig in response to dietary cholesterol. J Nutr 106: 515–528
10. Jondorf W, Maickel R, Brodie B, (1958) Inability of newborn mice and guinea pigs to metabolize drugs. Biochem Pharmacol 1: 352–354
11. Jukes TH (1979) Dr. Best, insulin, and molecular evolution. Can J Biochem 57: 455–458
12. Manin M, Tournaire C, DeLost P (1982) Measurement of the rate of secretion, peripheral metabolism, and interconversion of cortisol and cortisone in adult conscious male guinea pigs. Steroids 39: 81–88
13. National Survey of Laboratory Animal Facilities and Resources (1980) Prepared by: Committee on Laboratory Animal Facilities and Resources, USDHHS, PHS NIH Pub. No. 80–2091
14. Ostwald R, Shannon A (1964) Composition of tissue lipids and anemia of guinea pigs in response to dietary cholesterol. Biochem J 91: 146–154
15. Preston A, Dowdy R, Preston M, Freeman J (1976) Effect of dietary chromium on glucose tolerance and serum cholesterol in guinea pigs. J Nutr 106: 1391–1397
16. Prior J, Kurtz D, Aiegler D (1961) The hypercholesterolemic rabbits. Arch Pathol 71: 672–684
17. Rosenzweig J, Haurankoua J, Lesniak M, Brownstein M, Roth J (1980) Insulin is ubiquitous in the extrahepatic tissues of rats and humans. Proc Nat Acad Sci 77: 572–576
18. Rosenzweig J, Lesniak M, Samuels B, Yip C, Zimmerman A, Roth J (1980) Insulin in the extrapancreatic tissues of guinea pigs differs markedly from the insulin in their pancreas and plasma. Trans Assoc Am Physicians 93: 263–278
19. Sisk D (1976) In Wagner J, Manning P (eds), The Biology of the Guinea Pig. Academic Press, New York
20. Smith L (1966) Species variation in the amino acid sequence of insulin. Am J Med 40: 662–666
21. Swann A, Wiley MH, Siperstein MD (1975) Tissue distribution of cholesterol feedback control in the guinea pig. J Lipid Res 16: 360–366
22. Underwood E (1971) Trace Elements in Human and Animal Nutrition, 3rd ed. Academic Press, New York
23. Weir B (1974) In Rowlands I, Weir B (eds), The Biology of Hystricomorph Rodents. Academic Press, London
24. Wagner J (1976) In Wagner J, Manning P (eds), The Biology of the Guinea Pig. Academic Press, New York
25. Wilson J, Lindsey C (1965) Studies on the influence of dietary cholesterol or cholesterol metabolism in the isotopic steady state of man. J Clin Invest 44: 1805–1814
26. Wriston JC Jr (1984) Comparative biochemistry of the guinea pig: A partial checklist. Comp Biochem Physiol B 77: 253–278
27. Yamanaka W, Ostwald R (1968) Lipid composition of heart, kidney, and lung in guinea pigs made anemic by dietary cholesterol. J Nutr 95: 381–387
28. Yamanaka W, Ostwald R, French S (1967) Histopathology of guinea pigs with cholesterol induced anemia. Proc Soc Exp Biol Med 125: 303–306
29. Zimmerman A, Moule M, Yip C (1974) Guinea pig insulin. II. Biological activity. J Biol Chem 249: 4026–4029
30. Zimmerman A, Yip C (1974) Guinea pig insulin. I. Purification and physical properties. J Biol Chem 249: 4021–4025

4

The Hamster

K. JANE WARDROP, DVM, MS and GERALD L. VAN HOOSIER, JR, DVM

Hamsters possess a number of unique characteristics that make them highly suitable for research purposes. They have been used in dental research, immunologic, toxicologic, and carcinogenic studies, and hibernation experimentation. They have served as animal models for diseases including diabetes mellitus (in which there is a high incidence in some lines of the Chinese hamster) and myopathies (seen in certain Syrian hamster strains). Of the hamster species used in research, approximately 90 per cent are Syrian (Golden) hamsters (*Mesocricetus auratus*), with the remainder being primarily the Chinese (striped black) hamster (*Cricetus griseus*), the European hamster (*Cricetus cricetus*), and the Armenian hamster (*Cricetulus migratorius*) (62).

Hamster blood chemistry studies have received relatively little attention in the literature. Although normal values exist for a number of hamster blood constituents (see Appendix), the effects of disease or varying physiologic states on these values are not well documented. In this chapter, special effort is made to address those hamster blood chemistry values for which changes have been reported (71). Also, as blood biochemical values found in the literature pertain primarily to the more commonly used Syrian hamster, values presented will be those of the Syrian hamster unless otherwise stated.

SPECIMEN HANDLING

Collection of Specimen

Hamsters are among the smallest laboratory animals, and collection of blood can therefore be a frustrating task. If possible, samples should be obtained when activity and food intake are observed to be minimal. Another consideration is its hibernating habits. Hamsters are permissive hibernators, that is, under conditions of a decreased photoperiod and cool temperature ($<20°C$), hamsters will hibernate for 2 to 3 days, alternating with periods of arousal. This can cause variation in laboratory values and should therefore be noted before blood collection. The sex and strain of hamster also should be recorded, as differences in chemistry parameters due to these factors have previously been described (37).

A number of methods for collecting blood have been reported. Cardiac puncture, using a 3/8 of an inch 25-gauge needle, can ensure a good yield of blood. Five milliliters can be obtained from a 100-g hamster under exsanguinating conditions, and 1 to 2 ml can be obtained with no ill effects (39,70). This technique requires practice, as the heart of a hamster can be difficult to locate and can roll away from the needle. Also, repeated sampling using this method is impractical as the mortality rate can be high.

A technique using the large vein on the lateral surface of the thigh of the hamster has been described (50). A tourniquet is placed above the stifle and the hair over the vein is clipped. With the limb in extension, a 5/8 of an inch, 25-gauge needle is inserted into the vessel and blood is collected directly from the needle hub with a microhematocrit tube or capillary micro-container (microtainer capillary whole blood collector, capillary blood serum separator, Becton-Dickinson, Rutherford, NJ).

The orbital region is probably the most common site for obtaining blood in the hamster. This region is highly vascular and readily accessible. One technique for collecting blood from this area uses a tuberculin syringe fitted with a 23-gauge needle. The syringe is coated with a 1:1000 dilution of heparin. The animal is either anesthetized or held firmly to stabilize the head and neck area. With the eye slightly bulged, the needle is placed just beneath the upper eyelid, midway between the medial and lateral canthus of the eye. The needle is gently directed toward the back of the orbit for a distance of approximately 4 mm. The tip of the needle now lies in a venous channel and blood can be aspirated. As much as 3 ml of blood from an adult Syrian hamster can be removed with this technique; however, if repeated sampling is desired, a smaller volume (0.5 ml) is advised (44). In a slight variation, a microhematocrit tube can be placed at the medial canthus of the eye and thrust under the globe to the orbital venous plexus. Pressure on the area for hemostasis is required on completion of bleeding. There also is a technique described for bleeding at the posterior angle of the eye (55).

Preparation of Specimen for Laboratory Submission or Storage

Serum is used for most chemical analyses, as anticoagulants can interfere with test procedures. If an anticoagulant is used, heparin is preferred because of its lack of interference with most assay procedures. Heparin may elevate inorganic phosphorus values, however, and caution should be used when interpreting phosphorus values in heparin-preserved specimens (8). After collection, the whole blood sample is allowed to clot. The sample is then centrifuged at 850 to 1,000 g, and the serum is harvested. Anticoagulated blood samples are simply cen-

trifuged and the plasma is harvested. Both serum and plasma specimens may then be used immediately or refrigerated at 4°C for use within 24 to 48 hours. The sample also may be frozen at $\leq -20°C$. Care should be taken to consult appropriate reference charts before freezing, as certain analytes, especially enzymes, are unstable when frozen (32,39). The use of hemolyzed and lipemic samples should be avoided, as these conditions can seriously alter chemistry values (8,39). Also, serum obtained by cardiac puncture may be contaminated by enzymes (creatine phosphokinase, aspartate aminotransferase, lactate dehydrogenase, and alanine aminotransferase) found in high concentration in cardiac muscle (37).

HAMSTER CLINICAL CHEMISTRIES

Glucose

Glucose is the most commonly measured carbohydrate in the blood and can be affected by a number of parameters. Handling, feeding, and anesthesia can all influence serum glucose levels and should be minimized when possible. Sample handling is of primary importance when evaluating blood glucose concentrations, because glucose values can decrease when serum is left in contact with red cells. Samples should be centrifuged as soon as possible and the serum separated for analysis. Samples may also be collected in sodium fluoride (10 mg/ml of blood), which helps to prevent glycolysis and the resultant decrease in glucose concentration (46).

Thiobarbiturate anesthesia is reported to produce blood glucose concentrations as high as 300 mg/dl in adult male Syrian hamsters as compared to unanesthetized controls (control mean at 144.8 ± 17.3 mg/dl). (Unless otherwise specified, data in this chapter are presented as the mean $\pm$ standard deviation). Hyperglycemia in this study existed up to 5 hours after anesthetic induction and was not influenced by anesthetic duration. Because the liver was involved in the catabolism of the thiobarbiturate, the catabolic process may have caused an increase in gluconeogenesis or glycogenolysis, causing hyperglycemia (61). Hibernation can also have an effect on hamster blood glucose values, with higher glucose concentrations seen during hibernation (35). Circadian rhythms of plasma glucose concentration have been described in hamsters. The lowest glucose concentration occurred near the onset of the dark photoperiod in one study, and the higher concentrations occurred near the onset of the light photoperiod (12). Decreased blood glucose values were observed in a study using fibrosarcoma-bearing animals with 24-hour fasting samples in 28 animals averaging 38 ± 24 mg/dl. Nonfasting values averaged 109 ± 43.5 mg/dl. Control hamsters without fibrosarcomas had nonfasting glucose values of 174 ± 55 mg/dl and 24-hour fasting values of 123 ± 62.7 mg/dl (5).

Special note should be made of the Chinese hamster, which is a widely used animal model of diabetes mellitus. Certain lines of this hamster exhibit a high incidence of diabetes, ranging from mild to severe. Blood glucose values as high as 500 mg/dl have been reported in this condition. These hamsters may also be hypercholesterolemic, insulinopenic, and glucagonemic (11,24). A plasma glucagon value of 178 ± 13 pg/ml (61 ± 8 pg/ml for controls) and a plasma insulin value of 41 ± 8 μU/ml (118 ± 20 μU/ml for controls) in the diabetic Chinese hamster have been reported (72).

Urea Nitrogen

Urea nitrogen (often called blood urea nitrogen, although serum is generally used) is a commonly used indicator of renal function in most laboratory animals, including the hamster. Hamsters inoculated with *Leptospira pomona* have urea nitrogen concentrations as high as 424 mg/dl in association with renal lesions and renal failure (1). Dietary protein can affect urea nitrogen levels, with higher protein diets producing higher urea nitrogen values in the hamster (19). This finding is thought to reflect increased nitrogen metabolism from available protein rather than decreased removal by the kidneys. Published data on sex differences for urea nitrogen vary, with some studies showing higher values for the female (37). Hamsters can also develop kidney disease associated with increased urea nitrogen during the aging process; therefore, consideration should be given to age when assessing urea nitrogen values (19,54).

Creatinine

Creatinine is a nonprotein nitrogen compound formed during the metabolism of muscle

creatine. Creatinine is filtered by the glomerulus of the kidney and is used as a measure of renal function in laboratory animals. Neither sex nor age differences have been observed in the hamster. Elevations in serum creatinine have been reported in cases of nephrotic syndrome associated with renal amyloidosis (48).

Cholesterol

Hamster cholesterol concentrations tend to be the highest of those in laboratory rodents and rabbits, with a range of 112 to 210 mg/dl observed in one comparative study (33). Cholesterol biosynthesis from acetate-1C^{14} increases after phenobarbital administration, but this increased rate is not reflected by increased plasma cholesterol values (31). The photoperiod may also affect cholesterol in the hamster, with short photoperiods (10 light hours, 14 dark hours) reducing the cholesterol concentration in the blood (63,64). Exposure to cold environmental temperatures can produce the opposite effect, that is, hamsters housed outdoors in a cold environment exhibit moderate hypercholesterolemia when compared with hamsters housed under normal indoor temperature conditions (51,63). Hypercholesterolemia has also been reported in diabetic Chinese hamsters, alloxan-treated diabetic Syrian hamster, and hamsters with amyloidosis (24,25). A strain of golden hamsters displaying spontaneous hypercholesterolemia has been described (62). These hamsters develop a further increase in plasma cholesterol when exposed to a low environmental temperature (61).

Bilirubin

Bilirubin is a breakdown product of hemoglobin and is normally processed by the liver. It can be a useful indicator of liver function. Specimens obtained for bilirubin analysis should be protected for light (bilirubin is slowly oxidized under conditions of light exposure). Freezing also may alter bilirubin levels in serum (46).

Total Protein

Total protein concentrations in hamsters have been studied under a variety of conditions. A study evaluating plasma proteins from 500 normal male hamsters aged 4 weeks to 1 year reported the following significant changes with age (proteins were studied using a paper electrophoresis system): (1) a decrease in albumin concentration during the first year; (2) an increase in α_2 globulin concentration by 6 months; (3) a decrease in β-globulin concentration at 8 weeks; (4) an increase, decrease, and increase in the γ-globulin fibrinogen (hamster fibrinogen migrates in the γ-globulin range) concentration at 8 weeks, 6 months, and 1 year, respectively; and (5) a decrease in the albumin:globulin ratio with age. Total protein values for the study were low in comparison to other reported values (see Appendix), with an average of 4.5 ± 0.73 g/dl (30). Changes have also been noted in pregnant hamsters. Using cellulose acetate strips and Owens buffer, a decrease in the albumin fraction and an increase in α-globulins were shown in 15-day old pregnant hamsters (45). Hibernating hamsters have altered protein concentrations, with increased β-globulin, decreased γ-globulin, and increased albumin and total protein (56). Amyloidosis, which occurs with high frequency in hamsters greater than 18 months of age, is accompanied by a decrease in serum albumin concentration and an increase in globulin concentrations, particularly the γ-globulin fraction (25,38,40). Gamma-globulin concentrations also increase after experimentally induced inflammation and may be noted 3 days after insult (9).

Chinese hamsters with spontaneous hereditary diabetes mellitus have high α_2 proteins (10 to 30 per cent, control 3 to 8 per cent). Asymptomatic hamsters with an elevation in the α_2-globulin region were shown to subsequently develop chemical or clinical diabetes or both (27). Previously unknown plasma protein variants also were indentified in Chinese hamster lines (13).

Electrolytes

Little mention is made in the literature of differences in hamster plasma or serum calcium, phosphorus, sodium, and chloride values from those of other species. Similar to many species, immature hamsters do have higher serum phosphorus values than do adults (15). Serum magnesium levels in hamsters are reported to increase during hibernation (20). Hemolysis can affect potassium levels in the hamster, and potassium levels as high as 8 mEq/l have been obtained using hemolyzed specimens (5).

Blood Gas/Acid-Base

Arterial blood gases and pH were measured in awake, adult Syrian hamsters through aortic arch cannulation. In one study, using an ultra-micro blood gas analyzer (Instrumentation Laboratories, Inc., Lexington, MA), the following mean $\pm$ SD values were noted: PaO_2 of 71.8 ± 4.9 mm Hg, $PaCO_2$ of 41.1 ± 2.4 mm Hg, pH of 7.48 ± 0.03, and HCO_3^- of 29.9 ± 2.9 mEq/l (36). During exercise on a treadmill, the mean pH was unchanged, and the PaO_2 showed a mean increase of 12.9 ± 7.9 mm Hg. The $PaCO_2$ decreased 6.6 ± 2.6 mm Hg, and the HCO_3^- decreased 3.5 ± 2.3 mEq/l. Blood gases also were measured in hibernating and hypothermic hamsters. Two separate investigations have shown relatively little change in blood pH and HCO_3^- concentrations under the foregoing conditions, whereas venous PCO_2 decreased (34,65). In another report, a decrease in blood pH was seen with the induction of hypothermia (7).

Enzymes

Creatine Kinase

Creatine Kinase (CK) (creatine phosphokinase [CPK]; [EC 2.7.3.2]) catalyzes the phosphorylation of creatine by means of adenosine triphosphate and is a principal enzyme in muscle metabolism. It is found in skeletal muscle, heart, and brain. Creatine kinase levels in the Syrian hamster have been of particular interest to researchers, as this species does show a hereditary myopathy characterized by an elevation in CK concentrations (4,17,29). Values as high as 730 IU/l have been demonstrated in this disorder, with a control value of 23.2 IU/l (29).

Lactate Dehydrogenase

Lactate dehydrogenase (LDH) (EC 1.1.1.27) is another enzyme found principally in skeletal and cardiac muscle, liver, and kidney. The enzyme concentration was shown to increase in the hereditary myopathy of the hamster (29). Serum LDH values also were seen to rise following inoculation of hamsters with a sarcoma-inducing virus (18).

Alkaline Phosphatase

Alkaline phosphatase (EC 3.1.3.1) is found in many tissues, with principal sources being bone, liver, and intestine. Age-related changes are present in the hamster, with the more immature animal showing a two- to threefold elevation of the serum enzyme (15,18,60). In a study using hamsters as a model of virus-induced hepatitis, alkaline phosphatase appeared to be a more sensitive indicator of liver damage than bilirubin or alanine aminotransferase (56).

Transferases

Aspartate aminotransferase (AST), also known as glutamic oxalacetic transaminase (GOT) (EC 2.6.1.1), is an enzyme found in highest concentration in skeletal muscle, heart muscle, and liver. Serum AST values were shown to increase with neoplastic involvement of the liver and may also become elevated with hepatic metabolic change (18). Another transferase, alanine aminotransferase (ALT), also known as glutamic pyruvic transaminase (GPT) (EC 2.6.1.2), was shown to increase in hamsters in association with both acetaminophen-induced and viral-induced hepatic necrosis (16,47).

Hormones

Thyroid Hormones

Thyroid hormones have probably received more attention in the hamster because of the interest shown in hormones during hibernation in this species. Chronic exposure to a short photoperiod was shown to decrease plasma thyroid-stimulating hormone (TSH), thyroxine (T_4), and triiodothyronine (T_3) levels (28,65). Exposure to cold conditions produces a rise in T_3 levels and a concomitant decline in the serum T_4 level (64). Basal T_3 and T_4 also were shown to decrease with age. In one study using a standard radioimmunoassay, the mean plasma T_4 in 3-month-old hamsters was 6.75 ± 0.75 μg/dl. (Values reported as mean $\pm$ SEM.) The mean T_4 level in 20-month-old hamsters was 3.59 ± 0.16 μg/dl. Plasma T_3 levels were 62 ± 2 ng/dl in the 3-month-old hamsters, and 42 ± 3 ng/dl in the 20-

month-old hamsters. Older animals showed a lesser increase in the T_3 and T_4 levels after TSH administration. T_4 in hamster serum interacts only with albumin, and the binding is weaker than that seen in man with thyroxine-binding globulin (41). Pregnant hamsters may metabolize thyroid hormone differently, as a decrease in protein-bound iodine is seen during pregnancy (22).

Adrenal Hormones

The adrenal cortex of the hamster is anatomically similar to that of other species, containing a well-defined zona glomerulosa, zona fasciculata, and zona reticularis. Pituitary-adrenal function appears to be influenced by testosterone in the male hamster, and males have larger adrenal glands and a higher concentration of plasma steroids than do females (23). Exposure to cold does not appear to stimulate the pituitary adrenal axis (68). Peak adrenal secretory activity in the hamster occurs approximately 3 hours before the onset of the dark photoperiod (21).

Normal hamster cortisol concentrations are low in comparison with those of other species. One study, using a competitive protein-binding technique, showed a normal cortisol level of 0.45 ± 0.04 (SEM) μg/dl for the male hamster and 0.38 ± 0.09 (SEM) μg/dl for the female (23). Radioimmunoassay procedures also were used to determine plasma cortisol concentration. One study of the consummatory behavior in hamsters listed radioimmunoassay basal cortisol values at 0.8 ± 0.11 (SEM) μg/dl for males and 0.96 ± 0.16 (SEM) μg/dl for females (67). Another study gave a value of 0.33 ± 0.04 μg/dl for nonpregnant female hamsters. During pregnancy, plasma cortisol values increased sharply from about 0.3 μg/dl to more than 30 μg/dl at the end of gestation. Following parturition, the cortisol values decreased to basal levels. In this study, the hamsters responded readily to exogenous adrenocorticotrophic hormone (ACTH) stimulation (10). Administration of ACTH also will produce an increase in adrenal weight (3). Even exposure to a novel environment such as a new cage can elevate cortisol levels in hamsters, with males exhibiting a greater response than females (66).

Although early research suggested that cortisol was the predominant glucocorticoid secreted by the hamster in the basal state (49,69), more recent data suggest that the hamster adrenal cortex is capable of secreting both cortisol and corticosterone (2,43). Using sensitive radioimmunoassay procedures to measure each hormone separately, it was demonstrated that hamster plasma corticosterone concentrations were 3 to 4 times higher than cortisol concentrations under basal, daytime conditions. Following stimulation with ACTH or after acute stress, both hormones became elevated, with a relatively greater increase in cortisol. Only plasma cortisol concentrations became elevated following chronic stress (52). Glucocorticoid concentrations were also shown to exhibit a circadian pattern similar to that of other nocturnal rodents. When hamsters were housed under a 14:10 light-dark cycle, corticosterone concentrations predominated during the light phase and cortisol concentrations predominated near the onset of the dark phase (2).

Reproductive Hormones

Hamsters have been used frequently in the study of reproductive processes. The female hamster has a very regular 4-day estrous cycle and a gestation period of 16 days. Generally, the day of ovulation is designated as day 1 of the cycle, and day 4 corresponds to proestrus. Serum gonadotropins in 4-day cycling rodents show one luteinizing hormone (LH) surge and a biphasic follicle-stimulating hormone (FSH) release. In the hamster, the first FSH surge occurs concurrent with, or shortly after, the serum LH increase during the afternoon of proestrus, whereas a second FSH peak (without an increase in serum LH concentration) starts late in the evening of proestrus and peaks during the morning of estrus (14,26,52). The second increase in FSH concentration is thought to be responsible for the initiation and/or maintenance of follicular growth during the next cycle. Ovulation occurs approximately 9 to 10 hours after the peak concentration of LH. Maintenance of a functional corpora lutea in hamsters depends on a luteotropic complex of prolactin, FSH, and a small amount of LH (53).

For the first 3 days of the hamster cycle, there is an inverse relationship between progesterone and estradiol. Progesterone is the dominant hormone for the first 2 days of the cycle (the luteal phase), then it declines, only to rise again on

the afternoon of proestrus (day 4). This preovulatory rise is LH dependent. Serum estradiol levels are low for the first 2 days of the cycle, then rise and fall (follicular phase) on day 4 at 1400 to 1500 hours of proestrus. During the period of the luteal-follicular shift (days 2 through 3 of the cycle), there are no significant changes in serum LH or FSH concentrations (6,57,59). Changes in serum LH, FSH, estradiol, and progesterone concentrations are given in Table 4.1 for the cycling hamster.

Serum prolactin has also been measured by a radioimmunoassay procedure in the female hamster during the estrous cycle and during pregnancy. During the estrus cycle, maximum serum concentrations of prolactin occur each day in the afternoon, with the highest concentrations occurring at proestrus (454 ± 84 ng/ml at 1700 hours, day 4). Release during pregnancy is characterized by a daily surge, and the total amount released decreases as the pregnancy advances (58). Ether anesthesia and handling stress can induce significant elevations of serum prolactin in the female hamster (42).

REFERENCES

1. Abdu MTF, Sleight SD (1965) Pathology of experimental *Leptospira pomona* infection in hamsters. Cornell Vet 55: 74–86
2. Albers HE, Yogev L, Todd RB, Goldman BD (1985) Adrenal corticoids in hamsters: role in circadian timing. Am J Physiol 248: R434–R438
3. Alpert M (1950) Observations on the histophysiology of the adrenal gland of the golden hamster. Endocrinology 46: 166–176
4. Bajusz E, Homburger F (1966) Myopathies. Science 152: 1112–1113
5. Bannon PD, Friedell GH (1966) Values for plasma constituents in normal and tumor bearing golden hamsters. Lab An Care 16: 417–420
6. Bast JD, Greenwald GS (1974) Serum profiles of follicle stimulating hormone, luteinizing hormone and prolactin during the estrous cycle of the hamster. Endocrinology 94: 1295–1299
7. Beaton JR (1961) Note on blood metabolite and electrolyte levels in the hypothermic hamster. Can J Biochem Physiol 39: 1207–1208
8. Benjamin MM, McKelvie DH (1978) In Benirschke K, Garner FM, Jones TC (eds), Pathology of Laboratory Animals, Vol 2. Springer-Verlag, New York
9. Betts A, Tanguay R, Friedell GH (1964) Effect of necrosis on hemoglobin, serum protein profile and erythroagglutination reaction in golden hamsters. Proc Soc Exp Biol Med 116: 66–69
10. Brinck-Johnsen T, Brinck-Johnsen K, Kilham L (1981) Gestational changes in hamster adrenocortical function. J Steroid Biochem 14: 835–839

Table 4.1. Serum Steroid and Gonadotropin Levels in Cycling Hamsters[a]

Day/Hour	FSH (ng/ml)	LH (ng/ml)	Estradiol (pg/ml)	Progesterone (ng/ml)	Reference
1:0900	...	...	17.6 ± 1.1^{b}	5.1 ± 0.6	48
1:1500	427 ± 16	12.7 ± 1.1	...	...	59
2:0900	147 ± 11	11.0 ± 0.5	31.9 ± 6.3	5.2 ± 0.3	59, 48
3:0900	157 ± 9	11.8 ± 2.3	89.3 ± 9.4	1.5 ± 2	59, 48
4:0900	147 ± 8	12.7 ± 1.5	93.3 ± 10.3	0.6 ± 0.2	59, 48
4:1200	197 ± 11	16 ± 2	152.0 ± 11.9	1.4 ± 0.9	53, 48
4:1400	214 ± 16	40 ± 9	121.4 ± 14.9	3.5 ± 1.4	53, 48
4:1600	773 ± 104	$2,521 \pm 438$	101.7 ± 13.7	14.0 ± 1.2	53, 48
4:2000		Basal (10–30)	...	...	57
4:2200	95	...	...	...	57

[a] All values determined by radioimmunoassay. All hamsters on 14-hour light/10-hour dark schedule.
[b] Mean ± SEM.

11. Chang AY (1981) Biochemical abnormalities in the Chinese hamster (*Criceiulus griseus*) with spontaneous diabetes. Int J Biochem 1: 41–43

12. Cincotta AH, Meier AH (1984) Circadian rhythms of lipogenic and hypoglycaemic responses to insulin in the golden hamster (*Mesocricetus auratus*). J Endocrinol 103: 141–146

13. Copeland FJ, Ginsberg LC (1982) Major plasma glycoproteins of diabetic and nondiabetic Chinese hamsters. J Hered 73: 311–313

14. Coutifaris C, Chappel SC (1982) Intraventricular injection of follicle-stimulating hormone (FSH) during proestrus stimulates the rise in serum FSH on estrus in phenobarbital-treated hamsters through a central nervous system-dependent mechanism. Endocrinology 110: 105–113

15. Dent NJ (1977) The use of the Syrian hamster to establish its clinical chemistry and hematology profile. In Duncan WA, Leonard BJ (eds), Clinical Toxicology, XVIII. Excerpta Medica, Amsterdam-Oxford, pp 321–323

16. El-Hage AN, Herman EH, Ferrans VJ (1983) Examination of the protective effect of ICRF-187 and dimethyl sulfoxide against acetaminophen-induced hepatotoxicity in Syrian golden hamsters. Toxicology 28. 295–303

17. Eppenberger M, Nixon CW, Baker JR, Homburger F (1964) Serum phosphocreatine kinase in hereditary muscular dystrophy and cardiac necrosis of Syrian golden hamsters. Proc Soc Exp Biol Med 117: 465–468

18. Eugster AK, Albert PJ, Kalter SS (1966) Multiple enzyme determinations in sera and livers of tumor bearing hamsters. Proc Soc Exp Biol Med 123: 327–331

19. Feldman DB, McConnell EE, Knapka JJ (1982) Growth, kidney disease, and longevity of Syrian hamsters (*Mesocricetus auratus*) fed varying levels of protein. Lab An Sci 32: 613–618

20. Folk GE Jr, Riedesel HL, Hock RJ (1956) Serum magnesium changes with hibernation and winter rest of mammals. Anat Rec 125: 656

21. Frenkel JK, Cook K, Grady HJ, Pendleton SK (1965) Effects of hormones on adrenocortical secretion of golden hamsters. Lab Invest 14: 142, 156

22. Galton VA, Galton M (1966) Thyroid hormone metabolism in the pregnant Syrian hamster (*Mesocricetus auratus*). Acta Endocrinol 53: 130–138

23. Gaskin JH, Kitay JI (1970) Adrenocortical function in the hamster: sex differences and effects of gonadal hormones. Endocrinology 87: 779–786

24. Gerritsen GC (1982) The Chinese hamster as a model for the study of diabetes mellitus. Diabetes 31: 14–25

25. Gleister CA, Van Hoosier GL, Sheldon WG, Read WK (1971) Amyloidosis and renal paramyloid in a closed hamster colony. Lab An Sci 21: 197–202

26. Goldman BD, Porter JC (1970) Serum LH levels in intact and castrated golden hamsters. Endocrinology 87: 676–679

27. Green MN, Yerganian G (1963) Serum proteins in Chinese hamsters with spontaneous hereditary diabetes mellitus. Diabetes 12: 369

28. Hoffman RA, Davidson K, Steinberg K (1982) Influence of photoperiod and temperature on weight gain, food consumption, fat pads and thyroxine in male golden hamsters. Growth 46: 150–162

29. Homburger F, Nixon CW, Eppenberger M, Baker JR (1966) Hereditary myopathy in the Syrian hamster: Studies on pathogenesis. Ann NY Acad Sci 138: 14–27

30. House EL, Pansky B, Jacobs MS (1961) Age changes in blood of the golden hamster. Am J Physiol 200: 1018–1022

31. Jones AL, Armstrong DT (1965) Increased cholesterol biosynthesis following phenobarbitol induced hypertrophy of agranular endoplasmic reticulum in liver. Proc Soc Exp Biol Med 119: 1136–1139

32. Kaneko JJ (ed) (1980) Clinical Biochemistry of Domestic Animals. Academic Press, New York

33. Lee CC, Hermann RG, Froman RO (1959) Serum, bile, and liver total cholesterol of laboratory animals, toads, and frogs. Proc Soc Exp Biol Med 102: 542–544

34. Lyman CP, Hastings AB (1951) Total CO_2, plasma pH and PCO_2 of hamsters and ground squirrels during hibernation. Am J Physiol 167: 633–637

35. Lyman CP, Leduc EH (1953) Changes in blood sugar and tissue glycogen in the hamster during arousal from hibernation. J Cell Comp Physiol 41: 471–492

36. Matt KS, Soares MJ, Talamantes F, Bartke A (1983) Effects of handling and ether anesthesia on serum prolactin levels in the golden hamster. Proc Soc Exp Biol Med 173: 463–466

37. Maxwell KO, Wish C, Murphy JC, Fox JG (1985) Serum chemistry reference values in two strains of Syrian hamsters. Lab An Sci 35: 67–70

38. Mezza LE, Quimby FW, Durham SK, Lewis RM (1984) Characterization of spontaneous amyloidosis of Syrian hamsters using the potassium permanganate method. Lab An Sci 34: 376–380

39. Mitruka BM, Rawnsley HM (1981) Clinical Biochemistry and Hematological Reference Values in Normal Experimental Animals. Masson Publishing USA, Inc, New York

40. Murphy JC, Fox JH, Niemi SM (1984) Nephrotic syndrome associated with renal amyloidosis in a colony of Syrian hamsters. J Am Vet Med Assoc 185: 1359–1362

41. Neve P, Authelet M, Golstein J (1981) Effect of aging on the morphology and function of the thyroid gland of the cream hamster. Cell Tissue Res 220: 499–509

42. O'Brien JJ Jr, Lucey EC, Snider GL (1979) Arterial blood gases in normal hamsters at rest and during exercise. J Appl Physiol 46: 806–810

43. Ottenweller JE, Tapp WN, Burke JM, Natelson BH (1985) Plasma cortisol and corticosterone concentrations in the golden hamster (Mesocritus auratus). Life Sci 37: 1551–1558

44. Pansky B, Jacobs M, House EL, Tassoni JP (1961) The orbital region as a source of blood samples in the golden hamster. Anat Rec 139: 409–412

45. Peterson RP, Turbyfill CL, Soderwall AL, Yamanaka JS (1961) Electrophoretic serum protein patterns in pregnant hamsters (Abstr). Anat Rec 139: 264

46. Ringler DH, Dabich L (1979) In Baker HJ, Lindsey JR, Weisbroth SH (eds), The Laboratory Rat, Vol 1, Biology and Diseases. Academic Press, New York

47. Rollinson EA, White G (1983) Relative activities of acyclovir and BW 759 against Aujeszky's disease and equine rhinopneumonitis viruses. Antimicrob Agents Chemother 24: 221–226

48. Saidapur SK, Greenwald GS (1978) Peripheral blood and ovarian levels of sex steroids in the cyclic hamster. Biol Reprod 18: 401–408

49. Schindler WJ, Knigge KM (1959) Adrenal cortical secretion by the golden hamster. Endocrinology 65: 739–747

50. Schuchman SM (1980) In Kirk RW (ed), Current Veterinary Therapy, VII, Small Animal Practice. WB Saunders, Philadelphia

51. Sicart R, Sable-Amplis R, Bluthe E (1986) Marked elevation of HDL-cholesterol in cold-adapted golden hamsters. Experientia 42: 153–155

52. Siegel HI, Bast JD, Greenwald GS (1976) The effects of phenobarbital and gonadal steroids on periovulatory serum levels of luteinizing hormone and follicle-stimulating hormone in the hamster. Endocrinology 98: 48–55

53. Siegel HI, Greenwald GS (1978) The temporal pattern of LH, FSH, and ovulatory responsiveness to luteinizing hormone releasing hormone in the cyclic hamster. Proc Soc Exp Biol Med 158: 313–317

54. Slauson DO, Hobbs CH, Crain C (1978) Arteriolar nephrosclerosis in the Syrian hamster. Vet Pathol 15: 1–11

55. Sorg DA, Buckner B (1964) A simple method of obtaining venous blood from small laboratory animals. Proc Soc Exp Biol Med 115: 1131–1132

56. South FE, Jeffay H (1958) Alterations in serum proteins of hibernating hamsters. Proc Soc Exp Biol Med 98: 885–887

57. Stetson MH, Watson-Whitmyre M (1977) The neural clock regulating estrous cyclicity in hamsters: gonadotropin release following barbiturate blockade. Biol Reprod 16: 536–542

58. Talamantes F, Marr G, DiPinto MN, Stetson MH (1984) Prolactin profiles during estrous cycle and pregnancy in hamster as measured by homologous RIA. Am J Physiol 247: E126–E129

59. Terranova PF, Greenwald GS (1981) Alteration of the serum follicle-stimulating hormone to luteinizing hormone ratio in the cyclic hamster treated with antiluteinizing hormone: Relationship to serum estradiol, free antiluteinizing hormone and superovulation. Endocrinology 108: 1909–1914

60. Thomas RG, London JE, Drake GA, Jackson DE, Wilson JS, Smith DM (1979) The Golden Hamster—Quantitative Anatomy with Age. Los Alamos Scientific Laboratory, University of California (sponsored by US Government)

61. Turner TT, Howards SS (1977) Hyperglycemia in the hamster anesthetized with inactin (5-ethyl-5(1-methyl propyl)-2-thiobarbiturate). Lab An Sci 27: 380–382

62. Van Hoosier GL, Ladiges WC (1984) Biology and Diseases of Hamsters. In Fox JG, Cohen BJ, Loew FM (ed), Laboratory Animal Medicine, American College of Laboratory Animal Medicine Series. Academic Press, New York, 123–147

63. Vaughan MK, Brainard GC, Reiter RJ (1984) The influence of natural short photoperiodic and temperature conditions on plasma thyroid hormones and cholesterol in male Syrian hamsters. Int J Biometeorol 28: 201–210

64. Vaughan MK, Powanda MC, Richardson BA, King TS, Johnson LY, Reiter RJ (1982) Chronic exposure to short photoperiod inhibits free thyroxine index and plasma levels of TSH, T4, triiodothyronine (T3) and cholesterol in female Syrian hamsters. Comp Biochem Physiol 71A: 615–618

65. Volkert WA, Mussachia XJ (1970) Blood gases in hamsters during hypothermia by exposure to He-O_2 mixture and cold. Am J Physiol 219: 919–922

66. Weinberg J, Wong R (1986) Adrenocortical responsiveness to novelty in the hamster. Physiol Behav 37: 669–672

67. Weinberg J, Wong R (1983) Consummatory behavior and adrenocortical responsiveness in the hamster. Physiol Behav 31: 7–12

68. Wendler DH, Lyman CP (1954) Body temperature, thyroid and adrenal cortex of hamsters during cold exposure and hibernation, with comparisons to rats. Endocrinology 55: 300–315

69. Whitehouse BJ, Vinson GP, Janssens PA (1967) The

effect of blood-borne factors on adrenal steroid synthesis in the golden hamster (*Mesocricetus auratus nehring*). J Endocrinol 37: 139–146

70. Williams CSF (1976) Practical Guide to Laboratory Animals. Mosby, St. Louis

71. Wolford ST, Schroer RA, Gohs FX, Gallo PP, Brodeck M, Falk HB, Ruhren R (1986) Reference range data base for serum chemistry and hematology values in laboratory animals. J Toxicol Envir Health 18: 161–188

72. Wyse BM, Chang AY, Greenburg HS (1978) Glucose, insulin, and glucagon levels in nondiabetic and spontaneously diabetic Chinese hamsters. Diabetes 27: 514

5

The Rabbit

RICHARD R. FOX, PhD

Intermediate body and skeletal size, ear vascularization, immunologic response to antigens, timed ovulatory response, nest-building phenomena, response to presumptive teratogenic drugs, and the simplicity of care relative to the larger animals have given the rabbit a unique importance in biomedical research. The rabbit is large enough to provide adequate quantities of tissue for experimental work without pooling of samples, but it is small enough to be more economical than the dog or monkey. Blood samples can be taken from birth onward in sufficient quantity to run a series of biochemical tests to study the effect of age during the development of a particular pathologic condition. The rabbit provides an excellent mammalian model system to investigate placental transfer of drugs, metabolites, and steroids because both rabbits and humans have the same type of placentation (hemochorial), allowing the closest contact between maternal and fetal circulation. The rabbit, *Oryctolagus cuniculus*, unlike some other members of the order Lagomorpha, breeds well in the laboratory and adapts easily to the laboratory environment. Medlars II has had in its data bank since 1966 over 130,000 bibliographic citations linking the rabbit to studies in almost all areas of biomedical research. Major subject areas include genetics, blood, embryology, immunity, parasitology, physiology, neoplasms, anatomy and histology, growth and development, metabolism, and microbiology.

Rabbit blood chemistry studies have received a reasonable amount of attention in the literature (see Appendix) and the effects of varying physiologic states have partially been documented (27).

The well-documented practice of coprophagy, or reingestion, has many benefits for rabbits. It allows them to survive a week or more without food or water. It greatly improves utilization of a number of dietary constituents (23,25). It also may minimize the effect of fasting on various clinical chemistry measurements.

SPECIMEN HANDLING

Collection of Specimen

Repeated blood samples for clinical chemistry and hematologic determinations are easily obtained from the marginal ear vein or even the medial artery by simple drip method, vacuum ear bleeder (22), or a Vacutainer® (Becton, Dickinson & Co.) (6). Cardiac puncture, using a 1.5-inch 19-gauge needle, can also be performed repeatedly, but this takes considerable experience. In two experiments repeated samples were taken on days 10, 20, 30, 40, 50, 60, 90, and 120 with minimal problems (29,30). Alternatively, rabbits restrained with ketamine hydrochloride and clipped may be bled from the jugular vein using a 1-inch 20-gauge needle (Loeb, personal communication).

The rabbit can provide a large quantity of blood on a regular basis. An adult New Zealand White can easily be bled every 2 weeks and 25 to 30 ml taken with the vacuum ear bleeder (22). One report suggests that a volume of 50 to 60 ml can be collected in 2 minutes at weekly intervals (4). It should be realized that anesthesia can modify certain clinical chemistries (2).

Preparation of Specimen for Laboratory Submission or Storage

Serum is preferred for most analyses, as anticoagulants may interfere with some test procedures. Rabbit blood clots quickly at room temperature, so 30 to 45 minutes are adequate followed by centrifugation at approximately $1100 \times g$ to collect serum. Inadequate clotting time may result in fibrin clots in the serum. Rabbit blood may require more anticoagulant than that from some other species. We routinely have used 1,000 units of preservative-free heparin per milliliter of whole blood in producing washed red blood cells. Storage of frozen samples at $-20°C$ may be satisfactory for a short time, but $-70°C$ is recommended for long-term storage. When in doubt, the stability of the analyte under conditions of storage should be validated. The use of hemolyzed or lipemic samples should be avoided.

RABBIT CLINICAL CHEMISTRIES

Acetylators of Drugs and Environmental Carcinogens

An important metabolic step in the biotransformation of arylamines and hydrogens is N-acetylation via the cytosolic enzyme N-acetyltransferase (EC 2.3.1.5) located predominantly in the liver and small intestine. A difference in N-acetylation capacity between individuals is inherited as a simple autosomal Mendelian trait with two alleles at a common locus. The genetically determined acetylator status of an individual has important pharmacokinetic and toxicologic significance, because the frequency of a variety of drug-induced pathologic conditions has been shown to depend on acetylator phenotype or genotype.

The rabbit has been used most often as an animal model of the acetylation polymorphism. It has been known, for example in man and the rabbit, that large differences exist between rapid and slow acetylators for isoniazid, sulfamethazine, and 2-aminofluorene N-acetyltransferase activity, whereas smaller differences exist for N-acetyltransferase activity, p-aminosalicylic acid, and p-aminobenzoic acid. The presence of such differences among inbred strains of rabbits has enhanced their value to the scientific community (20,21,41).

Adrenal Hormones

Corticosterone is the major corticosteroid secreted in vivo in the rabbit. Normally the ratio of corticosterone to cortisol in adrenal venous blood is about 20:1 (34). Chronic treatment with ACTH will shift this ratio to unity. Strain differences in corticosterone levels following mild stress have been reported (34). Cortisol levels in rabbits vary with time of day (24,38).

Alkaline Phosphatase

Serum alkaline phosphatase levels are influenced by age in most species, but data on this in the rabbit are not available. Differences have been associated with breed (25) and strain (13). No differences due to sex or time of day have been observed (12,13). Bone diseases such as osteopetrosis will cause elevation of the serum alkaline phosphatase level (33).

Bilirubin

Serum bilirubin in the rabbit presents no unique features. Values of 1 mg/dl or less are in accord with reference values in other species. No real differences have been associated with sex or strain (14).

Blood Urea Nitrogen

Serum blood urea nitrogen levels (BUN) are commonly used to indicate the level of renal function, but they may be significantly altered by protein catabolism, protein synthesis or both. The time of day is extremely important as to the BUN levels observed, with peak values between 1600 and 2000 hours (12). Also, breed, strain, and sex can affect the measured levels (12,13,

Table 5.1. Rabbit (*Oryctolagus Cuniculus*) Reference Values for Some Uncommon Analytes[a]

Analyte	Sex[b]	Mean	SD	Reference
Acid phosphatase (IU)	M	110.3	14.3	37
Acid protease (μM of tyrosine/ml of serum/h)	M	1.29	0.15	37
Alpha-amino nitrogen (mM/l)	B	4.47	0.98	2
Cholesterol, free (mg/dl)	B	38	3	42
	B	22	13	3
	M	6.2	1.6	31
	F	11.9	3.3	31
Corticosterone (μg/dl) TO[c]	M	1.54	0.88	34
T22[d]	M	14.0	4.3	34
Cortisol (μg/dl) T22[d]	M	1.03	0.12	34
Growth hormone (ng/ml)	M	11.0	3.5	36
	F	12.2	4.0	36
Lipids, total (mg/dl)	B	243	89	3
	B	390	80	42
	F	328	16	25
Phospholipids, total (mg/dl)	B	78	33	3
	B	113	29	42
Neutral fat (mg/dl)	B	105	50	3
Total fatty acids (mg/dl)	B	169	66	3
Taurine (nM/ml)	B	101	26	19
Total iron binding capacity (μg/dl)	M	267	25.5	14
	F	256	24.4	14
Tryptophan (ng/ml)				
Total	B	14	2.5	24
Free	B	0.85	0.24	24

[a] For common analytes, see Appendix.
[b] B = either sex not specified or sexes combined.
[c] TO = initial baseline level.
[d] T22 = after 22 minutes of immobilization.

25). Tumors affecting kidney function will result in elevated BUN levels. These tumors may be spontaneous (16) or induced (10,11,15,17).

Cholesterol

Serum cholesterol levels are under the direct influence of the thyroid, liver, and steroid-producing organs. Cholesterol produced in the liver is circulated in both free and esterified forms to provide precursors for steroid production by both the adrenals and the gonads. Serum cholesterol levels rise rapidly after birth in a similar pattern to that observed for protein bound iodine. The levels peak at approximately 20 days and then fall slowly to adult levels which are reached at about 90 days (29). It has been reported that increased levels are later attained with increasing old age (32). Breed, strain, sex, and time of day (25,28,31) also influence greatly the cholesterol levels of rabbits. A threefold difference in the total cholesterol level was shown to be dependent on the strain (AX/J strain levels of 69 mg/dl versus OS/J levels of 22 mg/dl) (31). Females have greater adult levels than do males. This difference is not evident in adolescents (29). Peak levels of total cholesterol were observed between 1600 and 2000 hours (28). Fivefold differences in serum cholesterol levels (300 vs 1,500 mg/dl) were observed following 4 weeks of a dietary supplement of 0.5 per cent cholesterol, depending on the strain of rabbit used (47).

Complement

The rabbit appears to be the animal of choice as the source of complement for lymphocytotoxic testing of murine and human cells, a technique widely used in typing for tissue transplantation and in studies of tumor immunobiology. Experience has shown that only about 1 randomly bred rabbit in 40 gives serum that is suitable for high quality assays. The ideal complement for the lymphocytotoxic test should be uniform from rabbit to rabbit and have both a high titer and a low level of nonspecific cytotoxicity. Genetic differences associated with specific strains as sources of complement have been clearly demonstrated (7–9).

Components of Reproductive Tract Fluid

Kozma et al (25) presented an excellent review of the literature on this subject, including in tabular form a listing of the component, concentration in the reproductive tract fluid, and appropriate references. Although the critical experiments showing how these constituents vary with age, sex, strain, and the like were not reported, it would not be surprising if many of them did.

Electrolytes

Serum phosphorus levels are influenced physiologically by vitamin D metabolism parathormones, renal function, and level of ionized calcium present. Differences in levels have been associated with both strain and sex but not with time of day (5,12,13). Serum sodium and chloride vary depending on the breed of rabbit according to a review by Kozma et al (25). Serum calcium levels are elevated in tumor-bearing animals with VX_2 carcinoma (43).

Esterases

Although serum esterases are not usually part of a discussion on clinical chemistry, it is important to realize that genetic differences in esterases such as atropine or cocaine do exist (18,35,46) and that these differences can influence greatly the degradation of various drugs (45), pointing out the necessity of knowing the genotype of the breed or strain of rabbit used in drug testing.

Glucose

Glucose is the most commonly measured carbohydrate in the blood and is affected by a number of parameters. The genetic background, whether it be breed (25) or inbred strain (13), will affect the normal base level. The base serum level on fasting is reported to increase with increasing age (32). It has been stated that the rabbit can survive short periods (96 hours) of fasting and maintain its serum glucose levels

(25), probably because of coprophagy (23). In contrast, however, is the report on diurnal variations (12) in which a low of about 115 mg of glucose per deciliter of serum was observed 1 hour before and 3 hours after feeding values of 130 mg (females) and 145 mg (males) per deciliter of serum were obtained. Urethane and halothane anesthesia were reported to increase serum glucose levels in rabbits (2).

Growth Hormone

Serum growth hormone levels have been shown to vary threefold as a function of strain (36). These differences associated with strain were not correlated with body size but were based on genetic relationships among strains.

Protein Bound Iodine

Protein bound iodine (PBI) is used as an indicator of thyroid function. It primarily reflects the circulating levels of the thyroid hormones triiodothyronine (T_3) and tetraiodothyronine (T_4). The PBI in rabbits increases rapidly from its level at birth to a peak at about 20 days and then decreases to adult levels, which are obtained at approximately 60 days (29). The PBI levels also vary with strain, sex, and time of day (28,31). T_3 and T_4 levels have been shown to increase significantly during starvation (40).

Serum Iron and Total Iron Binding Capacity

Serum iron, total iron binding capacity, and the ratio of these in man have been used as diagnostic criteria for iron deficiency anemia, Hodgkin's disease, and the like. In rabbits these levels can be affected by sex, strain, and time of day (14). For example, serum iron levels vary significantly with the time of day; the low level appears to be at 0800 hours and the high at 2000 hours. Total iron binding capacity does not vary diurnally but does differ significantly with sex. Both parameters exhibit strain differences.

Taurine

Three groups of rabbits assayed for taurine levels had similar serum levels but marked variation in their levels in the aqueous humor (19). It was suggested that this difference was due in part to an inherited condition for buphthalmos in the rabbit.

Total Protein and Albumin

The breed (25) or strain (13) of rabbit can affect the level of total protein from a statistically significant standpoint, but the range is relatively narrow, as a biologically significant alteration in the total serum protein level is indicative of an abnormal physiologic state. Generally, alteration in total proteins is associated with kidney or liver disease. Total protein is also elevated when an animal is dehydrated or in shock and supportive fluid treatment is indicated. Time of day does not seem to be a factor in altering total protein levels (12).

The albumin fraction represents about 60 per cent of the total protein and appears to be greater in the female than in the male New Zealand White rabbit (26). The same investigators also show that females have a lower α-globulin fraction than do males, in contrast to a previous report in which no sex differences were observed (1). Extreme care must be exercised in defining the method used to quantitate serum albumin levels, as Quimby (personal communication) compared two test methods, bromcresol green versus cellulose acetate electrophoresis, and found that one yielded 50 per cent higher levels. Wostmann (44) reported that germ-free rabbits had greatly reduced amounts of α-globulin when compared with conventionally reared rabbits. Cold stress was reported to result in increases in total plasma proteins and β-globulins and a decrease in serum albumin (39).

Tryptophan

Plasma tryptophan is a precursor of 5-hydroxytryptamine (5-HT) of the brain, a biogenic amine with neurotransmitter functions. In the pineal gland, it has been implicated in the neural control of circadian rhythm. Tryptophan circulates in the blood mainly in bound form to albumin, and 10 to 20 per cent is present as free amino acid. Plasma-free tryptophan may be an important determinant of brain tryptophan concentrations. Both plasma tryptophan and free tryptophan vary diurnally and appear to vary in an inverse relationship (24).

ACKNOWLEDGEMENT

This work was supported in part by institutional funds of the Jackson Laboratory. The Jackson Laboratory is fully accredited by the American Association for Accreditation of Laboratory Animal Care.

REFERENCES

1. Allen RC, Watson DF (1958) Paper electrophoretic analysis of rabbit serum as an aid in the selection of experimental rabbits. Am J Vet Res 19: 1001–1003
2. Bito LZ, Eakins KE (1969) The effect of general anesthesia on the chemical composition of blood plasma of normal rabbits. J Pharmacol Exp Ther 169: 277–286
3. Boyd EM (1942) Species variation in normal plasma lipids estimated by oxidative micromethods. J Biol Chem 143: 131–132
4. Burke JG (1977) Blood collecting by the ear artery method. Lab An 6: 49
5. Buss SL, Bourdeau JE (1984) Calcium balance in laboratory rabbits. Mineral Electrolyte Metab 10: 127–132
6. Cohen CA (1955) A method for bleeding rabbits. Am J Clin Pathol 25: 604
7. Fox RR, Cherry M (1978) Effect of rabbit strain on activity level and cytotoxicity of serum complement. II. Comparison of five murine target cells. J Hered 69: 331–336
8. Fox RR, Cherry M, Shultz KL (1978) Effect of rabbit strain on activity level and cytotoxicity of serum complement. J Hered 69: 107–112
9. Fox RR, Cherry M, Shultz KL, Salvatore KJ (1979) Effect of rabbit strain on activity level and cytotoxicity of serum complement. III. Comparison of four tumor target cells. J Hered 70: 109–114
10. Fox RR, Diwan BA, Meier H (1975) Transplacental induction of primary renal tumors in rabbits treated with 1-ethyl-1-nitrosourea. J Nat Cancer Inst 54: 1439–1448
11. Fox RR, Diwan BA, Meier H (1977) Transplacental carcinogenic effects of combined treatment of ethylurea and sodium nitrite in rabbits. J Nat Cancer Inst 59: 427–429
12. Fox RR, Laird CW (1970) Biochemical parameters of clinical significance in rabbits. II. Diurnal variations. J Hered 61: 265–268
13. Fox RR, Laird CW, Blau EM, Schultz HS, Mitchell BP (1970) Biochemical parameters of clinical significance in rabbits. I. Strain variations. J Hered 61: 261–265
14. Fox RR, Laird CW, Kirshenbaum J (1974) Effect of strain, sex and circadian rhythm on rabbit serum bilirubin and iron levels. Proc Soc Exp Biol Med 145: 421–427
15. Fox RR, Meier H, Bedigian HG, Crary DD (1982) Genetics of transplacentally induced teratogenic and carcinogenic effects in rabbits treated with N-Nitroso-N-ethylurea. J Nat Cancer Inst 69: 1411–1417
16. Fox RR, Meier H, Crary DD, Myers DD, Norberg

RF, Laird CW (1970) Lymphosarcoma in the rabbit: Genetics and pathology. J Nat Cancer Inst 45: 719–729

17. Fox RR, Meier H, Pottathil R, Bedigian HG (1980) Transplacental teratogenic and carcinogenic effects in rabbits chronically treated with N-ethyl-N-nitrosourea. J Nat Cancer Inst 65: 607–614

18. Fox RR, Zutphen LFM van (1977) Strain differences in the prealbumin serum esterases of JAX rabbits. J Hered 68: 227–230

19. Harris TM, Nance CS, Sheppard LB, Fox RR (1983) Evidence for an hereditary defect in taurine transport in the ciliary epithelium of an inbred strain of rabbits. J Inherit Metab Dis 6: 163–166

20. Hein DW, Smolen TN, Fox RR, Weber WW (1982) Identification of genetically homozygous rapid and slow acetylators of drugs and environmental carcinogens among established inbred rabbit strains. J Pharmacol Exp Ther 223: 40–44

21. Hein DW, Smolen TN, Glowinski IB, Fox RR, Weber WW (1981) Identification of rapid and slow acetylators of arylamine drugs and carcinogens among established inbred rabbit strains (abstr) Pharmacologist 23: 200

22. Hoppe PC, Laird CW, Fox RR (1969) A simple technique for bleeding the rabbit ear vein. Lab An Care 19: 524–525

23. Hunt CE, Harrington DD (1974) In Weisbroth SH, Flatt RE, Kraus AL (eds), The Biology of the Laboratory Rabbit. Academic Press, New York

24. Hussein L, Goedde HW (1979) Diurnal rhythm in the plasma level of total and free tryptophan and cortisol in rabbits. Res Exp Med (Berl) 176: 123–130

25. Kozma C, Macklin W, Cummins LM, Mauer R (1974) In Weisbroth SH, Flatt RE, Kraus AL (eds), The Biology of the Laboratory Rabbit. Academic Press, New York

26. Kozma C, Pelas A, Salvador RA (1967) Electrophoretic determination of serum proteins of laboratory animals. J Am Vet Med Assoc 151: 865–869

27. Laird CW (1972) Representative values for animal and veterinary populations and their clinical significances. Hycel Inc., Houston

28. Laird CW, Fox RR (1970) Diurnal variations in rabbits: Biochemical indicators of thyroid function. Life Sci 9: 191–202

29. Laird CW, Fox RR (1970) The effect of age on cholesterol and PBI levels in the III/IIIc hybrid rabbits. Life Sci 9: 1243–1253

30. Laird CW, Fox RR, Mitchell BP, Blau EM, Schultz HS (1970) Effect of strain and age on some hematological parameters in the rabbit. Am J Physiol 218: 1613–1617

31. Laird CW, Fox RR, Schultz HS, Mitchell BP, Blau EM (1970) Strain variations in rabbits: Biochemical indicators of thyroid function. Life Sci 9: 203–214

32. Nasledova ID, Silnitsky PS (1972) [Some age peculiarities of lipid and carbohydrate metabolism and the state of the aortic wall in female rabbits]. Biull Eksper Biol Med 73: 19–22.

33. Pearce L (1948) Hereditary osteopetrosis of the rabbit. II. X-ray, hematologic, and chemical observations. J Exp Med 88: 597–620

34. Redgate ES, Fox RR, Taylor FH (1981) Strain and age effects on immobilization stress in JAX rabbits. Proc Soc Exp Biol Med 166: 442–448

35. Sawin PB, Glick D (1943) Atropinesterase, a genetically determined enzyme in the rabbit. Proc Nat Acad Sci 29: 55–59

36. Schindler WJ, Hutchins MO, Laird CW, Fox RR (1974) Effect of strain and sex variation on growth hormone in rabbit serum. Proc Soc Exp Biol Med 147: 820–822

37. Shtacher G (1969) Selective renal involvement in the early development of hypercalcemia and hypophosphatemia in VX-2 carcinoma-bearing rabbits: Studies on serum and tissues alkaline phosphatase and renal handling of phosphorus. Cancer Res 29: 1512–1528

38. Singh RK, Chansouria JPN, Udupa KN (1975) Circadian periodicity of plasma cortisol (17-OHCS) levels in normal, traumatized, corticotrophin and dexamethasone treated rabbits. Indian J Med Res 63: 793–798

39. Sutherland GB, Trapani IL, Campbell DH (1958) Cold adapted animals. II. Changes in the circulating plasma proteins and formed elements of rabbit blood under various degrees of cold stress. J Appl Physiol 12: 367–372

40. Takagi A, Isozaki Y, Kurata K, Nagataki S (1978) Serum concentrations, metabolic clearance rates, and production rates of reverse triiodothyronine, triiodothyronine, and throxine in starved rabbits. Endocrinology 103: 1434–1439

41. Weber WW, Hein DW, Glowinski IB, Fox RR, King CM (1982) Association of arylhydromatic acid N, O-Acetyltransferase (AHAT) and genetically polymorphic N-Acetyltransferase (NAT) in established inbred rabbit strains, pp 405–412. Invited paper presented at the WHO Conference on *Host Factors in Human Carcinogenesis* held at Cape Sunion, Greece, June 1981. In Bartsch H, Armstrong B (eds), IARC Sci. Publ. No. 39 Int. Assoc. Research Cancer, Lyon, France

42. Westerman MP, Wiggins RG III, Mao R (1970) Anemia and hypercholesterolemia in cholesterol-fed rabbits. J Lab Clin Med 75: 893–902

43. Wolfe HJ, Bitman WR, Voelkel EF, Griffiths HJ, Tashjian AH (1978) Systemic effects of the VX_2 carcinoma on the osseous skeleton. Lab Invest 38: 208–215

44. Wostmann BS (1961) Recent studies on the serum proteins of germ-free animals. Ann NY Acad Sci 94: 272–293

45. Zutphen LFM van (1974) Serum esterase genetics in rabbits. I. Phenotypic variation of the prealbumin esterases and classification of atropinesterase and cocainesterase. Biochem Genet 12: 309–326

46. Zutphen LFM van (1974) Serum esterase genetics in rabbits. II. Genetic analysis of the prealbumin esterase system, including atropinesterase and cocainesterase polymorphism. Biochem Genet 12: 327–343

47. Zutphen LFM van, Fox RR (1977) Strain differences in response to dietary cholesterol by JAX rabbits: Correlation with esterase patterns. Atherosclerosis 28: 435–446

6

The Dog

WALTER F. LOEB, VMD, PhD

The standard research dog is the beagle, bred and raised for laboratory use. The breed is fairly uniform and tends to be free of breed-related diseases except for coagulation factor VII deficiency, which is often asymptomatic and can be detected by the one-stage prothrombin time (46). Random or pound dogs are generally unacceptable for most research applications because of nonuniformity, lack of medical history, and the occurrence of undetectable diseases. Breeds of dogs other than the beagle, in particular the American Foxhound, are occasionally used for special purposes such as when a larger body size than that of the beagle is required.

Stress alters the results of various clinical chemistry determinations, as will be discussed in conjunction with specific analytes. It is therefore important, and results in the most uniform data, to acclimate the dogs well, house them in a stress-free environment, and handle them gently but firmly, especially when drawing blood samples.

Blood samples are best drawn from the jugular vein. The needle size is somewhat at the discretion of the person collecting the samples, but a 1-inch, 20-gauge or 1-inch, 21-gauge thin-walled needle is suitable. The dog is firmly but gently restrained by an assistant who turns the dog's head away from the person collecting the sample. The jugular vein is compressed and immobilized ventrally by the thumb of the person drawing the sample and stroked downward with the forefinger, making the vein turgid and easy to puncture. After the tip of the needle is seated well in the lumen of the vein, pressure on the vein is released, and the appropriate samples are collected. Alternatively samples may be withdrawn from the cephalic, femoral, or saphenous veins, but the smaller diameter of these veins and their tendency to collapse may limit sample availability. Canine erythrocytes are more fragile than those of some other species and excess suction should be avoided to prevent hemolysis.

Van Sluijs et al (82) compared capillary and venous blood samples with arterial samples for the measurement of acid-base and blood gases in dogs. They concluded that in dogs with pulmonary disease capillary samples may be substituted for arterial samples unless there is circulatory impairment in which instance an unacceptably large difference occurs between arterial and capillary values.

Lipemia, the presence of visibly detectable lipid in serum or plasma, is much more common in the dog than in other laboratory animals and may invalidate or interfere with analytic methodology. In the healthy dog, 12 hours of fasting renders the animal essentially physiologically nonabsorptive and free from physiologic lipemia. Unless otherwise indicated by the experimental design, serum or plasma lipid determinations should be performed under these conditions. The presence of lipemia in the fasting dog may occur in diabetes mellitus, acute pancreatitis, for a period of time after hepatic disease because of failure of synthesis of pre-beta lipoprotein, and in congenital dyslipo-proteinemia (4). Lipemic serum or plasma may be clarified by high speed centrifugation (65,000 × g for 10 minutes), but this should not be performed unless lipemia-free serum is unavailable because of uncertainty as to the relative partition of analytes between the aqueous and lipid layers.

The canine erythrocyte is a high sodium, low potassium cell, in contrast to man, the rat, or nonhuman primates whose erythrocytes are low in sodium and high in potassium (33). Therefore, hemolysis in canine serum or failure to remove serum from the erythrocytes does not elevate potassium to a degree comparable to that in high-potassium-erythrocyte species. Hemolysis does result in passage of lactic dehydrogenase, phosphorus, and some aspartate aminotransferase to the serum, as does failure to promptly separate serum from erythrocytes. The latter also results in glycolysis; the same good practices of promptly separating serum from cells after firm clotting should be applied in working with dog serum as with the serum of other species. Thixotropic silicone gel is of value in obtaining prompt, clean separation. After separation the serum should be transferred to a clean tube; the thixotropic gel should not be relied upon to form an impenetrable barrier. Conditions of storage before testing should be individually tested with respect to the analyte under consideration. Freezing at household refrigerator-freezer temperature (about −20°C) may be too slow or insufficiently cold to protect the analyte. Freezing may also result in cryoprecipitation of globulins, resulting in their loss from the supernatant serum.

Canine urine samples are best collected by catheterization, which is easy in male dogs and can readily be learned in females. Timed urine samples collected over long periods are sometimes collected in metabolism cages, but it is difficult to prevent the contamination of these samples with feces, food, or other debris.

FUNCTION STUDIES

Because of the dog's relatively large size among research animals and comparatively tractable behaviour, function studies have been utilized more extensively in the canine than in other laboratory animal species. By contrast to static clinical chemistry measurements which determine the concentration of an analyte under basal or otherwise standardized conditions, these function studies determine the animal's response to a specific biochemical challenge or stimulation. Numerous such studies have been proposed, the most extensively used among them being glucose tolerance, inulin and creatinine clearance, ACTH response and dexamethasone suppression, TSH stimulation, and ammonia tolerance. Some of these are briefly discussed in this and other chapters of this book. These studies have demonstrated the weaknesses of relying on single basal values of clinical chemical analyses in some instances. For example, it is well and extensively documented that many dogs with adrenocortical hyperfunction have basal serum cortisol values well within the reference range and that ACTH stimulation and/or dexamethasone suppression tests are required to discriminate such dogs from the euadrenocortical population. Past trends suggest that such function tests will be progressively standardized and simplified and will receive more extensive use in the evaluation of laboratory animals.

Glucose

The level of serum glucose in the dog is affected by numerous factors including absorptive or fasting state, the concentration of plasma insulin, epinephrine (74), cortisol, somatotropin, and thyroid and hepatocellular function. Unless serum or plasma is collected with an inhibitor of glycolysis such as sodium fluoride, it is essential to separate the serum from the cells as promptly as possible. At room temperature typical glycolysis by the erythrocytes in an uncentrifuged blood sample will result in a decreased determined glucose value of 15 mg/dl/h. Stress in the dog mildly elevates blood glucose, not extremely as in the cat or some nonhuman primates. Through cortisol, which undergoes marked circadian rhythm, glucose values may undergo circadian variation. In a study in which glucose is determined repeatedly, it is essential to collect all samples in the same fasting or absorptive state and at the same time of day. Historical serum glucose values in healthy fasting adult dogs are 60 to 90 mg/dl and postprandially up to 165 mg/dl (70–73,81). In the bitch, the estrus cycle does not affect baseline blood glucose or insulin values, but during estrus glucose tolerance is impaired.

Hyperglycemia has been observed in diabetic dogs treated with large doses of insulin; on reduction of the insulin dosage the magnitude of fluctuation and therefore of hyperglycemia may be reduced (26).

The use of glycosylated hemoglobin determination has proved a valuable aid in the long-term monitoring of blood glucose in man. Glycosylated hemoglobin is formed by the non-enzymatic coupling of the carbohydrate moiety to hemoglobin, and it reflects the long-term control of blood glucose. Chromatographic demonstration of hemoglobin A_{1c} has been validated in the dog (50,78,91). Mean hemoglobin A_{1c} in normal dogs was shown to be 2.95 per cent with 1 standard deviation of 0.38 per cent, whereas hyperglycemic diabetic dogs had a mean value of 4.97 per cent with 1 standard deviation of 1.6 per cent (90). Canine insulin can be measured validly by the human insulin radioimmunoassay (69,78).

Evaluation of Renal Function

Serum urea nitrogen and creatinine are conventionally measured in the dog to assess impairment of renal function despite their recognized insensitivity. Urea is produced from ammonia in the ornithine-arginine-citrulline cycle by hepatocytes, excreted in the glomerular filtrate, and partially resorbed passively with water in the renal tubules. A decreased concentration of serum urea is seen in dogs with severe hepatocellular dysfunction, portosystemic shunts, or biochemical defects in hepatic urea synthesis, which, like portosystemic shunts, may be congenital. Urea nitrogen levels become elevated when nephron function is reduced to 25 per cent of maximum. Elevations of blood urea nitrogen occur relatively readily in the dog, and terminally values may be higher than is typical in other species—as high as 400 mg/dl (27).

Watson et al (86) showed that plasma urea concentrations increased two to three times fasting values at approximately 8 hours after a meal of cooked or raw meat or "semimoist" dog food. Concentrations of creatinine increased to 140 per cent of baseline values 2 to 5 hours after a meal of cooked meat but were minimally affected by ingestion of raw meat or "semimoist" dog food.

Urine specific gravity or osmolality and increases in these parameters in response to water deprivation constitute a more sensitive evaluation of functional renal capacity than does measurement of urea nitrogen or creatinine.

Urine protein to creatinine ratio has been used to assess proteinuric disease, either on a 24-hour urine sample (12) or on a random voided sample (30). This ratio was shown to detect significant proteinuria with greater sensitivity than did 24-hour urine protein loss, and to correlate with urine protein per 24 hours. In healthy dogs the urine protein to creatinine ratio is generally less than 0.2 and invariably less than 0.4, whereas diseased dogs may have values in excess of 20 (12,30).

Urine gamma glutamyl transpeptidase, a marker of renal tubular necrosis, was shown to detect nephrotoxicity induced by gentamycin more sensitively than did serum creatinine, 24-hour endogenous creatinine clearance, or the presence of urinary casts (31).

The clearance of inulin and of either endogenous or exogenous creatinine has been used to determine the glomerular filtration rate in the dog, a more sensitive method for estimating diminished nephron function. Finco et al (27) devised a protocol for the simultaneous determination of inulin clearance and clearance of exogenous creatinine in the dog using constant infusion of 14C inulin and a single subcutaneous injection of creatinine. They demonstrated that this procedure determines glomerular filtration rate more validly than does endogenous creatinine clearance or other tests of renal function such as phenolsulfonphthalein clearance or sodium sulfanilate clearance.

Evaluation of Hepatic Disease

Relating the interpretation of clinical chemical determinations to anatomic-pathologic classifications of hepatic disorders leads to the conclusion that three general classes of information about the liver may be obtained; *leakage enzymes* provide sensitive evidence of injury to hepatocytes, including some indication of severity and subcellular localization. Numerous analytes are influenced by hepatocellular functions of synthesis and metabolism and reflect *liver function*. These include urea nitrogen, albumin, cholesterol, bilirubin, uric acid, ammonia, prothrombin, and fibrinogen. The evaluation generally tends to be insensitive and is compiled from the measurement of several analytes. *Impaired biliary function* and *flow* are reflected in altered alkaline phosphatase, gamma glutamyl transferase, total and direct reacting bilirubin, and urine urobilinogen. These three categories are not altogether mutually exclusive. Taken together each contributes specific information of value in the interpretation of hepatic disorders (45,79).

Leakage Enzymes

Numerous enzymes including alanine aminotransferase, aspartate aminotransferase, lactic dehydrogenase, sorbitol dehydrogenase, glutamate dehydrogenase, arginase, and creatine kinase are produced for intracellular utilization in cytosol or subcellular organelles and leak from the cells in which they were produced, as a function of injury to the organelles, increased plasma membrane permeability, or necrosis. Because of the liver's extensive functions of synthesis, it is a very rich source of the foregoing enzymes except creatinine kinase. Cardiac and skeletal muscle constitutes the principal source of creatine kinase and an important source of aspartate aminotransferase and lactic dehydrogenase. Serum levels of enzymes depend on the enzyme activity of the source tissue, localization of enzyme within the source cells, type of injury, mass of injured tissue, and rate of clearance of the specific enzyme in serum. These properties vary among species and are considered in detail in Chapter 11 (83).

In the dog, alanine aminotransferase (serum glutamic pyruvic transaminase) is present in liver cells in four times greater activity than that of any other tissue. Plasma clearance is biphasic with a first phase half-time of 17 hours and a second phase half-time of 61 hours. Combined with cytosol origin, these characteristics make alanine aminotransferase a very sensitive and rather specific enzyme for the detection of hepatocellular injury. Abdelkader and Hauge (1) compared the sensitivity and hepatospecificity of glutamate dehydrogenase and sorbitol dehydrogenase to those of alanine aminotransferase and aspartate aminotransferase in dogs

with a variety of hepatic diseases including hepatic neoplasms, chronic hepatitis, cirrhosis, fatty liver, and others. They concluded that glutamate dehydrogenase was the most sensitive and that the magnitude of elevation correlated with the extent of liver cell necrosis. Sorbitol dehydrogenase values correlated with those of alanine aminotransferase but were insensitive. Kraft et al (43) concluded that despite its mitochondrial localization, glutamate dehydrogenase is a sensitive indicator of hepatocellular injury, particularly in the centrilobular region in which it is concentrated, in contrast with alanine aminotransferase which is present in highest activity periportally.

Arginase and ornithine carbamoyltransferase are released only in necrosis. They are hepatospecific but insensitive, and they may be used in conjunction with the aforementioned enzymes to assess the severity of injury (5,43).

The other leakage enzymes just listed present few special advantages in evaluating liver cell injury in the dog. Lactic dehydrogenase, a ubiquitous enzyme having five major isoenzymes, may be used as a broad screen for tissue injury and, if elevated, localized somewhat as to source by determination of isoenzyme pattern (5).

Liver Function

Albumin, cholesterol, urea, and ammonia are considered elsewhere in this chapter. Uric acid is produced in purine metabolism. In the dog, it is converted to allantoin in the liver by uricase (urate oxidase). Hepatocellular dysfunction may result in elevation of serum uric acid caused by failure of this conversion. In our laboratories, serum uric acid levels over 1.0 mg/dl suggest hepatocellular dysfunction in the dog. The evaluation is quite insensitive.

Prothrombin (factor II) and fibrinogen are readily and conveniently measurable coagulation proteins produced by hepatocytes. Although detailed consideration of the factors altering their serum concentrations is beyond the scope of this book, hepatocellular dysfunction does result in decreased values. In our experience, the evaluation is insensitive; significantly reduced values related to hepatocellular failure occur only in conjunction with massive hepatic damage.

Bilirubin is a product of heme breakdown and

is conjugated, predominantly as diglucuronide, by hepatocytes before being excreted into the intestine by the biliary tree. Here it is converted by bacteria to urobilinogen which is partially resorbed and recycled or excreted in urine. Thus, bilirubin and its metabolic products are markers of both hepatocellular and biliary tree function. The dog is able to excrete bilirubin, especially bilirubin diglucuronide, very readily through the kidney. For this reason, hyperbilirubinemia and icterus are rare in the dog in the absence of impaired renal function, and measurement of serum bilirubin in the dog to detect hepatocellular or biliary tree impairment is less sensitive than it is in other species.

Evaluation of the Biliary Tree

Alkaline phosphatase activity in the dog is present predominantly in the intestine with lower activity in the kidney and very little activity in the liver; nevertheless, elevation of serum alkaline phosphatase in the dog is induced principally by biliary stasis, adrenocortical hyperfunction, or osteoblastic hyperactivity. Each of these induces a specific isoenzyme. Furthermore, the biliary or adrenocortical mechanism may induce massive elevation of serum activity (10 to 60 times the upper reference range values), whereas elevations due to osteoblastic hyperactivity are typically less extreme (5,20).

Marx et al (51) studied dogs with experimentally produced penetrating injuries of the small intestine or colon to identify clinical laboratory tests to detect intestinal perforation. Significantly elevated levels of alkaline phosphatase were observed in peritoneal lavage fluid 1 and 5 hours after injury. By contrast, the experimental animals did not have significantly different erythrocyte or leukocyte counts or amylase activity in their peritoneal lavage fluid than did the sham-operated control animals.

Gamma glutamyl transferase (transpeptidase) activity resides principally in the canine kidney and pancreas. Serum values are elevated in both cholestasis and adrenocortical hyperfunction but not in osteoblastic hyperactivity. Kraft et al (43) showed that gamma glutamyl transferase is less sensitive in detecting cholestasis than is alkaline phosphatase but frequently is valuable in determining the source of elevated alkaline phosphatase.

5′Nucleotidase was much more sensitive than alkaline phosphatase and somewhat more sensitive than gamma glutamyl transpeptidase in detecting biliary tree disease in dogs (1).

Because urobilinogen production and its ultimate excretion in the urine depends on the presence of bilirubin in the intestine, total obstruction of the biliary tree results in the absence of urobilinogen from urine. This marker is insensitive to partial cholestasis.

Ammonia and Bile Acids

Congenital or acquired portosystemic vascular shunts occur occasionally in the dog, resulting in failure to transport intestinal ammonia to the liver for conversion to urea. Massive hepatocellular dysfunction may also result in failure to convert ammonia to urea. Dogs affected with these disorders have increased levels of plasma ammonia and inappropriately low levels of serum urea. Signs of neurologic disease related to irritation of the central nervous system by ammonia frequently accompany hyperammonemia. In other dogs, inappropriately low serum urea levels in routine clinical chemistry profiles constitute the first evidence of this class of disease (32).

When plasma ammonia concentration is marginally elevated, the dog may be challenged by giving 100 mg of ammonium chloride per kilogram of body weight orally and determining plasma ammonia 30 minutes later. Following this challenge normal dogs had levels of 156 ± 71 μg/dl in contrast to dogs with portosystemic shunts, which had levels of $1,049 \pm 256$ μg/dl. The test should not be applied to dogs with basal hyperammonemia because of neurotoxicity of ammonia (32).

Measurement of serum bile acid concentration has recently been introduced into the evaluation of canine hepatobiliary disease (8,10,11,34,37,53). Enzymatic measurement may be made by spectrophotometry (11,34,53) or radioimmunoassay. In the healthy dog, fasting bile acids range from 0 to 5.1 μmol/l, whereas 2-hour postprandial values are 0 to 22 μmol/l (53). Greatest diagnostic sensitivity is achieved by measuring bile acids both on fasting and 2 hours postprandially. In the diagnosis of portosystemic venous anomalies this procedure is more sensitive than sulfobromophthelein (BSP) clearance and equal to the ammonia tolerance test (10).

Amylase and Lipase

The high incidence of spontaneous pancreatic disease in the dog has led to more extensive evaluation of serum amylase and lipase measurements in the canine than in other laboratory animal species. Increased activity of these enzymes in serum is reported to reflect acute injury to pancreatic acinar cells in acute pancreatitis or acute exacerbations of chronic pancreatitis. Studies by Nakashima et al (56) revealed that pancreatectomized dogs have approximately one half the activity of serum amylae of intact ones, that is, one half the serum amylase activity in healthy dogs is derived from the pancreas. These workers concluded that pancreatic amylase in the dog is removed by an extra urinary mechanism, explaining the absence of hyperamylasuria in the dog following pancreatitis, in contrast to postpancreatitis hyperamylasuria which is observed in man. Other workers have explained this paradox by speculating that the kidney in the dog inactivates amylase. The level of serum amylase is not influenced by diet. In dogs with spontaneous renal failure, amylase and lipase are elevated, though inconsistently. Amylase may be elevated to two and a half times basal values, and lipase to four times basal values. The magnitude of elevation is not correlated with the increase in serum urea nitrogen or creatinine clearance or to inulin clearance (85). Because vascular shock associated with pancreatitis may result in elevation of serum urea and creatinine levels, the combination of hyperamylasemia and/or hyperlipasemia with azotemia may be observed in either pancreatic or urinary tract disease. These two entities are not readily differentiated by usual clinical chemical parameters (67). The administration of dexamethasone elevates serum lipase levels, though not by inducing pancreatic lesions. In healthy dogs, the administration of dexamethasone decreased serum amylase activity, though this was variable in dogs with pancreatic disease (64).

Four isoenzymes of amylase may be demonstrated in dog serum by agarose gel electrophoresis. Isoenzyme 3 (counting from anode to cathode) was shown to be of pancreatic origin. Although the other enzymes of amylase also increased in experimentally induced pancreatitis, the greatest increase was found in isoamylase 3 (55). Serum levels of antiprotease were shown to decrease in dogs with spontaneous or experimentally induced acute pancreatitis (54).

Strombeck et al (80) investigated the diagnostic utility of determining serum amylase and lipase levels in dogs with pancreatic disease. They concluded that neither enzyme was specific for pancreatic acinar cell injury; elevated serum lipase levels were observed in some dogs that had renal or hepatic but not pancreatic disease. Nevertheless, these workers concluded that lipase determination had greater diagnostic value than did amylase determination. Low lipase values generally excluded the possibility of pancreatitis, whereas high values were frequently associated with pancreatitis.

Cholesterol

Cholesterol is principally synthesized de novo from acetate by the liver and to a lesser degree by other tissues. The dietary content of cholesterol significantly but modestly affects the serum concentration, more by serving as a regulator of hepatic synthesis than by direct absorption. In the dog, serum cholesterol is transported on low and high density lipoprotein. Although the measurement of serum cholesterol in the dog is regarded as diagnostically important, the controlling factors of cholesterol homeostasis are so numerous and complex that alterations, generally increases in serum cholesterol, may suggest any of several etiologic mechanisms. The influence of diet on serum cholesterol has already been mentioned. In studies this is rarely an unanticipated factor because diet is either kept constant among all test and control groups or, as in nutritional studies, dietary modifications are made to meet a specific research objective (4).

Esterification of cholesterol occurs principally in the liver. In hepatocellular disease, total cholesterol is increased though frequently only modestly so, and the esterified portion of the total cholesterol is decreased. Although measurement of free and esterified cholesterol is no longer widely used in the evaluation of liver function, hepatocellular dysfunction and cholestasis must be considered as causes of hypercholesterolemia.

Serum cholesterol may be elevated in uremic renal disease, in particular in nephrosis (4).

Thyroid function stimulates both the synthesis and the degradation of cholesterol. Although serum cholesterol is not generally altered in hyperthyroid states, many dogs with hypothyroidism have elevated levels of serum cholesterol. This relationship is not sufficiently consistent to recommend cholesterol as a valid measurement of thyroid function; conversely, however, hypothyroidism must be considered and evaluated as a mechanism leading to hypercholesterolemia (39).

Electrolytes, Blood Gases, Acid-Base Balance, and Proteins

Cornelius and Rawlings (18) surveyed the relationship of blood gas and acid-base analysis in dogs having a variety of spontaneous clinical illnesses. Primary metabolic acidosis was reported to be the most frequent abnormality, accompanying vomiting and diarrhea, dehydration, and polydipsia-polyuria. Arterial hypoxemia was observed in dogs with lower respiratory tract disease, dirofilariasis, and circulatory system disease.

In dogs exposed to thermal stress (40°C for 6 hours, 45°C for 90 minutes, or 50°C for 60 minutes at 20 ± 10 per cent humidity) dehydration developed with a much more pronounced rise in serum sodium, potassium, and chloride than the slight rise in packed cell volume (68).

Determination of blood pH and blood gases in dogs with acute gastric dilatation and volvulus yielded results no different from those in clinically normal dogs. This was interpreted to demonstrate that dogs with acute gastric dilatation and volvulus have simultaneous off-setting factors preventing metabolic acidosis (88).

As in other animal species, puppies have higher serum inorganic phosphorus levels than do adult dogs. Russo and Nash (75) investigated its possible relation to dietary intake or glomerular filtration rate and found it to be independent of both. Puppies given aluminum hydroxide gel to impair phosphorus absorption had serum inorganic phosphorus levels similar to those of puppies orally loaded with sodium phosphate.

In dogs with experimentally produced intestinal ischemia, an elevation of serum inorganic phosphorus 4 hours after the onset of ischemia was the most sensitive marker in detecting this abnormality (48).

Serum calcium may be elevated markedly in dogs with neoplastic disease, especially lymphoma or adenocarcinoma. This entity is termed pseudohyperparathyroidism. Its mechanism is not always identifiable, but it may be related to production by the tumor of a peptide having a parathyroid hormone-like action or to production of massive quantities of prostaglandin, especially PGE_2 (9,91).

Failure of dogs with seriously impaired renal function to normally excrete inorganic phosphorus results in stimulation of parathyroids (secondary renal hyperparathyroidism) which in turn produces demineralization of bone and steadily rising serum inorganic phosphorus. Serum calcium levels actually remain normal or nearly so until the agonal phase of the disease in which there may be hypocalcemia. Hypocalcemia is also observed occasionally in dogs with acute pancreatitis, apparently caused by the binding of calcium to soaps produced by the action of lipase of fats (9,36).

Meuten et al (52) demonstrated that in dogs as has been shown in other species, total serum calcium rises and falls with serum albumin. Therefore, in dogs with spontaneous or experimentally induced hypoalbuminemia, concurrent calcium values below the reference range should not be interpreted as an indication of disordered calcium metabolism.

Serum albumin (and therefore total serum protein) is often decreased in dogs with chronic hepatic dysfunction because of impaired synthesis and in dogs with glomerular renal disease because of loss as proteinuria. Most profound hypoalbuminemia and hypoproteinemia is observed in dogs with protein-losing enteropathies or malabsorption syndromes (76). Deysine et al (19) observed that dogs with severe clinical bacterial infections had a significantly decreased level of serum albumin. This hypoalbuminemia could be prevented by the administration of cortisone after, but not before, the onset of the infection. This was attributed to the stimulation of hepatic albumin synthesis by cortisone.

Adrenocortical Hormones

The high incidence of adrenocortical hyperfunction in the dog (Cushing's disease, Cushing's syndrome), which may be of primary adrenal, hypophyseal, or hypothalamic origin, has prompted numerous and extensive studies of the hypophyseal-adrenocortical axis in the canine species (22,24,25,66). Excitement markedly elevates plasma cortisol and, through cortisol, many other parameters, again demonstrating the need for well-conditioned dogs and gentle handling.

Olson et al (62) found no difference between canine serum and canine plasma anticoagulated with heparin or EDTA for the measurement of cortisol by radioimmunoassay. They reported that storage of the blood samples at 4°C for 40 hours, with serum or plasma in contact with the erythrocytes, did not alter measured cortisol values. Samples having high concentrations yielded reduced values when stored for 5 days at room temperature, though no changes were reported in samples having normal or reduced concentrations under similar conditions. In our laboratories, hemolysis reduced measured levels of cortisol in plasma.

As indicated earlier, basal cortisol levels are inadequate in discriminating euadrenocortical, hyperadrenocortical, and hypoadrenocortical (addisonian) dogs. Numerous function tests devised to aid in this consist of measuring the cortisol response to ACTH stimulation, including synthetic ACTH and to dexamethasone suppression (21,22,25,41,42,66). Dexamethasone, a synthetic adrenocortical steroid, is recognized by the normal canine cortisol-ACTH feedback loop and thus suppresses ACTH and indirectly cortisol production, though it does not cross-react in the radioimmunoassay for cortisol. Vigorous exercise resulted in marked elevation of plasma cortisol, but it did not alter maximum levels induced by ACTH stimulation (7).

Gordon et al (29) demonstrated a significant decrease in cortisol response to ACTH stimulation in the sodium-depleted dog. Beagles with glaucoma had significantly higher levels of serum cortisol than did control animals with normal intraocular pressure. It is not possible to assess the part played by stress in this effect (16). Adrenocortical response to hypoglycemia has been studied (40).

Experimental hemorrhagic shock in dogs resulted in an increase in plasma cortisol level, which peaked at five times the basal level before decreasing. Later, aldosterone levels rose to 10 times the basal value (38).

Thyroid Hormones

Thyroid function in the dog has been evaluated by measurement of total serum thyroxine (T_4), triiodothyronine (T_3), a test measuring the T_4 response to thyrotropic hormone (TSH), and free T_4. Normal canine T_4 levels are much lower than those in man. Therefore, early in the history of thyroxine measurement special procedures were devised to measure canine T_4.

Excellent anti-T_4 antibodies in current use no longer make this necessary, though it is important to use calibration standards and controls in the normal canine (2 μg/dl) rather than in the normal human (10 μg/dl) range (44). Measurement of canine T_3 by usual methods designed for human T_3 presents no special problems. Canine TSH cross-reacts very weakly with antibody to the human hormone and a species-specific TSH assay is required for valid results (39).

The presence of abnormal thyroxine- or triiodothyronine-binding factor, possibly autoantibody, can be detected in the solid phase radioimmunoassay of the hormones by spuriously high, irreproducible values and in charcoal separation assays by spuriously low values. Young et al (92) showed the factor to resist heat inactivation and the action of 8-anilino-1-naphthalene sulfonic acid, but to be precipitated by goat antibody to canine IgG.

Less uniform agreement exists as to the importance of the TSH stimulation test than the ACTH stimulation test. As for ACTH stimulation, various protocols have been devised for TSH stimualtion tests (58). Lorenz and Stiff (47) administered TSH to dogs intramuscularly at 0.4 U per kilogram of body weight. Failure of T_4 to increase from basal values by 100 per cent or more at 10 hours correlated well with clinical responsiveness to thyroid medication and was interpreted as evidence of hypothyroidism. In response to intravenous TSH triiodothyronine levels increase more rapidly than do thyroxine levels (57,87). The peak responses of T_3 and T_4 occur at 6 hours after intravenous administration of TSH (87). Repeated intravenous administration of TSH may result in anaphylaxis (87).

Alternatively, the pituitary-thyroid axis may be evaluated by the administration of thyrotropin-releasing hormone. Thyroxin is measured before and 6 hours after intravenous administration of thyrotropin-releasing hormone at a dose of 0.1 mg/kg. A normal response consists of doubling of the baseline value (49).

Serum levels of T_3 and T_4 were reduced by the administration of prednisone (90). Many dogs with spontaneous hyperadrenocorticism (Cushing's syndrome) have reduced basal levels of T_3 and T_4, but a significant increase in these hormone levels in response to TSH (65). In dogs with adenocarcinoma of the thyroid, T_3 as well as T_4 may be elevated (15). The thyroid hormones have been evaluated in hemorrhagic shock (84).

Sex Hormones

The concentration of plasma progesterone in heparinized whole canine blood was unaltered when stored at refrigerator temperature (4°C) for 5 days (63). The concentration of testosterone in canine serum stored at room temperature for 6 days did not change significantly, whereas in whole blood determined values increased significantly in 48 hours (28).

In male dogs testosterone and luteinizing hormone were determined at intervals for 1 year. Luteinizing hormone fluctuated cyclically without corresponding changes in testosterone. Testosterone levels remained constant through most of the year except in late summer when they rose (23). Levels of androgens and estradiol-17-beta were determined in dogs 8 months to 9 years of age. Levels of estradiol-17-beta were unaffected by age, but levels of androgens declined with age. In male dogs with feminizing syndrome and testicular atrophy, significantly reduced testosterone levels comparable to those in castrated males were observed (6,17).

The cyclic fluctuations of hormones in the bitch have been studied extensively, comparing levels in Labrador Retriever bitches during their first and second estrus cycles. Values for estrone, estradiol, and luteinizing hormone were significantly higher during the second cycle, whereas levels of progesterone were higher in the first cycle (13,14). Highest levels of testosterone in bitches occurred late in anestrus. The results of various workers with respect to the estrus cycle of the bitch are somewhat difficult to compare, because of lack of agreement as to the reference points in the cycle. Estradiol peaks about mid-proestrus, luteinizing hormone about the start of estrus, and progesterone about the start of diestrus (35,59,60). In bitches with intact ovaries, hysterectomy did not alter progesterone secretion (61).

Cerebrospinal Fluid

Bailey and Higgins (2) compared the protein content and cell count of canine cisternal cerebrospinal fluid (CSF) with those of canine lumbar CSF. Cerebrospinal fluid samples were collected from dogs first tranquilized with acepromazine followed by pentobarbital anesthesia. Cisternal CSF had a leukocyte count of 0 to 4 per microliter with a mean of 1.5 and a protein content of 3 to 23 mg/dl with a mean of 14. Lumbar CSF had a leukocyte count of 0 to 5 per microliter with a mean of 0.6. The protein content was 18 to 44 mg/dl with a mean of 28.7. There was no significant difference whether the cisternal or lumbar fluid was drawn first (2). Dogs with brain tumors generally had elevated CSF pressure (over 170 mm of water). Dogs with all types of brain tumors had elevated CSF protein, though the degree of elevation was loosely correlated with the type of tumor; it was most marked in dogs with choroid plexus papillomas and least in dogs with astrocytomas. Leukocyte counts in CSF varied widely with the type of tumor, being normal in dogs with oligodendroglioma and markedly elevated in those with meningioma (3).

REFERENCES

1 Abdelkader SV, Hauge JG (1986) Serum enzyme determination in the study of liver disease in dogs. Acta Vet Scand 27: 59–70

2. Bailey CS, Higgins RJ (1985) Comparison of total white blood cell count and total protein content of lumbar and cisternal cerebrospinal fluid of healthy dogs. Am J Vet Res 46: 1162–1165

3. Bailey CS, Higgins RJ (1986) Characteristics of cisternal cerebrospinal fluid associated with primary brain tumors in the dog: A retrospective study. J Am Vet Med Assoc 188: 414–417

4. Bartley JC (1980) Lipid metabolism and its disorders. In Kaneko JJ (ed), Clinical Biochemistry of Domestic Animals, 3rd Ed, Chap 2. Academic Press, New York

5. Boyd JW (1983) The mechanisms relating to increases in plasma enzymes and isoenzymes in diseases of animals. Vet Clin Path 12: 9–24

6. Brendler CB, Berry SJ, Ewin LL, McCullough AR, Cochran RC, Strandberg JD, Zirkin BR, Coffey DS, Wheaton LG, Hiler ML, Bordy MJ, Niswender GD, Scott WW, Walsh PC (1983) Spontaneous benign prostatic hyperplasia in the beagle. Age-associated changes in serum hormone levels, and the morpho-

logy and secretory function of the canine prostate. J Clin Invest 71: 1114–1123

7. Brzezinaka Z, Nazar K, Kozlowski S (1980) Effect of prolonged exhausting exercise on the adrenal cortex response to ACTH. Acta Physiol Pol 31: 567–569

8. Bunch SE, Center SA, Baldwin BH, Reimers TJ, Balazs T, Tennant BC (1984) Radioimunnoassay of Conjugated Bile Acids in Canine and Feline Sera. Am J Vet Res 45: 2051–2054

9. Capen CC, Martin SL (1980) Calcium-regulating hormones and diseases of the parathyroid glands. In Ettinger S (ed), Textbook of Veterinary Internal Medicine, 2nd Ed, Chap 66. Saunders, Philadelphia

10. Center SA, Baldwin BH, de Lahunta A, Dietze AE, Tennant BC (1985) Evaluation of serum bile acid concentrations for the diagnosis of portosystemic venous anomalies in the dog and cat. J Am Vet Med Assoc 186: 1090–1094

11. Center SA, Baldwin BH, Erb HN, Tennant BC (1985) Bile acid concentration in the diagnosis of hepatobiliary disease in the dog. J Am Vet Med Assoc 187: 935–940

12. Center SA, Wilkinson E, Smith CA, Erb H, Lewis RM (1985) 24-Hour urine protein/creatinine ratio in dogs with protein-losing nephropathies. J Am Vet Med Assoc 187: 820–824

13. Chakraborty PK, Panko WB, Fletcher WS (1980) Serum hormone concentrations and their relationships to sexual behaviour at the first and second estrous cycles of the Labrador bitch. Biol Reprod 22: 227–232

14. Chakraborty PK, Stewart AP, Seager SW (1983) Relationship of growth and serum growth hormone concentration in the prepubertal Labrador bitch. Lab An Sci 33: 51–55

15. Chastain CB, Hill BL, Nichols CE (1980) Excess triiodothyromine production by a thyroid adenocarcinoma in a dog. J Am Vet Med Assoc 177: 172–173

16. Chen GL, Gelatt KN, Gum GG (1980) Serum hydrocortisone (cortisol) values in glaucomatous and normotensive Beagles. Am J Vet Res 41: 1516–1518

17. Cochran RC, Ewing LL, Niswender GD (1981) Serum levels of follicle stimulating hormone, luteinizing hormone, prolactin, testosterone, 5-alpha-dihydrotestosterone, 5-alpha-androstane-3 alpha, 17-beta-estradiol from male Beagles with spontaneous or induced benign prostatic hyperplasia. Invest Urol 19: 142–147

18. Cornelius LM, Rawlings CA (1981) Arterial blood gas and acid-base values in dogs with various diseases and signs of disease. J Am Vet Med Assoc 178: 992–995

19. Deysine M, Leiblich N, Rubenstein R, Rosario E (1980) Effects of cortisone on decrease of serum albumin secondary to experimental infections. Surg Gynecol Obstet 151: 477–480

20. Eckersall PD, Nash AS (1983) Isoenzymes of canine plasma alkaline phosphatase: An investigation using isoelectric focusing and related to diagnosis. Res Vet Sci 34: 310–314

21. Eiler H, Oliver J (1980) Combined dexamethasone suppression and cosyntropin (synthetic ACTH) stimulation test in the dog: New approach to testing of adrenal gland function. Am J Vet Res 41: 1243–1246

22. Eiler H, Oliver JW, Legendre AM (1984) Stages of hyperadrenocortisonism: Response of hyperadrenocorticoid dogs to the combined dexamethasone suppression/ACTH stimulation test. JAVMA 185: 289–294

23. Falvo RE, DePalatis LR, Moore J, Kepic TA, Miller J (1980) Annual variations in plasma levels of testosterone and luteinizing hormone in the laboratory male mongrel dog. J Endocrinol 86: 425–430

24. Feldman EC (1981) Effect of functional adrenocortical tumors on plasma cortisol and corticotropin concentration in dogs. J Am Vet Med Assoc 178: 823–826

25. Feldman EC (1983) Comparison of ACTH response and dexamethasone suppression as screening tests in canine hyperadrenocorticism. J Am Vet Med Assoc 182: 506–510

26. Feldman EC, Nelson RW (1982) Insulin-induced hyperglycemia in diabetic dogs. J Am Vet Med Assoc 180: 1432–1437

27. Finco DR, Coulter DW, Barsanti JA (1981) Simple, accurate method for clinical estimation of glomerular filtration rate in the dog. Am J Vet Res 42: 1874–1877

28. Frankland AL (1985) Canine testosterone concentrations in samples stored at room temperature. Brit Vet J 141: 308–311

29. Gordon RD, Nicholls MG, Tree M, Fraser R, Robertson JI (1980) Influence of sodium balance on ACTH/adrenal corticosteroid dose-response curves in the dog. Am J Physiol 238: E543–551

30. Grauer GF, Thomas CB, Eicker SW (1985) Estimation of quantitative proteinuria in the dog, using the urine protein-to-creatinine ratio from a random voided sample. Am J Vet Res 46: 2116–2119

31. Greco DS, Turnwals GH, Adams R, Gossett KA, Kearney M, Casey H (1985) Urinary gamma-glutamyl transpeptidase activity in dogs with gentamycin-induced nephropathy. Am J Vet Res 46: 2332–2335

32. Hardy RM (1980) Diseases of the liver. In Ettinger S (ed), Textbook of Veterinary Internal Medicine, 2nd Ed, Chap 60. Saunders, Philadelphia

33. Harris JW, Kellermeyer RW (1970) The Red Cell. Harvard University Park Press, Cambridge

34. Hauge JG, Abdelkader SV (1984) Serum bile acids as an indicator of liver disease in dogs. Acta Vet Scand 25: 495–503

35. Holst PA, Phemister RD (1975) Temporal sequence of events in the estrous cycle the bitch. Am J Vet Res 36: 705–706

36. Jacob AI, Galvellas G, Canterbury J, Bourgoignie JJ (1982) Calcemic and phosphaturic response to parathyroid hormone in normal and chronically uremic dogs. Kidney Int 22: 21–26

37. Johnson SE, Rogers WA, Bonagura JD, Caldwell JH (1985) Determination of serum bile acids in fasting dogs with hepatobiliary disease. Am J Vet Res 46: 2048–2053

38. Kajihara H, Malliwah JA, Matsumura M, Taguchi K, Iijima S (1983) Changes in blood cortisol and aldosterone levels and ultrastructure of the adrenal

cortex during hemorrhagic shock. Pathol Res Pract 176: 324–340

39. Kaneko JJ (1980) Thyroid function. In Kaneko JJ (ed), Clinical Biochemistry of Domestic Animals, 3rd Ed., Chap 12. Academic Press, New York

40. Keller-Wood ME, Shinsako J, Keil LC, Dallman MF (1981) Insulin-inducted hypoglycemia in conscious dogs. I. Dose-related pituitary and adrenal responses. Endocrinology 109: 818–824

41. Kemppainen RJ, Thompson FN, Lorenz MD (1982) Effects of dexamethasone infusion on the plasma cortisol response of cosyntropin (synthetic ACTH) injection in normal dogs. Res Vet Sci 32: 181–183

42. Kemppainen RJ, Thompson FN, Lorenz MD (1983) Use of a low does synthetic ACTH challenge test in normal and prednisone-treated dogs. Res Vet Sci 35: 240–242

43. Kraft W, Ghermai AK, Winzinger H, Knoll L (1983) Comparison of serum AST, ALT, AP and GGT activities in the diagnosis of liver diseases in dogs. Berl Munch Tierarztl Wochenschr 96: 421 431

44. Larsson M, Lumsden JH (1980) Evaluation of an enzyme linked immunosorbent assay (ELISA) for determination of plasma thyroxine in dogs. Zentralbl Veterinaermed |A| 27: 9–15

45. Loeb WF (1982) Clinical biochemistry of liver disease. Mod Vet Pract 63: 629–631

46. Loeb WF, Wickum M (1973) Factor VII deficiency in Beagle dogs. Bull Soc Pharm Environ Path 1: 3–4

47. Lorenz MD, Stiff ME (1980) Serum thyroxine content before and after thyrotropin stimulation in dogs with suspected hypothyroidism. J Am Vet Med Assoc 177: 78–81

48. Lores ME, Canizares O, Rosello PJ (1981) The significance of elevation of serum phosphate levels in experimental intestinal ischemia. Surg Gynecol Obstet 152: 593–596

49. Lothrop CD, Tamas PM, Fadok VA (1984) Canine and Feline thyroid function assessment with the thyrotropin-releasing hormone response test. Am J Vet Res 45: 2310–2313

50. Mahaffey EA, Cornelius LM (1982) Glycosylated hemoglobin in diabetic and nondiabetic dogs. J Am Vet Med Assoc 180: 635–637

51. Marx JA, Moore EE, Bar-Or D (1983) Peritoneal lavage in penetrating injuries of the small bowel and colon: Value of enzyme determinations. Ann Emerg Med 12: 68–70

52. Meuten DJ, Chew DJ, Capen CC, Kociba GJ (1982) Relationship of serum total calcium to albumin and total protein in dogs. J Am Vet Med Assoc 180: 63–67

53. Meyer DJ (1986) Liver function tests in dogs with portosystemic shunts: Measurement of serum bile acid concentration. J Am Vet Med Assoc 188: 168–169

54. Murtaugh RJ, Jacobs RM (1985) Serum antiprotease concentrations in dogs with experimentally induced acute pancreatitis. Am J Vet Res 46: 80–83

55. Murtaugh RJ, Jacobs RM (1985) Serum amylase and Isoamylases and their origins in healthy dogs and dogs with experimentally induced acute pancreatitis. Am J Vet Res 46: 742–747

56. Nakashima Y, Akita H, Appert HE, Howard JM (1980) The contribution of pancreas and kidney in regulating serum amylase levels in dogs. Gastroenterol Jpn 15: 476–479

57. Oliver JW, Held JP (1985) Thyrotropin stimulation test—New perspective on the value of monitoring triiodothyronine. J Am Vet Med Assoc 187: 931–934

58. Oliver JW, Waldrop V (1983) Sampling protocol for thyrotropin stimulation test in the dog. J Am Vet Med Assoc 182: 486–489

59. Olson PN, Bowen RA, Behrendt MD, Olson JD, Neff TM (1982) Concentrations of reproductive hormones in canine serum throughout late anestrus, proestrus and estrus. Biol Reprod 27: 1196–1206

60. Olson PN, Bowen RA, Behrendt MD, Olson JD, Nett TM (1984) Concentrations of testosterone in canine serum during late anestrus, proestrus, estrus, and early diestrus. Am J Vet Res 45: 145–148

61. Olson PN, Bowne RA, Behrendt MD, Olson JD, Nett TM (1984) Concentrations of progesterone and luteinizing hormone in the serum of diestrous bitches before and after hysterectomy. Am J Vet Res 45: 149–153

62. Olson PN, Bowen RA, Husted PW, Nett TM (1981) Effects of storage on concentration of hydrocortisone (cortisol) in canine serum and plasma. Am J Vet Res 42: 1618–1620

63. Oltner R, Edgvist LE (1982) Changes in plasma progesterone levels during storage of heparinized whole blood from cow, horse, dog and pig. Acta Vet Scand 23: 1–8

64. Parent J (1982) Effects of dexamethasone on pancreatic tissue and on serum amylase and lipase activities in dogs. J Am Vet Med Assoc 180: 743–746

65. Peterson ME, Ferguson DC, Knitzer PP, Drucker WD (1984) Effects of spontaneous hyperadrenocorticism on serum thryoid concentrations of the dog. Am J Vet Res 45: 2034–2038

66. Peterson ME, Gilbertson SR, Drucker WD (1982) Plasma cortisol response to exogenous ACTH in 22 dogs with hyperadrenocorticism caused by adrenocortical neoplasia. J Am Vet Med Assoc 180: 542–545

67. Polzin DJ, Osborne CA, Stevens JD, Hayden DW (1983) Serum amylase and lipase activities in dogs with chronic primary renal failure. Am J Vet Res 44: 404–410

68. Rai UC, Ambwaney P (1980) Plasma volume and electrolyte changes during varied thermal stress. Indian J Med Res 72: 416–421

69. Reimers TJ, Cowan RG, McCann JP, Ross MW (1982) Validation of a rapid solid-phase radioimmunoassay for canine, bovine, and equine insulin. Am J Vet Res 43: 1274–1278

70. Renauld A, Sverdlik RC, Aguero A, Rodriguez RR, Foglia VG (1982) Serum insulin, free fatty acids and blood sugar during the estrous cycle of dogs. Horm Metab Res 14: 4–7

71. Renauld A, Sverdlik RC, Garrido D (1980) Blood sugar, serum insulin and serum free fatty acid responses to slow graded glucose in thyroxine-treated dogs. Acta Diabetol Lat 17: 189–197

72. Renauld A, Sverdlik RC, Garrido D (1982) Blood sugar, serum insulin and serum free fatty acid responses to graded glucose pulses in hypothyroid dogs. Acta Diabetol Lat 19: 97–105

73. Renauld A, von Lawzewitsch I, Pérez RL, Sverdlik R, Aguero A, Foglia VG, Rodriguez RR (1982) Effect of estrogens on blood sugar, serum insulin and serum free fatty acids, and pancreas cytology in female dogs. Acta Diabetol Lat 20: 47–56

74. Rottiers R, Mattheeuws D, Kaneko JJ, Vermeulen A (1981) Glucose uptake and insulin secretory responses to intravenous glucose loads in the dog. Am J Vet Res 42: 155–158

75. Russo JC, Nash MA (1980) Renal reponse to alterations in dietary phosphate in the young Beagle. Biol Neonate 38: 1–10

76. Sherding RG (1980) Disease of the small bowel. In Ettinger S (ed), Textbook of Veterinary Medicine, 2nd Ed., Chap 58. Saunders, Philadelphia

77. Smith JE, Wood PA, Moore K (1982) Evaluation of a colorimetric method for canine glycosylated hemoglobin. Am J Vet Res 43: 700–701

78. Stockham SL, Nachreiner RF, Krehbiel JD (1983) Canine immunoreactive insulin quantitation using, five commercial radioimmunoassay kits. Am J Vet Res 44: 2179–2183

79. Stogdale L (1981) Correlation of changes in blood chemistry with pathological changes in the animal's body: II. Electrolytes, kidney function tests, serum enzymes, and liver function tests. J.S. Afr Vet Assoc 52: 155–164

80. Strombeck DR, Farver T, Kaneko JJ (1981) Serum amylase and lipase activity in the diagnosis of pancreatitis in dogs. Am J Vet Res 42: 1966–1970

81. Vanhelder WP, Sirek A, Sirek OV, Norwich KH, Policova Z, Vanhelder T (1980) Diurnal episodic pattern of insulin secretion in the dog. Diabetes 29: 326–328

82. van Sluijs FH, deVries HW, DeBruijne JJ, van den Brom WE (1983) Capillary and venous blood compared with arterial blood in the measurement of acid-base and blood gas status of dogs. Am J Vet Res 44: 459–462

83. Visser MP, Krill MT, Muljtjens HM, Willems GM, Hermens WT (1981) Distribution of enzymes in dog heart and liver; significance for assessment of tissue damage from data on plasma enzyme activities. Clin Chem 27: 1845–1850

84. Vitek V, Shatney CH, Lang DJ, Cowley RA (1984) Relationship of thyroid hormone patterns to survival in canine hemorrhagic shock. Eur Surg Res 16: 89–98

85. Wagner AE, Macy DW (1982) Nephelometric determination of serum amylase and lipase in naturally occurring azotemia in dogs. Am J Vet Res 43: 697–699

86. Watson AD, Church DB, Fairbairn AJ (1981) Postprandial changes in plasma urea and creatinine concentrations in dogs. Am J Vet Res 42: 1878–1880

87. Wheeler SL, Husted PW, Rosychuk RAW, Allen TA, Nett TM, Olson PN (1985) Serum concentrations of thyroxine and 3,5,3'-triiodothyronine before and after intravenous or intramuscular thyrotropin administration in dogs. Am J Vet Res 46: 2605–2608

88. Wingfield WE, Twedt DC, Moore RW, Leib MS, Wright M (1982) Acid-base and electrolyte values in dogs with acute gastric dilation-volvulus. J Am Vet Med Assoc 180: 1070–1072

89. Woltz HH, Thompson FN, Kemppainen RJ, Munnell JF, Lorenz MD (1983) Effect of prednisone on thyroid gland morphology and plasma thyroxine and triiodothyronine concentrations in the dog. Am J Vet Res 44: 2000–2003

90. Wood PA, Smith JE (1980) Glycosylated hemoglobin and canine diabetes mellitus. J Am Vet Med Assoc 176: 1267–1268

91. Yarrington JT, Hoffman WE, Mach D, Hawker C (1981) Morphologic characteristics of the parathyroid and thyroid glands and serum immunoreactive parathyroid hormone in dogs with pseudohyperparathyroidism. Am J Vet Res 42: 271–274

92. Young DW, Sartin JL, Kemppainen RJ (1985) Abnormal canine triiodothyronine-binding factor characterized as a possible triiodothyronine autoantibody. Am J Vet Res 46: 1346–1350

7

The Nonhuman Primate

WALTER F. LOEB, VMD, PhD

Nonhuman primates used in biomedical research represent a range of species of Pongidae or apes, Cercopithecidae and Colobidae or Old World monkeys, Cebidae or New World monkeys, Callithricidae or Marmosets and Tamarines, and Lorsidae or prosimians. Some of the prosimians have an appearance more closely resembling the raccoon than they do the typical "monkey." Nonhuman primates range in size from adult marmosets, which may be smaller than adult rats, to baboons and gorillas, several times the weight of a man. Thus, they represent much greater diversity than is true of the individual species of laboratory animals discussed in the earlier chapters. It is important to understand that the term "monkey" is almost meaningless and does not define a specific species. For the immediate future, the use of primates in biomedical research may be less extensive than in the recent past because of the failure of primate research to demonstrate marked general superiority over that done in other laboratory animal species, public attitudes, high animal cost, and the difficulty in obtaining uniform and healthy animals. In the past, rhesus monkeys (*Macaca mulatta*) have been the most extensively used primates in research. Currently the slightly smaller and more docile cynomologus monkey (*M. fascicularis*) is most extensively used, whereas other genera such as baboons (*Papio*), Capuchins (*Cebus*), and mar-

mosets (*Saguinus* and *Callithrix*) are used for selected applications.

Blood for clinical chemistry may be collected from the femoral, saphenous, or median antecubital vein of animals that are manually restrained, restrained in squeeze cages, or chemically restrained with phencyclidine or ketamine (68). Some animals, in particular apes, may be trained to extend an arm from the cage for venipuncture. Restraint, whether physical or chemical, should be kept to a minimum consistent with handler safety and achievement of research objectives, and taken into consideration in the interpretation of analytic results (7,88,103). Compendia of clinical chemistry reference values have been prepared for various nonhuman primate species (10,16,31,49,50,51,52, 76,77,93,96). These values are tabulated in the appendix.

URIC ACID

Although of limited diagnostic significance, serum uric acid constitutes an informative example of biochemical relationships in primate phylogeny. In man and submammalian vertebrates, uric acid is the end product of purine metabolism, which it reflects as well as an insensitive indicator of renal function. In most subprimate mammals, the enzyme uricase (urate oxidase) in hepatocytes converts uric acid to the more soluble and readily excreted allantoin. In these species, serum uric acid is elevated in hepatic cellular dysfunction and a rather insensitive liver function test. Christen et al (13) studied hepatic urate oxidase and serum and urine uric acid in 10 species of Old World monkeys, New World monkeys, and prosimians. In Tupaia, Galago, and Nycticebos prosimians, they detected a high activity of stabile hepatic uricase similar to that in subprimate mammals, with resultant low serum uric acid. In New World monkeys, including Cebus, Lagothrix, and in marmosets (Saguinus), little hepatic uricase activity was observed; like man and great apes, these species had relatively high serum uric acid levels. In the Old World Papio and Macaca monkeys there was a high level of activity of hepatic uricase which was unstable and distinct from the uricase of phylogenically lower species, but a low concentration of serum uric acid.

GLUCOSE

Serum glucose concentration reflects numerous factors including gastrointestinal absorption, insulin, hepatic storage and release, glucagon, somatotropin, epinephrine, and cortisol. Through the latter two hormones, stress and excitement may produce significant elevation of serum glucose. Diabetes mellitus is not rare in nonhuman primates, but it should not be diagnosed on the basis of a single determination of elevated serum glucose, in particular if measured on a stressed animal (33,45). Variations among primate species with respect to anatomy and transit time of the gastrointestinal tract should be considered in determining the length of fasting required to render an animal nonabsorptive. The excitement of restraint appears to induce hyperglycemia much more readily and to a greater degree in Cebidae than in Cercopithecidae or Pongidae (18).

In fasting rhesus monkeys and baboons, Goodner et al (27) observed periodic oscillations of insulin, glucose, and glucagon. Glucose and insulin oscillated in phase with one another and out of phase with glucagon. In rhesus monkeys these oscillations had a periodicity of 9 minutes. Similar oscillations have not been observed in man.

Obese male rhesus monkeys have shown markedly elevated serum insulin values and mildly (statistically nonsignificant) elevated fasting serum glucose values when compared with nonobese control animals (34). Anticipation of feeding did not affect serum insulin levels in rhesus monkeys (64).

Glucose Tolerance

The response of the body's several glucose-regulating mechanisms to an administered challenge dose of glucose may be determined by glucose tolerance tests. The logarithmic decrease in the concentration of serum glucose, expressed by fractional turnover rate K, may be determined from the intravenous glucose tolerance test. It results principally from the deposition of glucose in hepatocytes as glycogen under the influence of insulin, but it is also influenced by all factors regulating serum glucose. The oral glucose tolerance test is additionally influenced by intestinal absorption, a factor not influencing the results of the intravenous glucose tolerance test. The value of K is derived from the formula, $C_t = C_o^{e-kt}$, where C_o is the concentration of glucose at time O, C_t is the concentration of glucose at the time t, and K is the constant for the percentage decrease of blood glucose per minute. From the foregoing formula a working formula may be derived:

$$K = \frac{0.6931}{T_{\frac{1}{2}}} \times 100.$$

Fulmer et al (22) developed an intravenous glucose tolerance test for evaluating glucose regulation in rhesus and African Green monkeys and studied the effect of chemical and physical restraint on glucose clearance coefficient K. Animals were fasted for 21 to 24 hours. After collection of a fasting blood sample for glucose determination, a dose of glucose of 0.75 g/kg was injected intravenously. Additional blood samples for glucose determination were collected at 10, 20, 30, 60, 90, and 120 minutes afer glucose injections. In man, K values in normal individuals are over 1.2; values below 1 are diagnostic of diabetes mellitus. In male and female rhesus or African Green monkeys studied by Fulmer et al (22), restrained with ketamine or anesthetized with pentobarbital, and in female rhesus monkeys manually restrained, K values ranged from 1.2 to 6.78 and did not differ significantly among methods of restraint within animal groups. Male rhesus and male and female African Green monkeys that were manually rather than chemically restrained had significantly decreased glucose clearance constants; K values were as low as 0.20. Female rhesus monkeys are more docile and tractable than male rhesus or African Green monkeys of either sex. Fulmer et al (22) concluded that the hormonal response to stress accounted for impaired glucose clearance in manually restrained primates. In permanently catheterized unrestrained squirrel monkeys, Ausman and Gallina (2) obtained K values of 7.75 ± 2.84. In a study of the oral glucose tolerance test, Streett and Jonas (88) concluded that ketamine impaired glucose absorption from the intestine. Meis et al (58) reported that during gestation cynomolgus monkeys had a decrease in fasting glucose and an increase in peak plasma insulin response to glucose challenge. Peak plasma insulin response remained elevated postpartum during lactation. Glucose clearance rates were unaffected.

UREA NITROGEN AND CREATININE

Measurements of serum urea nitrogen and creatinine are widely used in nonhuman primates principally to assess renal function. Urea nitrogen is formed in the liver from ammonia in the ornithine-arginine-citrulline cycle, is excreted through the glomerular filtrate, and partially resorbed passively with water in the renal tubules. Creatinine is formed in muscle as the irreversible anhydride of creatine, excreted in the glomerular filtrate, and generally not resorbed in the renal tubules. With respect to these analytes, nonhuman primates do not appear to present unique features. As in other species, extensive renal injury may occur before elevations of urea nitrogen and creatinine outside of reference range occur. Slight but progressive increase in serum creatinine signals progressive deterioration of renal function; thus, an animal's own earlier creatinine values may be of greater importance then the historical reference range in detecting early renal dysfunction. Because of the quantitative renal excretion of creatinine and its rather consistent rate of production, creatinine constitutes an endogenous substance suitable for clearance testing. The test requires measurement of serum creatinine and a timed urine sample for determination of volume and urine creatinine concentration. A more detailed discussion of the creatinine clearance

test is found in Chapter 14 entitled "Markers of Renal Function and Injury."

The diagnostic applicability of hepatocellular urea synthesis should not be overlooked. In hepatocellular dysfunction and in other conditions in which ammonia fails to undergo hepatocellular conversion to urea normally, serum urea nitrogen levels are disportionately low. Conversely, these animals have elevated levels of plasma ammonia. In our laboratories we observed a young chimpanzee (*Pan troglodytes*) that consistently had a serum urea nitrogen level of 3 mg/dl with normal creatinine and clinical chemical indicators of hepatocellular function. Our unconfirmed observations suggested that this animal had a congenital enzymatic defect of the ornithine-arginine-citrulline cycle, of which several types occur in man.

ENZYMES

Alanine Aminotransferase

Alanine aminotransferase (formerly termed serum glutamic pyruvic transaminase, SGPT) is a cytosol enzyme. In marmosets, Mohr et al (61) showed it to be in highest activity in the liver although cardiac muscle and kidney are also quite rich in it. In nonhuman primates, alanine aminotransferase is not as specific for liver cell injury as it is in the dog, rat, or mouse. Nevertheless, it is a sensitive indicator of hepatocellular injury. This and other leakage enzymes should be recognized as markers of hepatocellular injury, not of hepatocellular function. The cytosol origin of the predominant serum activity renders it a very sensitive enzyme which may be detected in the serum in significantly increased activity in the presence of cell membrane alteration without necrosis.

Aspartate Aminotransferase

Aspartate aminotransferase (formerly serum glutamic oxalacetic transaminase, SGOT) occurs in the same cells as two distinct isoenzymes, one mitochondrial, the other occurring in the cytosol. Mohr et al (61) reported that in marmosets the highest activity occurred in cardiac muscle. Although other tissues had activities only one third or one fourth that in cardiac muscle (by wet weight), other tissues comparatively rich in activity were the liver, skeletal muscle, kidney, and brain. The enzyme generally does not cross the blood-brain barrier; thus, except in massive brain necrosis, such as that in overwhelming cerebrovascular accident, enzyme from the brain does not contribute to activity measured in serum. Unlike alanine aminotransferase, cellular injury without concurrent necrosis generally does not result in elevation of serum aspartate aminotransferase.

Creatine Kinase

Creatine kinase (creatine phosphokinase) occurs in highest activity in skeletal muscle, cardiac muscle, and brain. The enzyme is a dimer composed of two types of monomers, designated M and B. Thus, there are three isoenzymes designated as BB or I, MB or II, and MM or III. Only Type III is found in skeletal muscle and only Type I in the brain. Cardiac muscle contains a mixture of Types II and III. In a study of experimental myocardial infarction in Capuchin monkeys, marked variation in total creatine kinase was observed. The total serum activity of creatine kinase was found to be related to the amount the animal struggled when being caught for blood collection rather than to the experimental manipulation.

Alkaline Phosphatase

Alkaline phosphatase measurement represents the joint enzymatic activity of a group of phosphomonoesterase isoenzymes determined at a pH of approximately 10. The method of Bessey, Lowry, and Brock as modified by Morgenstern has been optimized for man and is currently most widely used. Altering the pH, concentration of substrate, activators, and the like changes the contribution made by each of the constituent isoenzymes; thus, values obtained by one method cannot linearly be converted to another method. Tissues may be rich in alkaline phosphatase activity, but if the specific isoenzyme has a short serum half-life, it contributes little to the total activity.

In nonhuman primates, the so-called biliary and osteoblastic isoenzymes are the principal components of serum activity. The "biliary" isoenzyme is derived from cytomembranes; it is not a leakage enzyme, but one released and activated in biliary stasis. Young growing animals have higher serum osteoblastic alkaline phosphatase activity proportional to their growth rate. We have observed that male rhesus monkeys have serum alkaline phosphatase activity approximately one third higher than that of females; however, Beland et al (3) reported higher values in female squirrel monkeys than in male.

Amylase

Amylase activity in the tissues and serum of several species of nonhuman primates has been studied by McGeachin and Akin (53). All species studied except squirrel monkeys had high activities in the pancreas and parotid salivary gland and low activity in the liver. In squirrel monkeys low activity was observed in the parotid salivary gland. Except for the rhesus monkey, all other species studied, including great apes and squirrel monkeys, had serum amylase activity of 50 to 150 U/1, comparable to that in man. Rhesus monkeys had activities approximating 800 U/1, comparable to those of the dog or cat.

BILIRUBIN

After extensive review, Cornelius (14) concluded that bilirubin metabolism in nonhuman primates resembled that of man. Neonatal physiologic hyperbilirubinemia, comparable to that in human infants, is reported in the rhesus monkey. It may lead to kernicterus when hypoxia accompanies the hyperbilirubinemia. A model for Gilbert's syndrome in man has been oberved in clinically healthy Bolivian squirrel monkeys with serum concentrations of unconjugated bilirubin (indirect reacting) as high as 2 mg/dl and a delayed clearance of bilirubin and sulfobromophthalein (71).

SULFOBROMOPHTHALEIN

Sulfobromophthalein is a dye that, when administered at appropriate dosage, is totally cleared from the circulation of normal nonhuman primates by the liver. A delay in its clearance is therefore compatible with primary or secondary impairment of hepatic function.

A kinetic technique for measuring sulfobromophthalein clearance appropriate to rhesus monkeys was developed in our laboratories and later modified for application to cynomolgus monkeys. Afer injection of the dye, uniform mixing was complete in all animals by 3 minutes, in some as early as 1 minute. In some animals the exponential phase of clearance terminated as early as 6 minutes after dye injection. A baseline serum sample is collected before injection of dye. The 15 mg (0.3 ml) of sulfobromophthalein dye are injected intravenously in the rhesus monkey, 10 mg (0.2 ml) in the cynomolgus monkey. Carefully timed serum samples are collected at exactly 3 and 6 minutes or exactly 3 and 5 minutes after injection and the clearance half-time is determined. Healthy monkeys in our laboratories had clearance half-times of 2 to 6 minutes (48).

LIPIDS AND LIPOPROTEINS

Cholesterol, lipoproteins, and triglycerides have been studied very extensively in nonhuman primates, particularly with respect to models of atherosclerosis. Many of these studies were performed in animals fed experimental diets (62,69,81,85,86,91). Serum cholesterol and triglyceride levels increased with age in adult *Macaca mulatta* and *M. nemestrina*, consistent with observations in man and the rat (90). The spectrum of fatty acids in serum triglycerides in *M. mulatta* differed very slightly with age, though older animals had a significantly higher proportion of palmitic acid (44). In *M. nemestrina* there were age-related increases in high-density lipoprotein (HDL) cholesterol and decreases in low-density lipoprotein (LDL) cholesterol. In pregnancy, serum cholesterol is decreased in *M. mulatta*, *M. nemestrina*, and baboons. In *M. nemestrina* this is associated with a decrease in HDL cholesterol (56,80).

Determination of basal serum cholesterol and serum cholesterol following a high cholesterol diet challenge allows for the characterization of *M. mulatta* and other primate species into high and low cholesterol and high and low cholesterol responder categories, believed to be genetically controlled (6,20). In African green monkeys (*Cercopithicus aethiops*), the grivet subspecies responds to a high cholesterol challenge with a much more marked increase in both total serum cholesterol and HDL cholesterol than does the vervet subspecies (81).

In baboons, McGill et al (54) found a positive correlation between fatty streaks of the aorta and its main branches and the concentration of LDL cholesterol in the blood and a negative correlation between fatty streaks and the concentration of HDL cholesterol.

Brazilian squirrel monkeys on a lithogenic diet were highly susceptible to cholelithiasis, whereas Bolivian males are resistant. This was associated with HDL-2, which is high in the Brazilian subspecies and low in the Bolivian subspecies. The transport of cholesterol to bile is attributed to HDL-2 (70).

CALCIUM AND PHOSPHORUS

Nutritional secondary hyperparathyroidism in lemurs (*Lemur catta* and *L. varigatus*) associated with a diet high in phosphorus and low in vitamin D and calcium led to skeletal deformities and low serum calcium (as low as 2.6 mg/dl). Serum inorganic phosphorus was moderately elevated and alkaline phosphatase was unaffected. Correction of the diet for 6 months resulted in reversal of the abnormalities in serum chemical values (92).

SPECIFIC SPECIFICITY IN IMMUNOCHEMICAL PROTEIN MEASUREMENT

The widespread and growing use of immunochemical methods in clinical chemistry (radial immunodiffusion, radioimmunoassay, enzyme-linked immunosorbent assay, etc) presents a problem in the application of these methods to specimens from nonhuman species. The validity of the assay depends on the antibody uniquely binding the desired analyte. If human calibration standards are used, the binding affinity must be identical to the species in question in order to achieve accuracy. Even in validated heterologous systems, homologous standards should be used if possible. The absence of interfering or competitive contaminants is essential. Because amino acid sequences in proteins and polypeptides generally follow phylogeny, the close phylogenic relationship of nonhuman primates to man constitutes a distinct advantage of nonhuman primate specimens when compared, for example, to rodent specimens. Nonprotein analytes such as steroids present no similar problem of species specificity.

Holmberg et al (19,30) assayed the serum of a number of species of nonhuman primates by radial diffusion immunoassay for human C_3 of the complement cascade as well as measuring

CH_{50} a functional assay for total complement activity. Human calibration standards were used. Although immunoreactivity was observed in all higher primates studied (though not with serum from the Galago, a prosimian), poor correlation was obtained between the C_3 assay and the assay of CH_{50} which shows less immunologic species specificity. This finding suggests that although antibody to human C_3 may bind the C_3 of high nonhuman primates, the avidity of binding to the latter may be decreased. Thus, numerical results appear inaccurate, but relative concentrations among members of a single species may be valid.

The measurement of lemur (*L. catti*) and baboon luteinizing hormone by an ovine luteinizing hormone-antiovine, luteinizing hormone radioimmunoassay (used in several species) has been validated (66,89).

THYROID HORMONES

Thyroxine and triiodothyronine in the serum of nonhuman primates may be assayed by standard human radioimmunoassay methods. Kaack et al (36,37) demonstrated that in maturing squirrel monkeys thyroxine progressively decreases, whereas triiodothyronine values do not change. Much higher values for both thyroxine and triiodothyronine were observed in the Bolivian subspecies of *Saimiri sciureus* than in the Columbian subspecies. The administration of estradiol to intact female rhesus monkeys increased their serum thyroid stimulating hormone by decreasing its degradation (82).

CORTISOL

Serum cortisol levels are lower in infant and juvenile squirrel monkeys than in adults (35). A circadian periodicity has been demonstrated in many species. In the rhesus monkey cortisol levels are highest in the morning and lowest in the evening, whereas in the squirrel monkey values are highest at the start of the light period and lowest 4 hours after the onset of darkness (18,23,47,74,79,84,98). Serum concentrations of adrenal corticosteroids are five to ten fold higher in marmosets than in macaques and very loosely bound to transport protein (101).

Behavioral stress was shown to elevate plasma cortisol in rhesus and squirrel monkeys, resulting in data that may lead to erroneous interpret-ation of the dexamethasone suppression test (26,38,72). The stress of capture results in elevation of plasma cortisol for the following 60 minutes (7).

Diabetic rhesus monkeys have significantly higher plasma cortisol values than do non-diabetic monkeys (23).

In African green vervets, Meis and Rose (59) determined that feeding resulted in rapid elevation of cortisol, with a subsequent decrease to minimal values 5 hours after feeding. Timed feeding synchronized the circadian rhythm of cortisol. The relationship between dominance and resting serum cortisol was studied in male vervets. In stable groups dominant and subordinate males had similar serum cortisol values. However, in unstable groups, males achieving dominance had higher serum cortisol values than did subordinate males (55). In talapoin monkeys, dominant animals had cerebrospinal fluid cortisol concentrations that were proportionately higher with respect to serum cortisol than did subordinate animals (29).

SEX HORMONES AND GONADOTROPINS

Non human primates are extensively utilized in investigations of pituitary and sex hormone responses because of their similarity to humans in these respects.

High serum levels of testosterone of testicular origin are present in neonatal male rhesus and pigtail macaques. Females of similar age have testosterone levels comparable to castrated males and low levels of estradiol (78). Luteinizing hormone and follicle stimulating hormone levels are high in male rhesus monkeys during the first three months of life, decreasing thereafter to low or undetectable levels (21). In male chimpanzees, serum testosterone levels increase stepwise with age, from a mean juvenile value of 13 ng/dl at one to six years to an adolescent value of 178 ng/dl at seven to ten years, to an adult value of 397 ng/dl (57).

In male rhesus monkeys, testosterone, androstenedione, 5-α-dihydrotestosterone, and luteinizing hormone have a circadian periodicity. Peak values for testosterone, luteinizing hormone and 5-α-dihydrotestosterone occur at 2100 hours, however investigators do not concur as to the time of the lowest values. By contrast, androstenedione decreases in the evening and increases at night to reach peak values at 0700 hours. No difference in hormone levels was observed between young and old adults. An annual periodicity was observed for testosterone and 5-α dihydrotestosterone, with highest levels in the fall and winter and lowest levels in the spring. No similar annual rhythm was observed for androstenedione (11,18,24,25,28,67,73,79, 87). In the nocturnal male owl monkey (*Aotus trivirgatus*), lowest serum levels of testosterone are present during the dark period and five-fold higher levels are present during the light period, the reverse of patterns reported in diurnal primates (17). In *M. nemestrina* no annual periodicity in testosterone was observed but values rose when females were introduced into formerly all male groups (4). In male vervet African green monkeys, circadian rhythm was demonstrated for androgens, with peak values at 2100 to 0600 hours and for 17-β-estradiol with peak values at 2400 to 0600 hours (5). In squirrel monkeys under laboratory conditions plasma levels of total androgens (testosterone and dihydrotestosterone) are much higher than in Old World primates but neither circadian rhythm nor annual periodicity was observed (98).

During the breeding season, female squirrel monkeys (*S. sciureus*) have a periodicity of approximately 9 days for 17-β-estradiol and for progestins (100).

Measurements of estrogens and progesterone during the menstrual cycle have been reported in owl monkeys (*Aotus trivirgatus*) (8), capuchin monkeys (*Cebus apella*) (63), rhesus monkeys (*Macaca mulatta*) (32), stump tailed macaques (*M. arctoides*) (97), and baboons (*Papio cynocephalus*) (43). In a natural environment, the menstrual cycles of rhesus monkeys are ovulatory in fall and winter and anovulatory, with low levels of FSH and estradiol in spring and summer (94).

The endocrine profile of pregnancy in the patas monkey was studied by Winterer et al (99) who found it remarkably similar to its human counterpart. Plasma levels of estrone, estradiol, estriol, progesterone, aldosterone, and plasma renin activity were determined weekly from 4 to 6 weeks of gestation to parturition (day 167 ± 10). These studies suggested that the patas monkey may be a good model for human pregnancy toxemia. In female baboons, serum estradiol, the primary source of urine estrone increases in concentration during the course of pregnancy, and falls precipitously at parturition

(1). The hormonal changes associated with pregnancy have also been studied in the marmoset (*Callithrix jacchus*) (12).

Serum levels of hormones of Bolivian squirrel monkeys undergoing spontaneous abortion were investigated by Diamond et al (15). In pregnant animals progesterone levels remained above 100 ng/ml whereas chorionic gonadotropin and estradiol levels rose gradually from the onset of pregnancy to a peak at 50 days. In animals undergoing spontaneous abortion, hormone levels were observed to decline to one fifth or less of peak values. Weekly measurement of chorionic gonadotropin and estradiol identified those animals that aborted (15). In rhesus monkeys pregnant with live anencephalic fetuses, estradiol was significantly lower than in pregnant normal controls but estrone was not decreased, while following fetal death, both estradiol and estrone decreased significantly. Concentrations of cortisol and progesterone did not differ among the three groups (95).

Chorionic gonadotropin occurs in the serum and urine of pregnant female monkeys. The molecule consists of an alpha and a beta subunit. The structure of the alpha subunit is highly species specific; the beta subunit is immunologically similar among species. Antibody to the beta subunit of ovine luteinizing hormone is used in a hemagglutination inhibition assay and a radioimmunoassay which have been used in pregnancy diagnosis in *M. mulatta*, *M. arctoides*, *M. fascicularis*, *M. radiata*, and also in owl monkeys, squirrel monkeys, baboons, tamarins, marmosets, orangutans, gorillas, and chimpanzees. The duration of reliable positive reaction is brief; in *M. mulatta* and *M. arctoides* it occurs on days 20 to 24 of pregnancy and in *M. fascicularis*, on days 24-28 (9,46,75,102). Use of the hemagglutination inhibition test in rhesus monkeys was evaluated at 19 to 21 days after breeding. Pregnant females were detected with an accuracy of 73.3 per cent. Of 104 urine samples from non-pregnant intact females 11.5 per cent yielded a false positive result. Rarely, urine from males or ovariectomized females yielded false positive results (65).

EFFECTS OF AGE AND PERIODICITY

The effect of maturation and aging on clinical chemical parameters of primates has been investigated extensively. Kaack et al (35), studying squirrel monkeys, found that serum protein levels, in particular albumin, were lower at 30 days of age than at 6 months, when values approximated those found in the adult. Maturation was associated with a decline in cholesterol and thyroxine, though no significant change in triiodothyronine occurred. Kessler et al (41) determined that serum iron and magnesium levels were lower in aged male rhesus monkeys than in young adults, whereas globulin and triglycerides levels were higher. In females, magnesium and alkaline phosphatase levels were lower than in young adults, whereas globulin and uric acid levels were higher. The relationship of endocrine parameters to age from birth to adulthood was studied in *M. fascicularis* by Meusy-Dessolle and Dang (60). Testosterone, 5-α-dihydrotestosterone, delta-4-androstenedione, dehydroepiandrosterone, and estradiol-17-β were determined. The studies revealed a 3 to 4 month long neonatal period of testicular activity, a 29-month period of inactivity (infancy), a 43-month prepubertal phase of erratic values, and the attainment of adult values at about 5 years of age. Endocrine functions of aged male rhesus monkeys were measured by Kaler et al (39,40). Pulsatile secretion of growth hormone occurred in both aged and young males, though in the aged animals pulses were less frequent, and mean plasma growth hormone per 24 hours was lower. Testosterone pulses similarly showed lower frequency and amplitude in aged animals, whereas luteinizing hormone pulses were similar in young and aged animals. These observations led to the conclusion that aging in male rhesus monkeys was associated with decreased hypothalamic sensitivity to negative feedback by testosterone and decreased testicular response to luteinizing hormone.

Circadian rhythm of hematologic and clinical chemical parameters of the owl monkey, a nocturnal primate, were studied by Klein et al (42). The animals were housed in artificial lighting, 12 hours of light and 12 hours of dark. The serum protein zenith occurred at the second hour of the light phase and was 10 per cent higher than the nadir which occured at the second hour of the dark phase. The serum iron zenith occurred at the same time as the protein zenith, and it was 84 per cent higher than the nadir at the sixth hour of the light phase.

REFERENCES

1. Albrecht ED, Townsley JD (1978) Serum estradiol in mid- and late gestation and estradiol/progesterone ratio in baboons near parturition. Biol Reprod 18: 247–250
2. Ausman LM, Gallina DL (1978) Response to glucose loading of the lean squirrel monkey in unrestrained conditions. Am J Physiol 234: R20–24
3. Beland MD, Sehgal PK, Peacock WC (1979) Baseline blood chemistry determinations in the squirrel monkey (*Saimiri sciureus*). Lab An Sci 29: 195–199
4. Bernstein IS, Gordon TP, Rose RM, Peterson MS (1978) Influences of sexual and social stimuli upon circulating levels of testosterone in male pigtail macaques. Behav Biol 24: 400–404
5. Beattie CW, Bullock BC (1978) Diurnal variation of serum androgen and estradiol in 17-beta in the adult male green monkey (Cercopithecus sp.). Biol Reprod 19: 36–39
6. Bhattacharyya AK, Eggen DA (1983) Mechanism of the variability in plasma cholesterol response to cholesterol feeding in rhesus monkeys. Artery 11: 306–326
7. Blank MS, Gordon TP, Wilson ME (1983) Effects of capture and venipuncture on serum levels of prolactin, growth hormone and cortisol in outdoor compound-housed female rhesus monkeys (*Macaca mulatta*). Acta Endocrinol (Copenh) 102: 190–195
8. Bonney RC, Dixson AF, Fleming D (1979) Cyclic changes in the circulating and urinary levels of ovarian steroids in the adult female owl monkey (*Aotus trivirgatus*). J Reprod Fertil 56: 271–280
9. Boot R, Huis in't Veld LG (1981) Pregnancy diagnosis in *Macaca fascicularis*. J Med Primatol 10: 141–148
10. Burns KF, Ferguson FG, Hampton SH (1967) Compendium of normal blood values for baboons, chimpanzees and marmosets. Am J Clin Path 48: 484–494
11. Chambers KC, Resko JA, Phoenix CH (1982) Correlation of diurnal changes in hormones with sexual behavior and age in male rhesus macaques. Neurobiol Aging 3: 37–42
12. Chambers PL, Hearn JP (1979) Peripheral plasma levels of progesterone, oestradiol-17 beta, oestrone, testosterone, androstenedione and chorionic gonadotrophin during pregnancy in the marmoset monkey, *Callithrix jacchus*. J Reprod Fertil 56: 23–32
13. Christen P, Peacock WC, Christen AE, Wacker WEC (1970) Urate oxidase in primate phylogenesis. Eur J Biochem 12: 3–5
14. Cornelius CE (1982) The use of non-human primates in the study of bilirubin metabolism and bile secretions. Am J Primatol 2: 343–354
15. Diamond EJ, Aksel S, Hazelton JM, Barnet SB, Williams LE, Abee CR (1985) Serum hormone patterns during abortion in the Bolivian squirrel monkey. Lab An Sci 35: 619–623
16. DiGiacomo RF, McDonash BF, Gibbs CJ Jr (1975) The progression and evaluation of hematologic and serum biochemical values in the chimpanzee. J Med Primatol 4: 188–203
17. Dixon AF, Gardner JS (1981) Diurnal variations in

plasma testosterone in a male nocturnal primate, the owl monkey (*Aotus trivirgatus*). J Reprod Fertil 62: 83–86

18. Dubey AK, Puri CP, Puri V, Anand Kumar TC (1983) Day and night levels of hormones in male rhesus monkeys kept under controlled or constant environmental light. Experientia 39: 207–209

19. Ellingsworth LR, Holmberg CA, Osburn BI (1983) Hemolytic complement measurement in eleven species of nonhuman primates. Vet Immunol Immunopathol 5: 141–149

20. Flow DL, Cartwright TC, Kuehl TJ, Mott GE, Kraemer DC (1981) Genetic effects on serum cholesterol concentrations in baboons. J Hered 72: 97–103

21. Frawley LS, Neill JD (1979) Age related changes in serum levels of gonadotrophins and testosterone in infantile male rhesus monkeys. Biol Reprod 20: 1147–1151

22. Fulmer R, Loeb WF, Martin DP, Gard EA (1984) Effects of three methods of restraint on intravenous glucose tolerance testing in rhesus and African green monkeys. Vet Clin Pathol 13: 19–25

23. Garg SK, Chhina GS, Singh B (1978) Factors influencing plasma cortisol (11-hydroxycorticoids) levels in rhesus monkeys. Indian J Exp Biol 16: 1184–1185

24. Goncharov NP, Tavadyan DS, Vorontsov VI (1982) Circadian and seasonal rhythms of androgen content in the blood plasma of rhesus monkeys. Neurosci Behav Physiol 12: 501–505

25. Goncharov NP, Tavadyen DS, Voronstov VI (1981) Diurnal-seasonal rhythms of androgen in Macaca rhesus blood plasma. Probl Endokrinol Mosk 27: 53–57

26. Gonzalez CA, Coe CL, Levine S (1982) Cortisol responses under different housing conditions in female squirrel monkeys. Psychoneuroendocrinology 7: 209–216

27. Goodner CJ, Walike BC, Koerker DJ, Ensinck JW, Brown AC, Chideckel EW, Palmer J, Kalnasay L (1977) Insulin, glucagon, and glucose exhibit synchronous, sustained oscillations in fasting monkeys. Science 195: 177–179

28. Gordon TP, Bernstein IS, Rose RM (1978) Social and seasonal influences on testosterone secretion in the male rhesus monkey. Physiol Behav 21: 623–627

29. Herbert J, Keverne EB, Yodyingyuad U (1986) Modulation by social status of the relationship between cerebrospinal fluid and serum cortisol levels in male talapoin monkeys. Neurendocrinol 42: 436–442

30. Holmberg CA, Ellingsworth L, Osburn BI, Grant CK (1977) Measurement of hemolytic complement and the third component of complement in nonhuman primates. Lab An Sci 27: 993–998

31. Holmes AW, Passovog M, Capps RB (1967) Marmosets as laboratory animals. III. Blood chemistry of laboratory kept marmosets with particular attention to liver function and structure. Lab An Care 17: 41–47

32. Hotchkiss J, Dierschke DJ, Butler WR, Fritz GR, Knobil E (1982) Relation between levels of circulating ovarian steroids and pituitary gonadotropin content during the menstrual cycle of the rhesus monkey. Biol Reprod 26: 241–248

33. Howard CF (1982) Nonhuman primates as models for the study of human diabetes mellitus. Diabetes 31: 37–42

34. Jen IC, Hansen BC, Metzger B (1985) Adiposity, anthropometric measures, and plasma insulin levels of rhesus monkeys. Int J Obesity 9: 213–224

35. Kaack B, Brizzee KR, Walker L (1979) Some biochemical blood parameters in the developing squirrel monkey. Folio Primatol 32: 309–318

36. Kaack B, Walker L, Brizzee KR, Wolf RH (1979) Comparative normal levels of serum triiodothyronine and thyroxine in non-human primates. Lab An Sci 29: 191–194

37. Kaack B, Walker M, Walker L (1980) Seasonal changes in the thyroid hormones of the male squirrel monkey. Arch Androl 4: 133–136

38. Kalin NH, Shelton SE (1984) Acute behavioral stress affects the dexamethasone suppression test in rhesus monkeys. Biol Psychiatry 19: 113–117

39. Kaler LW, Gliessman P, Craven J, Hill I, Critchlow V (1986) Loss of enhanced nocturnal growth hormone secretion in aging rhesus males. Endocrinology 119: 1281–1284

40. Kaler LW, Gliessman P, Hess D, Hill J (1986) The androgen status of aging male rhesus macaques. Endocrinology 119: 566–571

41. Kessler MJ, Rawlins RG, London WT (1983) The hemogram serum biochemistry, and electrolyte profile of aged rhesus monkeys (*Macaca mulatta*). J Med Primatol 12: 184–191

42. Klein R, Bleiholder B, Jung A, Erkert HG (1985) Diurnal variaton of several blood parameters in the owl monkey, *Aotus trivirgatus griseimembra*. Folia Primatol 45: 195–203

43. Koyama T, DelaPena A, Hagino N (1977) Plasma estrogen, progestin, and luteinizing hormone during the normal menstrual cycle in the baboon: role of luteinizing hormone. Am J Obstet Gynecol 127: 67–72

44. Lacko AG, Davis JL (1979) Age-related changes in rat and primate plasma cholesterol metabolism. J Am Geriatr Soc 27: 212–217

45. Leathers CW, Schedewie HK (1980) Diabetes mellitus in a pigtailed macaque (*Macaca nemestrina*). J Med Primatol 9: 95–100

46. Lequin RM, Elvens LH, Bertens AMG (1981) Early detection of pregnancy in rhesus and stump-tailed macaques (*Macaca mulatta* and *Macaca arctoides*): Evaluation of two radioimmunoassays and a hemagglutination inhibition test. J Med Primatol 10: 189–198

47. Leshner AI, Toivola PT, Terasawa E (1978) Circadian variations in cortisol concentrations in the plasma of female rhesus monkeys. J Endocrinol 78: 155–156

48. Loeb W (1972) The kinetics of sulfobromophthalein clearance in the rhesus monkey. Lab An Sci 22: 383–396

49. Manning PJ, Lehner NDM, Feldner MA, Bullock BC (1969) Selected hematologic, serum chemical, and arterial blood gas characteristics of squirrel monkeys (*Saimiri sciureus*). Lab An Care 19: 831–837

50. McClure HN, Keeling ME, Guilloud NB (1972)

Hematologic and blood chemistry data for the chimpanzee (*Pan troglodytes*). Folio Primatol 18: 444–462

51. McClure HM, Keeling ME, Guilloud NB (1972) Hematologic and blood chemistry data for the gorilla (*Gorilla gorilla*). Folio Primatol 18: 300–316

52. McClure HM, Keeling ME, Gilloud NB (1972) Hematologic and blood chemistry data for the orangutang (*Pongo pygmaeus*). Folio Primatol 18: 284–299

53. McGeachin RL, Akin JR (1982) Amylase levels in the tissue and body fluids of several primate species. Comp Biochem Physiol A 72: 267–269

54. McGill HC Jr, McMahan CA, Kruski AW, Mott GE (1981) Relationship of lipoprotein cholesterol concentrations to experimental atherosclerosis in baboons. Arteriosclerosis 1: 3–12

55. McGuire MT, Brammer GL, Raleigh MJ (1986) Resting cortisol levels and the emergence of dominant status among male vervet monkeys. Hormones and Behavior 20: 106–117

56. McMahan MR, Clarkson TB, Sackett GP, Rudel LL (1980) Changes in plasma lipids and lipoproteins in *Macaca nemestrina* during pregnancy and the postpartum period. Proc Soc Exp Biol Med 164: 199–202

57. Martin DE, Swenson RB, Collins DC (1977) Correlation of serum testosterone levels with age in male chimpanzees. Steroids 29: 471–481

58. Meis PJ, Kaplan JR, Koritnik DR, Rose JC (1982) Effects of gestation on glucose tolerance and plasma insulin in cynomolgus monkeys (*Macaca fascicularis*). Am J Obstet Gynecol 144: 543–545

59. Meis PJ, Rose JC (1983) Plasma cortisol response to feeding in African green vervets. J Med Primatol 12: 49–52

60. Meusy-Dessolle N, Dang DC (1985) Plasma concentrations of testosterone, dihydrotestosterone, delta-4-androstenedione, dehydroepiandrosterone, and estadiol-17-beta in the crab-eating monkey (*Macaca fascicularis*) from birth to adulthood. J Reprod Fert 74: 347–359

61. Mohr JR, Mattenheimer H, Holmes AW, Deinhardt F, Schmidt FW (1971) Enzymology of experimental liver disease in marmoset monkeys. I. Patterns of enzyme activity in liver, other organs and serum of marmosets compared to man and other mammals. Enzyme 12: 99–116

62. Mott GE, McMahan CA, Kelley JL, Farley CM, McGill HC Jr (1982) Influence of infant and juvenile diets on serum cholesterol, lipoprotein cholesterol, and apolipoprotein concentrations in juvenile baboons (Papio sp.). Atherosclerosis 45: 191–202

63. Nagle CA, Denari JH, Guiroga S, Riarte A, Merlo A, Germino NI, G'omez-Argaña F, Rosner JM (1979) The plasma pattern of ovarian steroids during the menstrual cycle in capuchin monkeys (*Cebus apella*). Biol Reprod 21: 979–983

64. Natelson BH, Stokes, PE, Root AW (1982) Plasma glucose and insulin levels in monkeys anticipating feeding. Pavlov J Biol Sci 17: 80–83

65. Naqvi RH, Lindberg MC (1985) Evaluation of the subhuman primate pregnancy test kit for the detection of early pregnancy in the rhesus monkey (*Macaca mulatta*). J Med Primatol 14: 229–233

66. Norman RL, Brandt H, van Horn RN (1978) Radioimmunoassay for luteinizing hormone (LH) in the ring-tailed lemur (*Lemur catta*) with antiovine LH and ovine 125I-LH. Biol Reprod 19: 1119–1124

67. Plant RM (1982) A striking diurnal variation in plasma testosterone concentration in infantile male rhesus monkeys (*Macaca mulatta*). Neurendocrinology 35: 370–373

68. Porter WP (1982) Hematologic and other effects of ketamine and ketamine-acepromazine in rhesus monkeys (*Macaca mulatta*). Lab An Sci 32: 373–375

69. Portman OW, Alexander M, Neuringer M, Illingworth DR, Alam SS (1981) Effects of long-term protein deficiency on plasma lipoprotein concentrations and metabolism in rhesus monkeys. J Nutr 111: 733–745

70. Portman OW, Alexander M, Tanaka N, Osuga T (1980) Relationships between cholesterol gallstones, biliary function, and plasma lipoproteins in squirrel monkeys. J Lab Clin Med 96: 90–101

71. Portman OW, Roy Chowdhury J, Roy Chowdhury N, Alexander M, Cornelius CE, Arias IM (1984) A non-human primate model of Gilbert's syndrome. Hepatology 4: 175–179

72. Puri CP, Puri V, Anad Kumar TC (1981) Serum levels of testosterone, cortisol, prolactin and bioactive luteinizing hormone in adult male rhesus monkeys following cage-restraint or anesthetizing with ketamine hydrochloride. Acta Endocrinol (Copenh) 97: 118–124

73. Puri CP, Puri V, David GF, Kumar TC (1980) Testosterone, cortisol, prolactin and bioactive luteinizing hormone in day and night samples of cerebrospinal fluid and serum of male rhesus monkeys. Brain Res 200: 377–387

74. Quabbe HJ, Gregor M, Bumke-Vogt C, Härdel C (1982) Pattern of plasma cortisol during the 24-hour sleep wake cycle in the rhesus monkey. Endocrinology 110: 1641–1646

75. Rao AJ, Kotagi SG, Moudgal NR (1984) Serum concentrations of chornionic gonadotrophin, oestradiol-17 beta and progesterone during early pregnancy in the south Indian bonnet monkey (*Macaca radiata*). J Reprod Fertil 70: 449–455

76. Renquist DM, Montrey RD, Hooks JE, Manus AG (1977) Hematologic, biochemical, and physiologic indices of the sacred baboon (*Papio hamadryas*). Lab An Sci 27: 271–275

77. Robinson FR, Ziegler RF (1968) Clinical laboratory data derived from 102 *Macaca mulatta*. Lab An Care 18: 50–57

78. Robinson JA, Bridson WE (1978) Neonatal hormone patterns in the Macaque. I. Steroids. Biol Reprod 19: 773–778

79. Rose RM, Gordon TP, Bernstein IS (1978) Diurnal variation in plasma testosterone and cortisol in rhesus monkeys living in social groups. J Endocrinol 76: 67–74

80. Rudel LL, McMahan MR, Shah RN (1981) Pregnancy effects on non-human primate high density lipoprotein. J Med Primatol 10: 16–25

81. Rudel LL, Reynolds JA, Bullock BC (1981) Nutritional effects on blood lipid and HDL chol-

esterol concentrations in two subspecies of African green monkeys (*Cercopithecus aethiops*). J Lipid Res 22: 278–286

82. Sawhney RC, Rastogi I, Rastogi GK (1978) Effect of estrogens on thyroid function. I. Alterations in rhesus plasma thyrotropin and its kinetics. Endocrinology 102: 1310–1316

83. Slop AK, Ooms MP, Vreeburg JY (1979) Annual changes in serum testosterone in laboratory housed male stump-tail macaques (*M. arctoides*). Biol Reprod 20: 981–984

84. Socol ML, Manning FA, Murata Y, Challis J, Martin CB Jr (1978) Plasma cortisol in the chronic rhesus monkey preparation (*Macaca mulatta*). Am J Obstet Gynecol 132: 421–424

85. Srinivasan SR, Clevidence BA, Pargaonkar PS (1979) Varied effects of dietary sucrose and cholesterol on serum lipids, lipoproteins and apolipoproteins in rhesus monkeys. Atherosclerosis 33: 301–314

86. Srinivasan SR, Radhakrishnamurthy B, Foster TA, Berenson GS (1983) Divergent responses of serum lipoproteins to changes in dietary carbohydrate and cholesterol in cynomolgus monkeys. Metabolism 32: 777–786

87. Steiner RA, Peterson AP, Yu JY, Conner H, Gilbert M, terPenning B, Bremner WJ (1980) Ultradian luteinizing hormone and testosterone rhythms in the adult male monkey, *Macaca fascicularis*. Endocrinology 107: 1489–1493

88. Streett IW, Jonas AM (1982) Differential effects of chemical and physical restraint on carbohydrate tolerance testing in the non-human primates. Lab An Sci 32: 263–266

89. Su JH, Aso T, Motohashi T, Aochi H, Matsuoka M, Horie K, Nishimura T (1980) Radioimmunoassay method for baboon plasma gonadotropins. Endocrinol Jpn 27: 513–520

90. Szmanski ES, Kritchevsky D (1980) Serum lipid levels of young and old rhesus monkeys. Exp Gerontol 15: 365–367

91. Terpstra AH, Sanchez-Muniz FJ, West CE, Woodward CJ (1982) The density profile and cholesterol concentration of serum lipoproteins in domestic and laboratory animals. Comp Biochem Physiol [B] 71: 669–673

92. Tomson FN, Lotshaw RR (1978) Hyperphosphatemia and hypocalcemia in lemurs. J Am Vet Med Assoc 173: 1103–1106

93. Vondruska JF (1970) Certain hematologic and blood chemical values in adult stump-tailed macaques (*Macaca arctoides*). Lab An Care 20: 97–200

94. Walker ML, Wilson ME, Gordon TP (1984) Endocrine control of the seasonal occurrence of ovulation in rhesus monkeys housed outdoors. Endocrinology 114: 1074–1081

95. Walsh SW, Kittinger GW, Novy MJ (1979) Maternal peripheral concentrations of estradiol, estrone, cortisol, and progesterone during late pregnancy in rhesus monkeys (*Macaca mulatta*) and after experimental fetal anencephaly and fetal death. Am J Obstet Gynecol 135: 37–42

96. Wellde BT, Johnson AJ, Williams JS, Langbehn HR, Sadun EH (1971) Hematologic, biochemical, parasitologic parameters of the night monkey (*Aotus trivirgatus*). Lab An Sci 21: 575–580

97. Wilks IW (1977) Endocrine characterization of the menstrual cycle of the stump-tailed monkey (*Macaca arctoides*). Biol Reprod 16: 474–478

98. Wilson MI, Brown GM, Wilson D (1978) Annual and diurnal changes in plasma androgen and cortisol in adult male squirrel monkeys (*Saimiri sciureus*) studied longitudinally. Acta Endocrinol (Kbh) 87: 424–433

99. Winterer J, Palmer AE, Cicmanec J, Davis E, Harbaugh S, Loriaux DL (1985) Endocrine profile of pregnancy in the patas monkey (*Erythrocebus patas*). Endocrinology 116: 1090–1093

100. Wolf RC, O'Connor RF, Robinson JA (1977) Cyclic changes in plasma progestins and estrogens in squirrel monkeys. Biol Reprod 17: 228–231

101. Yamamoto S, Utsu S, Tanioka Y, Ohsawa N (1977) Extremely high levels of corticosteroids and low levels of corticosteroid binding macromolecule in plasma of marmoset monkeys. Acta Endocrinol (Kbh) 85: 398–405

102. Yoshida T (1983) Serum gonadotropin levels during the menstrual cycle and pregnancy in the cynomolgus monkey. Jpn J Med Sci Biol 36: 231–236

103. Zaidi P, Wickings EJ, Nieschlag E (1982) The effects of ketamine HCl and barbiturate anesthesia on the metabolic clearance and production rates of testosterone in the male rhesus monkey, *Macaca mulatta*. J Steroid Biochem 16: 463–466

PART B

Classes of Substances:
The Role of Species Specificity
in Their Measurement

8

Carbohydrate Metabolism

J. J. KANEKO, DVM, PhD, DVSc (Hon) and C. F. HOWARD, Jr, PhD

Laboratory animals play a significant role in biomedical research and their clinical chemistry is of particular importance in metabolic disease research. The growth of the field of clinical chemistry of laboratory animals has been a direct outgrowth of this emphasis, and in metabolic disease research, carbohydrate studies have been devoted to the fundamental as well as the medical and toxicologic aspects of carbohydrate metabolism. Animal models have historically played an important role in these studies. The prevalence of diabetes mellitus in the human population and the multifactorial nature of diabetes mellitus as expressed in its genetic aspects, pathogenesis, biochemistry, methods of detection, and management have resulted in a preponderance of carbohydrate studies in laboratory animals being directed towards diabetes. The multifactorial nature of diabetes mellitus also results in the use of a wide spectrum of laboratory animals, each being particularly well suited for the study of a particular aspect of the overall metabolic problem. Thus, at least a dozen or more species or strains within species have been used to study carbohydrate metabolism and diabetes in laboratory animals.

On the premise that the nonhuman primate is most closely related to humans for whom the ultimate value of most biochemical research is intended, a discussion of carbohydrate metabolism in the nonhuman primate will be presented first. Included are many of the related fundamental hormonal aspects of carbohydrate metabolism such as the action of insulin, which can now be regarded as crossing species lines. Following in order of similarities to spontaneous human diabetes, other laboratory animal species starting with the dog are discussed. In each section, species differences and appropriateness for certain types of carbohydrate metabolic studies are noted and discussed.

CARBOHYDRATE METABOLISM IN THE NONHUMAN PRIMATE

In the following sections, various aspects of carbohydrate management, as studied in primates, are discussed first, followed by results of experimental or spontaneous aberrations. Species differences are emphasized so that the appropriateness of a particular primate species for use as a model can be evaluated. There are several reviews on carbohydrate management in primates to which the reader is referred for complete details (55,57,58).

Only changes in blood metabolites, hormones, and hormone responses are presented here. Although urinalysis is commonly used to assess carbohydrate metabolism in humans, it is used less often in primates. It is difficult to sample primate urine, but blood can readily be withdrawn when the primate is handled.

73

Furthermore, urinary samples reflect metabolic clearances of its constituents, which occurred some time before the sample was taken. However, urinary components in diabetic primates do confirm the presence of progressive glucosuria and ketonuria as the diabetes becomes more severe.

Plasma Glucose

Plasma glucose in most primates is similar to that in nondiabetic humans when testing occurs under optimal conditions, that is, 60 to 100 mg/dl. The close similarity of primate to human values contributes to the usefulness of primates as models of human carbohydrate metabolism. Although most data are reported under fasting conditions, postprandial glucose can often be used for screening for carbohydrate metabolic aberrations. Dietary preparation and fasting times are discussed in the section on glucose tolerance testing.

Many experimental manipulations or spontaneous diseases are known to alter plasma glucose. Spontaneous or induced diabetes results in hyperglycemia (57,58). The basic criteria for diagnosis of human diabetes is a fasting plasma glucose concentration of 140 mg/dl or greater (112). This is an adequate guideline for primates, but carbohydrate metabolic impairment can often be suspected if the fasting plasma glucose is greater than 115 mg/dl when samples are taken under optimum conditions.

Alterations in plasma glucose due to experimental manipulations are usually transient unless the conditions are severe or prolonged. Neither ketamine nor sernylan sedation causes significant changes in plasma glucose (14,80). Extensive hemorrhage elevates plasma glucose during hypovolemia (48). Antibiotics have no effect on plasma glucose (6,7). Infection by a number of microorganisms, such as *Escherichia coli*, can either increase (28) or decrease (141,147) plasma glucose. Generally, however, the changes are minimal and plasma glucose returns to baseline within a few hours in primates that survive the infection. Many experimentally induced changes in plasma glucose are attributable either directly or indirectly to stress (143), and they are often secondary to insulin suppression by epinephrine (104). Primates often have plasma glucose of less than 50 mg/dl

without the apparent adverse reactions seen in humans.

Intravenous Glucose Tolerance Test

The intravenous glucose tolerance test (IVGTT) offers a more reliable means of evaluating glucometabolic status than does a single plasma glucose sample. Glucose clearance may appear unaffected during the early phases of spontaneous impairment or with minimal experimental manipulation; however, impairments due to insulin are often discernible in the early stages and therefore the IVGTT can be a sensitive indicator of metabolic aberrations (44). If other hormones and metabolites are measured during the IVGTT, further insight into glucose metabolic controls can be gained. There is a need to establish minimal guidelines for uniformity so that results among different investigators can be compared.

Pretest Diet

An adequate carbohydrate-containing diet should be given for several days before the test to assure that hormonal responses and glucose clearance accurately reflect metabolic capabilities. When both beta cells and peripheral tissues are capable of responding to the glucose load, then impaired clearance reflects metabolic impairment rather than transient tissue insensitivity. For the oral glucose tolerance test in humans, consumption of at least 150 g of carbohydrate per day for 3 or more days before the test is recommended, whereas some investigators advocate up to 300 g per day. A similar standard to primates would be the consumption of 2 to 4 g of carbohydrate per kilogram of body weight per day.

The common and most reasonable criterion to determine adequate nutrition is maintenance of weight and health. This implies adequate food intake, but it does not specifically address dietary preparation for glucose tolerance testing. The type of food consumed and the schedule of feeding before an IVGTT are usually reported, often in exact detail (4).

Pretest Fasting

Most investigators withhold food for 16 to 20 hours, usually overnight. The fasting time is often a matter of convenience, that is, food is removed at the end of the work day and the IVGTT is conducted the following morning.

An adequate fast is one that is beyond the postprandial state; 16 to 18 hours of fasting are generally sufficient. A fast of 24 hours or longer can place monkeys in a semistarved state in which time, beta, and peripheral cell responses to glucose may be impaired and the causes for delayed clearance would be obscured. An extended fast can be used to differentiate normal monkeys from those with incipient carbohydrate impairment (54).

Primates of many species can store food pellets in their buccal pouches. Generally, pellets soften and are masticated and swallowed with 1 to 2 hours. Thus, the term "food deprivation" is probably a more accurate term than "fast" for timing postprandial events, unless pellets have been expressed form the buccal pouches at a specific time.

Glucose Load

The glucose load most commonly used in humans and primates is 0.5 g of glucose per kilogram of body weight. Glucose loads have varied from as low as 0.075 g/kg to as high as 1.5 g/kg. Unless effects of the glucose load are being studied, an infusion of 0.5 g/kg is recommended.

Most investigators infuse the glucose in less than 1 minute, usually within 30 seconds. Because one advantage of measuring glucose clearance with the IVGTT is the ability to establish a zero time point, the glucose should be infused as rapidly as feasible. Longer infusion times can cause sustained insulin release. It is preferable to define the zero time as midway through the infusion.

Chemical and Physical Restraint

Most IVGTTs are conducted on awake monkeys by repeated venipuncture. Because stress can affect the clearance of glucose, a nonsedated, nonadapted monkey is often the least desirable subject for an IVGTT. Feral monkeys usually react more adversely to handling than do caged monkeys familiar with handlers.

If monkeys are to be sedated during the IVGTT, selection of the pharmacologic agent is critical. Many compounds, such as barbiturates

and atropine (29,98), cause impairment in insulin secretion and thereby contribute to apparent glucose intolerance. Ketamine hydrochloride appears to be the chemical agent of choice for the IVGTT (14,20,80). There are some effects on insulin secretion; however, variations in awake, nonsedated monkeys or from chair-adapted monkeys are minimal as compared to those with other pharmacologic agents.

Indwelling catheters are usually used in monkeys being tested while restrained in a chair or on a tether so that blood sampling can proceed without the repeated trauma of capture, handling, and venipuncture. Tolerance tests can be performed on adapted, awake monkeys that are unaware that tests are being performed. Results from tethered, quiescent monkeys likely provide the most accurate information on glucose clearance and hormone responses. Therefore, how well the species or the individual monkey tolerates the stress of testing should always be noted.

Sampling Times

Within minutes after infusion of the glucose load, there is equilibration of glucose throughout the circulatory system and into extracellular spaces. Glucose in excess of the renal threshold is mainly cleared by the kidneys (73). After equilibration and minimization of renal clearance, metabolic processes account for plasma glucose clearance.

The first blood samples are drawn soon after glucose infusion, usually between 5 and 15 minutes; some investigators sample after only 1 or 2 minutes others 30 minutes. Rapid, sequential sampling is best accomplished with catheterization. The IVGTT can extend from 1 to more than 3 hours, but 1 hour is usually sufficient to establish glucose clearance and insulin secretion.

The peak glucose concentration in non-diabetic monkeys occurs in the first sample; thereafter, glucose concentrations decrease.

Calculations

Rapidity of clearance is generally computed as:

$$K = \frac{0.693}{T_{\frac{1}{2}}} \times 100 = \%/min$$

where $T\frac{1}{2}$ is the time taken for the glucose concentration to decrease by one half (95). Alternately the $T\frac{1}{2}$ alone can be reported. Measurement of glucose clearance is accurate only if values result in a straight line when plotted on a semilog scale. Linearity often is not achieved until at least 5 to 10 minutes after infusion and seldom goes beyond 60 minutes. Calculations should be based on values in samples taken no sooner than 10 minutes after infusion and should not extend beyond the time taken for glucose concentrations to fall to fasting levels, generally not more than 30 to 45 minutes in nondiabetic primates.

Species Variations

In rhesus macaques (*Macaca mulatta*), glucose concentrations are usually between 150 and 250 mg/dl at 5 to 10 minutes (57,60,148) and decrease to below 100 mg/dl within 15 to 20 minutes in most monkeys; virtually all reach fasting levels within 60 minutes. Other Old World primates generally have slightly slower clearance rates. Pigtailed macaques (*M. nemestrina*) (90), Celebes crested macaques (*M. nigra*) (54), a Formosan rock macaque (*M. cyclopis*) (61), and chimpanzees (*Pan troglodytes*) (119) reach glucose levels of 250 to 350 mg/dl at 10 to 15 minutes and return to fasting levels within 60 minutes. When squirrel monkeys (*Saimiri sciureus*), a New World species particularly sensitive to stress, are trained, adapted, and tethered (4), glucose is at a maximum of 230 mg/dl and falls below 100 mg/dl within 20 minutes. When untrained, nonacclimated monkeys are studied, the return to fasting levels extends beyond 60 minutes (4).

Most K values in nondiabetic primates are between 2 and 3 per cent per minute, corresponding to $T\frac{1}{2}$ values of 20 to 35 minutes. Occasionally, K values of <2 per cent per minute have been observed in normal Old World monkeys (40), whereas in some species, normal values can exceed 5 per cent per minute. The K values in untrained squirrel monkeys are routinely <2 per cent per minute, whereas in trained, tethered monkeys the clearance can be increased to >8 per cent per minute (4). Variations in K values among investigators can reflect actual differences in clearance, but variations in the sampling times chosen for the cal-

culations also cause the apparent variabilities. Hence there is a need for standardization.

Impaired Glucose Tolerance

Monkeys with spontaneous diabetes have impaired glucose clearance and impaired insulin responses (45,57,58,59,60,137). Streptozotocin or alloxan can cause overt diabetes (67,113,151) as well as intermediate impaired states (66, 67,68,113). Experimental manipulations such as hemorrhage (48), immobilization (94), pregnancy (103), stress (143), adrenalectomy (51), or administration of atropine (29) or other pharmacologic agents also decrease the insulin response and glucose clearance. At times, glucose clearance is enhanced, such as after placement of a lesion in the central nervous system (27), when stress is minimized (4), or after administration of synthetic estrogens (11). Reactions to infections vary. Pneumococcal and salmonella endotoxemias (34) cause no changes in glucose clearance, whereas yellow fever infection impairs clearance (140). Venezuelan equine encephalitis virus impairs glucose clearance in young, but not in adult rhesus macaques (13). Coxsackie B_4 virus is most effective in producing impaired glucose tolerance in patas monkeys (*Erythrocepus patas*); it has only transient effects in rhesus, cynomologus (*M. fascicularis*), and squirrel monkeys (152). Neither cortisone (82) nor antibiotics (7) change glucose clearance in normal monkeys; traumatic injury to the head produces abnormalities of only a few hours' duration (92).

Advantages and Disadvantages of the Intravenous Glucose Tolerance Test

The IVGTT is the preferred analytic method for assessing glucose clearance in primates. Establishment of an exact zero time allows accurate calculation of the rate of clearance and the entire test can be completed within 60 to 90 minutes. If dietary preparation has been adequate, glucose clearance after the initial equilibration phase represents only metabolic activity, and the results are not complicated by absorptive processes or by secretion of hormones associated with the gastrointestinal tract. However, results of IVGTTs in primates cannot directly be compared with data on humans in whom the oral glucose tolerance test is the more common diagnostic tool.

Oral Glucose Tolerance Test

The oral glucose tolerance test (OGTT) has been used less commonly than the IVGTT as a diagnostic method of evaluating carbohydrate metabolic status in primates.

Pretest Diet

Recommendations for carbohydrate consumption as discussed for the IVGTT should be followed, that is, 2 to 4 g per kilogram per day for at least 3 days before the test. As with the IVGTT, an 18-hour or overnight fast is reasonable for most species and a fast of 24 hours or longer can impair clearance.

Glucose Administration

The most common procedure has been intubation and administration of the glucose load as a 50 per cent glucose solution, usually within 1 minute. Monkeys have been trained to drink the glucose solution within 3 minutes (4). The glucose load advocated for the OGTT in human beings is either a standard 100 g of glucose or 1.75 g of glucose per kilogram of body weight. Although the latter amount has been used in primates (54), glucose amounts of 2 or 4 g/kg are more common; other loads have been 1 or 1.5 g/kg and 100 g of glucose per square meter of body surface (78). Glucose at 4 g/kg gives higher peaks and clears more slowly than do loads of 2 g/kg (31). Some monkeys can accommodate glucose adequately, and their levels do not vary significantly throughout the period of measurement (135). Recommendations for standardization of oral loads are difficult, given the rationalization for the different doses already in use. Better diagnostic results might be obtained in primates with a dose of 2 to 4 g/kg. It seems reasonable to use concentrations most appropriate to the species being studied and consistent within each experimental condition.

Blood Sampling Times and Interpretation of the Oral Glucose Tolerance Test

Sampling usually begins within 10 minutes and continues for 2 to 3 hours. Plasma glucose concentrations and times of peak concentrations vary extensively among various studies, because tests are conducted under nonstandard conditions with different species and glucose loads. The highest glucose concentrations in nondiabetic monkeys are found in the first sample, regardless of when it is taken.

Few investigators have attempted to analyze OGTT mathematically. Summations or increments between the first few samples (31,78) or a weighted formula covering the entire time of the test (88) have been used. Most investigators simply graph their results, often with the means and standard errors for each value. This allows comparisons with the controls and subjective interpretations of the curves.

Species Variation and the Effects of Stress or Sedation

The macaque species generally has a greater ability to clear glucose than do New World squirrel monkeys (148). Proposals that there are subpopulations of squirrel monkeys with impaired clearance, as judged by differences in OGTTs (88), have not been borne out (4,148). Impairment in glucose clearance can be due, at least in part, to the stress of the OGTT. More of the cynomolgus macaques (*M. fascicularis*) that are feral have abnormal glucose clearance patterns than do those bred in the laboratory (53). The relative contribution of stress versus inherent glucose metabolic impairment has not always been differentiated adequately. Monkeys sedated with ketamine hydrochloride had abnormal OGTT compared to the same monkeys adapted to chair restraint and given an oral load of glucose without chemical restraint (135).

Impaired Tolerance

The peak level of glucose during the OGTT is higher in diabetic primates than in nondiabetic control animals, often in excess 500 mg/dl. The peak time is usually delayed and may not be reached for at least 2 hours. Spontaneously diabetic Celebes macaques (54), cynomolgus macaques (69), a hamadryas baboon (*Papio hamadryas*) (129), and rhesus macaques with a streptozotocin-induced diabetes (78) have elevated glucose concentrations through at least 2 hours of testing.

Advantages and Disadvantages of the Oral Glucose Tolerance Test

There is a large body of data on the OGTT in humans to which the OGTT results in primates could be compared. Several disadvantages exist which make direct comparisons difficult or meaningless. The glucose load varies considerably among laboratories. Though some investigators have trained monkeys to consume a glucose load, most prefer to intubate, which is itself stressful. Clearance of the oral glucose load can be affected by hormones associated with the gastrointestinal tract; apparently normal clearance could result from impaired absorption. Choice of a pharmacologic agent for chemical restraint may be even more critical for attaining valid results from the OGTT than from the IVGTT. No consistent mathematical treatment of the data has been presented for computing clearance. Glucose values are often at their peak during early sampling times in nondiabetic monkeys, whereas glucose levels in diabetic or impaired monkeys usually do not reach maximum levels until midway through or late in the OGTT. These differences in responses complicate attempts at mathematical analyses to quantitate the data. Thus, the interpretation of the OGTT remains a subjective rather than a quantitative evaluation.

Metabolites Other Than Glucose

Ketones

Ketone bodies have long been associated with abnormalities in carbohydrate metabolism. When glucose is unavailable (starvation) or cannot be utilized (insulin deficiency in diabetes), fatty acids are used for energy. Products of fatty acid metabolism generate the ketones β-hydroxybutyric acid, acetoacetic acid, and acetone), and these pass into the circulation and thence into the urine. Increased concentration of the various ketones usually indicates impaired carbohydrate metabolism.

Total ketones in normal rhesus macaques range up to 5 mg/dl after an overnight fast and may increase to greater than 50 mg/dl after 3 to 6 days of food deprivation. Diabetes after pancreatectomy raises ketone levels to as high as 730 mg/dl. Ketone bodies in adult baboons average 2.2 mg/dl, increase to 22 mg/dl after 3 days of starvation (39), and after pan-createctomy and withdrawal in insulin therapy, reach 11 to 75 mg/dl. Insulin therapy, hypophysectomy, or adrenalectomy return ketones to near normal levels of 2 to 5 mg/dl (38). The ratio of β-hydroxybutyric acid to acetoacetic acid in baboons increases from 1.5 to 4 with starvation (124).

Glycosylated Hemoglobins

Circulating glucose reacts nonenzymatically with hemoglobin to form glycosylated derivatives. The percentages of these glycosylated hemoglobins increase with increased glucose. Although hemoglobin A_{1c} (HbA_{1c}) is the most sensitive to glucose changes and is the most commonly measured, many assays measure total glycosylated hemoglobins (HbA_1).

Levels of HbA_{1c} serve as indicators of long-term glucose control, reflecting carbohydrate management and glucose responses to therapy, that is, HbA_{1c} levels gradually increase above baseline values to a maximum after several weeks of hyperglycemia; they return toward normal levels with institution of therapy and diminution of glucose levels. The HbA_{1c} can be assessed by chromatographic separation and quantification. Variations in pI of hemoglobin proteins require validation of the chromatographic procedure for each species. Total HbA_1 is measured by chromogenic reactions against the hemoglobin carbohydrate moieties.

Patterns of glycosylated hemoglobins in nondiabetic primates are similar to those in humans (2,49,118,131,132). Concentrations of HbA_1 in nondiabetic primates range from nondetectable levels to 5.6 per cent of the total hemoglobin; with onset of diabetes, HbA_1 achieves from 10 to 21 per cent (2,66,79). The HbA_{1c} fraction ranges from nondetectable levels to 2.6 per cent in nondiabetic primates and from < 5 per cent to > 13 per cent in diabetic primates (2,66,144). Nondiabetic Celebes black macaques average 2.6 per cent HbA_1, and the borderline diabetic primates have a small but significant increase to 3.5 per cent; diabetic primates average 7.9 per cent (56). Therefore, glycosylated hemoglobins can be used for long-term monitoring of glucose concentrations in impaired states and during therapy of primates as in other animals and humans.

Hormones of Glucose Homeostasis

Immunocross-reactivity in Immunoassays

Radioimmunoassay is the most common means by which protein hormones are measured. Biologic activity may or may not be identical to immunoreactivity. Because specific antisera and purified standards are seldom available for each primate species, immunoassays must depend on the ability of antibodies from various sources to cross-react with primate hormones.

Pituitary hormones from several primate species assayed with antisera against different human pituitary hormones give parallel reactions, but the primate hormones react to a lesser degree than do the human hormones (138). Several investigators have noted the differences in insulin immunocross-reactivity between Old and New World animal species. An antibody to pork insulin gives comparable degrees of cross-reactivity in rhesus macaques, chimpanzees, and humans, but the reactivity of squirrel and capuchin monkeys is negligible (96). Squirrel monkeys demonstrate about one third the insulin immunoreactivity of rhesus macaques during glucose tolerance tests (148). Some antibodies have been specifically developed against monkey insulin (148). The structure of rhesus monkeys' insulin is identical to that of human insulin (1907). Reactivities of insulin antisera with insulin of dogs, pigs, cows, Old World monkeys, and humans are generally equivalent (142); New World species, both monkeys and guinea pigs, generally have lower reactivities.

Even when absolute cross-reactivity is lacking, information on relative concentrations can be gained. For example, the amount of insulin measured in response to glucose in a primate may not be identical with a given standard, but the changes in amounts secreted and the factors controlling secretion can still be assessed. The term "hormone equivalent" should be used when specific primate standards and antisera are lacking, but it is seldom used.

Insulin

Serum insulin:

Insulin concentrations in fasting nondiabetic primates range from 5 to >90 μU/ml. Most species have concentrations between 20 and 50 μU/ml (57). Some variations between investigators are attributable to differences in antibodies used in the assays, but experimental conditions, such as sedation, length of fast, antecedent diet, and stress, also vary. Insulin values reported as picograms per milliliter can be multiplied by 24 for conversion to the more common microunits per milliliter.

Numerous investigators have reported the effects of various metabolites and hormones on insulin secretion. The reactions of beta cells to external stimuli are governed by the need to maintain metabolic homeostasis. Glucose and many other dietary metabolites enhance insulin secretion; the net goals are storage and utilization of the dietary components. Situations in which glucose is required by the body tend to suppress insulin secretion. For example, stress acts through epinephrine, cortisol, glucagon, and other catabolic hormones to minimize circulating insulin concentrations and allow greater availability of glucose.

Most responses of insulin that occur during fasting are the same as those that occur during glucose tolerance tests and in response to other hormones associated with carbohydrate homeostasis. These reactions are discussed in subsequent sections. More extensive lists of references on specific concentrations of insulin during experimental manipulations are available from comprehensive reviews (55,57,58). One report of interest is the enhancement of insulin secretion in rhesus macaques when a hypothalamic extract is infused (50).

Responses in the intravenous glucose tolerance test:

Islet cells in vitro secrete insulin biphasically in response to glucose. The initial phase is due to insulin readily released from the beta cells most sensitive in their response to the glucose stimulus. The second, more prolonged phase is the result of insulin synthesis, migration of granules to the plasmalemma, and release of insulin from cells reactive to sustained increases in glucose levels. Similar secretory responses can be seen in vivo in primate blood sampled repeatedly over the first few minutes (29). Insulin concentrations in the peripheral circulation increase to peak values within the first few minutes, decrease, and then increase again to a second peak by about 10 to 15 minutes to be followed by a second decrease. The biphasic secretory pattern becomes less evident as monkeys progress toward overt diabetes (46a). Insulin concentrations in the portal vein are greater and more readily reveal the biphasic secretory response to glucose.

Concentrations of insulin in most nondiabetic primate species usually reach maximum values after 5 to 10 minutes and thereafter diminish toward fasting concentrations (57). The peak concentration of insulin varies considerably; it is generally at least 100 to 200 μU/ml, but may exceed 500 μU/ml. The amount and duration of glucose infusion can also affect the secretory pattern. Some investigators do not find a biphasic secretory pattern, which may merely be a delay in the time of peak insulin concentrations (60,137). A glucose pulse of a few seconds can cause a single peak of insulin that decreases in less than 5 minutes (26).

Primate insulin responses in the IVGTT have seldom been analyzed. The amount of insulin in an early sample minus the fasting levels gives an indication of the acute insulin response (56). In one insulinogenic index, the total amount of insulin secreted during the IVGTT, minus the baseline value, is summed (10); the amount of glucose cleared can also be read into this index. Calculations of insulin secretion are complicated by variations in timing and amount of insulin at the peaks as well as by changes in the diminution rate. For consistency, the method should include delineation of insulin responses at different times during the IVGTT. A more accurate assessment of the insulin/glucose interactions can be obtained with the frequent sampling IVGTT (9). Assays of C-peptide can also be used to monitor and confirm residual insulin secretory capacities (119,128,137). Again, there are numerous problems of immunocross-reactivity when C-peptide assays designed for humans are used to assess primate C-peptide, that is, homologies between primate and human C-peptide are less than those between insulin molecules.

Priming of tissues by adequate insulin concentrations appears to be as much a prerequisite for glucose clearance as does the amount of insulin secreted during the early phases of the tolerance test.

The insulin response to glucose is minimal and delayed in impaired monkeys and is absent in diabetic monkeys. Streptozotocin and alloxan decrease or obliterate insulin secretory capabilities. Hemorrhagic shock (121) and atropine (29) lower the insulin response and impair glucose clearance. The early insulin increment is diminished during the second and third trimesters of pregnancy in rhesus macaques (105); there is no insulin response of the fetus to infused glucose (105). Gestational diabetes causes impaired insulin secretion and glucose clearance during but not after or before pregnancy (60,81). Progesterone (10) or pneumococcal infections (34) enhance insulin secretion during the IVGTT, but they do not change glucose clearance. Somatostatin (26) and epinephrine (85) both inhibit insulin secretion and thus cause impaired glucose clearance and hyperglycemia. Intestinal hormonal polypeptides stimulate insulin release, but glucose clearance is unaffected (139).

Responses in the oral glucose tolerance test:

Few investigators have examined insulin responses during the OGTT. The peak insulin response is reached between 30 and 60 minutes after the test is begun (4,78). Monkeys with streptozotocin-induced diabetes have minimal insulin responses to oral glucose (78). Data on other animals and on humans indicate greater insulin secretion in response to glucose in an OGTT than in response to the same amount of glucose infused in an IVGTT.

Glucagon

Glucagon has more amino acid homologies among the various animals species than do the different insulins. Immunocross-reactivity among various glucagon antisera appears to be adequate, although concentrations are usually much greater in primates than in humans (57). Concentrations in a few nondiabetic primates have been reported to be about the same as those in humans, that is 100 to 150 pg/ml. However, most primates have values of 200 to 300 pg/ml routinely, and some exceed 1,000 pg/ml (57). Whether these differences are due to varied immunoreactivities or to actual biologic concentrations is unknown.

In primates, as in other animals and humans, it is necessary to differentiate between alpha cell glucagon (mol wt = 3500) and several other immunoreactive glucagons with greater molecular weights, most of which are of gastrointestinal origin. Generally, care has been taken to assure that data on circulating immunoreactive glucagon are attributable to a specific molecular weight form. Although glucagon is also found in the gastric fundus in primates, the amount is far less than that in the pancreas (47). Furthermore, it may not be identical to the pancreatic alpha cell glucagon (16).

Glucagon secretion during the IVGTT is generally the reverse of insulin secretion. Concentrations decrease to minimal levels in about 10 minutes (34) and sustained infusion of glucose depresses glucagon until infusion ceases (26).

Glucagon secretion is also affected by other hormones. Increased glucagon during stress is probably due to the stimulatory effects of epinephrine because exogenous epinephrine immediately increases glucagon (25). Somatostatin inhibits both glucagon and insulin secretion (83). A hypothalamic extract acts in the reverse manner as somatostatin and increases glucagon secretion in rhesus macaques (50).

Glucagon concentrations increase after induction of overt diabetes with streptozotocin in rhesus macaques (67), but monkeys in an intermediate, carbohydrate-disturbed state have about the same concentrations of glucagon as their controls. The rhesus fetus secretes glucagon after infusion of L-DOPA, but it does not respond to arginine (24). Celebes macaques have substantially increased glucagon concentrations in the intermediate stages of diabetes; concentrations decrease with the onset of overt diabetes and extensive alpha cell loss (62).

Catecholamines

Circulating catecholamines have seldom been measured in primates. Catecholamines in rhesus macaques show cyclic oscillations with concentrations averaging 122 pg/ml in one instance (46b) and much higher, 150 to >800 pg/ml, in another (91). Metabolic roles of catecholamines have been established through both direct and indirect studies. Epinephrine infused into baboon decreases insulin and increases glucose (133) and glucagon (25). Pharmacologic agents that affect the sympathetic adrenergic system mimic catecholamines, and they probably are mediated through neural norepinephrine, that is, they suppress insulin and enhance glucagon secretion (25,85,104).

Cortisol

Cortisol is a stress hormone with a diurnal variation (5) and ultradian rhythms (52). Care is usually taken to measure acute responses or, when responses are examined longitudinally, to have appropriate controls from the same time of day. Concentrations in rhesus macaques and baboons generally range from 17 to 40 μg/dl when measured under control fasting conditions. Squirrel monkeys have high resting cortisol values of 400 to >670 μg/dl.

Numerous experimental conditions increase cortisol concentrations by 50 to 250 per cent. Hemorrhagic shock causes immediate elevations, but the response is abolished by adrenalectomy (121). The stress of handling increases cortisol concentrations in squirrel monkeys (15) and rhesus macaques (12). Protein malnutrition increases cortisol levels and obliterates differences in diurnal rhythms after 6 weeks (5). Pneumococcal infections (34) or exposure to cold (3) increase cortisol concentrations. Electrical stimulation of the ventromedial hypothalamus, with and without streptozotocin diabetes (32) or sedation with ketamine (80), has little effect on cortisol concentrations.

Growth Hormone

Although various postulates have been advanced for contributions of growth hormone (GH) to the diabetic state, there is as yet no understanding of a specific role for GH. The GH concentrations sometimes respond immediately to experimental manipulations, but there are generally only minor changes over long periods of time.

Under optimal, nonstressed conditions, GH concentrations in most primates vary from 2 to 14 ng/ml. Stress effects on GH often occur in conjunction with changes in other hormones. The GH concentrations increase upon capture and return to normal with adaptation to caging or chair restraint (15). Amphetamines (126), hypothalamic stimulation (32), pitressin or insulin (123), and hemorrhagic shock (21) increase GH concentrations in baboons and macaques; dopamine stimulation can be blocked by thyrotropin-releasing hormone (133). Although there may be some transient changes, the GH concentrations are not significantly affected by pneumococcal (34) or *E. coli* infections (28), central nervous system lesions (27), ketamine sedations (20), or circulating somatostatin (26). Hypothalamic lesions in squirrel monkeys diminish the response to the stress of capture and chair restraint (15) or to insulin-induced hypoglycemia (1). Only minor changes in the amount and periodicity of GH variations can be seen after a 96-hour fast (134). The GH does not respond to intravenous glucose in the fetus or the mother (105).

CARBOHYDRATE METABOLISM IN THE DOG

The dog is the only species in which the major counterparts of human diabetes mellitus types can be considered to have been well defined. The presence of spontaneous Type I (insulin-dependent diabetes mellitus, IDDM), Type II (Non-insulin-dependent diabetes mellitus, NIDDM), and a Type III comparable to the impaired glucose tolerance (IGT) type has been reported using most of the criteria for classification of the human disease (74,112). Recent important discoveries are the inherited Type I diabetes of Keeshond dogs (84) and in golden retrievers (145). Furthermore, the influence of obesity in the Type II diabetic dog has recently been defined (99).

Glucose

Plasma Glucose

It is well known that the blood glucose concentrations of all animals are affected by a wide variety of factors including presampling status, sampling procedure, handling of the blood sample after sampling, and reliability of the method employed. The most important presampling procedure in the dog is to develop a standard protocol of a 12- to 14-hour fast before sampling. This is most conveniently done by placing the dog on an overnight fast and obtaining the blood sample the following morning before feeding. In this way, the blood glucose sample is most likely to reflect the glucometabolic status of the dog; the sample itself will be clear and free of interfering substances such as lipids and will reflect basal conditions so that variations of concentration will be minimized. Furthermore, frequently handled and trained dogs are less likely to have variations due

to periods of excitement from unaccustomed handling and sampling. This also requires that the sampler be experienced and able to obtain a sample with minimal disturbance to the dog. Postsampling procedures also play an important part, in that glucose breakdown by red blood cells takes place very rapidly at about 10 per cent per hour at room temperature and occurs even more rapidly if the sample is contaminated by bacteria. Therefore, the plasma or serum must be separated from the red cells as soon as possible, or if unable to do so, the glucose in the blood sample must be protected from glycolysis by the red blood cells. This is best done by the addition of sodium fluoride (10 mg/ml of blood) and by refrigeration. Standard sodium fluoride containing evacuated tubes are ideal for this purpose.

Numerous methods for glucose determination in the plasma or serum have been developed, and the enzymatic methods are presently the methods of choice. The degree of accuracy among the glucose enzymatic methods is such that any of these may be employed with confidence. When these procedures become standardized, the fasting blood glucose concentration in the dog can be developed with a high degree of reliability. Performed in this way, a plasma glucose of 90 ± 12 mg/dl (SD) is a good reference value to be used for the dog. This is very close to that of the adult human and can be used in further decision-making processes (72).

Evaluation of Glucometabolic Status: Glucose Tolerance Tests

The glucose tolerance test is the first step in the functional evaluation of glucometabolic status in animals or human beings. Many variations exist in the tolerance test conducted for diagnostic purposes in clinical medicine, but for the purposes of glucometabolic evaluation of the laboratory dog, the need exists for establishing and defining a more narrowly reproducible result than is normally required in clinical medicine. Therefore, a standard form of glucose tolerance test should be used to obtain the most meaningful data for evaluating glucometabolic status in the laboratory dog. Generally, two forms of glucose tolerance test have been used in the dog or other animals: the OGTT and the IVGTT. It is well known that a high protein diet in a dog will generate a diabetic type or glucose intolerant curve (72). This term, glucose intolerance, describes the shape of the glucose curve in the OGTT or the shape and rate of disappearance of glucose in the IVGTT. In comparison to a normally tolerant curve, the curve expressing glucose intolerance describes one with a very high peak and a slow return to pre-infusion concentrations. In either test, it is of great importance to standardize the diet of the dog before performance of the test. The dog should be placed on a standard carbohydrate diet consisting of 100 to 200 g of carbohydrates per day or 5 to 10 per kilogram of body weight per day for at least 3 days before performance of the test to eliminate apparent glucose intolerance and promote reliability.

Oral glucose tolerance test:

The OGTT has been used infrequently in the dog primarily because of variations induced by excitement attending intubation and the gastrointestinal problems associated with oral infusion of 1.5 to 4 g of glucose per kilogram of body weight. The general procedure is to place the dog on a standard 3-day carbohydrate-containing diet, to take an overnight fasting sample, and then to give the glucose as a 50 per cent solution by intubation. Blood samples are taken at 30-minute intervals for 3 hours thereafter. Plasma glucose concentrations are then plotted on linear coordinates with time and subjectively compared to reference curves obtained for the procedure. The standard normal curve exhibits a peak at 30 minutes to 1 hour and returns to the fasting concentration within 2 to 3 hours. The height of the peak and the rate of return to normal are important subjective measures of the ability of the dog to metabolize the oral glucose load. The diabetic or glucose intolerant curve has a higher peak than does the standard and has not returned to the preinfusion concentration by the end of 3 hours. Thus, in addition to logistic problems which induce inaccuracies in the OGTT, the subjective nature of the evaluation of the OGTT curve makes it a less desirable test for evaluation of the glucometabolic status. Furthermore, insulin response by the pancreas is not adequately stimulated and this parameter cannot be evaluated by the OGTT.

Intravenous glucose tolerance test:

In the IVGTT, a standard dose of glucose is infused intravenously into the laboratory dog after a conditioning regimen similar to that for the OGTT. For this purpose a standard glucose load of 0.5 g/kg has been recommended as high enough to provoke maximal insulin response and permit reliable evaluations of glucose clearance (73,120). It has been shown that glucose infusions greater than 0.5 g/kg are rapidly excreted in the urine and do not directly reflect the glucometabolic status of the dog (73). In the standard IVGTT, a preinfusion of blood sample is taken and the standard glucose load of 0.5 g of glucose per kilogram of body weight is infused as a sterile 50 per cent solution in 30 seconds. Timing for the test is begun at the midpoint of the infusion period or 15 seconds after beginning infusion. Subsequent blood samples are taken at 5, 15, 25, 35, 45, and 60 minutes for plasma glucose determination and insulin if desired. The results of plasma glucose concentrations are plotted on semilogarithmic coordinates versus time from which the half-time ($T\frac{1}{2}$), the time required for the glucose concentration to fall by one half is calculated or graphically estimated between the 15- and 45-minute points. It is also well known that the plasma glucose disappearance rate is truly a curve and is only quasilinear at certain times. In the standard IVGTT described here, the best quasilinear straight line is observed between 15 and 45 minutes after infusion. The $T\frac{1}{2}$ is then calculated between 15 and 45 minutes and the K value may then be determined from the relationship:

$$K = \frac{0.693}{T\frac{1}{2}} \times 100 = \%/min$$

The K value is described as the fractional turnover rate, glucose turnover rate, glucose disappearance rate, glucose clearance rate, glucose disappearance coefficient, or simply the K value. With this standard method the normal $T\frac{1}{2}$ in the dog is 25 ± 8 minutes (range 15 to 45) and with a K value greater than 1.5 per cent per minute. The diabetic curve with its slower rate of glucose disappearance results in a half-time longer than 45 m which calculates into a K value of less than 1.5 per cent per minute (72).

The standard IVGTT has a number of advantages. First, the dog is more physically tolerant of the intravenous procedure than of the oral intubation procedure, and no sedation or anesthesia is required. It has been shown (98) that atropine has no effect; however, pentobarbital anesthesia markedly decreases glucose disappearance and insulin response in the IVGTT. Second, the K value (or $T_{\frac{1}{2}}$) can readily be calculated by computer, knowing the plasma glucose concentrations at any of several times between 15 and 45 minutes and the quantified data can provide a more precisely defined measure of carbohydrate intolerance. Third, the IVGTT has a higher degree of reproducibility than does the OGTT, which is one of its most distinct advantages. Fourth, additional areas of diagnostic significance can be discerned from the IVGTT; the 5-minute peak is inordinately high and the 60-minute value has not returned to baseline in carbohydrate metabolic failure. Fifth, the IVGTT also has the added advantage of time over the OGTT, because only 60 minutes are required for completion.

The intravenous glucose tolerance test and the insulin response:

A significant advantage of the standard IVGTT in the dog is its ability to generate information related to the insulin response by the pancreas to the glucose load. The glucose load in the standard IVGTT is adequate to invoke a maximal insulin response in the dog. The insulin response to a glucose load in humans follows a biphasic curve with one peak in the early phases, between 3 and 7 minutes, and a second peak at 20 to 40 minutes. In the dog an early initial peak of insulin is also observed at 3 to 7 minutes after infusion, but a second insulin peak has not been clearly discerned. It is now generally regarded that the early insulin peak is the result of an acute release of insulin from the pancreas stimulated by the acute hyperglycemia and that the second peak is the result of the de novo synthesis of insulin by the stimulated pancreatic beta cells.

These data obtained from the IVGTT play an important role in the classification of the various forms of diabetes. The IVGTT and its insulin response form the basis for the classification of several types of spontaneous diabetes mellitus in the dog. Three types, Type I, Type II, and Type III, have been classified on the basis of their IVGTT, fasting insulin, insulin peak response, total insulin secretion, and insulinogenic index (74) and are closely similar to

the similarly classified human types of diabetes. Type I (IDDM, insulin-dependent diabetes mellitus or juvenile diabetes), Type II (NIDDM, noninsulin-dependent diabetes mellitus or adult diabetes), and chemical (IGT, inappropriate glucose tolerance or chemical diabetes) are the comparable forms in human beings (112). Type I canine diabetes does not have as high a prevalence in the young as does human Type I (IDDM), but canine Type II does have as high a prevalence in the adult as does human Type II (NIDDM). Canine Types II and III tend frequently to be associated with obesity in older dogs as is true of their human counterparts. This close similarity of types of canine diabetes to the important types of human diabetes indicates that the spontaneously diabetic dog will be of even greater value in the study of carbohydrate metabolic disorders of human beings than previously. The obvious potential exists for the study of various types of diabetes with particular reference to the development of degenerative changes in a more natural environment. In this regard, renal functional impairment as evidenced by impaired creatinine and urea clearances in spontaneous canine diabetes has been reported (76).

Obesity and glucometabolic status:

It has also long been known that there is a relationship between obesity and the development of Type II diabetes (NIDDM) in humans. Most recently, the influence of obesity on the degree of diabetes in Type II canine diabetes was statistically defined and a linear correlation established (99). Statistical treatment of the data has shown that the degree of obesity is the most important factor influencing severity of the diabetes in Type II canine diabetes. These data define for the first time the statistical significance of the influence of obesity on the degree of diabetes and explains the improvement of the diabetic state which occurs on weight reduction. It is now also known that obesity itself has a profound direct correlation on the degree of glucose intolerance in the obese nondiabetic dog as well as in the obese Type II canine diabetic. This provides further evidence of the importance of nonobesity in all animals, and it could well explain the natural history of diabetes in the genetically prone obese individual who develops Type III diabetes (IGT) which later progresses to the obese Type II (NIDDM) diabetes. It is in these patients that the diabetes can be ameliorated by weight reduction often to the point at which exogenous insulin or oral hypoglycemic agents are not needed.

Other carbohydrate tolerance tests:

Several other tolerance tests have been developed but are not widely used for the general evaluation of glucometabolic status. These have been used only in special clinical circumstances and in the evaluation of pancreatic cell tumors. The insulin tolerance ($0.1 \ \mu/kg$) test has been used primarily for the clinical detection of insulin resistance and has been supplanted by insulin receptor studies (122). The epinephrine tolerance test has been used as an index of the availability of liver glycogen in suspected von Gierke's disease (glycogenosis; glucose-6-phosphatase deficiency), but the definitive diagnosis is based upon hepatic cell enzyme assay (141). The tolbutamide test has been used to evaluate insulin release by the pancreas as has the leucine-induced hypoglycemia test. The glucagon tolerance test has been used to evaluate the responsiveness of the pancreatic alpha cells (72).

Experimental diabetes:

Historically the most common method of inducing diabetes in dogs has been the use of phloridzin or alloxan. Alloxan has been used extensively for the induction of diabetes since its first report (30). Alloxan has since been used to induce diabetes in rabbits, rats, dogs, hamsters, sheep, pigeons, monkeys, mice and cats. Generally there is rapid and complete loss of beta cells within 18 and 24 hours after injection and severe, often permanent hyperglycemia develops. The specific mode of beta cell injury by alloxan is still unclear, but the major disadvantages of alloxan are the extrapancreatic lesions which include damage to the kidneys, adrenals, thyroids, pituitary, and liver. If the animal survives the initial insult, much of the pathology is reversible. However, these extrapancreatic lesions remain the major handicap of alloxan and explain the reluctance of many investigators to use it.

Streptozotocin, an antibiotic from *Streptomyces acromogenes*, has been found to be capable of inducing a more reproducible form of Type I (IDDM) diabetes mellitus with limited side effects. Mild diabetes with minimal renal injury can be produced using 20 mg of streptozotocin per gram (75). Permanent diabetes mellitus has been produced in dogs, cats, rats, and mice, and because of its reduced side effects, it has become the drug of choice in the induction of diabetes. A combination of alloxan (50 mg/kg) and streptozotocin (30 mg/kg) has also been used in the experimental induction of Type I (IDDM) diabetes in the dog (64,127). Because genetically reproducible diabetes mellitus has not been readily available, the experimentally produced Type I diabetic dog continues to remain a valuable laboratory model for the evaluation of diabetes. Streptozotocin-induced diabetes mellitus has all the features of Type I (IDDM) diabetes of human beings and is most amenable to acute studies. However, the study of long-term effects of diabetes are more amenable to the spontaneously diabetic dog, in particular now that at least two types comparable to the human types have been characterized. These spontaneously diabetic Type I dogs will certainly provide the opportunity to study the natural history of diabetes in a more natural environment and to study the chronic progressive pathologic lesions such as the microangiopathies, retinopathies, nephropathies, and vasculitides that occur in advanced and severe diabetes in humans.

Certain hormones, such as growth hormone, have been used to produce experimental diabetes. It has long been known that anterior pituitary extracts could produce transient diabetes and later permanent diabetes (153). The active diabetogenic agent was subsequently identified as growth hormone (18). Although extremely important from an endocrine viewpoint, the chemical methods are more amenable and should be used to produce experimental diabetes.

Ketones

In the severe forms of diabetes with progressive decreases in carbohydrate utilization, lipid metabolism increases to compensate as an energy source. The rate of lipid utilization increases progressively as the diabetes progresses in severity through increased mobilization of body fat depots. The mobilization of lipid intensifies as the activity of the hormone-

sensitive lipases increase. Thus, hypertriglyceridemia, hyperlipoproteinemia, and hypercholesterolemia all increase in direct relation to the degree of lipid mobilization. Concurrent with increased lipid metabolism by the
liver, there is increased ketogenesis, ketonuria,
and eventually ketoacidosis. Ketosis is now
known to occur as a result of overproduction of
ketone bodies by the liver and underutilization
of ketone bodies by the peripheral tissues. Insulin deficiency, whether absolute or relative (insu-
lin-resistant), remains the major and quite likely
the only hormonal abnormality directly responsible for all the subsequent hormonal and metabolic derangements of diabetes mellitus (72).
Thus, although total triglycerides, cholesterol,
and lipoproteins are important in the study of
diabetes, they are secondary to failure of glucose
metabolism in the diabetic animal. However, the
diabetic dog offers another means of study of the
effects of aberrant lipid metabolism on various
organ systems in relation to carbohydrate
metabolism. It also follows that because the
ketone bodies are strongly dissociated organic
acids, ketoacidosis is an overriding concern in
advanced diabetes and mechanisms of its control could be studied in the diabetic dog.

Glycosylated Hemoglobins

Within the past few years, a great deal of interest
has been generated in the "glycosylated hemoglobin" or HbA_{1c} assay as an index of long-
term glycemic control. The hemoglobins in the
erythrocyte, when first formed, are not linked to
glucose. However, the red cell is freely per-
meable to glucose and a fraction of the hemoglobins, the HBA_1s, are bound to glucose by a
slow, nonenzymatic, relatively irreversible
mechanism. This means that the glycosylated
fractions (HbA_{1a}, HbA_{1b}, and HbA_{1c}) bind to
glucose during the lifetime of the red cell. Of
these, HbA_{1c} is the fraction that binds glucose
in direct proportion to the blood glucose concentration. Because the binding is tight, it
remains bound over the lifespan of the red cell
and can be used as an index of the average
plasma glucose concentration over the previous
30 to 60 days.

The HbA_{1c} assay, then, is a means of monitoring a patient's blood glucose control by sampling as infrequently as once a month or two
rather than on a very frequent basis as must

often be done in diabetic patients. Hemoglobin
A_{1c} concentrations of approximately 3 to 6 per
cent are very closely correlated with a normal
blood glucose level having been maintained over
the past several months (150), and significantly
higher levels are associated with persistence of
hyperglycemia during the last several months.
This indirect method of monitoring blood glucose has been clearly documented recently (111)
as a valuable means to monitor glucose control.
This process has important implications because
it was shown by many that the control of blood
glucose within narrow limits is highly beneficial
to the health and survival of the patient. Other
serum proteins also have been employed in a
manner similar to hemoglobin (101) but do not
seem likely to replace HbA_{1c} as an effective glucose monitor.

Hormones Influencing Carbohydrate Metabolism

The hormones involved in carbohydrate metabolism in the dog are essentially the same as those
found to be of importance in primates or
rodents, and these have already been covered in
the previous section. The use of serum insulin
responses to a glucose load has already been
discussed in relation to classification of canine
diabetes into its Type I (IDDM), Type II
(NIDDM), and Type III (IGT). However, the
precise mechanism of hormone binding to receptor sites may ultimately explain its mechanism
of action.

Glucagon is a hyperglycemic hormone, synthesized and released by the pancreatic alpha
cells in response to hypoglycemia, and in this
way it is a principal insulin antagonist. Glucagon has been employed as a function test by
measuring its blood glucose response in the dog,
but no reliable method for hormone assay in the
dog is yet available. Among other hormones of
concern in carbohydrate metabolism, cortisol
and growth hormone have among their many
actions an antagonism to insulin and are therefore hyperglycemic. Epinephrine, through its
action on cyclic AMP, is glycogenolytic and
hyperglycemic. It also suppresses insulin release
and stimulates glucagon release by the pancreatic cells. Somatostatin is a hormone originally isolated from the hypothalamus, now
known to be present in the pancreas and intestinal tract, and thought to exercise a hypoglycemic effect through its antagonism to

growth hormone (117). Somatostatin also suppresses both insulin and glucagon. Thus, although the overriding concern of carbohydrate metabolism in the laboratory dog remains the study of glycometabolic status in diabetes mellitus and insulin action, the potential remains for the study of a wide variety of additional hormones and chemicals that directly or indirectly are involved in glucose homeostasis.

Inheritance of Diabetes

The genetics of inherited diabetes mellitus in Keeshond dogs was studied over an extended period of 10 years by Kramer (personal communication, 1987). The gene symbol dm was used to designate the gene. Their findings indicated incomplete penetrance and inheritance as a single Mendelian autosomal recessive. This finding is important because it establishes the heritable nature of diabetes in a laboratory animal species in which types of diabetes similar to those in humans have been discerned.

CARBOHYDRATE METABOLISM OF THE CAT

The laboratory cat has been used considerably less than the laboratory dog in the study of carbohydrate metabolic status. The incidence of spontaneous diabetes in the cat is also considerably less than that in the dog (125), so that historically the cat has been used considerably less than the laboratory dog in the study of carbohydrate metabolism. A significant and frequently cited study in which the cat played an important role was that of the development of experimental growth hormone-induced diabetes in the cat (18). Spontaneously diabetic cats, however, do not seem to be markedly different from the dog except for an unusually high incidence of hyperbilirubinemia reported in a group of diabetic cats. A later report (106) indicates that hyperbilirubinemia is not frequent in the cat, although serum ALP and AST remained elevated in 11 of 12 cats whereas only 2 had mild hyperbilirubinemia. Furthermore, the problem of assay of cat insulin has not been definitively resolved. Although it is well established that the diabetic cat responds to exogenous glucose or insulin as do other animals, lack of cross-reactivity with common insulins has precluded insu-

lin assay and extensive use of the cat as a model of diabetes.

Conversely, diabetes mellitus associated with pancreatic islet cell amyloidosis occurs significantly only in human beings and in the cat (35,65). Therefore, the cat would be uniquely suited as a model for the study of pancreatic amyloidosis in humans.

CARBOHYDRATE METABOLISM OF THE LABORATORY RODENT

Perhaps the laboratory rat of various strains has been the most extensively studied laboratory animal species in relation to carbohydrate metabolism. Presently, there are a number of strains and several species that can be characterized into the two major types of diabetes mellitus. The Chinese hamster and Wistar BB rat in addition to the Type I diabetic dog have been studied widely as animal models of Type I (IDDM) diabetes. The fatty (fa) rat, at least six mice strains, and more recently the guinea pig and vole have been studied as models of Type II (NIDDM) diabetes. These animals are generally characterized by obesity and subsequent diabetes.

Carbohydrate Metabolic Models Characterized by Insulin Deficiency (Type I, IDDM)

The Chinese Hamster

There are only a limited number of laboratory animals that can serve as models of Type I (IDDM) diabetes. Of these, the Chinese hamster has been studied most widely as the earliest model recognized for its close similarity to Type I diabetes and characterized by insulinopenia and hyperketonemia (102). The diabetes of the Chinese hamster is now recognized to have a homozygous recessive mode of inheritance. The Chinese hamster has a number of characteristics that attest to its close similarity to human Type I diabetes (IDDM). They are not obese, they are insulinogenic, their pancreatic insulin content is low, and they are prone to ketosis (36). They exhibit a markedly decreased insulin response to a glucose load, and both the first and second phase of the insulin response curve are decreased (37) as is cyclic AMP (115). Hepatic glucogenesis is increased, as evidenced by an increase in the gluconeogenic enzymes in the liver (22,23). Pancreatic glucagon varies, but in the perfused pancreas, excess glucagon is released (41). The decreased level of pancreatic somatostatin also attests to the close similarity to human Type I diabetes (IDDM). There does not appear to be any lymphocytic infiltration of the pancreas or other evidence of autoimmunity.

The Syrian Hamster

An interesting model of the rubella virus-induced Type I diabetes has been developed (116) by infecting neonatal Syrian hamsters with rubella virus passed through isolated pancreatic beta cells. They develop classic signs of Type I diabetes. The authors suggest the development of an autoimmune process followed by diabetes.

The Wistar BB Rat

More recently the Wistar BB rat, discovered in 1974 (109,110), has been studied extensively as an animal model of Type I (IDDM) diabetes. This model was discovered by a commercial breeder (Biobreeders, hence BB) in a Wistar strain. Similar to the Chinese hamster, the BB rat is nonobese, markedly hyperglycemic (257 to 752 mg/dl), glycosuric, hypoinsulimenic (0 to 1 ng/ml), hyperketonemic, and ketonuric. There was no insulin response to arginine or tolbutamide injections. Pancreatic insulin is very low and hyperlipidemia is marked, consisting of triglyceridemia and hypercholesterinemia is present. There is severe beta cell destruction. Additionaly, there is inappropriately normal glucagonemia and hyperresponsiveness of glucagon to arginine (114). Unlike in the Chinese hamster, the OGTT performed with 2.5 g of glucose per kilogram of body weight via gastric lavage and sampling at 0, 60, and 120 minutes was useful as an indicator of the severity of spontaneous diabetes. Thus, with the Chinese hamster and the Type I diabetic dog, the Wistar BB rat now provides a third spontaneous model for the study of Type I (IDDM) diabetes (97).

A major focus of interest in the diabetic Wistar BB rat is that its diabetes is spontaneous Type I with islet cell autoimmunity. Immunoglobulins or sera from diabetic rats were toxic to islet cells, bound to islet cells, and inhibited insulin secretion from normal rat islet cells (87). This is accompanied by lymphopenia, but re-

cently (93) a nonlymphopenic line was also uncovered.

The Nonobese Diabetic Mouse

The nonobese diabetic mouse is another laboratory rodent that develops spontaneous Type I diabetes. The basic defect in nonobese diabetic mice, based on results of perfusion studies of the pancreas, appears to be a defect in the initial phase of the insulin response to glucose stimulation by the beta cells (77).

Carbohydrate Metabolic Models Characterized by Obesity (Type II, NIDDM)

Much of the study of carbohydrate metabolism relative to diabetes mellitus has been in animal models characterized by obesity, hyperglycemia, hyperinsulinemia, and other signs that place them in the Type II (NIDDM) form. Diabetes mellitus in the obese laboratory rodent has been defined as two general forms. The first form is characterized by the obese (ob/ob) mouse (71,100), yellow (Ay/Ay) mouse (19), New Zealand obese (NZO) mouse (33), diabetic (KK) mouse (108), Wellesley hybrid mouse (17), and the fatty (fa/fa) rat (154). In these models there is significant obesity accompanied by hyperglycemia and hyperinsulinemia as well as corresponding hyperplasia of the beta cells and a general absence of ketonuria. Most exhibit glucose intolerance and often marked (10 to 30 times normal) hyperinsulinemia. Thus the hyperglycemia, hyperinsulinemia, and beta cell hyperplasia that accompany obesity may well be the precursor of Type II (NIDDM) diabetes in its natural history in which obesity predisposes a genetically at-risk animal.

The more typical Type II (NIDDM) diabetes is exemplified in the diabetic (db/db) mouse (63), the spiny mouse (42), and the sand rat (43,44). These animals are similar to the obese animals in that they are also obese, hyperglycemic, and hyperinsulinemic, and have beta cell hyperplasia. They are also glucose intolerant. Marked insulin resistance is a further characteristic and is associated with a loss of insulin receptors in tissues (8,70,130). Eventually there is beta cell exhaustion, leading to sustained hyperglycemia, insulinopenia, and ketoacidosis.

Other laboratory animals have been reported as models of diabetes mellitus, but there are insufficient data with which to characterize their type. This group includes the South African hamster (*Mystromys albicaudatus*) or white-tailed rat (136) and the spontaneously diabetic New Zealand white rabbit (146). They are glycosuric, ketonuric, hyperglycemic, and insulinopenic, have beta cell lesions, and because they are not obese, they may well be models of Type I (IDDM) diabetes. The guinea pig is unique in that its diabetes appears to be contagious, it exhibits hyperglycemia, glycosuria, and ketonuria, it is glucose intolerant, and it has beta cell hyperplasia (89). Other interesting models potentially useful for glucometabolic studies are the tuco-tuco (149) and recently the Japanese field vole (86).

SUMMARY

At the present time, there is no paucity of animal models of diabetes mellitus and new models are reported periodically. Although uncovering additional models may not seem of itself to be contributing towards the overall elucidation of diabetes, certainly it does point to its almost universal occurrence in mammals. The occurrence of diabetes in many of our domestic animals has not been included because of the focus of this chapter on the laboratory animal species Through the use of these animals the inheritance of diabetes is no longer in question, though the details may yet be unclear. The provocative effect of obesity is now more clearly defined through the use of the obese diabetic laboratory animal, the dog, and nonhuman primate. The natural history of the progressive biochemical deterioration has similarly been more clearly defined. These obese animals are now generally regarded to be models of human Type II (NIDDM) diabetes mellitus. The identification of this type in the dog now offers the opportunity to study Type II (NIDDM) diabetes in a more natural (for the dog) setting than in a laboratory environment. Type I (IDDM) diabetes also has been identified in the dog and offers a similar opportunity to study a model of human Type I (IDDM) diabetes in a more natural environment. However, other more readily available models of Type I (IDDM) diabetes, such as the Chinese hamster or the Wistar BB rat, will continue to be important animals for the study of this type of diabetes as well. Importantly, the more clearly defined types of diabetes and improved biochemical technology augur well for the future of diabetes research in all the available animal models of diabetes.

REFERENCES

1. Abrams RL, Parker ML, Blanco S, Reichlin S, Daughaday WH (1966) Hypothalamic regulation of growth hormone secretion. Endocrinology 78: 605–613
2. Alperin JB, Dow PA, Stout LC (1979) A comparison of hemoglobin A_{1c} in human and baboon blood. Acta Haematol 61: 334–338
3. Arora RB, Tariq M, Siddiqui HH (1971) Effect of experimental cold injury on the levels of blood lipids, cortisol and glucose in monkeys. Pharmacol Res Commun 3: 107–111
4. Ausman LM, Gallina DL (1978) Response to glucose loading of the lean squirrel monkey in unrestrained conditions. Am J Physiol 234: R20–R24
5. Bajaj JS, Khardori R, Deo MG, Bansal DD (1979) Adrenocortical function in experimental protein malnutrition. Metabolism 28: 594–598
6. Bandyopadhyay A, Banerjee S (1971) Some metabolic effects of cloramphenicol in rhesus monkeys. Indian J Biochem Biophys 8: 176–178
7. Banerjee S, Kumar KS, Bandyopadhyay A (1967) Effect of oxytetracycline and tetracycline on glucose tolerance and serum lipids. Proc Soc Exp Biol Med 125: 618–620
8. Baxter D, Lazarus NR (1975) The control of insulin receptors in the New Zealand obese mouse. Diabetologia 11: 261–267
9. Beard KC, Bergman RN, Ward WK, Porte D Jr (1986) The insulin sensitivity index in nondiabetic man. Correlation between clamp-derived values. Diabetes 35: 362–369
10. Beck P (1969) Progestin enhancement of the plasma insulin response to glucose in rhesus monkeys. Diabetes 18: 146–152
11. Beck P, Venable RI, Hom DI (1975) Mutual modification of glucose-stimulated serum insulin responses in female rhesus monkeys by ethinyl estradiol and nortestosterone derivatives. J Clin Endocrinol Metab 41: 44–53
12. Blank MS, Gordon TP, Wilson ME (1983) Effects of capture and venipuncture on serum levels of prolactin, growth hormone and cortisol in outdoor compound-housed female rhesus monkeys (*Macaca mulatta*). Acta Endocrinol 102: 190–195
13. Bowen GS, Rayfield EJ, Monath TP, Kemp GE (1980) Studies of glucose metabolism in rhesus monkeys after Venezuelan equine encephalitis virus infection. J Med Virol 6: 227–234
14. Brady AG, Koritnik DR (1985) The effects of ketamine anesthesia on glucose clearance in African green monkeys. J Med Primatol 14: 99–107
15. Brown GM, Schalch DS, Reichlin S (1971) Hypothalamic mediation of growth hormone and adrenal stress response in the squirrel monkey. Endocrinology 89: 694–703
16. Bryant MG, Bloom SR (1979) Distribution of the

gut hormones in the primate intestinal tract. Gut 20: 653–659

17. Cahill GF Jr, Jones EE, Lauris V, Steinke J, Soldner JS (1967) Studies on experimental diabetes in the Wellesley hybrid mouse. II. Serum insulin levels and response of peripheral tissues. Diabetologia 3: 171–174

18. Campbell J, Davidson IWF, Lei HP (1950) The production of permanent diabetes by highly purified growth hormone. Endocrinology 46: 588–590

19. Carpenter KJ, Mayer J (1958) Physiologic observations on yellow obesity in the mouse. Am J Physiol 193: 499–504

20. Castro MI, Rose J, Green W, Lehner N, Peterson D, Taub D (1981) Ketamine · HCl as a suitable anesthetic for endocrine, metabolic, and cardiovascular studies in *Macaca fascicularis* monkeys. Proc Soc Exp Biol Med 168: 389–394

21. Cerchio GM, Moss GS, Popovich PA, Butler E, Siegel DC (1971) Serum insulin and growth hormone response to hemorrhagic shock. Endocrinology 88: 138–143

22. Chang AY (1981) Biochemical abnormalities in the Chinese hamster (*Cricetulus griseus*) with spontaneous diabetes. Int J Biochem 13: 41–43

23. Chang AY, Schneider DI (1970) Rate of gluconeogenesis and levels of gluconeogenic enzymes in liver and kidney of diabetic and normal Chinese hamsters. Biochem Biophys Acta 222: 587–592

24. Chez RA, Mintz DH, Epstein MF, Fleischman AR, Oakes GK, Hutchinson DL (1974) Glucagon metabolism in nonhuman primate pregnancy. Am J Obstet Gynecol 120: 690–696

25. Chideckel EW, Goodner CJ, Koerker DJ, Johnson DG, Ensinck JW (1977) Role of glucagon in mediating metabolic effects of epinephrine. Am J Physiol 232: E464–470

26. Chideckel EW, Palmer J, Koerker DJ, Ensinck J, Davidson MB, Goodner CJ (1975) Somatostatin blockade of acute and chronic stimuli of the endocrine pancreas and the consequences of this blockade on glucose homeostasis. J Clin Invest 55: 754–762

27. Cornblath M, Levitsky LL, Kling A (1971) Response to intravenous glucose in juvenile macaque monkeys. Diabetes 20: 156–161

28. Cryer PE, Herman CM, Sode J (1971) Carbohydrate metabolism in the baboon subjected to gram-negative (*E. coli*) septicemia. I. Hyperglycemia with depressed plasma insulin concentrations. Ann Surg 174: 91–100

29. Daniel PM, Henderson JR (1975) The effect of atropine on insulin release caused by intravenous glucose in the rhesus monkey. Acta Endocrinol 78: 736–745

30. Dunn JS, Sheehan HL, McLethchie NGB (1943) Necrosis of islets of Langerhans produced experimentally. Lancet 1: 484–487

31. Gallina DL, Ausman LM (1979) Selected aspects of the metabolic behavior of the squirrel monkey, in Hayes KC (ed), Primates in Nutritional Research. Academic Press, New York, pp 225–247

32. Garg SK, China GS, Singh B (1983) Effects of stimulation of hypothalamic "feeding areas" on endocrines and metabolism in normal and diabetic monkeys. Primates 24: 260–265

33. Gates RJ, Hunt MI, Smith R, Lazarus NR (1972) Return to normal of blood glucose, plasma insulin, and weight gain in New Zealand obese mice after implantation of islets of Langerhans. Lancet 2: 567–570

34. George DT, Rayfield EJ, Wannemacher RW (1974) Altered glucoregulatory hormones during acute pneumococcal sepsis in the rhesus monkey. Diabetes 23: 544–549

35. Gepts W, Toussaint D (1967) Spontaneous diabetes in dogs and cats: A pathological study. Diabetologia 3: 249–265

36. Gerritsen GC, Dulin WE (1967) Characterization of diabetes on the Chinese hamster. Diabetologia 3: 74–84

37. Gerritsen GC, Clands MC (1974) Characterization of Chinese hamsters by metabolic balance, glucose tolerance and insulin secretion. Diabetologia 10: 493–499

38. Gilbert C, Gillman J, Savage N (1960) Persistence of the hyperglycaemia and reduction in the lipaemia and ketonaemia of diabetic baboons (*Paipi ursinus*) following bilateral adrenalectomy. S Afr J Med Sci 25: 77–80

39. Gillman J, Gilbert C, Savage N (1959) Serum lipid, blood glucose and liver fat in normal fasting baboons with a consideration of some of the controlling endocrine factors. S Afr J Med Sci 24: 115–124

40. Goldzieher JW, Chenault CB, de la Pena A, Dozier TS, Kraemer DC (1978) Comparative studies of the ethynyl estrogens used in oral contraceptives. VI. Effects with and without progestational agents on carbohydrate metabolism in humans, baboons, and beagles. Fertil Steril 30: 146–153

41. Grodsky GM, Frandel BJ, Gerich JR, Gerritsen GC (1974) The diabetic Chinese hamster: *in vitro* insulin and glucagon release; the "chemical diabetic"; and the effect of diet on ketonuria. Diabetologia 10: 521–528

42. Gutzeit A, Rabinovitch A, Studer PP, Trueheart PA, Cerari E, Renold AE (1974) Decrease intravenous glucose tolerance and low plasma insulin response in spring mice (*Acomys cohirinus*). Diabetologia 10: 667–670

43. Hacket DB, Mirat E, Lebovitz HE, Schmidt-Nielson K, Horton ES, Kinney TD (1967) The sand rat (*Psammonys abesus*) as an experimental animal in studies of diabetes mellitus. Diabetologia 3: 130–134

44. Haines HB, Hacket DB, Schmidt-Nielson K (1965) Experimental diabetes mellitus induced by diet in the sand rat. Am J Physiol 208: 297

45. Hamilton CL, Ciaccia P (1978) The course of development of glucose intolerance in the monkey (*Macaca mulatta*). J Med Primatol 7: 165–173

46a. Hansen BC, Bodkin NL (1986) Heterogeneity of insulin responses: Phases leading to type 2 (non-insulin-dependent) diabetes mellitus in the rhesus monkey. Diabetologia 29: 712–719

46b. Hansen BC, Schielke GP, Jen KLC, Wolfe RA, Movahed H, Pek SB (1982) Rapid fluctuations in plasma catecholamines in monkeys under undisturbed conditions. Am J Physiol 242: E40–E46

47. Helmstaedter V, Feurle GE, Forssman WG (1977) Relationship of glucagon-somatostatin and gastrin-somatostatin cells in the stomach of the monkey. Cell tissue Res 177: 29–46

48. Hiebert JM, Celik Z, Soeldner JS, Egdahl RH (1973) Insulin response to hemorrhagic shock in the intact and adrenalectomized primate. Am J Surg 125: 501–507

49. Higgins PJ, Garlick RL, Bunn HF (1982) Glycosylated hemoglobin in human and animal red cells. Diabetes 31: 743–748

50. Hill DE, Mayes S, Dibattista D, Martin JM (1977) Hypothalamic regulation of insulin release in rhesus monkeys. Diabetes 26: 726–731

51. Hoffman FG, Knobil E, Greep RO (1954) Effects of saline on the adrenalectomized rhesus monkey. Am J Physiol 178: 361–366

52. Holaday JW, Martinez HM, Natelson BH (1977) Synchronized ultradian cortisol rhythms in monkeys: Persistence during corticotropin infusion. Science 198: 56–58

53. Honjo S, Kondo Y, Cho F (1976) Oral glucose tolerance test in the cynomolgus monkey (*Macaca fasicularis*). Lab An Sci 26: 771–776

54. Howard CF Jr (1972) Spontaneous diabetes in *Macaca nigra*. Diabetes 21: 1077–1090

55. Howard CF Jr (1975) Diabetes and lipid metabolism in nonhuman primates. Adv Lipid Res 13: 91–134

56. Howard CF Jr (1982) Correlations of hemoglobin A_{1c} and metabolic status in nondiabetic spontaneously diabetic, and diabetic macacus rhesus. Diabetes 31: 1105–1108

57. Howard CF Jr (1983) Diabetes and carbohydrate impairment in nonhuman primates. In Dukelow WR (ed), Nonhuman Primate Models for Human Diseases. CRC Press, Boca Raton, Fla, pp 1–36

58. Howard CF Jr (1984) Diabetes mellitus: Relationships of nonhuman primates and other animal models to human forms of diabetes. In Hendrickx AG (ed), Advances in Veterinary Science and Comparative Medicine. Academic Press, New York, pp 115–149

59. Howard CF Jr, Fang TY (1984) Islet cell cytoplasmic antibodies in *Macaca nigra*. Diabetes 33: 219–223

60. Howard CF Jr, Kessler MJ, Schwartz S (1986) Carbohydrate impairment and insulin secretory abnormalities among *Macaca mulatta* from Cayo Santiago. Am J Primatol 11: 147–162

61. Howard CF Jr, Palotay JL (1975) Spontaneous diabetes mellitus in *Macaca cyclopis* and *Mandrillus leucophaeus*: Case Reports. Lab An Sci 25: 191–196

62. Howard CF Jr, van Bueren A (1981) Immunoreactive glucagon in nondiabetic and diabetic *Macaca nigra*. Horm Metab Res 13: 203–206

63. Hummel KP, Dickie MM, Coleman DL (1966) Diabetes, a new mutation in the mouse. Science 153: 1127–1128

64. Issekutz B, Issekutz TB, Elaki D, Barkow I (1974) Effect of insulin infusions on the glucose kinetics in alloxan-streptozotocin diabetic dogs. Diabetologica 10: 323–328

65. Johnson KH, Hayden DW (1979) Diabetes mellitus in cats with amyloidosis of pancreatic islets. In Andrews EJ, Ward BC, Altman NH (eds), Spontaneous Animal Models of Human Disease VI. Academic Press, New York, pp 118–121

66. Jonasson O, Jones CW, Bauman A, John E, Manaligod J, Tso MOM (1985) The pathophysiology of experimental insulin-dependent diabetes in the monkey. Implications for pancreatic transplantation. Ann Surg 201: 27–39

67. Jones CW, Reynolds WA, Hoganson GE (1980) Streptozotocin diabetes in the monkey. Plasma levels of glucose, insulin, glucagon and somatostatin, with corresponding morphometric analysis of islet endocrine cells. Diabetes 29: 536–546

68. Jones CW, West MS, Hong DT, Jonasson O (1984) Peripheral glomerular basement membrane thickness in the normal and diabetic monkey. Lab Invest 52: 193–198

69. Jones SM (1974) Spontaneous diabetes in monkeys. Lab An 8: 161–166

70. Kahn CR, Neville DM Jr, Gordon P, Freychet P, Roth J (1972) Insulin receptor defect in insulin resistance: Studies in the obese hyperglycemic mouse. Biochem Biophys Res Commun 48: 135–142

71. Kahn CR, Neville DM Jr, Roth J (1973) Insulin receptor interaction in the obese hyperglycemic mouse. J Biol Chem 248: 244–250

72. Kaneko JJ (1980) Carbohydrate metabolism and its disorders. In Kaneko JJ (ed), Clinical Biochemistry of Domestic Animals. Academic Press, New York, pp 2–51

73. Kaneko JJ, Mattheeuws D, Rottiers RP, van Der Stock J, Vermeulen A (1978) The effect of urinary glucose excretion on the plasma glucose clearances and plasma insulin responses to intravenous glucose loads in unanesthetized dogs. Acta Endocrinol 87: 133–138

74. Kaneko JJ, Mattheeuws D, Rottiers RP, Vermeulin A (1977) Glucose tolerance and insulin response in diabetes mellitus of dogs. J Small An Pract 18: 85–94

75. Kaneko JJ, Mattheeuws D, Rottiers RP, Vermeulin A (1978) Renal function insulin secretion and glucose tolerance in mild streptozotocin diabetes in the dog. Am J Vet Res 39: 807–809

76. Kaneko JJ, Mattheeuws D, Rottiers RP, Vermeulin A (1979) Renal clearance, insulin secretion and glucose tolerance in spontaneous diabetes mellitus in the dog. Cornell Vet 69: 375–383

77. Kano Y, Kanatsuna T, Kakamura N, Kitagawa Y, Mori H, Kajiyama S, Nakano K, Kondo M (1986) Defect of the first-phase insulin secretion to glucose stimulation in the perfused pancreas of the non-obese diabetic (NOD) mouse. Diabetes 35: 486–490

78. Kaul CL, Talwalker PK, Grewal RS (1980) Oral glucose tolerance test in normal sympathectomized and streptozotocin induced diabetic rhesus monkeys: Effect on plasma immunoreactive insulin, free fatty acids and blood lactate. Indian J Exp Biol 18: 623–626

79. Kemnitz JW, Engle MM, Perelman RH, MacDonald MJ, Eisele SG, Farrell PM (1980) Effects

of experimentally induced diabetes mellitus on reproductive function and food intake in female *Macaca mulatta*. Antropologica Contemporana 3: 220

80. Kemnitz JW, Kraemer GW (1982) Assessment of glucoregulation in rhesus monkeys sedated with ketamine. Am J Primatol 3: 201–210

81. Kessler MJ, Howard CF Jr, London WT (1985) Gestational diabetes mellitus and impaired glucose tolerance in an aged *Macaca mulatta*. J Med Primatol 14: 237–244

82. Knobil E, Hofmann FG, Greep RO (1953) Effects of large doses of desoxycorticosterone acetate, cortisone acetate and ACTH in intact monkeys. Proc Soc Exp Biol Med 82: 691–694

83. Koerker DJ, Halter JB (1982) Glucoregulation during insulin and glucagon deficiency: Role of catecholamines. Am J Physiol 243: E225–233

84. Kramer JW, Nottingham S, Robinetto J, Lenz G, Gylvester S, Dessoriky MI (1980) Inherited, early onset, insulin-requiring diabetes mellitus of keeshond dog. Diabetes 29: 558–565

85. Kris AO, Miller RE, Wherry FE, Mason J (1966) Inhibition of insulin secretion by infused epinephrine in rhesus monkeys. Endocrinology 78: 87–97

86. Kudo H, Oki Y (1984) *Microtus* species as new herbivorous laboratory animals: Reproduction; bacterial flora and fermentation in the digestive tracts; and nutritional physiology. Vet Res commun 8: 77–91

87. Laborie C, Sai P, Feutren G, Debray-Sachs M, Quiniou-Debrie MC, Poussier P, Marliss EB, Assan R (1985) Time course of islet cell antibodies in diabetic and nondiabetic BB rats. Diabetes 34: 904–910

88. Lang CM (1966) Impaired glucose tolerance in the squirrel monkey (*Saimiri sciureus*). Proc Soc Exp Biol Med 122: 84–86

89. Lang CM, Munger BL (1976) Diabetes mellitus in the guinea pig. Diabetes 25: 434–443

90. Leathers CW, Schedewie HW (1980) Diabetes mellitus in a pig-tailed macaque (*Macaca nemestrina*). J Med Primatol 9: 95–100

91. Levin BE, Goldstein A, Natelson BH (1978) Ultradian rhythm of plasma noradrenaline in rhesus monkeys. 279: 164–166

92. Lewis HP, King LR, Raminez R, Brielmaier J, McLaurin RL (1969) Glucose intolerance in monkeys following head injury. An Surg 170: 1025–1028

93. Like AA, Guberski DL, Buter L (1986) Diabetic Biobreeding/Worcester (BB/Wor) rats need not be lymphopenic. J Immunol 136: 3254–3258

94. Lipman RL, Raskin R, Love T, Triebwasser J, Lecocq RF, Schmire JJ (1972) Glucose intolerance during decreased physical activity in man. Diabetes 21: 101–107

95. Lundbaek K (1962) Intravenous glucose tolerance as a tool in definition and diagnosis of diabetes mellitus. Br Med J 2: 1507–1513

96. Mann GV, Crofford OB (1970) Insulin levels in primates by immunoassay. Science 169: 1312–1313

97. Marliss EB, Nakhoda AF, Poussier P, Sima AA (1982) The diabetic syndrome of the "BB" Wistar rat: Possible relevance to Type I (insulin dependent) diabetes in man. Diabetologia 22: 225–232

98. Mattheeuws D, Rottiers R, Kaneko JJ, Vermeulin A (1980) Glucose assimilation and insulin secretion in IVGTT in normal dogs: Influence of atropine and pentobarbital. Horm Metab Res 12: 553–554

99. Mattheeuws D, Rottiers R, Kaneko JJ, Vermeulin A (1984) Diabetes mellitus in dogs: Relationship of obesity to glucose tolerance and insulin response. Am J Vet Res 45: 98–103

100. Mayer J, Bates MW, Dickie MM (1951) Hereditary diabetes in genetically obese mice. Science 113: 746–747

101. Mayer TK, Freedman ZR (1983) Protein glycosylation in diabetes mellitus: A review of laboratory measurement and their clinical utility. Clin Chem Acta 127: 147–184

102. Meier H, Yerganian GA (1959) Spontaneous diabetes mellitus in the Chinese hamster (*Cricetulus griseus*). Proc Soc Exp Biol Med 100: 810–815

103. Meis PJ, Kaplan JR, Koritnik DR, Rose JC (1982) Effects of gestation on glucose tolerance and plasma insulin in cynomolgus monkeys (*Macaca fascicularis*). Am J Obstet Gynecol 144: 543–545

104. Miller RE, Soeldner JS (1969) Suppression of portal venous insulin concentration by epinephrine in the conscious monkey. Diabetologia 5: 179–182

105. Mintz DH, Chez RA, Hutchinson DL (1972) Subhuman primate pregnancy complicated by streptozotocin induced diabetes mellitus. J Clin Invest 51: 837–847

106. Moise NS, Reimer TJ (1983) Insulin therapy in cats with diabetes mellitus. JAVMA 182: 158–164

107. Naithani G, Steffens G, Tager HS, Buse G, Rubenstein AH, Steiner DF (1984) Isolation and amino acid sequence determination of monkey insulin and proinsulin. Hoppe-Seyler's Z Physiol Chem 365: 571–575

108. Nakamura M, Yamada K (1967) Studies on a diabetic (KK) strain of the mouse. Diabetologia 3: 212–221

109. Nakhooda AF, Like AA, Chappel CI, Murray FT, Marliss EB (1977) The spontaneously diabetic Wistar rat. Metabolic and morphologic studies. Diabetes 26: 100–112

110. Nakhooda AF, Lide AA, Chappel CI, Wei CN, Marliss EB (1978) The spontaneously diabetic Wistar rat (the "BB" Rat): Studies prior to and during development of the overt syndrome. Diabetologia 14: 199–207

111. Nathan DM, Singer DE, Hurxthal K, Goodson JD (1984) The clinical information value of the glycosylated hemoglobin assay. N Engl J Med 310: 341–346

112. National Diabetes Data Group (1979) Classification and diagnosis of diabetes mellitus and other categories of glucose intolerance. Diabetes 28: 1039–1057

113. Pitkin RM, Reynolds WA (1970) Diabetogenic effects of streptozotocin in rhesus monkeys. Diabetes 19: 85–90

114. Poussier P, Nakhooda AF, Grose M, Marliss EM (1983) Arginine induced glucagon secretion in the spontaneously diabetic BB Wistar rat. Metabolism 32: 487–491

115. Rabinovitch A, Renold AE, Cerasi E (1976) Decreased cyclic AMP and insulin response to glucose in pancreatic islets of diabetic Chinese hamsters. Diabetologia 12: 581–587

116. Rayfield EJ, Kell KJ, Yoon JW (1986) Rubella virus-induced diabetes in the hamster. Diabetes 35: 1278–1281

117. Reichlin S (1983) Somatostatin. N Engl J Med 309: 1495–1501

118. Richter NA (1986) Percentage of glycosylated hemoglobin and serum concentration of glucose in the blood of Japanese macaques and in three exotic ruminant species. Am J Vet Res 47: 1783–1784

119. Rosenblum IY, Barbolt TA, Howard CF Jr (1981) Diabetes mellitus in the chimpanzee (*Pan troglodytes*). J Med Primatol 10: 93–101

120. Rottiers R, Mattheeuws D, Kaneko JJ, Vermeulin A (1981) Glucose uptake and insulin secretory responses to intravenous glucose loads in the dog. Am J Vet Res 42: 155–158

121. Ryan NT, George BC, Harlow CL, Hiebert JM, Egdahl RH (1977) Endocrine activation and altered muscle metabolism after hemorrhagic shock. Am J Physiol 233: E439–E444

122. Sakamoto C, Williams JA, Roach E, Goldfine ID (1984) *In vitro* localization of insulin binding to cells of the rat pancreas (41827). Proc Soc Exp Biol Med 175: 487–502

123. Sakuma M, Knobil E (1970) Inhibition of endogenous growth hormone secretion by exogenous growth hormone infusion in the rhesus monkey. Endocrinology 86: 890–897

124. Savage N, Howard H (1970) The effect of starvation and a subsequent glucose load on the concentrations of the ketone bodies in the blood of the baboon (*Papio ursinus*). Int J Biochem 1: 24–28

125. Schaer M (1977) A clinical survey of thirty cats with diabetes mellitus. J Am An Hosp Ass 13: 23–27

126. Smith GP, Russ RD, Stokes P, Duckett GE, Root AW (1977) Plasma GH response to D- and L-amphetamine in monkeys. Horm Metab Res 9: 339–340

127. Smith JE, Wood PA, Moore K (1982) Evaluation of a colorimetric method for canine glycosylated hemoglobin. Am J Vet Res 43: 700–701

128. Snyder G, Reynolds WA, Hoversten G, Christ D, Jonasson O (1977) C-peptide levels in the streptozotocin-diabetic and pancreatectomized monkey. Diabetes (Suppl 1) 26: 258

129. Sokoloverova IM (1960) Spontaneous diabetes in a monkey. In Utkin IA (ed), Theoretical and Practical Problems of Medicine and Biology in Experiments on Monkeys. Pergamon Press, New York, pp 171–183

130. Soll AH, Kahn CR, Neville DM Jr, Roth J (1975) Insulin receptor deficiency in genetic and acquired obesity. J Clin Invest 56: 769–780

131. Solway J, McDonald M, Bunn HF, Aun F, Cole R, Soeldner JS (1979) Biosynthesis of glycosylated hemoglobins in the monkey. J Lab Clin Med 93: 962–972

132. Srinivas M, Ghosh K, Shome DK, Virdi JS, Kumar S, Mohanty D, Das KC (1986) Glycosylated hemoglobin (Hb A$_1$) in normal rhesus monkeys (*Macaca mulatta*). J Med Primatol 15: 361–365

133. Steiner RA, Illner P, Marques P, Williams D, Shen L, Edwards L, Gale CC (1977) Inhibition of dopamine-induced release of growth hormone by thyrotropin-releasing hormone. Am J Physiol 233: E430–E433

134. Stewart JK, Koerker DJ, Goodner CJ, Gale CC, Steiner RA (1981) Effects of fasting on growth hormone secretion in the male baboon. Endocrinology 108: 1186–1189

135. Streett JW, Jonas AM (1982) Differential effects of chemical and physical restraint on carbohydrate tolerance testing in nonhuman primates. Lab An Sci 32: 263–266

136. Stuhlman RA, Arivastava PK, Schmidt G, Vorbeck ML, Townsend VF (1974) Characterization of diabetes mellitus in South African hamsters (*Mystromys albicaudatus*). Diabetologia 10: 685–690

137. Tanaka Y, Ohto H, Kohno M, Cho F, Honjo S (1986) Spontaneous diabetes mellitus in cynomolgus monkeys (*Macaca fascicularis*). Exp An 35: 11–19

138. Tashjian AH Jr, Levine L, Wilhelmi AE (1965) Immunochemical relatedness of porcine, bovine, ovine and primate pituitary growth hormones. Endocrinology 77: 563–573

139. Turner DS, Etheridge L, Jones J, Marks V, Meldrum B, Bloom SR, Brown JC (1974) The effect of the intestinal polypeptides, IRP and GIP, on insulin release and glucose tolerance in the baboon. Clin Endocrinol 3: 489–493

140. Wakeman M, Morrell CA (1931) Chemistry and metabolism in experimental yellow fever in *Macacus rhesus*. Arch Int Med 48: 301–312

141. Walvoort THC (1983) Glycogen storage diseases in animals and their potential value as models of human disease. Inherited Metabolic Dis 6: 3–16

142. Wherry FE, Miller RE, Mason JW (1966) Insulin levels in monkey plasma determined by immunoassay. Metabolism 15: 163–172

143. White JAM, Bolstridge MC, Downing JH, Wessels BC, Klomass HJ (1973) Effects of stress on the results of glucose tolerance tests performed on vervet monkeys (*Cercopithecus pygerythrus* F Cuvier). J S Afr Vet Assoc 44: 379–381

144. Widness JA, Schwartz R, Reynolds WA, Chez RA (1978) Hemoglobin AIC in the glucose-intolerant, streptozotocin-treted or pancreatectomized Macaque monkey. Diabetes 27: 1182–1188

145. Williams M, Gregory R, Schall W, Gossain V, Bull R, Padgett G (1981) Characterization of naturally occurring diabetes in a colony of Golden Retrievers. Fed Prod 40: 740

146. Wilson HK, Boyed AE 3rd, Bolton WE, Conaway HH (1982) Somatostatin secretion in diabetic rabbits. Metabolism 31: 428–432

147. Wilson MF, Brackett DJ, Archer LT, Beller-Todd BK, Tompkins P, Hinshaw LB (1982) Survival characteristics during septic shock in 39 baboons. Adv Shock Res 7: 13–23

148. Wilson RB, Martin JM, Kelly H, Newberne PM (1971) Plasma and pancreatic insulin concentrations in adult squirrel and rhesus monkeys. Diabetes 20: 151–155

149. Wise PH, Wis BJ, Hime JM, Forrest E (1972) The

diabetic syndrome in the tuco-tuco (*Cytenomys tala-rum*). Diabetologia 8: 165–172

150. Wood PA, Smith JE (1980) Glycosylated hemo-globin and canine diabetes mellitus. JAVMA 176: 1267–1268

151. Yasuda H, Harano Y, Koshugi K, Nakano T, Suzuki M, Tsuruoka Y, Taniguchi Y, Nishmori T, Kikkawa R, Shigeta Y (1984) Development of early lesions of microangiopathy in chronically diabetic monkeys. Diabetes 33: 415–420

152. Yoon J-W, London WT, Curfman BL, Brown RL, Notkins AL (1986) Coxsackie virus B_4 produces transient diabetes in nonhuman primates. Diabetes 35: 712–716

153. Young FG (1937) Permanent experimental diabetes produced by pituitary (anterior lobe) injections. Lancet 2: 372–374

154. Zucker LM, Zucker TF (1961) Fatty, a new mutation in the rat. J Hered 52: 275–278

9

Lipids and Lipoproteins

RICHARD M. CARROLL, PhD and ELAINE B. FELDMAN, MD

The importance of the measurement of circulating lipids and lipoproteins in laboratory animals relates to the lipid hypothesis that elevations in blood lipids induce atherosclerosis and are directly implicated in atherogenesis. Presumably dietary excesses or imbalances lead to hyperlipidemia, which in some as yet unexplained way is atherogenic.

It was thought originally that atherosclerosis was peculiarly a disease of humans and was rarely observed in laboratory animals or in animals in the wild. This apparently is not so, as spontaneous atherosclerosis is observed in aged animals.

The development of animal models for atherosclerosis depends on: the lipid and lipoprotein levels and distribution unique to the species; genetic variations within the species; and the susceptibility of the species to increased or altered blood lipids and lipoproteins in the direction of atherogenesis which can be induced by a variety of diets, drugs, and other perturbations.

In this chapter we will compare with the human the animal models of hyperlipidemia in nonhuman primates and the laboratory rat and also describe in some detail the lipids and lipoproteins of rabbit, dog, swine, and some other species for which data are available (Table 9.1).

LIPIDS AND LIPOPROTEINS

Lipids are transported in plasma in the form of lipoproteins. Lipoproteins are classified according to their physical and chemical properties (Table 9.2). The plasma lipids include cholesterol, free and esterified, triglycerides, and phospholipids. The lipoproteins are chylomicrons, very low-density lipoproteins (VLDL), low-density lipoproteins (LDL), and high-density lipoproteins (HDL). All lipoproteins contain specific and different amounts of the various lipids and have specific protein components termed apolipoproteins, or apoproteins (39).

In the human plasma cholesterol levels (40) vary with age, increasing from puberty to about the fourth decade in males and increasing to about the fifth decade in females. Values in females are generally lower than those in males until the middle or later years. Mean levels of plasma cholesterol range between 170 and 230 mg/dl. About two thirds of the plasma cholesterol is transported as LDL. The LDL cholesterol levels parallel total cholesterol levels. Levels of HDL cholesterol average about 45 mg/dl in men and 9 to 17 mg/dl more in women. Lipid risk factors in atherosclerosis include the absolute levels of plasma cholesterol and LDL

Table 9.1. Representative Values of Circulating Lipids in Common Species of Laboratory Animals[a]

Species	Total Cholesterol (mg/dl)	HDL Cholesterol (mg/dl)	Triglycerides (mg/dl)
Rhesus monkey	148 (90–200)	65 (22–174)	56 (35–250)
Other macaques	150 (147–226)	49 (30–150)	30 (20–200)
Patas monkey	95 (60–140)	44 (20–60)	50 (25–200)
African green monkey	150 (134–173)	76 (63–76)	45 (25–150)
Baboon	175 (132–239)	94 (71–122)	30 (15–45)
Squirrel monkey	203 (130–290)	89 (12–80)	100 (50–250)
Other New World Monkeys	143 (130–227)	36 (30–60)	90 (50–300)
Rat	58 (44–86)	34 (20–80)	39 (39–128)
New Zealand white rabbit	78 (18–304)	39 (12–200)	76 (45–170)
Dog	153 (60–185)	113 (51–125)	36 (15–70)
Swine	102 (80–115)	35 (29–46)	36 (32–41)
Pigeon	400 (357–538)	196 (105–264)	80 (74–200)
Mouse	95 (50–120)	74 (25–100)	214 (100–300)
Guinea pig	45 (27–75)	3 (1–5)	20 (11–75)
Hamster	112 (112–210)	45 (30–100)	50 (25–150)

[a] Values are means and ranges for adults, males, or sex unspecified, fasting, ingesting a variety stock diet.

cholesterol and inverse correlations with the level of HDL cholesterol and the ratio of HDL to total cholesterol or HDL to LDL cholesterol. Genetic and dietary factors influence these levels as do some diseases such as hypothyroidism, diabetes mellitus, pancreatitis, obstructive liver disease, renal disease, and some drugs and hormones especially thyroid hormone and gonadal hormones. Dietary factors that influence plasma cholesterol levels include the total level of calories in the diet and the cholesterol intake (20).

Circulating triglyceride levels average about 100 mg/dl in young adults, are somewhat lower in women, and increase 50 to 75 per cent with age (40). Triglyceride levels are influenced by genetic and dietary factors (calories, fat, carbohydrate, and alcohol) and diseases (pancreatitis and diabetes mellitus).

The human diet, which is associated with the development of atherosclerosis, contains about 200 mg of cholesterol per 1,000 kcal and is a high fat diet. About 40 per cent of calories are derived from fat with about 15 per cent of calories from saturated fat, polyunsaturated fats contributing about 9 per cent of calories, and the remainder from monounsaturated fat (73).

Chylomicrons

Chylomicrons are formed when triacylglycerol esters of long chain fatty acids are ingested. They are present in plasma only after a fatty meal is eaten and not in the fasting state. Therefore, serum lipids should be measured in samples drawn 12 to 18 hours after the last meal. In some instances animals that are normally nibblers, such as the rat, are trained to eat meals in an eating pattern similar to that of humans. Chylomicrons in plasma will produce turbidity. Plasma is turbid when levels of triglycerides exceed 200 mg/dl; chylomicrons are usually not present unless triglyceride levels approach 1,000 mg/dl. Chylomicrons can also be observed by electrophoresis on a variety of supporting media.

The chylomicron is a large particle that floats at the density of serum and is the primary transporter of exogenous triglyceride. This lipoprotein particle consists predominantly of triglyceride with small amounts of phospholipids, esterified and free cholesterol, and its specific apolipoproteins (Table 9.2). Chylomicrons are absorbed from the small intestine into the lymphatics and into the circulation to be removed by the action of lipoprotein lipase, an enzyme located in the capillary endothelium of extrahepatic tissues. The lipolytic action of lipoprotein lipase produces the chylomicron remnant that is taken up by the liver which has receptors that recognize one of the apolipoprotein constituents. This recognition system varies among species.

Very Low-Density and Low-Density Lipoprotein

The VLDL is produced in the liver and is distinguished from the intestinal particle or chy-

Table 9.2. Plasma Lipoproteins in Human Subjects

Class	Particle Diameter (nm)	Flotation Density	Electrophoretic Mobility	Apoproteins	Chemical Composition				
					Surface			Core	
					Proteins	Phospholipids	Cholesterol (%)	Cholesterol Esters	Triglycerides
Chylomicrons	80–500	0.93	α2	B, E, A-I, A-IV, C	2	7	2	3	86
VLDL	30–80	0.95–1.006	pre-β	B, E, C	8	18	7	12	55
IDL	25–35	1.006–1.019	Slow pre-β	B, E	19	19	9	29	23
LDL	22	1.019–1.063	β	B	22	22	8	42	6
HDL₂	10	1.063–1.125	α1	A-I, A-II, C, E	40	33	5	17	5
HDL₃	7.5	1.125–1.210	α1	A-I, A-II, C	55	25	4	13	3

Adapted from Havel EJ, Goldstein JL, Brown MD (1980). Lipoproteins and lipid transport, In Metabolic Control and Disease, 8th ed. Bondy PK, Rosenberg LE (eds). WB Saunders, Philadelphia, p 398.
Reproduced with permission from Feldman EB (39), p 48.

lomicron by the molecular weight or size of the B apolipoprotein which both contain. The intestinal particle contains an apolipoprotein B of approximately half the molecular weight of the apolipoprotein B produced in the liver. The VLDL is the main transporter of endogenous triglyceride produced from carbohydrate precursors. The VLDL particle being somewhat smaller and containing somewhat less triglyceride than the chylomicron makes the plasma diffusely turbid, whereas the chylomicrons float as a creamy layer on top of the plasma. The VLDL particles contain more protein and more cholesterol than do the chylomicrons (Table 9.2). The VLDL is also removed from plasma by way of the activity of lipoprotein lipase. Removal of triglyceride from VLDL by lipoprotein lipase generates LDL (39,40).

The LDL is about 50 per cent cholesterol with more protein and less triglyceride than VLDL (Table 9.2). The LDL is taken up by peripheral tissues and liver by a specific cell surface lipoprotein receptor. The LDL is the most atherogenic of the lipoproteins through a mechanism as yet unclear.

Intermediate-Density Lipoprotein

Intermediate-density lipoprotein (IDL) is intermediate in the catabolism of VLDL to LDL. The IDL is enriched in the proportion of cholesterol to triglyceride compared to VLDL (Table 9.2). Atherogenic diets may give rise to the so-called β-VLDL which is related to IDL (52). The β-VLDL is cholesterol rich, contains apolipoproteins B and E, and interacts with the LDL receptor and the chylomicron (and VLDL) remnant receptor. A variety of atherogenic diets induce β-VLDL in several species (90; see Table 9.7).

High-Density Lipoprotein

The HDL is a small particle generated in the intestine or the liver. This particle is about half protein and half lipid with the predominant lipid component phospholipid (Table 9.2). In many animal species HDL is the primary transporter of cholesterol in plasma (Table 9.1). The HDL consists of subfractions among which the protein content and cholesterol content can vary. The cholesterol to triglyceride ratio increases in HDL as the dietary cholesterol is increased. Feeding cholesterol results in the production of specific HDL particles which differ from the usual in that they are enriched in cholesteryl esters, are larger, float at a lower density, and are enriched in apolipoprotein E. Nascent HDL may also be generated from surface constituents of triglyceride-rich lipoproteins during lipolysis.

Diets high in cholesterol or fat generally reduce HDL cholesterol concentrations in laboratory animals such as monkeys, rabbits, dogs, and swine.

TECHNIQUES OF ANALYSIS

In this section, methods for the quantitative analysis of plasma lipids and lipoproteins will be discussed. An enormous number of analytic techniques for lipid and lipoprotein analysis have been published. Rather than review the literature we will provide brief descriptions of reference methods and techniques we have found useful in our laboratory.

In many instances the methods described for plasma lipids may be applicable to analysis of lipids from other sources; however, caution should be exercised when these methods are extrapolated to analyze samples of other origins.

Plasma Lipids

The main constituents of plasma lipids are cholesterol (free, unesterified), cholesteryl esters with fatty acids, phospholipids (mostly lecithin or phosphatidylcholine, also phosphatidylethanolamine, sphingomyelin, phosphatidylserine and phosphatidylinositol), triglycerides (triacylglycerol), and unesterified or free fatty acids. Small amounts of mono- and diglycerides, bile acids, and other sterols are also present. Determination of individual lipids or lipid classes in many instances can be carried out on plasma or plasma extracts without further purification; however, in certain instances further purification of individual lipids is required.

The first step in purification of individual lipids is to prepare a total lipid extract. The two most widely used procedures are those involving ethanol-ether (3:1, v/v), introduced by Bloor (17), and chloroform-methanol (2:1, v/v), introduced by Folch et al (48).

In the chloroform-methanol procedure, plasma samples are extracted in 20 to 30 volumes of chloroform-methanol at room temperature. After filtration to remove protein precipitates, the extract is equilibrated with 0.2 volumes of water, 0.05 per cent sulfuric acid, and 0.01 per cent sodium chloride or other salt and allowed to stand overnight at 4°C to permit phase separation. The lower phase containing the lipids can then be used for lipid analysis.

Care must be taken in handling lipid extracts because unsaturated fatty acids are oxidized rapidly. Lipid samples should be kept on ice during handling, solvent evaporation should be carried out in a nitrogen atmosphere at 50°C or lower, and purified samples should be stored in solvents such as benzene, hexane, or chloroform at $-15°$ to $-20°C$ in a nitrogen atmosphere. Also to be avoided are water (samples can be dehydrated with sodium sulfite), excessive light and heat, and contamination by lipids from hands, rubber tubing, stopcock grease and lubricants, and the like.

Plasma lipids or lipid classes can be separated from total lipid extracts by thin layer chromatography on silica gel G or H (111). High quality thin layer plates can be purchased from commercial suppliers or prepared in the laboratory. Separation of phospholipids, cholesterol, unesterified fatty acids, triglycerides, and cholesteryl esters is readily accomplished using a solvent system consisting of petroleum ether, diethyl ether, and acetic acid (80:20:1, v/v/v) (111). Individual phospholipids can be separated using a solvent system consisting of chloroform, methanol, and aqueous ammonia (65:35:5) (140). Visualization of lipids following separation can be achieved by spraying the plates with water or with aqueous solutions of rhodamine 6G (0.001 per cent) or 2',5'-dichlorofluorescein (0.03 per cent in 0.01 N sodium hydroxide). With the latter two reagents, spots are visualized with short wave ultraviolet light. Iodine vapor, which is more sensitive for unsaturated than saturated lipids, also can be used as a general detection reagent. If the fatty acid composition of the individual lipids is to be determined, exposure to iodine vapor should be avoided because it may destroy the polyunsaturated fatty acids.

Following thin layer chromatography the lipid spots can be recovered from the plates by aspiration or by scraping the spots with a razor blade. The lipids can be eluted with chloroform-methanol in the case of cholesterol, unesterified fatty acids, glycerides, and cholesteryl esters. Quantitative recovery of individual phospholipids requires the use of chloroform, methanol, and aqueous ammonia (65:35:5, v/v/v). Once eluted, the lipids can be dried under nitrogen and resuspended in solvents suitable for the analytic procedures described in the remainder of this section. The correlation between certain lipid and lipoprotein concentrations and heart disease has prompted many epidemiologic studies. To compare results of studies carried out in different laboratories, many laboratories have adopted the methodology used by the Lipid Research Clinics (94). These procedures provide good reference methods for setting up analytic techniques.

Appropriate reference standards of varying purity are available from commercial sources. Accreditation and monitoring of quality control are customary for many laboratories, such as the College of American Pathologists, Communicable Disease Center.

Cholesterol

The reference method used for the determination of cholesterol was that of Abell et al (1). The plasma samples are saponified by incubation with alcoholic potassium hydroxide. The resulting free cholesterol is extracted with petroleum ether, an aliquot of the extract is dried, and cholesterol is determined spectrophotometrically by a modified Liebermann-Burchard reagent. This method does not lend itself well to determinations in large numbers of samples and may be replaced by newer enzymatic procedures (4).

Measurement of cholesterol using cholesterol oxidase is relatively simple, accurate, and rapid. Cholesterol is oxidized by atmospheric oxygen in the presence of cholesterol oxidase, producing hydrogen peroxide. In the presence of horseradish peroxidase, hydrogen peroxide yields oxygen which reduces phenol and aminoantipyrine to form a reddish purple color, which is read in a spectrophotometer. Cholesterol esterase is also included in the reagent to convert cholesteryl esters to free cholesterol. Free cholesterol alone can be measured if cholesterol esterase is omitted from the reagent; however, because many of the commercially available cholesterol oxidase preparations are con-

taminated with cholesterol esterase, they are unsuitable for measurement of free cholesterol.

The enzymatic procedure is more specific for cholesterol than are chemical methods, and it may yield slightly lower plasma cholesterol concentrations than do chemical methods.

Triglycerides

Plasma triglycerides are most often determined by analysis of glycerol released by saponification of triglycerides. Many of the procedures used are modifications of the procedure described by Van Handel and Zilversmit (145) which requires extraction of total lipids from plasma and removal of phospholipids by adsorption with zeolite. The lipid extract is then saponified to release glycerol, and the glycerol is oxidized to formaldehyde with periodic acid. The formaldehyde, when reacted with chromotropic acid, gives a violet compound which is measured spectrophotometrically.

As with cholesterol analysis, enzymatic procedures for triglyceride analysis are rapidly replacing the older chemical methods (133). In the enzymatic procedures triglycerides are hydrolyzed by lipase. The resulting glycerol is phosphorylated by glycerol kinase to form glycerol-1-phosphate which is oxidized by glycerol-1-phosphate dehydrogenase to form dihydroxyacetone phosphate and NADH. The NADH is reacted with 2-(p-iodophenyl)-3-(p-nitrophenyl)-5-phenyltetrazolium chloride in the presence of the enzyme diaphorase. The resulting red formazan is measured spectrophotometrically. This procedure is much faster and subject to less interference than are the chemical methods; however, plasma glycerol will interfere with the enzymatic determination. This difficulty can be corrected by running the reaction in the absence of lipase.

Phospholipids

Plasma phospholipids are usually measured by determining the amount of lipid phosphorus present in total lipid extracts from plasma (11).

Unesterified Fatty Acids

Plasma unesterified fatty acids, which are normally present in small amounts, are determined by titration of extracted plasma (36).

Fatty Acid Composition

When a fatty acid deficiency is present or the effects of dietary fat on lipid metabolism are being studied, it may be desirable to determine plasma fatty acid composition.

Long chain saturated and unsaturated fatty acids present in cholesteryl esters, glycerides, and phospholipids are usually determined by gas-liquid chromatography of fatty acid methyl esters (14). Total lipid extracts of plasma and the fatty acid methyl esters of the total lipid extract or of individual lipid classes are prepared. The transmethylation can be accomplished by using boron trifluoride in methanol, methanolic-HCl, or methanol-sulfuric acid (111). Detailed descriptions of methods for gas-liquid chromatography of fatty acid methyl esters are presented elsewhere (111) and will not be discussed here. Appropriate pure standards of a variety of methyl esters of fatty acids are available from commercial sources.

Plasma Lipoproteins

Lipoproteins (Table 9.2) are complex macromolecules composed primarily of lipid (phospholipids, glycerides, cholesterol, cholesteryl esters, and unesterified fatty acids) and protein (apolipoproteins). The apolipoproteins are the primary determinants of the metabolic fate of the individual lipoprotein particles and maintain the solubility of lipoprotein lipids in the aqueous environment of the plasma. The ratio of lipid to protein determines the hydrated density of the lipoprotein particle. The plasma lipoproteins are named according to their hydrated densities: VLDL, d < 1.006 g/ml; IDL, d = 1.006 to 1.019 g/ml; LDL, d = 1.019 to 1.063 g/ml, and HDL, d = 1.063 to 1.21 g/ml. The HDLs have been subdivided further into HDL_1, d = 1.063 to 1.125 g/ml, HDL_2, d = 1.125 to 1.21 g/ml, and very high-density lipoproteins (VHDL), d > 1.25 g/ml.

The techniques described in this section primarily were developed and applied to the isolation and characterization of human plasma lipoproteins. The characteristics of animal lipoproteins may be different from those of human lipoprotein. Caution should be exercised in equating results with animal lipoproteins to the data obtained in humans based on any single technique.

Blood Samples

The concentrations of all plasma lipoproteins depend to some degree on the subjects' antecedent and current diet. To minimize dietary variation, blood samples should be collected after a 12 to 18 hour fast, which improves accuracy and reproducibility of the data and allows valid comparisons with published data.

Lipoproteins, which are relatively stable, become increasingly unstable as they are separated from the milieu of the plasma proteins. The stability of the lipoproteins is improved by the addition of the chelating agent ethylenediamine tetraacetic acid (EDTA) to all solutions containing lipoproteins. We recommend that blood be collected in test tubes containing EDTA to give a final plasma concentration of 10^{-4} to 10^{-3}M.

To further reduce changes in lipoproteins the blood samples should be cooled by placing them on ice following collection, and the plasma separated promptly and stored at 0 to 4°C. The lipoprotein isolation should be performed promptly, preferably within several days. The plasma should not be frozen and certainly not thawed and refrozen repeatedly.

Lipoprotein Isolation

Ultracentrifugation:

Lipoproteins are isolated routinely by sequential preparative ultracentrifugation. The original lipoprotein fractionation in the preparative ultracentrifuge was described by DeLalla and Gofman (35), but it has been replaced by procedures using NaCl, NaBr, and KBr to achieve desired densities rather than the $NaNO_3$ and D_2O used by the earlier investigators. The classic method of Havel et al (58) has been used in numerous studies. In this procedure density adjustments to 1.063 g/ml are made with solutions containing NaCl and KBr and to densities of 1.125 and 1.21 g/ml with solid KBr. To minimize sample dilution we prefer to add solid KBr directly to the sample using the equation reported by Radding and Steinberg (119):

$$X = V_i(d_f - d_i)/1 - Vd_f$$

where X is the gram of solid KBr to be added for adjustment, V_i is the initial volume of solution to be adjusted, d_f is the final density desired, d_i is the initial density, and V is the partial specific volume of KBr.

Adjustments of plasma to densities of 1.063 and 1.21 g/ml using the foregoing procedures permit the fractionation of LDL and HDL, which can be collected by tube slicing; however, subfractionation of VLDL is more difficult. These procedures require 18 to 36 hours of repeated ultracentrifugation at high speed. Swinging bucket or fixed angle rotors have been used. The temperature of the runs has varied from 4° to 37°C and may influence isolation (41,106).

To avoid these difficulties investigators (31,81,82) have used density gradient ultracentrifugation and obtained separation by differences in the flotation velocity of the different lipoprotein particles in a single spin. A density gradient procedure using this technique for isolation of VLDL has been reported by Lindgren et al (82). A recent two-step ultracentrifugal procedure was used to separate lipoproteins in a variety of animals (62).

Chromatography:

Alternatively various chromatographic separation methods have been applied to lipoprotein analysis. These methods are advantageous in that the lipoproteins are not subjected to multiple high-speed centrifuge runs; therefore, they are more likely to be isolated in their native state. In the procedure of Rudel et al (128), the density of 10 ml of plasma is adjusted to 1.225 g/ml by the addition of 3.52 g of solid KBr, giving a final volume of approximately 11 ml. Ten milliliters of the sample are placed in a 13-ml ultracentrifuge tube and carefully overlayered with an additional 3 ml of NaCl adjusted to a density of 1.225 g/ml with solid KBr. The plasma is then placed in an SW-40 rotor (Beckman) and spun in an ultracentrifuge for 40 hours at 40,000 rpm at 15°C. The lipoprotein fraction, which contains all of the plasma lipoproteins, is collected by tube slicing and chromatographed on a 1.5 by 90 cm column containing BioGel® A-15m. This procedure not only is more rapid than stepwise ultracentrifugation but also separates small molecular weight proteins from the lipoprotein particles.

More recently, affinity chromatography using antisera specific for apolipoproteins was used to isolate lipoproteins (151). These techniques are very useful for detailed studies of lipoprotein composition, but they are not amenable to routine use in laboratories that must process large numbers of samples.

Electrophoresis:

The foregoing techniques are necessary if detailed studies on individual lipoproteins are to be carried out. In many instances the goal is to quantitate the cholesterol concentration in the individual lipoproteins; for this purpose simpler techniques may be applied. The simplest and most widely used is lipoprotein electrophoresis (56). Methods for the electrophoretic separation of plasma lipoproteins in a variety of media have been available for many years. The most widely used of these are paper (51), cellulose acetate (29), polyacrylamide (108), and agarose (113).

The best solution and greatest sensitivity are attained with agarose gels prepared on a photographic film base by the procedure of Noble (113). Briefly, electrophoresis is carried out in 0.5 per cent agarose in 0.05 M barbital buffer, pH 8.6, containing 0.4 per cent bovine serum albumin. Plasma samples are applied to the plate and a small amount of bromphenol blue in 1.0 per cent albumin is spotted between the plasma samples. Electrophoresis is carried out for 90 minutes at 100 mA. The gel is removed and placed in a fixative (acetic acid-ethanol-water, 4:60:20) for 1 hour. The gel is then dried and stained in a saturated solution of Oil Red O in 60 per cent ethanol at 37°C. Oil Red O has high specificity for lipid with greatest uptake by cholesteryl esters, intermediate uptake by triglycerides, and minimal uptake by free cholesterol and certain phospholipids. Because the composition of each lipoprotein class is different, it is not surprising that the staining of each lipoprotein is different. Therefore, electrophoretic methods are useful when effects that result in marked changes in the concentration of a particular lipoprotein are sought, but they are not useful as a quantitative method.

Precipitation:

The methods of lipoprotein quantitation using the ultracentrifuge are excellent, however, they are not always available in many laboratories. A rapid and simple method of lipoprotein separation uses anionic polysaccharides, such as heparin or dextran sulfate, and divalent metal ions, such as Ca, Mg, or Mn, to precipitate the apo B containing lipoproteins VLDL and LDL (146).

The HDL cholesterol in the supernatant is measured and this value is subtracted from the total plasma cholesterol to give the VLDL plus LDL cholesterol concentration. In many clinical laboratories this technique is applied routinely in the determination of HDL cholesterol, but the information is limited because of a lack of separation of VLDL and LDL for quantitation. All these techniques were developed using human plasma, and their application to determinations in plasma samples of laboratory animals should be checked carefully.

An excellent review of precipitation methods for determining HDL cholesterol has been published (146). By the addition of a single ultracentrifugation step to the precipitation method the total lipoprotein profile can be obtained. In the procedure used, aliquots of plasma of up to 5.6 ml are placed in a series of 6-ml polyallomer ultracentrifuge tubes. The tubes are capped and placed in a Ti 50.3 ultracentrifuge rotor, and the plasma is centrifuged for 18 hours at 40,000 rpm at 15°C. The turbid upper layer (approximately 2 ml), containing the VLDL is removed by tube slicing, and the cholesterol concentration of the infranatant is determined by the enzymatic method described previously. The HDL cholesterol concentration of the plasma is then determined by adding 0.1 ml of a solution containing 0.1 per cent dextran sulfate and 1.1 M magnesium sulfate to 1.0 ml of plasma, precipitating the VLDL and LDL. The cholesterol in the supernatant is measured. The VLDL cholesterol is calculated by subtracting the value of the infranatant cholesterol from the total plasma cholesterol. The LDL cholesterol is calculated by subtracting the HDL cholesterol from the infranatant cholesterol concentration.

Apolipoproteins

Recent studies in the human have shown that certain apolipoproteins in plasma may be better indicators of the risk of heart disease than are the lipids. This finding has led to the development of assay procedures for measuring plasma apolipoproteins in a number of species, particularly apo B, apo A-I, and apo A-II.

Immunoassay procedures including radioimmunoassay (137), radial immunodiffusion (93), and rocket immunoelectrophoresis (34) have been employed. The radial immunodiffusion method provides a rapid and simple method for apoprotein quantitation. The results of an international survey of apoproteins A-I and B were published recently (33).

Polyacrylamide gel electrophoresis (PAGE) methods have been used to study the apoproteins of individual lipoprotein classes. Molecular weight of apoproteins can be determined using sodium dodecylsulfate (SDS), PAGE (149). The protein solution is denatured by heating to 100°C in the presence of excess SDS and sulfhydryl reagent in order to cleave the disulfide bonds. Under these conditions most proteins bind SDS in a constant weight ratio. The intrinsic charges of the protein are insignificant compared to the negative charges of the SDS, and the protein migrates strictly according to its size. The polyacrylamide concentration must be varied according to the molecular weight of the protein.

Urea also has been used as a dissociating agent for electrophoresis of apoproteins. High (8M) urea concentrations are necessary, and a sulfhydryl reagent is also required for complete denaturation of the proteins containing disulfide bonds. Urea-PAGE has the advantage of not affecting the intrinsic charge of the protein, so separation of the proteins is based on both size and charge. Urea is not as good a solubilizer as SDS, and much of the protein may not enter the gel.

The most powerful technique used for examining apoprotein composition is isoelectric focusing (147). This technique, which separates proteins based on their isoelectric point, is carried out for apoproteins in the presence of urea. Before the sample is applied to the gel, the protein is dissolved in a buffer containing urea and a sulfhydryl reagent. This is important in breaking the apo E/A-I complex. Recently isoelectric focusing was used to study the genetic variation in human apo E and apo A-I (155).

PLASMA LIPIDS AND LIPOPROTEINS IN SELECTED SPECIES OF LABORATORY ANIMALS

Old World Primates

Old World monkeys are phylogenetically closer to man than are New World monkeys and may represent the best models for studying human arterial disease. Plasma lipoproteins have been studied more completely in rhesus monkeys (*Macaca mulatta*) than in any other species of Old World monkey under a variety of techniques and dietary conditions. Extensive studies on the structure of rhesus monkey LDL and HDL have been carried out (45,46,79,135).

Rhesus Monkeys

Rhesus monkey LDL is similar in composition to human LDL but differs in density (45). Ultracentrifuge studies have identified three LDL subfractions in the 1.019 to 1.063 g/ml density range. The mean densities of the three subfractions were: LDL-I, 1.027 g/ml; LDL-II, 1.036 g/ml; and LDL-III, 1.050 g/ml. Rudel et al (132) also isolated an LDL subfraction similar to LDL-III which cross-reacted with antisera to human lipoprotein a (LP(a)), and they suggested that it is analogous to human lipoprotein a. Rhesus LDL has a protein that is similar to human apo-B which makes up 95 per cent of the LDL protein. LP(a) is found in varying amounts in human plasma at density interval of 1.055 to 1.085 g/ml. The protein moiety is composed of 65 per cent apo-B, 20 per cent apo-LP(a), and albumin.

Rhesus HDL can be divided into subclasses by ultracentrifugation (135). HDL$_2$ has a hydrated density interval of 1.063 to 1.125 g/ml and HDL$_3$ a density interval of 1.125 to 1.21 g/ml. The chemical compositions of rhesus HDL$_2$ and HDL$_3$ are similar to those of human HDL, although some differences in phospholipid content have been reported (46). The primary difference in human and rhesus HDL lies in the HDL$_2$-HDL$_3$ distributions; rhesus HDL exhibits increased quantities of HDL$_2$ (136). Homologues to human apo A-I and apo A-II are present in rhesus monkey HDL, but they differ from human apoproteins in amino acid composition.

Gard and Feldman (53) reported data of an extensive study of rhesus monkeys fed a stock diet or a high fat, high cholesterol diet (15 per cent lard, 0.5 or 0.25 per cent cholesterol w/w) and followed over 7 years. In monkeys fed the control stock diet, serum total cholesterol and HDL cholesterol levels were significantly higher in adult females than in adult males (Table 9.3).

In rhesus offspring total serum cholesterol and HDL cholesterol levels were similar in both sexes up to $3\frac{1}{2}$ years of age. After 28 days of pregnancy, the total serum cholesterol levels decreased by 75 to 98 mg/dl, with HDL cholesterol decreasing 34 to 53 mg/dl.

In adults ingesting the 0.5 per cent cholesterol diet, levels of total serum cholesterol increased fourfold in males and 2.5-fold in females. Mean HDL cholesterol increased in females and decreased in males. Lower cholesterol intake (0.25 per cent) resulted in total serum cholesterol levels decreasing 36 per cent in males and 30 per cent in females from levels on the higher (0.5 per cent cholesterol intake; HDL cholesterol levels in both sexes were increased to values exceeding those with the control diet.

Serum triglyceride levels were not affected significantly by these diets and no differences were observed between sexes or with pregnancy.

Lipoprotein fractionation (ultracentrifugation) indicated that on the control diet VLDL, LDL, and HDL cholesterol levels were 5, 35, and 59 per cent respectively, of the total cholesterol; HDL$_3$ carried 60 per cent of the HDL cholesterol. With the 15 per cent lard, 0.25 per cent cholesterol diet VLDL, LDL, and HDL cholesterol values were 3, 81, and 15 per cent respectively, of the total cholesterol; HDL$_1$ increased, with variable response in the other HDL subfractions (25). Switching monkeys to a 20 per cent butter, 0.1 per cent cholesterol (0.3 mg/kcal) diet after an interval on the stock diet resulted in levels of plasma lipids and lipoproteins similar to those with a 15 per cent lard, 0.25 per cent cholesterol diet.

The rhesus monkey has been used frequently as a model for studying diet-induced hypercholesterolemia and atherosclerosis (38,46,79, 110,127,132). Although the experimental design differed in the type and amount of fat and the amount of cholesterol fed to induce hypercholesterolemia, the outcome of the studies is similar. Diet-induced hypercholesterolemia results in redistribution of lipoprotein cholesterol so that the largest percentage shifts from HDL to LDL with increases also in IDL. These increases are due to increased plasma cholesteryl ester. The hypercholesterolemia also depends on the type of fat ingested. Polyunsaturated or monounsaturated oils such as safflower and corn oil tend to moderate the degree of hypercholesterolemia pro-

Table 9.3. Serum Lipid Levels in Rhesus Monkeys (mean ± standard error)

Category	Diet	Number	Total Cholesterol (mg/dl)	HDL Cholesterol (mg/dl)
Adult, male	Control	13	147 ± 6.2	66 ± 3
Adult, female	Control	16	164 ± 5.8	84 ± 3
Adult, male	15% lard 0.5% cholesterol	27	619 ± 36	58 ± 6
Adult, female	15% lard 0.5% cholesterol	22	438 ± 38	88 ± 10
Adult, male	15% lard 0.25% cholesterol	24	398 ± 25	75 ± 8
Adult, female	15% lard 0.25% cholesterol	24	308 ± 32	96 ± 7
Offspring, male	Control	20	156 ± 7	70 ± 4
Offspring, female	Control	20	147 ± 7	66 ± 3

Table 9.4. Characteristics and Composition of Serum Lipoproteins of the Rhesus Monkey (*M. mulatta*)[a]

	VLDL	Remnant			LDL	HDL	
	I	II_A	II_{B50}	II_{B100}	III	IV_{front}	IV_{back}
Diameter (nm)	65	40	30	30	24	< 12	< 12
Protein (%)	5	9	18	26	21	45	48
Phospholipid (%)	12	16	22	20	23	28	27
Free cholesterol (%)	5	5	9	7	9	4	3
Triglyceride (%)	46	58	13	10	5	3	3
Cholesteryl ester (%)	31	13	39	36	42	20	19

[a] Data calculated from Rudel et al (127). Lipoproteins were isolated by agarose column chromatography. Values in columns represent percentage of composition.

duced by dietary cholesterol, and saturated fats such as coconut oil and lard exacerbate the hypercholesterolemia.

Rudel et al (128) separated and characterized rhesus lipoproteins using agarose column chromatography. Seven fractions were obtained with this technique; their characteristics are summarized in Table 9.4. These results consistently indicate a close resemblance between rhesus monkey and human lipoproteins.

The same workers also examined the effect of dietary cholesterol on plasma lipoprotein cholesterol distribution in rhesus monkeys fed high fat (45 per cent of calories as lard) diets with or without the addition of 1 mg/kcal of cholesterol. The addition of cholesterol increased total cholesterol from 165 to 836 mg/dl, reduced HDL cholesterol from 83 to 28 mg/dl, and increased LDL cholesterol from 51 to 622 mg/dl, IDL cholesterol from 25 to 106 mg/dl, and VLDL cholesterol from 3 to 64 mg/dl. Similar changes

also were observed in other Old World primates (129).

Other Macaques

Rudel and Pitts (130) reported on male-female variability in response to cholesterol-induced hyperlipoproteinemia in cynomolgus monkeys (*M. fascicularis*). They fed three diets to the animals: the basic diet with 40 per cent of calories as fat with no added cholesterol and two test diets with cholesterol added at 0.4 and 0.6 mg/kcal. The LDL concentrations in both males and females increased in response to dietary cholesterol. However, the LDL concentration in males increased the size of the LDL particles, whereas the LDL concentration in the females increased the number of LDL particles. Plasma HDL (total lipoprotein) decreased from 565 to 140 mg/dl in males and from 534 to 204 mg/dl in females. The compositions of cynomolgus LDL and HDL are similar to those of the rhesus monkey. Similar responses to dietary cholesterol also were reported in the pigtailed macaque (*M. nemestrina*) (100).

The effect of dietary ethanol on plasma lipids also was examined in the pigtailed macaque (78). Administration of ethanol had no effect on plasma lipids in animals on a low cholesterol diet, but it increased serum cholesterol from 594 to 949 mg/dl in animals fed a high cholesterol diet. Similarly, ethanol did not cause changes in plasma triglycerides in animals on a low cholesterol diet, but it increased triglycerides from 96 to 200 mg/dl in animals fed a high cholesterol diet.

Patas Monkey

Apart from the rhesus monkey, the most extensive studies of blood lipids in Old World primates have been conducted in the patas monkey (*Erythrocebus patas*). Using a preparative electrophoretic technique Mahley et al. (91) isolated lipoproteins that had the following density ranges: VLDL, d < 1.006 g/ml; LDL-I, d = 1.02 to 1.06 g/ml; LDL-II, d = 1.05 to 1.085 g/ml; and HDL, d = 1.07 to 1.21 g/ml. The VLDL makes up only 1 per cent of the total lipoprotein and contains more phospholipid and less cholesterol than does human VLDL. The principal apoprotein of patas monkey VLDL is similar in some respects to human apo B, and analogues to apo-E and apo-Cs were also observed.

The LDL-I and LDL-II overlapped in density, had similar chemical compositions, but could be distinguished by their apoprotein content. The LDL-II contained small amounts of apo E and apo A-I in addition to apo B which was the principal component of LDL-I. Further study of LDL-II showed that it cross-reacted with human Lp(a) and appears to be its homologue in the patas monkey. As in other primates, HDL in the patas monkey is the major lipoprotein class, resembling human HDL in size and composition. Detailed characterization of high-density lipoproteins in cholesterol-fed hyper- and hyporesponding patas monkeys was reported by Melchior et al (102).

African Green Monkey

Two subspecies of the African green monkey, the grivet (*Cercopithecus anthiops aethiops*) and the vervet (*C. aethiops pygerythrus*), are often obtained in shipments from commercial suppliers. Although some differences in the plasma lipoprotein responses to dietary cholesterol and fat have been demonstrated between the subspecies, detailed studies of the composition of the lipoproteins of the African green monkey (*C. aethiops*) have been reported only in the vervet subspecies (114,115,131). Rudel et al found HDL apoproteins similar in amino acid composition to human apo A-I, A-II, C-II, C-III, and serum amyloid protein. Apo A-I in this species constituted 69 per cent of HDL protein. Apo A-II constituted 11 per cent of the HDL protein and existed as a monomer. Apo C-II acted as a potent stimulator of lipoprotein lipase, as in the human, but it was chemically distinct from human apo C-II in its amino acid composition and sialic acid content.

Baboons

The effects of diet and heredity on serum lipoproteins in the baboon (genus *Papio*) were studied by McGill et al (86,98). As in many other primates, HDL is the major lipoprotein class and resembles human HDL (15,47). The plasma VLDL is relatively triglyceride poor and found in lower concentration than is VLDL in human plasma (18). The baboon LDL contains larger amounts of triglyceride than does human LDL (18). The major LDL protein is similar and cross-reacts with antisera to human apo B (18, 76). Baboon HDL apoprotein composition is also similar to that of man (15). The major proteins of baboon HDL appear to be homologous to human apo A-I and apo A-II and have a similar amino acid composition. Analogues to human apo C-I, C-II, and C-III also have been reported in baboon HDL (15).

New World Monkeys

Even though New World monkeys are easier to handle, breed readily in captivity, and are less expensive to maintain than are Old World monkeys, their lipids and lipoproteins have not been studied extensively. Lofland et al. (83) reported on blood lipids in six species of New World monkeys. The results, summarized in Table 9.5 show that most plasma cholesterol is carried in the VLDL + LDL fraction, as in the human. Proportions of VLDL + LDL cholesterol to

Table 9.5. Values of Serum Lipids in Six Species of New World Monkey[a]

Species	Total Cholesterol (mg/dl)	VLDL+LDL Cholesterol (mg/dl)	HDL Cholesterol (mg/dl)	Triglycerides (mg/dl)
Saimiri sciureus (squirrel)	225 ± 18	124 ± 15	102 ± 12	62 ± 13
Ateles geoffrey (spider)	160 ± 16	141 ± 14	18 ± 6	74 ± 8
Cebus apella	98 ± 11	76 ± 10	22 ± 21	97 ± 10
Cebus albifrons	90 ± 4	67 ± 3	23 ± 7	62 ± 4
Lagothrix lagothrix (woolly)	133 ± 12	118 ± 12	15 ± 24	108 ± 25
Saquinus nigricollis (marmoset)	69 ± 4	50 ± 3	19 ± 7	95 ± 7

[a] Values are means and standard errors. Data are adapted from references 83 and 134.

total cholesterol range from 71 per cent in the squirrel monkey to 92 per cent in the woolly monkey.

The effect of dietary cholesterol on lipoprotein cholesterol distribution was examined (129) in spider monkeys. In the spider monkey, contrary to the human, cholesterol increased from 160 to 213 mg/dl on a diet containing 0.5 mg of cholesterol per 100 mg. There was a shift of plasma cholesterol from the LDL into the HDL fraction. The HDL cholesterol increased from 19 to 105 mg/dl whereas the LDL cholesterol decreased from 131 to 100 mg/dl. Similar changes also were seen in the squirrel monkey (129).

The effect of dietary cholesterol on lipoproteins has also been examined by other investigators using analytic ultracentrifugation (129). With increasing dietary cholesterol, VLDL, LDL, and HDL concentrations increased, with the greatest increase occurring in LDL. The increase in HDL concentration was largely due to increases in the HDL_3 subfraction. This is in contrast to humans who have higher levels of HDL_2.

Little information is available concerning composition and metabolism of plasma lipoproteins in New World monkeys. Illingworth and Portman (63) separated apoproteins of VLDL and HDL by electrophoresis. Patterns for both squirrel monkey VLDL and HDL was found to be different from those of lipoproteins in the human.

Apes

The chimpanzee, gorilla, and orangutan are phylogenetically closest to man. We might expect that their lipids and lipoproteins would closely resemble those of humans; however, only the chimpanzee has been studied to any degree. The effects of dietary fat and cholesterol on plasma lipids and lipoproteins have been reported (16,124). The plasma total cholesterol level and lipoprotein cholesterol distribution are similar to those of the human, with a larger proportion of the total cholesterol found in HDL in the chimpanzee (40 per cent). Most chimpanzee HDL is of the HDL_2 subclass rather than HDL_3 as found in man. Unlike the other species studied, the chimpanzee has as part of its HDL a dimeric apo A-II as well as a counterpart to human apo A-I (16,136). These apoproteins are comparable to human apo A-I and apo A-II in molecular weight and amino- and carboxyterminal amino acids (16,136).

Rats

Detailed information will be provided on lipids and lipoproteins of the rat in view of its popularity as an experimental animal. Most data have been collected in male rats, mainly young adults. Scant information is available about changes in lipids and lipoproteins with sex and age. The hooded Long-Evans rat has about a 20 per cent higher cholesterol level than does the Wistar rat and is even more susceptible to increases with cholesterol feeding (67).

The rat is relatively resistant to the induction of hyperlipidemia and atherosclerosis. In contrast to the human and some laboratory animals, other manipulations in addition to a high fat/high cholesterol diet are needed to raise serum lipid levels appreciably, such as feeding of bile acids and propylthiouracil (60,72,109,144). In general, the higher the level of cholesterol and cholic acid in the diet, the higher the serum cholesterol. Cholesterol feeding regimens have ranged between 0.45 and 4.0 per cent of the diet with cholic acid fed at levels of 0.15 to 1.35 per cent of the diet. On these regimens serum total cholesterol levels increase up to 14-fold.

Most manipulations of plasma lipids in the rat relate to alterations in the composition of the diet. With the common stock diet, serum total cholesterol levels in the rat are reported to range from about 44 to 78 mg/dl (104). Approximately three quarters of the circulating cholesterol is esterified—a figure approximately that in the human. Fasting serum triglyceride levels range from 39 to 87 mg/dl (104). The serum phospholipid to cholesterol ratio in the rat is somewhat higher than that in man, in whom it approximates 1·1·1. In contrast to the human, approximately 60 per cent of the total cholesterol in the rat is transported as HDL cholesterol. Also, in contrast to the human in whom HDL_3 is the major carrier of HDL cholesterol, the rat is devoid of this component and HDL_2 is the major fraction (88). HDL_1 (d = 1.05 g/ml) is present in the rat and may contaminate LDL (85). This HDL_1 has apo E and resembles HDL_c, a lipoprotein produced in some species fed diets high in cholesterol (32). Rat HDL overall is richer in apo E than is human HDL.

With semisynthetic or purified diets (7), the cholesterol levels of the rat are slightly increased over those with the stock diet, ranging from 51 to 116 mg/dl (101). Serum triglyceride levels in rats fed these diets are increased and range from 94 to 221 mg/dl. Phospholipid levels do not differ from those observed with the stock diet. Various forms of fiber have been added to the semipurified diet with a minor decline in the serum lipid levels of the rat, which then resemble those observed with the stock diet. Deleting fat or protein from the diet causes only minor variations in serum lipid levels. When the protein is provided at differing levels or from different animal or vegetable sources, there are minor changes in serum lipids, with the lowest levels observed with 20 per cent egg albumin compared to casein and soy protein (24). Feeding excess histidine or tyrosine induces hypercholesterolemia (107). With choline deficiency, serum total cholesterol levels were decreased to 35 mg/dl; with a 5 per cent choline diet, serum cholesterol levels increased to 108 mg/dl (5). At least a threefold increase in triglycerides was observed with a diet of 60 per cent sucrose rather

Table 9.6. Effects of Dietary Fats on Serum Lipids in the rat[a]

Diet	Total Cholesterol (mg/dl)	HDL Cholesterol (mg/dl)	Triglycerides (mg/dl)
Semipurified	71 (51–116)	...	128 (94–221)
10%			
Trilaurin	72 ± 1	...	...
Trimyristin	...	...	63 ± 4
Tripalmitin	59 ± 1	...	45 ± 2
Tristearin	59 ± 1	49 ± 2	37 ± 8
Triolein	77 ± 1	56 ± 2	59 ± 4
Safflower oil	80 ± 1	31 ± 3	40 ± 0.1
Coconut oil	98 ± 5	...	...
Corn oil	60–74	...	68 ± 3
Soybean oil	133 ± 4.7	...	137 ± 7
15%			
Tripalmitin	43 ± 2	22 ± 1	83 ± 9
Tristearin	83 ± 4	58 ± 2	62 ± 4
Triolein	97 ± 4	60 ± 2	80 ± 6
Safflower oil	84 ± 2	41 ± 3	59 ± 4
Butter	99	...	...
Lard	75 ± 4.7	...	...
Cottonseed oil	80 ± 5.5	...	...
Corn oil	105	...	...
Cholesterol, 0.1%	86 ± 30	...	...

[a] Values are means ± standard error (n = 18) or range.

than the usual complex carbohydrate sources (142).

Most dietary manipulations in the rat have dealt with variations in the level of dietary fat and the nature of the fat fed (Table 9.6). It was initially reported that increasing fat from the usual low fat level to 10 and even 20 per cent of the diet (w/w) did not alter plasma cholesterol. Data from our laboratory and that of others indicate that even with an increase to only 10 per cent of the diet, ingestion of some saturated fats will raise plasma cholesterol in the rat (44,121) (Table 9.6). In the rat, in contrast to the human, monounsaturated fat, namely triolein, has a definite serum cholesterol-raising effect (43). When the fat level is increased to 15 per cent w/w, the cholesterol-elevating effect of both saturated fats and triolein is increased (42), whereas the modest cholesterol increase produced with safflower oil (also differing from cholesterol-lowering effect in the human) is relatively unchanged (99). Supplementing stock diets with 10 per cent fish oil resulted in plasma cholesterol and triglyceride levels of about 50 and 70 mg/dl, respectively, with HDL cholesterol of 36 mg/dl (6).

Serum triglyceride levels increase with 10 per cent trimyristin, but not with feeding of other fats at the 10 per cent level. When dietary fat is increased to 15 per cent w/w, however, serum triglyceride levels double and are highest with a diet in which about 68 per cent of the fatty acids are saturated (42).

When natural fats such as lard, butter, or corn oil are fed to rats at 15 per cent of the diet, serum cholesterol levels increase the most with butter and corn oil (71). Cholesterol fed at 0.1 per cent of the diet produces serum cholesterol levels in a similar range. When cholesterol at 1 per cent w/w is added to diets containing 9 to 10 per cent fat, serum cholesterol levels are increased by 67 to 100 per cent over the stock diet, with the greater effect when the dietary fat is saturated (109). When the dietary fat level is raised to 25 per cent, the dietary cholesterol level raised to 1 to 3 per cent, and cholic acid added at 0.5 or 1 per cent of the diet, serum cholesterol levels increased to a range of 350 to 700 mg/dl when the fat is saturated (109). With polyunsaturated fat sources, serum cholesterol levels are less elevated approximating 300 mg/dl (88). The highest cholesterol levels in the rat are achieved when these diets are combined with an antithyroid drug such as propylthiouracil at 0.1 per cent, with the serum cholesterol level reported at 2,000 mg/dl (109). These dietary manipulations have less effect on triglyceride levels, which rarely reach 200 mg/dl.

Dietary magnesium or copper deficiency produces hyperlipidemia (80,120). Feeding an excess of zinc has variable effects (80).

Hypothyroid rats have an increased serum cholesterol level of 88 ± 16 mg/dl (n = 4); with a 1 per cent cholesterol diet the serum cholesterol level increased to 119 ± 25 mg/dl (n = 7) (13). Lipid-lowering drugs (clofibrate and halofenate) have been effective in the rat (10,126). Administration of polychlorinated biphenyls causes hypercholesterolemia (107).

Diseases may influence serum lipid levels in the rat. There is a form of genetic hypercholesterolemia in which the plasma cholesterol level in rats fed the stock diet is double the normal (118). Triglycerides are elevated by 50 per cent in Sprague-Dawley rats from the Ivanovas Sieve Colony, double with fructose, and increase 10-fold with Triton® (84). In the germ-free rat total cholesterol increases about 20 mg/dl (69). In streptozotocin-induced diabetes in rats fed a diet of 10 per cent lard, 2 per cent cholesterol, and 1 per cent cholic acid, the highest cholesterol levels reported were $1,555 \pm 159$ mg/dl (9). These diabetic rats fed a high sucrose diet had triglyceride levels of 586 mg/dl, whereas diabetic rats fed a chow diet had mean serum triglyceride levels of 1,881 mg/dl and cholesterol of 181 mg/dl (153). Among genetically obese hyperlipoproteinemic Zucker fatty rats (fa/fa), the females had serum cholesterol levels that ranged from 180 to 323 mg/dl, serum triglycerides from 218 to 250 mg/dl, and HDL cholesterol averaged 48 mg/dl. In male fatty rats mean values were 148 mg/dl for serum cholesterol, 401 mg/dl for serum triglycerides, and 333 mg/dl for serum phospholipids (152).

As the male rat ages, serum cholesterol levels double from the 1 to 3-month levels to 9 months and triple by 18 months of age. Triglyceride levels increase fivefold by 9 months of age and steadily thereafter (23). Female rats appear more susceptible than male rats to the cholesterol-elevating effects of a high fat/high cholesterol diet; the increase is threefold in females compared to twofold in males.

The compositions of plasma lipoproteins of the rat resemble the human but are not the same. Both VLDL and LDL are higher in triglyceride and lower in cholesterol than are the respective lipoproteins in the human (77,87,116) (Table 9.7). The apolipoprotein composition of lipoproteins and distribution among lipoproteins in the rat are presented in Table 9.8 (9,57).

Rabbits

The serum lipid values of rabbits that ingest the stock diet resemble those of rats (Table 9.1). With a semisynthetic diet, however, serum cholesterol levels increase two- to three-fold, a more marked response than that in the rat (55). The circulating cholesterol level of the rabbit increases readily with a variety of dietary manipulations. Sucrose added to the diet triples cholesterol but has less effect on triglycerides (138). The rabbit is very sensitive to the addition of cholesterol to the diet. Thus, feeding the rabbit 1 g of cholesterol per day increases serum cholesterol levels to over 1,000 mg/dl, averaging about 1,400 mg/dl (21,125). When cholesterol is combined with 5 per cent saturated fat in the

Table 9.7. Characteristics and Composition of Serum Lipoproteins of the Rat

	VLDL	β-VLDL	Remnant	LDL	HDL$_1$	HDL
Diameter (nm)	57	...	44	25	20	10
Protein (%)	9	5	10	25	32	45
Phospholipid (%)	13	22	14	25	32	27
Free cholesterol (%)	5	—[a]	6	14	12	9
Triglyceride (%)	70	14	63	19	3	1
Cholesteryl ester (%)	3	—[a]	7	19	23	18

[a] Sum of percentage of free cholesterol and cholesteryl ester β-VLDL = 58. β-VLDL is described in section on intermediate-density lipoprotein.

diet, serum cholesterol levels increase to about 1,800 mg/dl (141). With cholesterol and fat feeding, serum triglyceride levels increase three- to sixfold and phospholipid levels increase four- to eightfold (141). Combining cholesterol and sucrose feeding increases the serum cholesterol level only slightly over that observed with the refined carbohydrate diet alone and does not influence serum triglyceride levels (138). Soy protein in the rabbit has a cholesterol-lowering effect compared to that of casein (24). The vitamin E-deficient rabbit shows a 60 per cent increase in plasma cholesterol, primarily as LDL cholesterol (32).

Even higher levels of serum cholesterol are achieved in the rabbit fed cortisone along with cholesterol, reaching about 2,000 mg/dl. Cortisone, either alone or in combination with epinephrine, has a minimal effect on the rabbit's serum cholesterol; epinephrine by itself has none (37).

Serum total cholesterol levels are twice as high in males compared with female rabbits (96). Serum cholesterol levels in the Japanese white rabbit are half the values in the New Zealand white rabbit (96).

With gestation the serum cholesterol level falls one quarter to one half the pre-pregnancy value. With lactation and feeding a diet of 15 per cent lard plus 1 per cent cholesterol, serum cholesterol levels increase to 2,500 to 2,800 mg/dl. The suckling rabbit has a cholesterol level of 219 mg/dl, which decreases rapidly with weaning to the stock diet and is at the usual stock diet levels after feeding for 1 month (122).

The Watanabe heritable hyperlipidemic rabbit is a model of familial hypercholesterolemia in the human (148). This mutant was identified in 1973. In the homozygous form, serum total cholesterol values average 500 mg/dl and may approach 1,000 mg/dl. Serum triglyceride levels of 100 to 700 mg/dl are observed with phospholipid levels of approximately 800 mg/dl. All of these rabbits develop atherosclerosis by 5 months of age. Ninety per cent of total cholesterol is transported as LDL with minimal amounts of HDL cholesterol (143).

High-density lipoprotein is the major transporter of cholesterol in the rabbit fed the stock diet, carrying about two thirds of the total cholesterol. The composition of the rabbit VLDL resembles that of the human more closely than that of the rat (123). Rabbit LDL is relatively lower in cholesterol and higher in triglycerides than is human LDL, whereas HDL is higher in triglycerides (125).

With cholesterol feeding, VLDL increases 20- to 40-fold and LDL 4- to 5-fold; VLDL and LDL cholesterol is enriched in cholesteryl esters and apo E and resembles the lipoproteins of Type 3 hyperlipoproteinemia in the human.

Table 9.8. Apoproteins of the Rat

Lipoprotein	A-I	A-II	B	C	A-IV	E
Composition of Lipoproteins (%)						
VLDL	0.1		31	53	<0.1	15
HDL	61		1	20	9	9
Distribution into Lipoproteins (%)						
VLDL	8		71	14	18	15
LDL	10		29	8	13	10
HDL	82		...	78	67	63

This so-called β-VLDL is similar in composition to β-VLDL of the rat but has even more cholesteryl ester and less triglyceride. HDL cholesterol levels decline with cholesterol feeding (125).

Dog

The total cholesterol level of the dog fed a stock diet is higher than that of rats and rabbits, resembling that of the human (Table 9.1). Phospholipid levels of the dog are proportionally higher in relation to cholesterol than are those of the human. The major transporter of cholesterol in the dog is HDL. In the dog VLDL resembles that in other species, LDL is relatively higher in triglyceride and lower in cholesterol, and HDL is relatively lower in protein and higher in phospholipid (139). Both HDL_1 and HDL_2 have been described in normal dogs, with the former isolated in the density range of human LDL (89). The latter is the predominant canine plasma lipoprotein, transporting approximately 85 per cent of the total cholesterol. The canine apoprotein patterns are similar to those of man.

The dog is relatively resistant to the induction of hypercholesterolemia, but it does develop atherosclerosis. Early (1946) regimens used cholesterol and thiouracil. Cholesterol feeding (1 per cent) to hypothyroid dogs also fed cholic acid induced hypercholesterolemia and β-VLDL. Plasma cholesterol levels ranged from 250 to 1,500 mg/dl, with triglycerides variably unchanged or increased to 100 to 500 mg/dl (90). The β-VLDL is less enriched in cholesterol in the dog than in other species, with cholesterol averaging about 30 per cent of the β-VLDL composition. The β-VLDL of the dog is relatively higher in triglyceride (87). Feeding euthyroid dogs a diet of 5 per cent cholesterol and 16 per cent coconut oil produced plasma cholesterol levels averaging 1,300 mg/dl with plasma triglycerides of 182 mg/dl. Substitution of 4 per cent safflower oil for coconut oil (reduced in the diet to 12 per cent) resulted in significantly lower plasma cholesterol levels of 330 mg/dl (97). The total cholesterol in the dog is decreased with clofibrate and increased with epinephrine (10).

Swine

The serum lipoproteins of the pig resemble those of the human but may separate at somewhat different densities (3). As in man, LDL is the main carrier of cholesterol. Feeding of saturated fat doubles serum total cholesterol and HDL cholesterol (70,95). An increase in the ratio of polyunsaturated to saturated fat in the diet decreases serum cholesterol. With gestation the serum cholesterol decreases 10 per cent depending on the breed and the food intake. Serum triglyceride levels increase 50 per cent with gestation. Exercise lowers serum cholesterol by one sixth (50). Recent studies in piglets examined the interactions of dietary protein and fiber, with a greater reduction in cholesterol-induced hypercholesterolemia by soy fiber in conjunction with soy protein than by casein (30). Cod liver oil-supplemented pigs fed a high-cholesterol (2 per cent)/high fat (30 per cent) diet w/w showed a similar fivefold increase over baseline in plasma cholesterol as did controls fed the atherogenic diet (150). Genetically obese pigs are no more susceptible to diet-induced hypercholesterolemia than are lean pigs (117).

In the minipig, serum lipid levels are similar to those of other breeds of swine: cholesterol (mean), 109 mg/dl (range 89 to 133); triglycerides (mean) 92 mg/dl (range 20 to 154) (92). Feeding various high fat (20 per cent cottonseed oil, dairy products, and eggs) and 1 to 2 per cent cholesterol diets with 0.5 per cent cholic acid increased serum cholesterol levels three- to sixfold with no change in serum triglycerides (2,66,92). Plasma cholesterol levels increased faster and reached a higher level in minipigs than in domestic swine fed an 11.2 per cent egg yolk—0.5 per cent cholesterol diet (66). Citrus pectin feeding reduced hypercholesterolemia 50 per cent (2). The serum lipoproteins of minipigs are relatively enriched in cholesterol compared to those of the human (92). Their β-VLDL resembles that of the dog in composition. The pig is a good animal model of atherosclerosis.

Others

Rodents

Serum cholesterol levels in the guinea pig resemble those of the rat and rabbit. In contrast to other herbivores in which HDL is the major transporter of serum cholesterol, in the guinea pig plasma cholesterol is primarily transported (80 per cent) as LDL (104). The HDL accounts

for less than 5 per cent of the total serum cholesterol. In contrast to some other species, feeding cholesterol to the guinea pig increases HDL
cholesterol.

Total serum cholesterol is somewhat higher
in mice, gerbils, and golden hamsters and even
higher in Chinese hamsters compared to rats
(Table 9.1). With an atherogenic diet, the serum
total cholesterol in the mouse can double (105).
In inbred strain C 57 BR/cd J fed a similar diet,
plasma total cholesterol increased fivefold (19).
In the gerbil, in contrast to the rat, a 20 per cent
safflower oil diet lowered serum total cholesterol
to 67 ± 4 mg/dl (SEM) from the usual 104 ± 5
mg/dl (112). Coconut oil increased cholesterol
levels in the gerbil to 59 ± 6 mg/dl. Feeding 0.1
per cent cholesterol to the gerbil increased cholesterol approximately 2.25-fold; increasing
dietary cholesterol to 0.5 per cent and adding 20
per cent fat raised total serum cholesterol to 400
to 500 mg/dl (103). Serum phospholipids are
relatively high in mice and low in guinea pigs.
There is a paucity of lipoprotein data in the
mouse (22) and the hamster. The principal apolipoproteins of murine serum are homologous
to human and rat apo A-I, A-II, B, and C-III
(49). Apo E increased in mice on an atherogenic
diet (19). With feeding of an 0.5 per cent cholesterol diet, VLDL, LDL, and HDL cholesterol
levels increased in the gerbil.

Birds

Avian species, particularly the chicken (*Gallus
domesticus*), have been of considerable interest
as animal models for studying the mechanisms
of estrogen-induced hyperlipidemia (61). However, there are substantial differences between
avian and human lipid transport. Birds, unlike
humans, absorb exogenous fat as VLDL
through the portal vein rather than as chylomicrons through the lymphatic system (27).

Despite these differences there have been a
number of studies on the qualitative and quantitative aspects of chicken lipoproteins. Chapman et al (28) characterized and compared
chicken and human lipoproteins. In pooled sera
they found mean total serum cholesterol and
triglyceride concentrations of 101 and 457
mg//dl, respectively, with a range for serum
cholesterol of 58 to 125 mg/dl and triglycerides
240 to 672 mg/dl. They determined lipoprotein
distributions by analytic ultracentrifugation; the

major lipoprotein fraction was VLDL followed
by LDL and HDL. Wide variations in lipoprotein distributions reported by other investigators may be attributable to differences in sex,
age, and hormone status of the chicken (27). The
low VLDL concentrations found in immature
chickens may increase to 2,000 mg/dl with onset
of egg production (154), and similar levels can be
obtained in males treated with diethylstilbestrol
(26).

The VLDL of chickens is smaller and more
dense than human VLDL (28). The LDL tends
to be larger and less dense than human LDL,
resembling IDL of other species (104).

The apoproteins of chicken VLDL, LDL
(54,65), and HDL (64,75) have been studied
extensively. A counterpart to human apo B
is the major protein component of chicken
VLDL and LDL. Immunologic cross-reactivity
between chicken and human VLDL and LDL
has been demonstrated (54). The other apoproteins of chicken VLDL and LDL do not
resemble those of human and may be involved
in egg formation (12).

Several studies have reported the properties
of chicken HDL (59,68,75). Comparison of
chicken HDL and human HDL_2 and HDL_3
showed that HDL in immature birds resembled
HDL_3 (74), whereas that of the rooster was more
like HDL_2 (75). The major protein of chicken
HDL resembles human apo A-I (64,75). Comparison of N- and C-terminal amino acid
sequences of chicken and human apo A-I
showed little homology. A protein similar in
electrophoretic mobility to human apo A-II also
was reported (75).

Studies were also carried out in the turkey
(*Meleagris galapavo galapavo*), goose (*Anser
anser*, quail (*Coturnix coturnix japonica*), and
pigeon (*Columba species*). Of these, the pigeon
has received considerable attention because of
differences in breeds in their susceptibility to
atherosclerosis. The characteristics of lipoproteins in these species have been reviewed in
detail (27). Plasma lipoproteins in White Carneau and Show Racer pigeons were characterized recently by Barakat and St. Clair (8).

REFERENCES

1. Abell LL, Levy BB, Brodie BB, Kendall FE (1952)
   A simplified method for the estimation of total chol-

esterol in serum and determination of its specificity. J Biol Chem 195: 357–366

2. Ahrens F, Hagemeister H, Pfeuffer M, Barth CA (1986) Effects of oral and intracecal pectin administration on blood lipids in minipigs. J Nutr 116: 70–76

3. Alexander C, Day CE (1973) Distribution of serum lipoproteins of selected vertebrates. Comp Biochem Physiol 46B: 295–312

4. Allain CC, Pool NS, Chan CSG, Richmond W, Fu PC (1974) Enzymatic determination of total serum cholesterol. Clin Chem 20: 470–475

5. Ashworth CT, Wrightsman F, Buttram V (1961) Hepatic lipids. Arch Pathol 72: 620–624

6. Balasubramaniam S, Simons LA, Chang S, Hickie JB (1985) Reduction in plasma cholesterol and increase in biliary cholesterol by a diet rich in n-3 fatty acids in the rat. J Lipid Res 26: 684–689

7. Balmer J, Zilversmit DB (1974) Effects of dietary roughage on cholesterol absorption, cholesterol turnover, and steroid excretion in the rat. J Nutr 104: 1319–1328

8. Barakat HA, St. Clair RW (1985) Characterization of plasma lipoproteins of grain and cholesterol-fed white Carneau and Show Racer pigeons. J Lipid Res 26: 1252–1268

9. Bar-On H, Roheim PS, Eder HA (1976) Serum lipoproteins and apolipoproteins in rats with streptozotocin-induced diabetes. J Clin Invest 57: 714–721

10. Barrett AM, Thorp JM (1968) Studies on the mode of action of clofibrate: Effects on hormone-induced changes in plasma free fatty acids, cholesterol, phospholipids and total esterified fatty acids in rats and dogs. Brit J Pharm Chemo 32: 381

11. Bartlett GR (1959) Phosphorus assay in column chromatography. J Biol chem 234: 466–468

12. Bengtsson G, Marklund SE, Olivecrona T (1977) Protein components of very low density lipoproteins from hens' egg yolk. Eur J Biochmem 79: 211–223

13. Best, MM, Duncan CH (1956) Effects of sitosterol on the cholesterol concentration in serum and liver in hypothyroidism. Circulation 14: 344–348

14. Blaton VH, Peeters H (1972) In Nelson GJ (ed), Blood Lipids and Lipoproteins: Quantitation, Composition and Metabolism. Wiley-Interscience, New York

15. Blaton V, Vercaemst R, Rosseneu M, Mortelmans J, Jackson RL, Gotto AM Jr, Peeters H (1977) Characterization of baboon plasma high density lipoproteins and of their major apoproteins. Biochemistry 16: 2157–2663

16. Blaton V, Vercaemst R, Vandecasteele H, Caster H, Peeters H (1974) Isolation and partial characterization of chimpanzee plasma high density lipoproteins and their apoproteins. Biochemistry 13: 1127–1135

17. Bloor WR (1914) A method for the determination of fat in a small amount of blood. J Biol Chem 17: 377–383

18. Bojanovski D, Alaupovic P, Kelley JL, Stout C (1978) Isolation and characterization of the major lipoprotein density classes of normal and diabetic baboons (*Papio anubis*) plasma. Atherosclerosis 31: 481–487

19. Breckenridge WC, Roberts A, Kuksis A (1985) Lipoprotein levels in genetically selected mice with increased susceptibility to atherosclerosis. Arteriosclerosis 5: 256–264

20. Caggiula AW, Orchard TJ, Kuller LH (1983) In Feldman EB (ed), Nutrition and Heart Disease, Contemporary Issues in Clinical Nutrition, Vol 6. Churchill-Livingstone, New York

21. Camejo G, Bosch V, Lopez A (1974) The very low density lipoproteins of cholesterol-fed rabbits. Atherosclerosis 19: 139–152

22. Camus M-C, Chapman MJ, Forgez P, Laplaud PM (1983) Distribution and characterization of the serum lipoproteins and apoproteins in the mouse, *Mus musculus*. J Lipid Res 24: 1210–1228

23. Carlson LA, Froberg SO, Nye ER (1968) Effect of age on blood and tissue lipid levels in the male rat. Gerontologia 14: 65–79

24. Carroll KK (1978) The role of dietary protein in hypercholesterolemia and atherosclerosis. Lipids 13: 360–365

25. Carroll RM, Russell BS, Gard E, Feldman EB (1983) High density lipoprotein subfractions regulate serum levels in rhesus monkeys. Arterisosclerosis 3: 477a

26. Chan L, Jackson RL, O'Malley BW, Means AR (1976) Synthesis of very low density lipoproteins in the cockerel. J Clin Invest 58: 368–379

27. Chapman MJ (1980) Animal lipoproteins: Chemistry, structure, and comparative aspects. J Lipid Res 21: 789–853

28. Chapman MJ, Goldstein S, Laudot MH (1977) Characterization and comparative aspects of the seven very low and low density lipoproteins and their apoproteins in the chicken (*Gallus domesticus*). Biochemistry 46: 3006–3015

29. Charman RC, Landowne RA (1967) Separation of human plasma lipoproteins by electrophoresis on cellulose acetate. Anal Biochem 19: 177–179

30. Cho BHS, Eqwim PO, Fahey GC Jr (1985) Plasma lipid and lipoprotein cholesterol levels in swine. Atherosclerosis 56: 39–49

31. Chung BH, Wilkinson T, Geer JC, Segrest JP (1980) Preparative and quantitative isolation of plasma lipoproteins: Rapid, single discontinuous density gradient ultracentrifugation in a vertical rotor. J Lipid Res 21: 284–291

32. Chupukcharoen N, Komaratat P, Wilairat P (1985) Effects of vitamin E deficiency on the distribution of cholesterol in plasma lipoproteins and the activity of cholesterol 7α-hydroxylase in rabbit liver J Nutr 115: 468–472

33. Cooper GA, Smith SJ, Wiebe DA, Kuchmak M, Hannon WH (1985) International Survey of Apolipoproteins A-I and B measurements (1983–1984). Clin Chem 31: 223–228

34. Curry MD, Gustafson A, Alaupovic P, McConathy WJ (1978) Electroimmunoassay, radioimmunoassay and radial immunodiffusion assay evaluated for quantification of human apolipoprotein B. Clin Chem 24: 280–286

35. DeLalla O, Gofman J (1954) Ultracentrifugal analysis of serum lipoproteins. Methods Biochem Res 6: 2–63

36. Dole VP, Meinertz H (1960) Microdetermination of long-chain fatty acids in plasma and tissues. J Biol Chem 235: 2959–2599

37. Dury A, Diluzio NR (1955) Effects of cortisone and epinephrine exhibition on lipid components and phospholipid turnover in plasma, liver and aorta of rabbits. Am J Physiol 182: 45–50

38. Erschow AG, Nicolosi RJ, Hayes KC (1981) Separation of the dietary fat and cholesterol influences on plasma lipoproteins of rhesus monkeys. Am J Clin Nutr 34: 830–840

39. Feldman EB (1983) In Feldman EB (ed), Nutrition and Heart Disease, Contemporary Issues in Clinical Nutrition, Vol 6. Churchill-Livingstone, New York

40. Feldman EB (1983) In Feldman EB (ed), Nutrition in the Middle and Later Years. Wright-PSG, Boston

41. Feldman EB, Russell BS, Chen R, Johnson J, Forte T, Benett Clark S (1983) Dietary saturated fatty acid content affects lymph lipoproteins: Studies in the rat. J Lipid Res 24: 967–976

42. Feldman EB, Russell BS, Hawkins CB, Forte T (1983) Intestinal lymph lipoproteins in rats fed diets enriched in specific fatty acids. J Nutr 113: 2323–2334

43. Feldman EB, Russell BS, Schnare FH, Miles BC, Doyle EA, Moretti-Rojas I (1979) Effects of tristearin, triolein and safflower oil diets on cholesterol balance in rats. J Nutr 109: 2226–2236

44. Feldman EB, Russell BS, Schnare FH, Moretti-Rojas I, Miles BC, Doyle EA (1979) Effects of diets of homogeneous saturated triglycerides on cholesterol balance in rats. J Nutr 109: 2237–2246

45. Fless GM, Scanu AM (1975) Physiochemical characterization of rhesus low density lipoproteins. Biochemistry 14: 1783–1790

46. Fless GM, Wissler RW, Scanu AM (1976) Study of abnormal plasma low density lipoproteins in rhesus monkeys with diet-induced hyperlipidemia. Biochemistry 1: 5799–5805

47. Flow BL, Mott GE (1984) Relationship of high density lipoprotein cholesterol to cholesterol metabolism in the baboon (Papio sp.). J Lipid Res 25: 469–473

48. Folch J, Lees M, Sloane-Stanley GH (1957) A simple method for the isolation and purification of total lipids from animal tissues. J Biol Chem 226: 497–509

49. Forgez P, Chapman MJ, Rall SC Jr, Camus M-C (1984) The lipid transport system in the mouse, Mus musculus: Isolation and characterization of apolipoproteins B, A-I, A-II and C-III. J Lipid Res 25: 954–966

50. Forsythe WA, Miller ER, Curry B, Bennink MR (1981) Aerobic exercise effects on lipoproteins and tissue lipids in young pigs. Atherosclerosis 38: 327–337

51. Fredrickson DS, Levy RI, Lees RS (1967) Fat transport in lipoproteins—an integrated approach to mechanisms and disorders. New Engl J Med 276: 32–44

52. Gallo LL (1983) In Feldman EB (ed), Nutrition and Heart Disease, Contemporary Issues in Clinical Nutrition, Vol 6. Churchill-Livingstone, New York

53. Gard E, Feldman EB (1984) Final Report. Data analysis of lipids and lipoproteins in macaca mulatta (rhesus monkeys). NO1-HV-5-3031. Litton Bionetics, Inc., Kensington, MD

54. Goldstein S, Chapman MJ (1976) Comparative immunochemical studies of the serum low density lipoproteins in several animal species. Biochem Genet 41: 883–896

55. Hamilton RMG, Carroll KK (1976) Plasma cholesterol levels in rabbits fed low fat, low cholesterol diets. Atherosclerosis 24: 47–62

56. Hatch FT, Lees RS (1968) Practical methods for plasma lipoprotein analysis. Adv Lipid Res 6: 2–63

57. Havel RJ (1978) In Gotto AM Jr, Miller NE, Oliver MF (eds), High Density Lipoproteins and Atherosclerosis. Elsevier, New York

58. Havel RJ, Eder HA, Bragdon JH (1977) The distribution and chemical composition of ultracentrifugally separated lipoproteins in human serum. J Clin Invest 34: 1345–1353

59. Hearn V, Bensadoun A (1975) Plasma lipoproteins of the chicken, Gallus domesticus. Int J Biochem 6: 295–301

60. Hegsted DM, Andrus SB, Gotsis A, Portman OW (1957) The quantitative effects of cholesterol, cholic acid and type of fat on serum cholesterol and vascular sudanophilia in the rat. J Nutr 63: 273–288

61. Hillyard LA, Entenman C, Chaikoff IL (1956) Concentration and composition of serum lipoproteins of cholesterol-fed and stilbestrol-injected birds. J Biol Chem 223: 359–368

62. Hollanders B, Mougin A, Diaye F, Hentz E, Aude X, Girard A (1986) Comparison of the lipoprotein profiles obtained from rat, bovine, horse, dog, rabbit and pig serum by a new two-step ultracentrifugal gradient procedure. Comp Biochem Physiol 84: 83–89

63. Illingworth DR, Portman OW (1973) Secretion of newly synthesized apo low density lipoprotein (LDL) into the plasma of squirrel monkeys. Circulation 47–48,(suppl IV); 111

64. Jackson RL, Lin H-Y, Chan L, Means AR (1976) Isolation and characterization of the major apo lipoprotein from chicken high density lipoproteins. Biochim Biophys Acta 420: 342–349

65. Jackson RL, Lin H-Y, Chan L, Means AR (1977) Amino acid sequence of a major apoprotein from hen plasma very low density lipoproteins. J Biol Chem 252: 250–253

66. Jacobsson L (1986) Comparison of experimental hypercholesterolemia and atherosclerosis in Göttingen minipigs and swedish domestic swine. Atherosclerosis 59: 205–213

67. Jeffery F, Redgrave TH (1982) Chylomicron catabolism differs between hooded and albino laboratory rats. J Lipid Res 23: 154–160

68. Kelley JL, Alaupovic P (1976) Lipid transport in the avian species. Part 1. Isolation and characterization of apolipoproteins and major lipoprotein density classes of male turkey serum. Atherosclerosis 24: 155–175

69. Kellogg TF (1974) Steroid balance and tissue cholesterol accumulation in germ-free and conventional rats fed diets containing saturated and polyunsaturated fats. J Lipid Res 15: 574–579

70. Kim DN, Lee KT, Reiner JM, Thomas WA (1974) Restraint of cholesterol accumulation in tissue pools associated with drastic short-term lowering of serum cholesterol levels by clofibrate or cholestyramine in hypercholesterolemic swine. J Lipid Res 15: 326–331

71. Kim JJ, Hamilton RMG, Carroll KK (1976) Effects of diet on catabolism and excretion of [26-^{14}C] cholesterol in rats. Can J Biochem 54: 272–279

72. Kim KS, Ivy AC (1952) Factors influencing cholesterol absorption. Am J Physiol 171: 302–318

73. Kritchevsky D (1983) In Feldman EB (eds), Nutrition and Heart Disease, Contemporary Issues in Clinical Nutrition, Vol 6. Churchill-Livingstone, New York

74. Kruski AW, Narayan KA (1973) The effect of dietary supplementation of cholesterol and its subsequent withdrawal on the liver lipids and serum lipoproteins of chickens. Lipids 7: 742–749

75. Kruski AW, Scanu Am (1975) Properties of rooster serum high density lipoprotein. Biochim Biophys Acta 409: 26–38

76. Kushwaha RS, Barnwell GM, Carey KD, McGill HC Jr (1986) Metabolism of apolipoprotein B in selectively bred baboons with low and high levels of low density lipoproteins. J Lipid Res 27: 497–507

77. Lasser NL, Roheim PS, Edelstein D, Eder HA (1973) Serum lipoproteins of normal and cholesterol-fed rats. J Lipid Res 14: 1–8

78. Leathers CW, Bond MG, Bullock BC, Rudel LL (1981) Dietary ethanol and cholesterol in *Macaca nemestrina* serum lipid and hepatic changes. Exp Mol Pathol 35: 285–299

79. Lee JA, Morris MD (1976) The effect of cholesterol feeding on primate serum lipoproteins. I. Low density lipoprotein characterization from rhesus monkeys with high serum cholesterol. Biochem Med 16: 116–126

80. Lefevre M, Keen CL, Lonnerdal B, Hurley LS, Schneeman BO (1985) Different effects of zinc and copper deficiency on composition of plasma high density lipoproteins in rats. J Nutr 115: 359–368

81. Lindgren FT, Freeman NK, Ewing AM (1967) Ultracentrifugal analysis of serum lipoprotein. Prog Biochem Pharmacol 2: 475–599

82. Lindgren FT, Jensen LC, Hatch FT (1972) In Nelson GJ (eds), Blood Lipids and Lipoproteins: Quantitation, Composition, and Metabolism. Wiley-Interscience, New York

83. Lofland HB, St. Clair RW, MacNintch JE, Pritchard RW (1967) Atherosclerosis in New World primates: Biochemical studies. Arch Pathol 83: 211–214

84. Lovati MR, Franceschini G, Allievi L, Dall Aglio E, Zavaroni I, Sirtori CR (1986) Endogenous hypertriglyceridemia in a nonobese rat model: Plasma lipoproteins and dietary sensitivity. Metabolism 35: 436–440

85. Lusk LT, Walker LF, Dubien LH, Getz GS (1979) Isolation and partial characterization of high density lipoprotein HDL$_1$ from rat plasma by gradient centrifugation. Biochem J 183: 83–90

86. McGill HC Jr, McMahon CA, Kushwaha RS, Mott GE, Carey KD (1986) Dietary effects on serum lipoproteins of dyslipoproteinemic baboons with high HDL. Arteriosclerosis 6: 651–663

87. Mahley RW (1978) In Dietschy JM, Gotto AM Jr, Oniko JA (eds), Disturbances in Lipid and Lipoprotein Metabolism. American Physiological Society, Bethesda, MD

88. Mahley RW, Holcombe KS (1977) Alteration of the plasma lipoproteins and apoproteins following cholesterol feeding in the rat. J Lipid Res 18: 314–324

89. Mahley, RW, Weisgraber KH (1974) Canine lipoproteins and atherosclerosis. I. Isolation and characterization of plasma lipoproteins from control dogs. Circ Res 35: 713–721

90. Mahley RW, Weisgraber KH, Innerarity T (1974) Canine lipoproteins and atherosclerosis. II. Characterization of the plasma lipoproteins associated with atherogenic and nonatherogenic hyperlipidemia. Circ Res 35: 722–733

91. Mahley RW, Weisgraber KH, Innerarity T (1976) Atherogenic hyperlipoproteinemia induced by cholesterol feeding in the patas monkey. Biochemistry 15: 2979–2985

92. Mahley RW, Weisgraber KH, Innerarity T, Brewer HB Jr, Assmann G (1975) Swine lipoproteins and atherosclerosis. Changes in the plasma lipoproteins and apoproteins induced by cholesterol feeding. Biochemistry 14: 2817–2823

93. Mancini G, Carbonara AO, Heremans JF (1965) Immunochemical quantitation of antigens by single radial immunodiffusion. Intern J Immunochem 2: 235–254

94. Manual of Laboratory Operations, Lipid Research Clinics Program, Lipid and Lipoprotein Analysis, DHEW Publication No. (NIH) 75–628 (1972)

95. Marsh A, Kim DN, Lee KT, Reiner JM, Thomas WA (1972) Cholesterol turnover, synthesis and retention in hypercholesterolemic growing swine. J Lipid Res 13: 600–615

96. Massaro ER, Zilversmit DB (1977) Controlling factors in the maintenance of plasma cholesterol concentration in the rabbit. J Nutr 107: 596–605

97. McCulllagh KG, Ehrhart LA, Bittkus A (1976) Experimental canine atherosclerosis and its prevention. Lab Invest 34: 394–405

98. McGill HC, Mott GE, Kuehl TJ (1980) In Lauer RM, Shekelle RB (eds), Childhood Prevention of Atherosclerosis and Hypertension. Raven Press, New York

99. McGovern RF, Quackenbush FW (1973) Influence of dietary fat on bile acid secretion of rats after portal injection of ^{3}H-cholesterol and [4-^{14}C] cholesteryl esters. Lipids 8: 473–478

100. McMahan MR, Rhyne AL, Lofland HB, Sackett GP (1980) Effects of sex, age and dietary modification on plasma lipids and lipoproteins of *Macaca nemestrina*. Proc Soc Exp Biol Med 164: 27–34

101. McNamara DJ, Proca A, Edwards KDG (1982) Cholesterol homeostasis in rats fed a purified diet. Biochim Biophys Acta 711: 252–260

102. Melchior GW, Baker HN, Abee CR, Roheim PS (1984) Density gradient characterization of the high density lipoproteins in cholesterol-fed-hyper- and

hyporesponding patas monkeys Erythrocebius patas). J Lipid Res 25: 979–990

103. Mercer NJH, Holub BJ (1979) Response of free and esterified plasma cholesterol levels in the mongolian gerbil to the fatty acid composition of dietary lipid. Lipids 14: 1009–1014

104. Mills GL, Taylaur CE (1971) The distribution and composition of serum lipoproteins in eighteen animals. Comp Biochem Physiol 40B: 489 501

105. Morrisett JD, Kim HS, Patsch JR, Datta SK, Trentin JJ (1982) Genetic susceptibility and resistance to diet-induced atherosclerosis and hyperlipoproteinemia. Arteriosclerosis 2: 312–324

106. Morrisett JD, Pownall HJ, Jackson RL, Gotto AM Jr, Taunton OD (1977) Effects of polyunsaturated and saturated fat diets on chemical composition and thermotropic properties of human plasma lipoproteins. American Oil Chemists Society, Champaign

107. Nagaoka S, Masaki H, Aoyama Y, Yoshida A (1986) Effects of excess dietary tyrosine or certain xenobiotics on the cholesterogenesis in rats. J Nutr 116: 726–732

108. Narayan KA, Creinin HL, Kummerow FA (1966) Disc electrophoresis of rat plasma lipoproteins. J Lipid Res 7: 150 157

109. Nath N, Wiener R, Harper AE, Elvehjem CA (1957) Diet and cholesterolemia. J Nutr 63: 289–307

110. Nelson CA, Morris MD (1977) Effects of cholesterol feeding on primate serum lipoproteins. II. Low density lipoprotein characterization from rhesus monkeys with a moderate rise in serum cholesterol. Biochem Med 17: 320–332

111. Nelson GJ (1972) In Nelson GH (ed), Blood Lipids and Lipoproteins: Quantitation, Composition, and Metabolism. Wiley-Interscience, New York

112. Nicolosi RJ, Marlett JA, Morello AM, Flanagan SA, Hegsted DM (1981) Influence of dietary unsaturated and saturated fat on the plasma lipoproteins of Mongolian gerbils. Atherosclerosis 38: 359–371

113. Noble RP (1968) Electrophoretic separation of plasma lipoprotein in agarose gel. J Lipid Res 9: 693–700

114. Parks JS, Rudel LL (1979) Isolation and characterization of high density lipoprotein apoproteins in the non-human primate (vervet). J Biol Chem 254: 6716–6723

115. Parks JS, Rudel LL (1985) Alteration of high density lipoprotein subfraction distribution with induction of serum amyloid A protein (SAA) in the nonhuman primate. J Lipid Res 26: 82–91

116. Pasquali-Ronchetti I, Calandra S, Baccarani-Contri M, Montagriti M (1975) The ultrastructure of rat plasma lipoproteins. J Ultrastructure Res 53: 180–192

117. Pond WG, Yen J-T, Mersmann HJ, Haschek WM (1986) Comparative effects of dietary protein and cholesterol-fat content on genetically lean and obese pigs. J Nutr 116: 1116–1124

118. Prescott MF, Muller KR (1983) Endothelial regeneration in hypertensive and genetically hypercholesterolemic rats. Arteriosclerosis 3: 206–214

119. Radding CM, Steinberg D (1960) Studies on the synthesis and secretion of serum lipoprotein by rat liver slices. J Clin Invest 39: 1560–1569

120. Rayssiguier Y, Gueux E (1986) Magnesium and lipids in cardiovascular disease. J Am Coll Nutr 5: 507–519

121. Reiser R, Williams MC, Sorrels MF, Murty NL (1965) Dietary myristate and plasma cholesterol concentration. J Am Oil Chem Soc 42: 1155

122. Roberts DCK, Huff MW, Carroll KK (1979) Influence of diet on plasma cholesterol concentrations in suckling and weanling rabbits. Nutr Metab 23: 476–486

123. Rodriguez JL, Chiselli GC, Torreggiani D, Sirtori CR (1976) Very low density lipoproteins in normal and cholesterol-fed rabbits: Lipid and protein composition and metabolism. Atherosclerosis 23: 73–83

124. Rosseneu M, Declercq B, Vandamme D, Vercaenst R, Soeteway F, Peeters H, Blaton V (1979) Influence of oral polyunsaturated and saturated phospholipid treatment on the lipid composition and fatty acid profile of chimpanzee lipoproteins. Atherosclerosis 32: 141–153

125. Roth RI, Gaubahz JW, Gotto AM Jr, Patsch JR (1983) Effect of cholesterol feeding on the distribution of plasma lipoproteins and on the metabolism of apolipoprotein E in the rabbit. J Lipid Res 24: 1–11

126. Rothfeld B, Karmen A, Hunter C (1970) Some effects of CPIB in the rat. Biochem Med 3: 344–354

127. Rudel LL, Greene DG, Shah R (1977) Separation and characterization of plasma lipoproteins of rhesus monkeys (Macaca mulata). J Lipid Res 18: 734–744

128. Rudel LL, Lee JA, Morris MD, Felts JM (1974) Characterization of plasma lipoproteins separated and purified by agarose column chromatography. Biochem J 139: 89–95

129. Rudel LL, Lofland H (1976) Circulating lipoproteins in nonhuman primates. Primate Med 9: 224–266

130. Rudel LL, Pitts LL II (1978) Male-female variability in the dietary cholesterol-induced hyperlipoproteinemia of cynomolgus monkeys (Macaca fascicularis). J Lipid Res 19: 992–1003

131. Rudel LL, Reynolds JA, Bullock BC (1981) Nutritional effects on blood lipid and HDL cholesterol concentrations in two subspecies of African green monkeys (Cercopithecus aethiops). J Lipid Res 22: 278–285

132. Rudel LL, Shah R, Greene DG (1979) Study of atherogenic dyslipoproteinemia induced by dietary cholesterol in rhesus monkeys (Macaca mulatta). J Lipid Res 20: 55–65

133. Sampson EG, Demers LM, Kreig AF (1975) Faster enzymatic procedure for serum triglycerides. Clin Chem 21: 1983

134. Sathanur R, Radhakrishnamurthy B, DalFeres E Jr, Berenson G (1979) Serum α-lipoprotein responses to variation in dietary cholesterol, protein, and carbohydrate in different nonhuman primate species. Lipids 14: 559–565

135. Scanu AM, Edelstein C, Vitello L, Jones R, Wissler R (1973) The serum high density lipoproteins of Macaca rhesus. I. Isolation, composition and properties. J Biol Chem 248: 7648–7652

136. Scanu AM, Edelstein C, Wolf RH (1974) Chim-

panzee (*Pan troglodytes*) serum high density lipoproteins. Isolation and properties of their two major
apolipoproteins. Biochim Biophys Acta 351: 341–
347

137. Schonfeld G, Lees RS, George PK, Pfleger B (1974)
Assay of total plasma apolipoprotein B concentration in human subjects. J Clin Invest 53: 1458–
1467

138. Sharma C, Srinivasan SR, Radhakrishnamurthy B,
Berenson GS (1981) Effect of exogenous cholesterol
on plasma lipids and hepatic enzymes in rabbits fed
different carbohydrate diets. Biochem Med 26: 249–
257

139. Sherrill BC (1980) Rapid hepatic clearance of the
canine lipoproteins containing only the E apoprotein by a high affinity receptor. J Biol Chem 255:
1804–1807

140. Skipski VP, Peterson RF, Barclay M (1964) Quantitative analysis of phospholipids by thin-layer chromatography. Biochem J 90: 374–378

141. Stange E, Agostini B, Papenberg J (1975) Changes
in rabbit lipoprotein properties by dietary cholesterol, and saturated and polyunsaturated fats.
Atherosclerosis 22: 125–148

142. Story JA, Czarnecki SK, Tepper SA, Kirtchevsky
D (1981) Dose response to dietary cholesterol in the
rat. Nutr Rep Int 24: 465–470

143. Tanzawa K, Shimada Y, Kuroda M, Tsujita Y,
Arai M, Watanabe W (1980) WHHD-rabbit, a low
density lipoprotein receptor-deficient animal model
for familial hypercholesterolemia. FEBS Letts 118:
81–84

144. Thomas WA, Jones R, Scott RF, Morrison E,
Goodale F, Imai H (1963) Production of early
atherosclerotic lesions in rats characterized by proliferation of "modified smooth muscle cells." Exp
Mol pathol Suppl 1: 40–61

145. Van Handel E, Zilversmit DB (1957) Micromethod
for the direct determination of serum triglycerides.
J Lab Clin Med 50P: 152–157

146. Warnick GR, Cheung MC, Albers JJ (1979) Comparison of current methods for high density lipoprotein cholesterol quantitation. Clin Chem 25:
596–604

147. Warnick GR, Mayfield C, Albers JJ, Hazzard WR
(1979) Gel isoelectric focusing method for specific
diagnosis of familial hyperlipoproteinemia type 3.
Clin Chem 25: 279–284

148. Watanabe Y (1980) Serial inbreeding of rabbits with
hereditary hyperlipidemia (WHHL-rabbit). Atherosclerosis 36: 261–268

149. Weber K, Osborn M (1969) The reliability of molecular weight determinations by dodecyl sulfate polyacrylamide gel electrophoresis. J Biol Chem 244:
4406–4411

150. Weiner BH, Ockene IA, Levine PH, Cuenoud HF,
Fisher M, Johnson BF, Daoud AS et al (1986) Inhibition of atherosclerosis by cod-liver oil in a hyperlipidemic swine model. New Engl J Med 315: 841–
846

151. Wichman A (1979) Affinity chromatography of
human plasma low- and high-density lipoproteins.
Biochem J 181: 691–698

152. Wilson JN, Wilson SP, Eaton RP (1984) Dietary
fiber and lipoprotein metabolism in the genetically
obese Zucker rat. Arterisclerosis 4: 147–153

153. Young NL, McNamara DJ, Saudek CD, Krasovsky
J, Lopez DR, Levy G (1983) Hyperphagia alters
cholesterol dynamics in diabetic rats. Diabetes 32:
811–819

154. Yu JY-L, Campbell LD, Marquardt RR (1976)
Immunological and compositional patterns of lipo-
proteins in chicken (*Gallus domesticus*) plasma.
Poultry Sci 55: 1626–1631

155. Zannis VI, Breslow JL (1979) Characterization of a
unique human apolipoprotein E variant associated
with type III hyperlipoproteinemia. J Biol Chem
255: 1759–1762

10

Specific Proteins

PREFACE

In this chapter, the discussion of specific proteins is organized into four sections based primarily on function: Immunoglobulins, the Complement System, Transport Proteins, and Acute Phase Reactants. Occasionally, a protein fills more than one functional category; however, for the sake of brevity, these will be discussed in only one section but comments will be made on those characteristics that a particular protein shares with proteins of another section. The Transport Protein section does not include a discussion of ceruloplasmin, which is represented in the section on Acute Phase Reactants. Haptoglobulin and certain complement components (C3, C4, C2, and Factor B) are acute phase reactants covered in the sections Transport Proteins and the Complement System, respectively. In each section, the author(s) explores the molecular biology, biosynthesis, function, analysis, and interpretation of each protein; however, the style of individual authors varies slightly.

The quantitation of many of the specific proteins to be discussed is not standard practice in most laboratory animal clinical pathology laboratories despite the fact that they are commonly measured and aid in the diagnosis of human disease. The careful characterization and quantitation of these proteins in animals, associated with previous research activities, allow them to be easily integrated by the veterinary clinical chemist into the diagnostic laboratory.

Investigations involving living animals are being scrutinized with increasing emphasis on maximizing the amount of data collected on individual animals and reducing the number of experimental subjects. The measurement of various specific proteins in research protocols, particularly those easily quantitated using micromethodology, may document more completely the pathogenesis of various diseases, extend the range of body systems potentially at risk from injury by unknown (toxic) substances, and allow investigators to monitor individual animals and predict a fatal outcome before clinical signs become obvious.

As will be seen on numerous occasions, naturally occurring deficiencies, mutations, and neoplasms in laboratory animals have precipitated research that has added significantly to our current body of knowledge and in some instances has directly benefited animal and man.

A. Immunoglobulins

RICHARD B. BANKERT, VMD, PhD and PAUL K. MAZZAFERRO, PhD

BIOCHEMISTRY OF IMMUNOGLOBULINS

General Considerations

Immunoglobulins from all species possessing such molecules share some common structural features. (For a review see reference 148.) The basic functional unit consists of four polypeptide chains (two light and two heavy chains) linked by interchain disulfide bridges. Each chain can be further subdivided into structural domains, each containing at least one intrachain disulfide bond. The domain containing the amino-terminus of each polypeptide chain is termed the variable-region domain, and the domains subsequent to this are referred to as constant-region domains. The ligand-binding ability of immunoglobulins resides within the variable portion of the polypeptide chains. The diversity of amino acid sequences found within this region of the polypeptide chains (both H and L) accounts for the great variability in antigen-binding specificities exhibited by immunoglobulins. In contrast, the constant-region domains, so named because of their relatively constant amino acid composition between immunoglobulins of different specificities, mediate other effector functions associated with the immunoglobulin molecule such as complement fixation, protein A binding, opsonization, placental/intestinal transport, passive cutaneous anaphylaxis and attachment to mast cells, basophils, macrophages, and lymphocytes. (For a review see reference 110.)

Immunoglobulin heavy chains are composed of four to five domains including the variable-region domain. Heavy chains have been further classified on the basis of different structural determinants located in the constant-region domains. Five basic classes or isotypes (IgM, IgG, IgA, IgE, and IgD) have been defined and are represented in most of the species to be discussed. In contrast, immunoglobulin light chains are composed of only two structural domains and are classified as the kappa or lambda type chain; again, this classification is based on determinants found in the constant region of the polypeptide chain. Various aspects of these heavy and light chain isotypes will be discussed as they pertain to individual species of laboratory animals.

Much of the recent information on the structural aspects of immunoglobulin molecules has come from the laboratories of molecular geneticists studying the immunoglobulin gene. Most of the work in this area was done on either mouse or human lymphocytes. Because the human work (92,175) corroborates that in the mouse, the mouse system (3,95) will be used as a general example of the structure of immunoglobulin genes.

Immunoglobulins are composed of only two different polypeptide chains (heavy and light

118

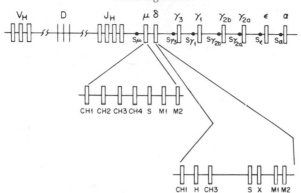

Figure 10.A.1. Diagram of murine immunoglobulin heavy-chain gene loci. The variable (V_H), diversity (D), junction (J_H), and constant-region genes (μ, δ, γ, ε, α) are shown within these loci. The μ and δ constant-region portions are expanded to show individual coding segments for the protein domains (CH1–CH3,4), the hinge (H) region, and membrane (M1,M2) and secreted (S,γ) tail pieces of the immunoglobulin molecule. Also shown are the switch sites ($S\mu$,$S\gamma3$), which allow placement of VDJ gene segments adjacent to the various heavy-chain gene regions.

chains); however, at the genetic level the genes encoding these polypeptides are highly segmented (Figure 10.A.1). Figure 10.A.1 demonstrates that each domain is coded for by one or more segments of DNA, with special purpose areas such as the hinge region or the hydrophobic tail of immunoglobulin (allowing insertion into the membrane) also encoded by separate gene segments. The heavy chain variable-region domain is encoded by three separate minigene segments (V_H, D, and J_H) in the germline DNA. The V_H and D regions of DNA contain many different minigene segments that can be used to construct the variable-region domain, whereas the J_H region contains only four possible segments for use. Sometime during maturation of the B-lymphocyte a recombinational event occurs at the level of the DNA to join one V_H segment with one D segment and one J_H segment to form a functional VDJ minigene adjacent to the mu minigene segment (Figure 10.A.2). Other rearrangements of the genome also can occur to place the VDJ segment close to other heavy chain constant-region minigenes (isotype switching). The VDJ and constant-region segments are joined at the level of transcription by RNA splicing to remove the intervening sequences of RNA between individual segments.

The light chain genes have a similar structural basis with the exception that a D-region segment has not been described, so that only a VJ recombination occurs at the DNA level (18,30,184,185,209).

Isolation of Immunoglobulins

The isolation of immunoglobulin G and M from the serum of animals has classically been performed using a combination of ion-exchange chromatography and gel permeation chromatography often on an immunoglobulin fraction precipitated from the serum with either ammonium or sodium sulfate (88,89,109). Good separation of rabbit (126), guinea pig (123), and hamster (38,39) IgG/IgM can be obtained with these procedures, including separation of the IgG subclasses. Mouse (55,56), rat (21,132), and dog (217) IgG and IgM can be separated by similar procedures, although incomplete separation of the IgG subclasses may occur, especially that of the IgG2a and IgG2b subclasses of the mouse which are notoriously similar in structure (57). The IgA class can also be isolated by similar techniques and elutes later than IgG from a DEAE ion-exchange column. However, because of the low concentration of this isotype in the serum, often colostrum, milk, or other secretion products are used as the starting material from which IgA is isolated (37,107,207). As is commonly done with the other isotypes, immunoglobulins E and D cannot be isolated in pure form from the serum because of their low concentrations and elution properties from DEAE and gel permeation columns (80,102,162,183,194). Consequently, these isotypes have been isolated in pure form only when specific gammopathies (ie, IgE or IgD myelomas) have made available a relatively large

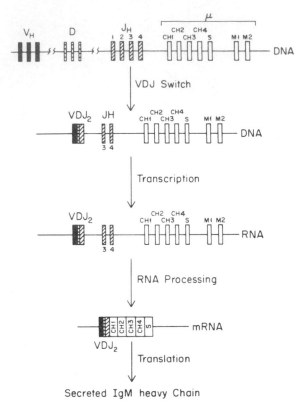

Figure 10.A.2. Diagram of events occurring at the DNA and RNA level leading to formation of an IgM molecule. Nascent DNA undergoes a rearrangement early in the development of B-cells to yield a VDJ gene combination. The DNA is then transcribed into a precursor RNA molecule, which undergoes further processing and removal of intervening sequences between the VDJ gene segment and the various constant-region genes. The mRNA product is then translated into its protein product, in this case a secreted IgM molecule.

amount of either isotype in the serum of the animal.

Immunoglobulin Light Chains

Two classes of light chain molecules have been described for most of the vertebrate species: the kappa and lambda isotypes. Their distribution among different species is shown in Table 10.A.1. The molecular weight of the light chains from a variety of species has been calculated to be between 20,000 and 25,000 (93). Structurally, the light chains from phylogenetically related species (ie, primates) are similar on the basis of their cross-reactivities with antisera raised against a single species within the same order (93). Immunodiffusion analysis of cross-reactivity between anti-human L-chain antisera and rhesus monkey or chimpanzee light chains showed commonalities among the light chains.

Similar cross-reactivities between other primate species have been noted using light chain inhibition of radioimmune precipitation assays (194). The degree of cross-reactivity followed the phylogenetic relatedness of the species tested. Similar structural correlates of relatedness have been noted by Hood et al (93) following peptide and sequence analysis of light chains from a variety of species including the dog, cat, mouse, guinea pig, rat, baboon, and human. Additionally, disc polyacrylamide gel electrophoresis of light chains from different animal species showed the same heterogeneity of banding patterns (six to eight bands), indicating their structural relatedness (39).

Immunoglobulin G

This isotype exhibits the greatest degree of diversity with respect to the number of subclasses

Table 10.A.1. Expression of Kappa and Lambda Immunoglobulin Light Chain Isotypes in the Sera of Various Species[a]

| Order | Species | Percentage of Light Chains in the Serum | |
		Kappa	Lambda
Lagomorpha	Rabbit	70–90	10–30
Rodentia	Mouse	95	5
	Rat	95	5
	Guinea pig	70	30
Carnivora	Dog	10	90
	Cat	10	90
Primates	Human	70	30
	Rhesus	50	50
	Baboon	50	50
Perissodactyla	Horse	5	95
	Mule	5	95

[a] Data derived from Grant JA, Saunders B, Hood L (1971) Biochemistry 10: 3123, and Hood L, Grant JA, Sox HC (1969). In Steryl J, Riha I (eds) Developmental Aspects of Antibody Formation and Structure, Vol 1. Academic Press, New York, p 283.

defined for each species. Four subclasses have been defined for human, dog, mouse, rat, and horse IgG, whereas rabbit, hamster, and guinea pig have only two known subclasses. Nonhuman primates also probably have four distinct subclasses of IgG similar to human immunoglobulins. Antisera specific for the four human subclasses have identified similar molecules in the sera of chimpanzees, gorillas, and orangutans (4,5,215). However, gibbons and all lower primates did not share determinants with human immunoglobulins which were recognized by the antihuman antisera (210). Baboons were shown to possess four IgG subclasses based on antigenic differences in the Ig heavy chain localized to the Fc region of the molecule (45). These determinants were not shared with human immunoglobulins, but they were found on immunoglobulin from other ceropothecid monkeys including the mandrill, gelada, and talapoin (46).

The classes and subclasses of immunoglobulins from a variety of species are shown in Table 10.A.2. and arranged for comparison with their human Ig counterparts. In general, structural and functional correlates of the human Ig subclasses can be found in the other species; however, some species appear to lack specific subclasses that can be correlated with their human IgG counterparts.

All of the IgGs share similar structural and biochemical characteristics. They are composed of two light and two heavy chains and exist in the serum in monomeric form (7S). The heavy chains are joined by interchain disulfide bridges. Guinea pig and mouse IgG have three such linkages between the heavy chains, whereas the rabbit IgG has only a single disulfide link similar to that found in human IgM and IgD. However, IgG from other species may be more variable in the number of interchain disulfide bridges as evidenced by the human IgG subclasses which have 2 to 15 such linkages between the chains (151).

The intact IgG molecules can be cleaved by various enzymes to yield specific peptide fragments. Treatment with papain cleaves the IgG molecule into three fragments of approximately equal molecular weight (45 to 50 K). Two of the fragments formed contain an intact antigen-binding region (light-chain plus two heavy-chain domains) and are termed the Fab portion of the molecule. The third fragment is termed the Fc portion and is composed entirely of heavy-chain domains from the carboxy-terminal end of the molecule. The Fc portion of rabbit immunoglobulins, isolated in this way, were found to crystallize from solution, indicating the homogeneity of the product (170). The Fc portion from guinea pig IgG also gives crystallizable fragments (153); however, Fc regions from other species including dog, mouse, and rat do not easily crystallize from solution. This finding is not unexpected because the various IgG subclasses have been shown to bear subclass-specific determinants in their Fc regions while expressing common determinants in their Fab portions (9,38,137,202); thus, Fc fragments prepared from the aforementioned species would be somewhat heterogeneous and not likely to crystallize easily. In contrast, rabbit IgG is composed almost entirely of a single IgG subclass (IgG1) and therefore would yield a very homogeneous preparation of Fc fragments for crystallization.

Pepsin treatment of IgG from most species, including the rabbit (149,150), guinea pig (154), hamster (38), and human (151), yields a single large fragment termed $F(ab')_2$ (mol wt 95 Kilodaltons (Kd)) which includes the hinge region for the original molecule and some smaller fragments of the Fc portion of the molecule that are nonfunctional and are not rec-

Table 10.A.2. Classes and Subclasses of Immunoglobulins

Species	Immunoglobulin Class and Subclass				
Human	IgG1, IgG2, IgG3, IgG4	IgA1, IgA2	IgM1, IgM2	IgE	IgD
Ape	IgG[a]	IgA	IgM	IgE	IgD
Monkey	IgG[b]	IgA	IgM[c]	IgE	IgD
Mouse	IgG2a, IgG2b, IgG3, IgG1	IgA1, IgA2	IgM	IgE	IgD
Rat	IgG2a, IgG2b, IgG2c, IgG1	IgA	IgM	IgE	IgD
Hamster	IgG2, -[d], -, IgG1	IgA	IgM	IgE	...
Guinea pig	IgG2, -, -, IgG1	IgA	IgM	IgE	...
Rabbit	IgG2, -, -, IgG1	IgA1, IgA2	IgM	IgE	IgD
Dog	IgG2a, IgG2b, IgG2c, IgG1	IgA	IgM	IgE	...

Source: Adopted from Wang AC (1976) In Fudenberg HH, Stites DP, Caldwell JL, Wells JV (eds) Basic and Clinical Immunology, Lange, Los Altos, CA.

[a] Using antisera specific for human subclasses, four corresponding subclasses have been identified in the chimpanzee, gorilla, and orangutan.

[b] Four subclasses have been identified in the baboon based on γ-chain differences; however, these determinants are not shared with the human subclasses.

[c] Two distinct types have been reported in the rhesus monkey after immunization.

[d] Hyphen indicates the absence of a subclass corresponding to the human IgG subclasses.

ognized by Fc-specific antisera. However, mouse IgG was shown to be sensitive to treatment with pepsin and does not give a high yield of the F(ab')$_2$ fragment; instead, the molecule is digested into smaller fragments. This sensitivity to pepsin digestion is presumed to reflect unfolding or denaturation of the molecule caused by the low pH required for proteolytic activity of the enzyme (73).

The various IgG subclasses have been defined using subclass-specific antisera; however, they also differ in their functional properties (to be discussed later) and in some of their biochemical properties. Hamster (38) and guinea pig (16) IgG migrates as a slow and a fast component in electrophoresis. Immunochemical analysis of these bands has shown them to be the IgG2 and IgG1 subclasses, respectively. The dog (107), rat (21,22), and mouse (57,58) immunoglobulins, each having four IgG subclasses, show a more complex banding pattern after electrophoresis. The IgG1 molecule of each species migrates the fastest, whereas the IgG2a and IgG2b molecules migrate the slowest and are inseparable with this technique.

The IgG1 (IgGd) subclass of the dog differs from the IgG of other species in that this molecule will not cause precipitation of multideterminant antigens from solution. This unique property is shared with the IgGT subclass found in the horse; however, structural analysis of both molecules does not show any commonality to account for this property (74).

Immunoglobulin M

Immunoglobulin M or γ macroglobulin from all species exists as a pentamer of the basic 7S subunit characteristic of immunoglobulins. This 19S molecule has a molecular weight in the range of 900,000 to 1,000,000. The 7S chains are linked by a J-chain disulfide bonded to the penultimate half-cystine residue of the heavy chains (136). Classically, the IgM structure can be broken into its component parts by reduction of the J-chain disulfide links with 2-mercaptoethanol. The 7S unit of IgM is characteristically heavier than its IgG counterpart, having a molecular weight of 190,000 daltons (d) (8,39,58,107,116,117,123). This is due in part to the IgM molecule containing an extra heavy-chain domain (four heavy-chain domains in IgG, five in IgM) and to the higher proportion of carbohydrate associated with the heavy chain (10 to 11 per cent carbohydrate for IgM vs 2 to 3 per cent for IgG) (151). This higher content of carbohydrate allows IgM to be separated from IgG by a lentil lectin affinity column which preferentially binds the IgM molecules. Proteolytic digestion of IgM with papain or pepsin will yield Fab and F(ab')$_2$ fragments, respectively, as found for IgG; however, the Fc portion is usually digested and cannot be isolated in an intact form as with IgG (179).

The J chain is associated with IgM molecules from most species including the human, dog, rabbit, mouse, horse, guinea pig, and rat. (For a review see reference 44.) The molecular weight of the J chain is between 14,000 and 16,000 d depending on the species from which it is isolated and the procedure used for analysis (44). The J chain also has been shown to be a highly conserved molecule throughout the vertebrates. There is a high degree of sequence homology and cross-reactivity of anti-J chain antisera between widely divergent species.

IgM has been found in virtually all vertebrates tested and is thought to be the most evolutionarily conserved immunoglobulin class. Generally, this class does not show any subclass diversity; however, human IgM is known to exhibit two forms (IgM1 and IgM2) and it has been suggested that the rhesus monkey may also have two forms of IgM (116).

Immunoglobulin A

This immunoglobulin class is primarily found in bodily secretions such as saliva, bile, colostrum/milk, and tears. Furthermore, the predominant phenotype of lymphoid cells found in the lamina propria is that of the IgA-containing B-cell. The serum form of IgA exists as a four-chain 7S monomer (mol wt 150,000 d) or as polymers of this basic unit in association with the J chain (mol wt 15,000 d) (44). The secreted form is typically a dimer (or larger polymer) of the 7S monomer linked by both a J chain and a secretory component (SC, mol wt 70,000 d). The J chain is structurally the same as that associated with IgM and binds the IgA molecule at the penultimate half-cystine on the heavy chains. The secretory component, which has a high carbohydrate content (15 to 20 per cent), is also associated with the heavy chains; however, the exact location of this association is not clear. The secretory component is derived from a transmembrane protein expressed on the surface of epithelial cells (139,140). This protein has structural homologies with the immunoglobulin molecule (141,219) and is used to transport IgA or IgM from the basolateral surface of the cell, across the intracellular matrix (as an endocytotic vesicle), to the luminal surface where a proteolytic event cleaves the protein yielding the soluble secretory piece in association with the polymeric immunoglobulin molecules (144,145,176,189,199). In most species the secretory component is disulfide bonded to the IgA molecule; however, in the rabbit there is strong evidence that there is only a non-covalent association of the chains for some IgA molecules, albeit a strong association (37,81,204). Rat (24) and hamster (19,78) IgA may lack a secretory component as indicated by immunochemical studies. However, biochemical evidence (ie, a larger sedimentation coefficient and resistance to reduction with 2-mercaptoethanol) suggests that IgA from these species contains a secretory component as well. Polymers of the basic 7S molecules were demonstrated in the secretions of both rats and hamsters. A 15.2S molecule, similar to that found in human urine (20) also was isolated from the external secretions of hamsters (19). Dog, mouse, guinea pig, and primate (baboon and rhesus monkey) IgA appears to have properties similar to those of human IgA both structurally and in the heterogeneity of electrophoretic patterns that can be obtained. Serum IgA in the dog exists as an 11S dimer; this is unlike most species, including the human, which express predominantly the 7S monomeric form (208). Serum IgA from BALB/c mice has an unusual disulfide structure in which the light chains are linked to each other, but not to the heavy chains (1,75). Thus, under denaturing conditions H_2 and L_2 molecules can be isolated separately. In contrast, New Zealand black mice have a normal disulfide-linked structure (216). These two structural forms of mouse IgA correspond to similar structural features found in the human IgA1 molecule and the A_2m (151) allotype of the IgA2 molecule, respectively.

Subclasses of IgA have been defined for only a few species including the human, mouse, and rabbit. Each species has two IgA subclasses labeled IgA1 and IgA2.

Immunoglobulin E

Reaginic antibody (IgE) has been reported in most species including the rat (43,115), mouse (142,172,177), guinea pig (49), rabbit (178,221), monkey (102), dog (165), and human (103). This molecule exists in the serum of most species as a four-chain monomer with a sedimentation coefficient of 8S corresponding to molecular weight of 185 to 200 Kd. An 11S dimeric form of IgE also was reported in the serum of guinea pigs. IgE molecules are heat labile, losing their reaginic activity after exposure to 56°C for 1 hour, and they persist (>6 days) in the skin for relatively long periods after passive transfer. The low concentration of IgE in serum has precluded direct isolation and characterization of this molecule. Therefore, most of what is known about the structure of IgE has been obtained from IgE myeloma proteins as found in certain humans, mice, and rats with specific gammopathies. However, the physical and functional properties that are known for each species appear to be similar to the model IgE molecules isolated from humans and mice. (For a review see references 17,104,105, and 147.) The functional properties of IgE will be discussed.

Immunoglobulin D

This immunoglobulin represents an oddity among the isotypes in that no clear effector functions have been assigned to the IgD molecule; however, it does serve as a receptor on the surface of B-lymphocytes (reviews in references 194 and 203) and has been found in the milk of rats (156). The role of this receptor in B-cell activation or tolerance is unclear; however, Putman et al (173) suggested that proteolytic fragments of IgD, produced following ligand binding, may serve as immune modulators in a manner analogous to the action of proteolytic fragments of complement. The extremely low concentrations of IgD found in the serum (< 1 μg/ml) have made it a difficult molecule to identify and study. An immunoglobulin thought to correspond to the human IgD molecule has been identified in only a few other species including the mouse (2,134), rat (13,183), nonhuman primate (124,130), and rabbit (190). Subclasses of IgD have not yet been identified in any species.

The structure and biochemistry of mouse and human IgD have been studied extensively owing to the availability of IgD myeloma proteins from these species. Primate IgD appears to be structurally similar to human IgD which is composed of four heavy-chain domains and two light-chain domains. The first and second constant-region domains are separated by a hinge region similar to that found in IgG and IgA molecules. However, IgD is unique in that this region is highly extended (64 amino acid residues) in the human (173), which makes the hinge more susceptible to proteolytic enzymes. In contrast, mouse IgD has been shown to lack an extended hinge region and also is missing the second constant-region domain (205). However, the molec-

ular weight of the heavy chain reported for mouse IgD (70,000 d) is comparable to human IgD (70,000 d) due to a larger content of carbohydrate (70,135,167,191). The human IgD molecule is also known to have a single disulfide link between each of the heavy- and light-chain portions as well as one disulfide link between the two heavy chains in the lower half of the hinge region. Because this region is absent from mouse IgD, Putman et al (173) have hypothesized that mouse IgD does not contain an interheavy chain disulfide bridge and may exist as an HL monomer. However, strong noncovalent bonds may form a stable H_2L_2 molecule as well.

TECHNIQUES FOR THE QUANTITATION OF IMMUNOGLOBULIN CLASSES AND SUBCLASSES

All of the techniques available for the quantitation of immunoglobulins rely on class or subclass specific antisera for detecting the various isotypes. Thus, the ability to quantitate immunoglobulins from different species depends on the availability of species specific anti-immunoglobulin antisera. These antisera are prepared by purifying the immunoglobulin class or subclass of interest and immunizing a second species of animal (ie, a rabbit or goat) with the product. The antisera are made isotype specific by adsorbing the unwanted specificities on an affinity column conjugated with immunoglobulin containing all of the known light- and heavy-chain isotypes except for the relevant isotype. The specificity of this adsorbed antisera is checked against a battery of known isotype standards in the assay system of interest. Often myeloma proteins are used in place of normal serum immunoglobulin because myeloma proteins are more easily isolated and can be obtained in larger quantities. These proteins have proved to be extremely useful for developing antiserum to the rare isotypes (ie, IgE and IgD). However, myelomas have not been described in all species for all of the different classes and subclasses of immunoglobulin. Complete sets of myeloma proteins have been described for the human, mouse, and rat (with the exception of an IgD myeloma in rats), whereas other species of laboratory animals lack more than one myeloma protein representing a specific class or subclass of immunoglobulin.

Quantitation of the major isotypes (IgG and

Table 10.A.3. Sensitivity of Various Assays Used for Detecting Immunoglobulin Isotypes

Technique Used	Sensitivity (units/ml)
Quantitative precipitation	Mid microgram range
Radial immunodiffusion	Mid-low microgram range
Radioimmunoassay	Low nanogram range
Enzyme immunoassay	Low nanogram range

IgM) in the serum can be accomplished using a variety of immunoassay techniques because the concentration of these isotypes is reasonably high and assay sensitivity is therefore not a prime consideration. (For the sensitivity range of various techniques, see Table 10.A.3). Quantitative immunoprecipitation (66) and radial immunodiffusion (157) may be used to analyze these immunoglobulin isotypes. Of these two assays, radial immunodiffusion is the more sensitive technique, and methods for extending its range of sensitivity by the addition of a radiolabeled second antibody (182) or by enhancing the contrast and intensity of precipitin lines in the gel (85,188) have been described. These enhancements have allowed the detection of IgD and IgE in serum.

Rocket immunoelectrophoresis (157), another popular technique used for quantitation of antibodies to a variety of different antigens, is a less useful technique for quantitating immunoglobulin isotypes. This assay involves electrophoresis of the antigen preparation into an agar gel containing anti-antigen antibody. The technique relies on selecting an optimal pH of the buffer system that allows migration of the antigen into the gel while maintaining a neutral net charge on the anti-antigen antibodies, thus preventing their migration into the gel. In this way, precipitin arcs can form in the agar. However, for quantitation of isotypes both the antigen and antibody in the assay system are immunoglobulins; therefore, optimizing conditions for electrophoresis that would allow migration into the gel of one immunoglobulin species (ie, the immunoglobulin isotype of interest) while maintaining a neutral charge on the second immunoglobulin species (ie, the anti-isotype antisera in the agar) would be very difficult, if not impossible.

Radioimmunoassays and enzyme immunoassays offer more sensitivity in detecting the various immunoglobulin classes and subclasses than do the previously discussed techniques (101). This increase in sensitivity may be necessary when assaying for the presence of certain immunoglobulin isotypes (ie, IgE and IgD) that are normally present in very low concentration in the serum. These assays are also advantageous when a large number of different samples are to be assayed. As with the previously mentioned assays, the quality and sensitivity of the radioimmunoassay and enzyme immunoassay depend on the specificity and affinity of the isotype-specific antisera used in the assay. The isotype of interest is quantitated by assaying the ability of an unknown isotype sample to inhibit the binding between a radiolabeled (or enzyme-labeled) immunoglobulin isotype standard and anti-isotype antisera. These results are then compared with a standard curve to obtain the quantity of isotype in the assay sample.

PHYSIOLOGY AND EFFECTOR FUNCTIONS OF IMMUNOGLOBULINS

Placental/Gut Transfer of Immunoglobulins

Transfer of immunoglobulins from the mother to the fetus or newborn is an important mechanism of passive protection from disease for the newborn animal. Immunoglobulins may be transferred either prenatally, postnatally, or both. Prenatal transfer of immunoglobulin occurs in the human (69), monkey (11,174), rabbit (31), guinea pig (122), rat (74,82), mouse (87), and dog (32). Transfer is transplacental in each of these species with the exception of the rabbit and guinea pig which transfer immunoglobulin across the yolk sac. In addition to transplacental transfer of immunoglobulin in rats, the yolk sac may also be involved in transport of maternal immunoglobulin to the fetus (214). Postnatal transfer of maternal immunoglobulin G across the intestinal epithelium occurs in the rat, mouse and dog for 21, 16, and 10 days, respectively, following birth (32,33,79,138). There is no evidence of postnatal transfer of immunoglobulin in the guinea pig, rabbit, monkey, and human, however, high levels of maternal IgA are found in the intestinal lumen of neonates. IgG appears to be the only class of immunoglobulins transferred from mother to young except in rabbits which may also transport some IgM (214). There also may be differences in the transfer efficiency of certain IgG subclasses depending on the species investigated. Mouse IgG3 is transferred much more readily than the other IgG subclasses (76), whereas in the human and guinea pig all IgG subclasses are transferred equally well (35,195).

Complement Fixation

Fixation of complement by immunoglobulins is an important property of antibody molecules, which may lead to cell lysis, Arthus reaction, and/or enhanced opsonic activity and cytophilic binding. The classical pathway of complement activation uses all nine components (1,4,2,3, and 5 to 9 respectively), whereas the alternate pathway involves activation of the third and fifth to ninth components, respectively. (For a review of these pathways, please refer to the section on complement in this chapter and to references 72 and 143.) The IgG and IgM isotypes of all species appear to fix complement by the classical pathway; however, there may be subclass differences. Human IgG4, mouse IgG1 and IgG3, and guinea pig and hamster IgG1 do not fix complement through this pathway. In addition, a subpopulation of noncomplement-fixing IgM has been described for human, rabbit, and guinea pig immunoglobulins (195). The IgA, IgE, and IgD isotypes also do not fix complement through the classical pathway for any of the species considered here.

The alternate pathway of complement activation in the human involves only the two IgA subclasses, whereas the other isotypes are unable to fix complement through this pathway. In contrast, IgG1 and IgG2 in guinea pigs and IgG1 in mice and rabbits can fix complement through the alternate pathway (195). Aggregated IgD and IgE in many species also activate the alternate pathway.

Cytophilic and Opsonizing Activity

Antibodies that are cytophilic for macrophages presumably function to focus the phagocytic activities of the macrophage on the intruding organism or particle (opsonic activity). In the hamster (171), both the IgG1 and IgG2 subclasses bind to macrophages, with IgG1 having a higher affinity for binding than does IgG2. However, IgG2 exhibits more opsonic activity than does the IgG1 subclass. In contrast, only

Table 10.A.4. Binding Affinity of IgG Antibody to Protein A[a]

Species	Relative Binding Affinity
Human	1
Rabbit	1
Guinea pig	1
Dog	0.21
Mouse	1.33×10^{-2}
Rat	$<6 \times 10^{-4}$

[a] Numbers based on the amount of IgG required to inhibit binding of ^{125}I-labeled protein A to immobilized rabbit IgG as reported by: Langone JJ (1978) ^{125}I protein A: A tracer for general use in immunoassay. J Immunol Methods 24: 269–285.

the IgG2 subclass of guinea pig and mouse is cytophilic for macrophages (29,121,206), whereas all four human IgG subclasses (96) bind macrophages (IgG1, IgG3 > IgG2, and IgG4). The IgM isotype of mouse and man has also been shown to have opsonic activity when complexed with complement.

Protein A Binding

Staphylococcal protein A binds to IgG from a variety of mammalian species (120). The protein A molecule has four known binding sites available for interaction with the Fc portion of immunoglobulin molecules and can therefore form immune complexes of protein A and antibody in the serum. These immune complexes have been shown to fix complement as well as classical antigen-antibody complexes in serum (63,64). The relative effectiveness of protein A binding to IgG from different species is shown in Table 10.A.4. In addition to IgG, the IgA2 subclass of human immunoglobulin and IgM from the human, rabbit, mouse, and rat exhibit low levels of binding to protein A as well (71). Within the IgG subclasses of different species there also may be heterogeneity in the affinity of binding to protein A. The IgG1 subclass of mice and IgG3 subclass of humans both do not bind to protein A, whereas all subclasses of IgG in the guinea pig (IgG1, and IgG2) bind protein A equally well. Protein A binding presumably can play a physiologic role in protection against disease; however, there is no direct evidence for this.

Immediate Hypersensitivity Reactions

Immunoglobulin classes that can bind to either mast cells or basophils are termed homocytotropic antibodies and are capable of mediating immediate hypersensitivity reactions by causing release of histamine and other vasoactive agents from these cell types following binding of a ligand to the antibody molecule. Two types of antibody appear responsible for this reaction. Reaginic or IgE antibody can be demonstrated by the Prausnitz-Kunstner test and is heat labile, but long lived (11 to 15 days) in the skin after passive transfer. Most mammalian species, including the human (109), monkey (102), dog (165), rat (43,115), mouse (142,172,177), guinea pig (49), and rabbit (178,221), exhibit reaginic reactivity. In contrast, the second type of homocytotropic antibody is heat stable and has a short half-life (<1 day) in the skin after passive transfer. In the guinea pig, rat, and mouse this antibody belongs to the IgG1 subclass (195), whereas in the hamster the IgG2 subclass exhibits this activity (40). In contrast, none of the human IgG subclasses appears to be homocytotropic (195) and IgG exhibiting this activity has not been described for dogs, rabbits, and monkeys.

The homocytotropic antibodies bind to both mast cells and basophils in most species. In rats, IgG1 and IgE compete for the same cellular receptors although IgE has a higher affinity of binding (10, 119).

Heterologous sensitization of skin by various antibody classes can also be demonstrated. Human IgG1, IgG3, and IgG4, mouse IgG2a, and IgG2 of rats and rabbits will sensitize guinea pig skin in the reverse passive cutaneous anaphylaxis test (163,201). A similar reaction can also be elicited by monkey and dog IgG but not horse IgG when passively transferred to the guinea pig (164).

IMMUNOGLOBULIN METABOLISM AND ANTIBODY CONCENTRATIONS

Normal values for the half-life of immunoglobulin in serum and average levels of antibodies expressed in the serum of a number of laboratory animals are tabulated at the end of this chapter. The differences in serum concentrations between species reflect differences in immunoglobulin synthesis and catabolism in these animals. In a normal antigenic environment, immunoglobulin synthesis in man (23,192) and guinea pig (186) ranges from 25 to 35 mg/kg/day; whereas mice (15,59,97), rats

(41,111), and rabbits (7,36) synthesize from 50 to 130 mg/kg/day. In addition, the half-life of IgG in serum appears to be more variable between species than do other isotypes. The reported half-time survival of IgG in serum is 4.5 days in the mouse (15,59), 5.5 days in rats (41,111), 6 days in rabbits (7,36), 6.6 days in rhesus monkeys (48), 8 days in dogs (48) and guinea pigs (186), 12 days in baboons (42), and 20 to 25 days in humans (23,192). Differences in metabolism also exist between the various classes and subclasses of immunoglobulin. IgM has a predominantly intravascular distribution and a decreased survival rate in the serum (one tenth to one half the half-time survival rate of IgG). Similarly, IgA in mice has a half-time survival rate one quarter that of IgG (60). Subclass variations in the serum survival rate of mouse IgG (60) similar to that found within the human IgG subclasses (196) also exist in other species.

One factor that can alter the catabolic rate of immunoglobulin is the serum concentration. This effect has been shown to be variable between different classes of immunoglobulin. The catabolic rate of mouse and human IgA is independent of the serum concentration (12,60,193,196,198). In contrast, the catabolic rate of human IgD is inversely proportional to its serum concentration (181). Thus, as the concentration of IgD increases, the catabolic rate decreases.

A third metabolic relationship has been observed for the IgG class of immunoglobulins in both humans and mice. The rate of catabolism for this isotype is directly proportional to its serum concentration (15,60,61,97,128,181,192, 218). Thus, as the concentration of IgG increases in the serum, the catabolic rate increases as well. However, not all species show these same relationships between catabolic rate and immunoglobulin concentration. In rabbits the effect of immunoglobulin serum concentration on the catabolic rate is less clear, and several reports indicate that there is no direct correlation between the two parameters when immunoglobulin is passively transferred or elicited in vivo following hyperimmunization (7,98). In contrast, Catsoulis et al (36) reported an increase in the catabolic rate of IgG in hyperimmunized rabbits. Neonatal rabbits that exhibit low levels of serum IgG also showed a prolonged survival time of this isotype in their serum compared with adult values (47,99). Thus,

the serum IgG concentration can affect the catabolic rate; however, other factors may be
involved as well.

The situation in guinea pigs is better defined.
There is no change in the catabolic rate of IgG
over a wide range of serum concentrations
(100,186,187). This is in contrast to findings in
the latter species and shows that broad gen-
eralities cannot be made about this relationship
between species.

The major factor affecting the serum concentration of immunoglobulins is antigenic
stimulation. At one extreme are animals that
have been raised in a germ-free environment.
These animals are "immunologically virgin"
and express very low levels of immunoglobulin
in their serum (15,186,196). At the opposite
extreme are animals that have been exposed to
a high pathogen environment or that have been
hyperimmunized. These animals may have
serum levels of immunoglobulin that are 5 to
10 times the levels found in normal animals.
(Normal serum values of immunoglobulin for a
variety of species are given at the end of this
chapter.)

Specific classes or subclasses of immunoglobulin may be preferentially elicited by
different antigenic stimuli or disease states.
Expression of the IgG3 subclass in mice and
IgG2 subclass in humans has been predominantly associated with anti-carbohydrate
or anti-bacterial immunity (169,180,220). The
IgG2 isotype found in mice, guinea pigs, and
hamsters often increases more rapidly than does
IgG1 after antigenic stimulation of the animals
with protein antigens (38,171). Similarly, anti-
nuclear antibodies obtained from a lupus dog
were predominantly of the IgG2a,b isotypes
with lower levels of IgG1 and IgM being expressed (108). This distribution of isotypes is
also found in human patients with lupus.

IgM antibody often appears only transiently
in the serum following a primary exposure to
antigen; however persistent serum titers of this
isotype have been obtained in the hamster after
immunization with SRBC (65), in the rabbit
after immunization with streptococcal antigens
(34), and in mice immunized with dextran
(83,131). Thus, IgM can become a dominant
isotype in the serum of most species after
exposure of the animal to specific antigens or by
using immunization protocols that favor such
expression.

The serum and particularly the secreted level
of IgA is often increased by antigens that are
encountered orally or come in contact with the
intestinal mucosa. Thus, dogs (86) and mice
(26,94) immunized orally with *Vibrio cholera*
showed increased levels of IgA in the serum and
secretions. Similarly, rats immunized orally with
Escherichia coli 06 (84) or infected with tape-
worms (82) and rabbits immunized orally with
respiratory syncytial virus (168) showed increased titers of IgA in their secretions. (For
reviews on the secretory immune system see
references 90,133, and 155.)

The circulating levels of IgE are also influenced by various antigenic stimuli. The levels of
this isotype often are elevated in animals
infected with parasites or afflicted with a variety
of allergic disorders. (For reviews see references
14,25,166, and 200.) Protein antigens, when
injected with the appropriate adjuvant, will also
elicit high titers of reaginic antibody (125,212).
The mechanism(s) by which different antigens
preferentially elicit expression of one isotype
over another is not well understood, although
presumably there is a survival advantage for the
animal in preferentially expressing a particular
isotype(s) in response to different antigenic
stimuli.

The most dramatic shift in serum immunoglobulin concentration occurs with various
monoclonal gammopathies such as multiple
myeloma which has been found in humans, nonhuman primates, dogs, mice, and rats. These
gammopathies result in expansion of a single
clone of neoplastic B-cells secreting copious
amounts of antibody. Often the monoclonal
antibody product may represent greater than 90
per cent of the total immunoglobulin expressed
in serum. These abnormalities are clearly evident following cellulose acetate electrophoresis
of the serum proteins. The normally diffuse
banding region occupied by immunoglobulin
will contain a single, darkly stained band representing the neoplastic product and a fainter
diffusely stained region representing the normal
complement of immunoglobulin in the serum.
The large amounts of pure antibody that can be
isolated from the serum have allowed a variety
of biochemical and functional analyses to be
carried out on specific isotypes that are normally
expressed only at low levels (ie, IgE, and IgD)
and have thus proved to be extremely useful to
immunologists.

COMPONENTS (ISOTYPE, ALLOTYPE, AND IDIOTYPE)

Although the basic structural characteristics of immunoglobulins are very similar, this family of glycoproteins exhibits substantial heterogeneity in amino acid sequences in both the constant and variable regions of the light and heavy chains. These differences often reflect only one or a few amino acid substitutions and are most commonly detected by appropriate antisera that contain antibodies (ie, antiantibodies) that are able to recognize subtle differences between molecules. Three major serologically and structurally defined markers are found on immunoglobulin of most of the species that have been studied: isotypes, allotypes, and idiotypes. Because isotypes are presented in some detail in the section on biochemistry, this section will focus on the latter two components of immunoglobulins.

Allotypes are allelic variants of immunoglobulin light and heavy chains that segregate in a simple Mendelian fashion among outbreeding members of a species. Many of the currently studied immunoglobulin allotypes are analogous in many respects to the allelic forms of other proteins such as the hemoglobin chains. However, there are some interesting exceptions that have a very complex pattern of inheritance and expression. These more complex systems will be discussed later as individual species differences are considered. Several good reference articles on allotypes are available (91,113,127,129,146,152).

Idiotypes are antigenic determinants located exclusively in the variable region of the light and heavy chains. In contrast to the allotypes that are typically found on all immunoglobulins of a given isotype, the idiotypic determinants represent individual and specific markers, with each antibody or myeloma protein having its own unique set of idiotypic determinants. Idiotypes on immunoglobulins may be thought of as being analogous to fingerprints of individuals because both can be used to distinguish unique entities. A more complete discussion of idiotypy will be presented following the section on allotypes.

Immunoglobulin Allotypes

The genetically determined antigenic differences in the serum immunoglobulin of all of the spec-

ies to be covered are attributed to amino acid substitutions caused by mutations in the corresponding structural genes. Unlike genetic variants of other proteins, allotype variations do not appear to affect antibody specificity or any known biologic function of immunoglobulin. The fact that allotypy does not affect antibody specificity is not surprising because most allotypic determinants are located completely within the constant region of the light or heavy chain and the antibody combining site is completely within the variable region. The rabbit is one exception to the generalization regarding the placement of the allotypic determinant, because it is now well established that several allotypes are found in the variable region of rabbit immunoglobulin heavy chains.

When animals are bred, each expressing a different allele at a given locus, the heterozygous offspring expresses both allotypes in the serum immunoglobulins. This codominant expression of allotypes is seen in all species studied and occurs with both heavy- and light-chain allotypes. Thus, in an animal that is heterozygous for both heavy- and light-chain alleles, all four alleles are seen in the serum. Because it is generally agreed that an antibody-producing cell expresses only one of two possible parental heavy-chain alleles and one of two parental light-chain alleles (allelic exclusion), the serum contains a mixture of symmetrical immunoglobulin molecules, that is, both heavy chains have the same allotypic determinant and both light chains have the same allotypic determinant on any given antibody molecule. Genetic studies using immunoglobulin allotypes as markers revealed that genes coding for heavy chains and light chains were not linked and that kappa and lambda light-chain genes were also unlinked. Furthermore, studies with rabbit heavy-chain allotypes led investigators to hypothesize that the variable- and constant-region genes represent a gene family on the same chromosome. These conclusions based solely upon studies with allotypes have subsequently been verified by somatic cell geneticists and molecular biologists.

Methods of Detecting Allotypes

Allotypes are typically identified by antibodies that are able to recognize individual allotypic determinants. Anti-allotypic antibodies are generally elicited by injecting the immunoglobulin (or antibody-antigen complexes) of a donor individual that bears the allotype into a recipient of the same species that lacks the allotype. Although anti-allotypic antibodies can be raised by immunizing across species ie, mouse immunoglobulin into rabbit, rabbit antisera must then be adsorbed with mouse sera that do not contain the reference allotype. Prolonged immunization is frequently required to elicit allotype-specific antibodies, but the response can be enhanced by immunization with antibody-antigen complexes in Freund's complete adjuvant. Antisera specific for human allotypes are obtained from multiparous women, from patients who have received blood transfusions, or from patients recovering from various diseases.

Immunoprecipitin tests in agar gel (158) can be employed to detect allotypic specificities in some species, in particular rabbits. Because some allotypes are manifested by only minor structural changes in the polypeptide chain, anti-allotypic antisera often detect only one or two unique antigenic determinants. In such cases there is an insufficient development of a lattice formation that is required for an allotype-antiallotype precipitate to form. Therefore, other detection methods such as hemagglutination inhibition and radioimmunoassays using solid-phase adsorption or fluid phase second antibody precipitations are used (53,67,118). The radioimmunoassays have a distinct advantage in that they are quantitative and the proportions of allotypic markers can be detected in test sera. Several typical radioimmunoassays have been described (67,118).

Rabbit Allotypes

Allotypic determinants in the rabbit were first discovered by Oudin in 1956 (159). Since this original discovery, numerous allotypes have been identified and characterized. The allotype gene loci are designated by small italicized letters (*a*, *b*, *c*, etc) and the individual determinants (allotypes) at each locus are designated by nonitalicized letters and numbers (a1, a2, a3, etc). The numbers are assigned consecutively in order of their discovery, regardless of the positions of the loci coding for the determinant. Each species has a different nomenclature that will be covered as each is discussed. A representative list of the rabbit allotypes and their location within a particular heavy or light chain of immunoglobulin

Table 10.A.5. Rabbit Immunoglobulin Allotypes

Locus	Chain Location	Alleles
a	Variable heavy H chain	a1, a2, a3, a100–a103
x	Variable heavy H chain	x32, x⁻
y	Variable heavy H chain	y33, y⁻
n	Constant μH chain	Ms16, Ms17
d	Constant γH chain	d11, d12
e	Constant γH chain	e14, e15
f	Constant α_1H chain	f69–f73
g	Constant α_2 H chain	g74–g77
t	Secretory component of IgA	t61, t62
b	Constant κ L chain	b4, b5, b6, b9
c	Constant λ L chain	c7, c21

is presented in Table 10.A.5. Note that allotypes have been found in the constant region of κ(b)(50) and λ(c)(51) light chains, and the constant regions of λ (d and e, these may be identical), α_1 (f), α_2 (g), and μ (Ms) heavy chains. It is of particular interest that a few loci code for allotype determinants detected in the variable region (*a*, *x*, and *y*) of the rabbit heavy chain. These variable region allotypes are found on immunoglobulin of all of the isotypes.

The *a* and *b* loci constitute an exceptional case (152). These are so-called complex allotypes because when the chains carrying these allotypes were sequenced, no single allotype-specific residue could be identified as was the case with most other allotypes. The determinants coded for by the *a* and *b* loci consisted of a multitude of amino acid residues. The a1, a2, and a3, and b4, b5, b6, and b9 loci may represent a tightly linked cluster. If b4, b5, b6, and b9 were alleles, a single individual should not possess more than two of them and this is usually true. However, several investigators have reported rabbits transiently expressing three alleles. This may occur with greater frequency after hyperimmunization with a single antigen such as ovalbumin. Although the transitory and latent allotypes may be explained by regulatory genes that alter the expression of structural genes within a cluster, the issue currently remains unresolved.

Rabbits heterozygous for the *a* and *b* loci exhibit a preferential expression of each allele, that is, a101 > a1 > a3 > a2 > a100 and b4 > b6 > b5 > b9. This order may change in the presence of an infectious disease or after immunization with different antigens. The allelic genes in the *a* locus control the synthesis of 70 to 90

Table 10.A.6. Mouse and Rat Immunoglobulin Allotypes

Locus	Chain	Alleles	Allotypic Determinants
Mouse allotypes			
Igh–1	γ2a	1a–1h; 1j–1m	1–8; 26–30
Igh–2	α	2a–2d; 2f	12, 13, 14, 15, 17, 35
Igh–3	γ2b	3a, 3b, 3d–3g	4, 9, 11, 16, 22, 23, 31–34
Igh–4	γ 1	4a, 4b, 4d	8, 18, 19, 42
Igh–5	δ	5a, 5b	36, 37
Igh–6	μ	6a, 6b, 6e	38–41
Rat allotypes			
RI–1	κ	1a, 1b	...

per cent of rabbit heavy chains (52). Nearly all molecules of rabbit IgG are precipitated by a combination of anti-b or anti-c locus allotypes, indicating that if another light-chain locus exists, it must code for a very small proportion of rabbit light chains (213). Because these two genes segregate independently, it was correctly speculated that they exist on separate chromosomes (68). It also was noted that the genes coding for the light-chain allotypes were not linked to the genes controlling markers on rabbit heavy chains (51,112,158).

Mouse and Rat Allotypes

The recommended nomenclature for allotypes in mice designates the loci by Igh or Igl (h and l for heavy and light chains, respectively) with a number assigned in the order of discovery (Igh-1, Igh-2, Igh-3, etc). The allotypic determinants are also designated consecutively in order of their discovery and are separated from the locus by a period (Igh-1.1, Igh-1.2, Igh-1.3, etc). Mouse heavy-chain allotypes and their isotype association are listed in Table 10.A.6. All of the loci listed here code for determinants found in the constant region of the molecule. With more sensitive radioimmunoassay methods, it has been possible to identify markers in the variable Fd portion of the heavy chain (197). Most of the allotypic determinants in the mouse, however, are on the constant region and they are restricted to a single Ig class and subclass. As noted in Table 10.A.6 there are exceptions, namely, determinant 4 is shared by IgG2a and IgG2b and determinant 8 is shared by IgG1 and IgG2a.

The heavy-chain allotype loci in the mouse are closely linked genes. Specific combinations

of alleles at these loci (haplotypes) are designated in Table 10.A.7 and the distribution of the alleles among selected inbred strains is illustrated in Table 10.A.8. For a more complete listing of the allotype distribution in the mouse, guinea pig and rabbit, consult the FASEB biological handbook (6). The mouse Igh-1 locus is unusually polymorphic with 12 alleles (Table 10.A.8). The allotypes at this locus are very complex and resemble those of the rabbit *a* and *b* loci.

No serologically defined allotypic variants have been identified in the kappa light chains, but intraspecies differences of V-regions have been detected by other means (ie, isoelectric focusing and peptide mapping).

Allotypes similar to those of inbred strains have been observed in wild mice. However, the wild mice exhibit new haplotypes that suggest that recombinational events have occurred within the Igh locus.

Contrary to the lack of allotypic variants in the mouse kappa light chain, rats exhibit two alleles of this gene. The locus in the rat is termed RI-1 and there are two allotypes: RI-1a found in the DA inbred strain and RI-1b found in the LEW strain. These two markers are also considered to be complex allotypes because they differ by 11 amino acid substitutions.

Nonhuman Primate Allotypes

The first human allotype was discovered using an indirect method based on inhibition of hemagglutination similar to the one just described (77). The genetic locus was termed Gm because the determinant was found on the gammaglobulins. Many of the Gm markers presently recognized in human IgG have been identified

Table 10.A.7. Igh Haplotypes of Mouse

Prototype Strain	Igh Haplotype	Gene Loci Encoding Allotypic Determinants (Ig Chain in Parentheses)					
		Igh-1 (γ2a)	Igh-2 (α)	Igh-3 (γ2b)	Igh-4 (γ1)	Igh-5 (δ)	Igh-6 (μ)
BALB/c	a	1, 6, 7, 8, 26, 28, 29, 30	12, 13, 14	9, 11, 22, 31, 33, 34	8, 19	36	38, 39
C57BL	b	2, 27, 29	15	9, 16, 22, 33, 34	42	37	40, 41
DBA/2	c	3, 8, 29	35	9, 11, 22, 31, 33, 34	8, 19	36	...
AKR	d	4, 6, 7, 8, 26, 29	13, 17	4, 23, 31, 32, 33, 34	8, 19	36	...
A	e	4, 6, 7, 8, 26, 28, 29, 30	13, 17	4, 23, 31, 32, 33	8, 19	36	39, 41
CE	f	5, 7, 8, 26, 30	14	9, 11, 31, 32	8, 19	36	...
RIII	g	3, 8, 26	35	9, 11, 31	8, 19	36	...
SEA	h	1, 6, 7, 8, 28, 29	12, 13, 14	9, 11, 22, 31, 33, 34	8, 19	36	38, 39
CBA	j	1, 6, 7, 8, 28, 29, 30	12, 13, 14	9, 11, 22, 31, 33, 34	8, 19	36	38, 39
KH-1	k	3, 5, 7, 8	35	9, 11, 25	8, 19	...	...
KH-2	l	3, 5, 8	35	9, 11, 22	8, 19	...	...
Ky	m	1, 2, 6, 7, 8	15	9, 16, 22	8, 19	...	...
NZB	...	4, 6, 7, 8, 26, 28, 24, 30	13, 17	4, 23, 31, 32, 33	8, 19	36	39, 41

in nonhuman primates (210,211). Human allotypes identified so far have all been located on the constant region of heavy or light chains. Six human heavy-chain loci have been identified, G1m, G2m, G3m, Mm, A2m, and Km, encoding allotypes on γ_1, γ_2, γ_3, μ, α_2 and κ chains, respectively. Markers associated with G1m and G3m and light chain have been observed in nonhuman primates. Several of the allotypic markers for the human were found to be isotypic in primates because all gorillas, dwarf chimpanzees, and chimpanzees tested were positive for two of the allotypic markers that are associated with the G1m locus in humans (152).

Several human IgG3 allotypic markers are found in all gorillas but only in part of the chimpanzee population. Chimpanzees also appear to be polymorphic in the Km locus.

Immunoglobulin Idiotypes

Immunoglobulins typically represent an enormously heterogeneous set of glycoproteins. This heterogeneity is a reflection of amino acid differences that are most prevalent in the amino-terminal (variable region) end of the molecules. These differences represent individual antigenic determinants, termed idiotypic determinants, and the entire set of idiotypic determinants are referred to as the idiotype. Each clone of antibody-producing cells secretes an antibody having a single idiotype. Antibodies can be raised to the idiotypic determinants in a number of ways. Most commonly, anti-idiotype antibodies are produced by repeated immunization of an animal with a homogeneous immunoglobulin (either a monoclonal antibody or a myeloma protein) followed by adsorption of the resulting antiserum with normal serum or other hybridomas/myelomas with identical constant regions but different variable regions.

Since several excellent review articles documenting the molecular structure, the genetic regulation and the biologic and functional significance of idiotypes are available (27,28,54,62,106,114,160,210), our focus in this section will be limited to a few generalizations about idiotypes and anti-idiotype antibodies that apply to all of the species that produce antibodies. First, it should be recognized that antibodies may be directed to virtually any exposed determinant in the variable region and that most anti-idiotypic antibody preparations

Table 10.A.8. Distribution of Alleles (Igh Haplotypes) at the Igh Loci

Igh Haplotype	Prototype Strain	Locus (chain)					
		Igh–1 (γ2a)	Igh–2 (α)	Igh–3 (γ2b)	Igh–4 (γ1)	Igh–5 (δ)	Igh–6 (μ)
a	BALB/c	a	a	a	a	a	a
b	C57BL	b	b	b	b	b	b
c	DBA/2	c	c	a	a	a	...
d	AKR	d	d	d	a	a	...
e	A	e	d	e	a	e	e
f	CE	f	f	f	a	a	...
g	RIII	g	c	g	a	a	...
h	SEA	h	a	a	a	a	...
j	CBA/H	j	a	a	a	a	a
k	KH–1 (wild)	k	c	a	a	...	...
l	KH–2 (wild)	l	c	a	a	...	...
m	Ky	m	b	b	b	...	...
...	NZB	e	d	e	a	a	c

(with the exception of monoclonal anti-idiotype antibodies) have multiple specificities. These antibodies may be directed at idiotypic determinants within or outside the antibody-combining site. If the antibodies are directed against determinants within the site, then antigen can block the binding of the anti-idiotype antibody to the target immunoglobulin. These antibodies are called site-specific anti-idiotypic antibodies, and all others are called non-site-specific.

The best characterized idiotypes are those reported in mice (62,114). It has been demonstrated with conventional as well as monoclonal antibodies that some preparations of idiotype-specific reagents can recognize a single amino acid interchange within the variable region. In spite of this exquisite resolving power of anti-idiotype antibodies, conclusions regarding structural identity of antibodies cannot be based solely on the binding of the antibody to two separate antibody samples, because it is well established that antibodies of different isotypes may share a common idiotype and antibodies with the same isotype may share only partial identity with any particular idiotype (ie, micro-heterogeneity within the V-region).

Idiotypes are most often associated with antibodies of a single specificity. The first notable exception to this was reported by Oudin and Cazenave (161), and since then many interesting exceptions to this general rule have been reported.

Idiotypes have been divided into private and public idiotypes based on the distribution of idiotypes within a species. Originally, it was thought that an idiotype was unique and restricted to a single antibody clone derived from a single individual. This type of idiotype, also referred to as a minor, individual, or private idiotype, does exist at least in principle. However, it is now recognized that other idiotypes can be shared between individuals, and these are called public, major, or cross-reactive idiotypes. The private idiotype may represent a single clonal product, whereas a public idiotype may be a manifestation of an entire family of related antibodies that differ at various positions throughout the V-region of the light or heavy chain. Both private and public idiotypes may be inherited from generation to generation. Idiotype sharing among individuals is therefore much more frequent within inbred strains than within outbred animals. All animals of a given strain may produce antibodies, a portion of which cross-react idiotypically in response to a given antigen, but antibodies from another strain specific for the same antigen may show little or no cross-reactivity. These intrastrain idiotypic cross-reactions are typically unpredictable; however, examples of a genetic linkage between the gene coding for an idiotype and the gene coding for a heavy-chain allotype have been documented.

The most commonly used methods for detecting and quantitating idiotypes are direct or indirect quantitative precipitation and radioimmunoassays.

The concept of idiotype has led to a number

of valuable contributions regarding the genetics and biology of antibodies and antibody-producing cells. Among these contributions include: (a) their use as markers with which one can quantitatively follow the expression of an individual clone or family of related clones of antibody-producing cells within a heterogeneous population of antibody-producing cells, (b) the recognition that a clone of cells can switch from IgM to IgG secretion, (c) the broad range of idiotypic specificities of antibody directed against a single antigen or hapten reflecting a great diversity within the antibody repertoire, (d) alterations in the degree of idiotype cross-reactivity in an antibody population as a function of time after immunization, leading to the speculation that somatic mutations may occur during an immune response, and (e) the suggestion by Jerne and others that B or T lymphocytes' recognition of idiotypes displayed on the membrane of immunocompetent cells may play a role in immune regulation (28). Relevant to the last statement, it has been demonstrated that the administration of anti-idiotype antibody either in vitro or in vivo can suppress the synthesis of antibodies that bear the reference idiotype (28).

REFERENCES

1. Abel CA, Grey HM (1968) Studies on the structure of mouse γ A myeloma proteins. Biochemistry 7: 2682–2696
2. Abney ER, Parkhouse RME (1974) Candidate for immunoglobulin D present on murine B lymphocytes. Nature 252: 600–602
3. Adams JM, Kemp DJ, Bernard O, Gough N, Webb E, Tyler B, Gerondakis S, Cory S (1981) Organization and expression of murine immunoglobulin genes. Immunol Rev 59: 5–32
4. Alepa FP, Terry WD (1965) Genetic factors and polypeptide chain subclasses of human immunoglobulin G detected in chimpanzee serums. Science 150: 1293–1294
5. Alepa FP (1968) Antigenic factors characteristic of human immunoglobulin G detected in sera of non-human primates. Primates in Med 1: 1–9
6. Altman PL, Katz DD (eds) (1979) Inbred and genetically defined strains of laboratory animals, Part 1 and 2. FASEB, Bethesda
7. Andersen SB, Bjorneboe M (1964) Gamma globulin turnover in rabbits before and during hyperimmunization. J Exp Med 119: 537–546
8. Arnason BG, DeVaux SC, Relyveld EH (1964) Role of the thymus in immune reactions in rats. IV. Immunoglobulins and antibody formation. Int Arch Allergy Appl Immunol 25: 206–224

9. Askonas BA, Fahey JL (1962) Enzymatically produced subunits of proteins formed by plasma cells in mice. II. β_{2a}-myeloma protein and Bence Jones proteins. J Exp Med 115: 641–653
10. Bach MK, Block KJ, Austen KF (1971) IgE and IgA antibody mediated release of histamine from rat peritoneal cells. I. Optimum conditions for in vitro preparation of target cells with antibody and challenge with antigen. J Exp Med 133: 752–771
11. Bangham DR (1960) The transmission of homologous serum protein to the foetus and the amniotic fluid of the rhesus monkey. J Physiol 153: 265–289
12. Barth WF, Wochner RD, Waldman TA, Fahey JL (1964) Metabolism of human gamma macroglobulins. J Clin Invest 43: 1036–1048
13. Bazin H, Platteau B, Beckers A, Pauwels R (1978) Differential effect of neonatal injections of anit-μ or anti-δ antibodies on the synthesis of IgM, IgE, IgA, IgG1, IgG2a, IgG2b, IgG2c immunoglobulin classes. J Immunol 121: 2083–2087
14. Becker EL (1971) Nature and classification of immediate type allergic reactions. Adv Immunol 13: 267–313
15. Bell S, Fahey J (1964) Relationship between γ-globulin metabolism and low serum γ-globulin in germ free mice. J Immunol 93: 81–87
16. Benacerraf B, Ovary Z, Bloch KJ, Franklin EC (1963) Properties of guinea pig 7S antibodies. I. Electrophoretic separation of two types of guinea pig 7S antibodies. J Exp Med 117: 937–949
17. Bennich H, Johansson SGO (1971) Structure and function of human immunoglobulin E. Adv Immunol 13: 1–55
18. Bernard O, Hozumi N, Tonegawa S (1978) Sequences of mouse immunoglobulin light chain genes before and after somatic changes. Cell 15: 1133–1144
19. Bienenstock J (1970) Immunoglobulins of the hamster. II. Characterization of the γA and other immunoglobulins in serum and secretions. J Immunol 104: 1228–1235
20. Bienenstock J, Tomasi TB (1968) Secretory γA in normal urine. J Clin Invest 47: 1162–1171
21. Binaghi RA, Boussac-Aron Y (1975) Isolation and properties of a 7S rat immunoglobulin different from IgG. Eur J Immunol 5: 194–197
22. Binaghi RA, Sarandon deMerlo E (1966) Characterization of rat IgA and its non-identity with the anaphylactic anitbody. Int Arch Allergy Appl Immunol 30: 589–596
23. Birke G, Liljedahl SD, Olhagen B, Plantin LO, Ahlinder S (1963) Catabolism and distribution of gammaglobulin. A preliminary study with ^{131}I-labeled gammaglobulin. Acta Med Scand 173: 589–603
24. Bistany TS, Tomasi TB Jr (1970) Serum and secretory immunoglobulins of the rat. Immunochemistry 7: 453–460
25. Bloch KJ (1967) The anaphylactic antibodies of mammals including man. Progr Allergy 10: 84–150
26. Bloom L, Rowley D (1979) Local immune response in mice to V. cholerae. Aust J Exp Biol Med Sci 57: 313–323

27. Bona CA (1981) In Immunology, Dixon FJ, Kunkel HG (eds). Academic Press, New York

28. Bona CA, Kohler H (eds) (1983) Immune Networks, Vol 418. New York Academy Science, New York

29. Boyden SV (1964) Cytophilic antibody in guinea-pigs with delayed-type hypersensitivity. Immunology 7: 474–483

30. Brack C, Tonegawa S (1977) Variable and constant parts of the immunoglobulin light chain gene of a mouse myeloma cell are 1250 nontranslated bases apart. Proc Natl Acad Sci, USA 74: 5652–5656

31. Brambell FWR, Hemmings WA, Henderson M, Parry HJ, Rowlands WT (1949) The route of antibodies passing from the maternal to the fetal circulation in rabbits. Proc Roy Soc B 136: 131–144

32. Brambell FWR (1958) The passive immunity of the young mammal. Biol Rev 33: 488–531

33. Brambell FWR (1966) The transmission of immunity from mother to young and the catabolism of immunoglobulins. Lancet ii. 1087–1093

34. Braun DG, Jaton J-C (1974) Homogeneous antibodies: Induction and value as probe for the antibody problem. Cur Top Microbiol Immunol 66: 29–76

35. Caretti N, Ovary Z (1969) Transmission of γ G-antibodies from maternal to fetal circulation of the mouse. Proc Soc Exp Biol Med 130: 509–512

36. Catsoulis EA, Franklin EC, Oratz M, Rothschild MA (1964) Gamma globulin metabolism in rabbits during the anamnestic response. J Exp Med 119: 615–631

37. Cebra JJ, Robbins JB (1966) γ A-immunoglobulin from rabbit colostrum. J Immunol 97: 12–24

38. Coe JE (1968) The immune response in the hamster. I. Definition of two 7S globulin classes: 7S γ_1 and 7S γ_2. J Immunol 100: 507–515

39. Coe JE (1970) The immune response in the hamster. II. Studies on IgM. Immunology 18: 223–236

40. Coe J, Peel L, Smith RF (1971) The immune response in the hamster. V. Biologic activities of 7S γ_1 and 7S γ_2 globulins. J Immunol 107: 76–82

41. Cohen S (1957) Turnover of some chromatographically separated serum protein fractions in the rat. S Afr J Med Sci 23: 245–256

42. Cohen S (1956) Plasma-protein distribution and turnover in the female baboon. Biochem J 64: 286–296

43. Conrad DH, Bazin H, Sehon AH, Froese A (1975) Binding parameters of the interaction between rat IgE and rat mast cell receptors. J Immunol 114: 1688–1691

44. Cunningham-Rudles C (1978) In Good RA, Day SB (eds), Comprehensive Immunology, Vol 5, Chap 5. Plenum Medical Book, New York

45. Damian RT, Greene ND, Kalter SS (1971) IgG subclasses in the baboon (*Papio cynocephalus*). J Immunol 106: 246–257

46. Damian RT, Luker MF, Greene ND, Kalter SS (1972) The occurrence of baboon-type IgG subclass antigenic determinants within the order primates. Folia Primatol (Basel) 17: 458–474

47. Deichmiller MP, Dixon FJ (1960) The metabolism of serum proteins in neonatal rabbits. J Gen Physiol 43: 1047–1059

48. Dixon FJ, Talmage DW, Maurer PH, Deichmiller M (1952) The half-life of homologous gamma globulin (antibody) in several species. J Exp Med 96: 313–318

49. Dobson C, Rockey JH, Soulsby EJL (1971) Immunoglobulin E antibodies in guinea pigs: Characterization of monomeric and polymeric components. J Immunol 107: 1431–1439

50. Dray S, Dubiski S, Kelus AS, Lennox ES, Oudin J (1962) A notation of allotypy. Nature (Lond) 195: 785–786

51. Dray S, Young GO, Gerald L (1963) Immunochemical identification and genetics of rabbit γ-globulin allotypes. J Immunol 91: 403–415

52. Dray S, Nisonoff A (1965) In Molecular and Cellular Basis of Antibody Formation, Sterzl J (ed). Academic Press, New York, p 175

53. Dubiski S, Good PW (1972) Population genetics of the heavy chain immunoglobulin allotypes in the rabbit. Proc Soc Exp Biol Med 141: 486–489

54. Eichman K (1978) Expression and function of idiotypes on lymphocytes. Adv Immunol 26: 195–254

55. Fahey JL (1962) Chromatographic studies of anomalous γ, β 2A and γ_1-macroglobulins and normal γ-globulins in myeloma and macroglobulinemic sera. J Biol Chem 237: 440–445

56. Fahey JL, McLaughlin C (1963) Preparation of antisera specific for 6.6S γ-globulins, β_{2a}-globulins, γ_1-macroglobulins and for Type I and II common γ-globulin determinants. J Immunol 91: 484–497

57. Fahey JL, Wunderlich J, Mishell R (1964) The immunoglobulins of mice. II. Two subclasses of mouse 7S γ_2-globulins: γ_{2a} and γ_{2b}-globulins. J Exp Med 120: 243–251

58. Fahey JL, Wunderlich J, Mishell R (1964) The immunoglobulind of mice. I. Four major classes of immunoglobulins: 7S γ2-, 7Sγ1-, γ1a (β_{2a})- and 18S γ_1M-globulins. J Exp Med 120: 223–242

59. Fahey JL, Barth WF, Law LW (1965) Normal immunoglobulins and antibody response in neonatally thymectomized mice. J Natl Cancer Inst 35: 663–678

60. Fahey JL, Sell S (1965) The immunoglobulins of mice. V. The metabolic (catabolic) properties of five immunoglobulin classes. J Exp Med 122: 41–58

61. Fahey JL, Robinson AG (1963) Factors controlling serum γ-globulin concentration. J Exp Med 118: 845–868

62. Fleischman JB, Davie JM (1984) In Paul W (ed), Fundamental Immunology. Raven Press, New York

63. Forsgren A, Sjoquist J (1966) "Protein A" from *S. aureus*. I. Pseudoimmune reaction with human γ-globulin. J Immunol 97: 822–827

64. Forsgren A, Sjoquist J (1967) "Protein A" from *Staphylococcus aureus*. III. Reaction with rabbit γ-globulin. J Immunol 99: 19–24

65. Fugman RA, Sigel MM (1968) Immunologic and immunochemical studies in the hamster. I. Role of the antigen in eliciting IgG- and IgM-associated antibodies. J Immunol 100: 1101–1111

66. Garvey JS, Cremer NE, Susodorf DH (eds) (1977) Methods in Immunology, 3rd ed., WA Benjamin, Inc., Reading, MA, p 273–288

67. Gilman AM, Nisonoff A, Dray S (1964) Symmetrical distribution of genetic markers in individual rabbit γ-globulin molecules. Immunochemistry 1: 109–120

68. Gilman-Sachs A, Mage RG, Young GO, Alexander C, Dray S (1969) Identification and genetic control of two rabbit light chain immunoglobulin allotypes at a second light chain locus the c locus. J Immunol 103: 1159–1167

69. Gitlin D, Kumate J, Urrusti J, Morales C (1964) The selectivity of the human placenta in the transfer of plasma proteins from mother to fetus. J Clin Invest 43: 1938–1951

70. Goding JW, Herzenberg LA (1980) Biosynthesis of lymphocyte surface IgD in the mouse. J Immunol 124: 2540–2547

71. Goding JW (1978) Use of staphylococcal protein A as an immunological reagent. J Immunol Methods 20: 241–253

72. Good RA, Day NK (eds), (1977) Comprehensive Immunology, Vol 2. Biological Amplification Systems in Immunology. Plenum Press, New York

73. Gorini G, Medgyesi GA, Doria G (1969) Heterogeneity of mouse myeloma G globulins as revealed by enzymatic proteolysis. J Immunol 103: 1132–1142

74. Grant JA, Harrington JT, Johnson JS (1972) Carboxy-terminal amino acid sequences of canine immunoglobulin G subclasses. J Immunol 108: 165–168

75. Grey HM, Sher A, Shalitin N (1970) The subunit structure of mouse IgA. J Immunol 105: 75–84

76. Grey HM, Hirst JW, Cohn M (1971) A new mouse immunoglobulin: IgG3. J Exp Med 133: 289–304

77. Grubb R (1956) Agglutination of erythrocytes coated with "incomplete" anti-RH by certain rheumatoid arthritic sera and some other sera. Acta Pathol Microbiol Scand 39: 195–197

78. Haakenstad AO, Coe JE (1971) The immune response in the hamster. IV. Studies on IgA. J Immunol 106: 1026–1034

79. Halliday R (1955) The adsorption of antibodies from immune sera by the gut of the young rat. Proc Roy Soc B 143: 408–413

80. Halliwell REW, Swartzman RM, Montgomery PC, Rockey JH (1975) Physiochemical properties of canine IgE. Transpl Proc 7: 537–543

81. Halpern MS, Koshland ME (1970) Novel subunit of secretory IgA. Nature 228: 1276–1278

82. Hammerberg B, Musoke AJ, Williams JF, Leid RW (1977) Uptake of colostral immunoglobulins by the suckling rat. Lab An Sci 27: 50–53

83. Hansburg D, Briles DE, Davie JM (1976) Analysis of the diversity of murine antibodies to dextran B1355. I. Generation of a large, pauciclonal response by a bacterial vaccine. J Immunol 117: 569–575

84. Hanson LA, Ahlstedt S, Andersson B, Carlsson B, Cole MF, Cruz JR, Dahlgren U, Ericsson TH, Jalil F, Khan SR, Mellander L, Schneerson R, Eden CS, Soderstrom T, Wadsworth C (1983) Mucosal immunity. Ann NY Acad Sci 409: 1–21

85. Harrington JC, Fenton JW II, Pert JH (1971) Polymer-induced precipitation of antigen-antibody complexes: "Precipilex" reactions. Immunochemistry 8: 413–421

86. Heddle RJ, Rowley D (1975) Dog immunoglobulins. I. Immunochemical characterization of dog serum, parotid, saliva, colostrum, milk and small bowel fluid. Immunology 29: 185–195

87. Hemmings WA, Morris IG (1959) An attempt to affect the selective adsorption of antibodies from the gut in young mice. Proc Roy Soc B 150: 403–409

88. Herbert GA, Pelham PL, Pittman B (1973) Determination of the optimal ammonium sulfate concentration for the fractionation of rabbit, sheep, horse and goat antisera. Appl Microbiol 25: 26–36

89. Herbert GA (1974) Ammonium sulfate fractionation of sera: Mouse, hamster, guinea pig, monkey, chimpanzee, swine, chicken and cattle. Appl Microbiol 27: 389–393

90. Heremans JF (1975) The secretory immune system. A critical reappraisal. In Neter E, Milgrom F (eds), The Immune Systems and Infectious Diseases. Karger Basel, London, p 376–385

91. Herzenberg LA, Herzenberg LA (1978) In Weir DM (ed), Handbook of Experimental Immunology–Immunochemistry, Vol 1. Blackwell Scientific Publications, pp 12.1–12.33

92. Honjo T, Nakai S, Nishida Y, Kataoka T, Yamawaki-Kataoka Y, Takahashi N, Obata M, Shimizu A, Yaoita Y, Nikaido T, Ishida N (1981) Rearrangements of immunoglobulin genes during differentiation and evolution. Immunol Rev 59: 33–67

93. Hood L, Gray WR, Sanders BB, Dreger WJ (1967) Light chain evolution. Cold Spring Harbor Symp Quant Biol 32: 133–146

94. Horsfall DJ, Rowley D (1979) Intestinal antibody to V. cholerae in immunized mice. Aust J Exp Biol Med Sci 57: 75–85

95. Huang H, Crews S, Hood L (1981) In Hildemann WH (ed), Frontiers in Immunogenetics. Elsevier/North Holland Inc, New York

96. Huber H, Fudenberg HH (1968) Receptor sites of human monocytes for IgG. Int Arch Allergy Appl Immunol 34: 18–31

97. Humphrey JH, Fahey JL (1961) The metabolism of normal plasma proteins and gamma-myeloma protein in mice bearing plasma-cell tumors. J Clin Invest 40: 1696–1705

98. Humphrey JH, McFarlane AS (1954) Rate of elimination of homologous globulins (including antibody) from the circulation. Biochem J 57: 186–191

99. Humphrey JH (1961) The metabolism of homologous and heterologous serum proteins in baby rabbits. Immunology 4: 380–387

100. Humphrey JH, Turk JL (1961) Immunological unresponsiveness in guinea pigs. I. Immunological unresponsiveness to heterologous serum proteins. Immunology 4: 301–309

101. Hunter WM (1978) In Weir D (ed), Handbook of Experimental Immunology, Vol I, Chap 14. Blackwell Scientific, London

102. Ishizaka K, Ishizaka T, Tada T (1969) Immunoglobulin E in the monkey. J Immunol 103: 445–453

103. Ishizaka K, Ishizaka T (1967) Identification of γE-antibodies as a carrier of reaginic activity. J Immunol 99: 1187–1198

104. Ishizaka K, Ishizaka T (1971) IgE and reaginic hypersensitivity. Ann NY Acad Sci 190: 443–456

105. Ishizaka K, Ishizaka T (1971) Immunoglobulin E and homocytotropic properties. In Amos B (ed), Progress in Immunology, Vol 1. Academic Press, New York, pp 859–874

106. Janeway C, Servary EE, Wigzell H (eds) (1981) Immunoglobulin Idiotypes. Academic Press, New York

107. Johnson JS, Vaughan JH (1967) Canine immunoglobulins. I. Evidence for six immunoglobulin classes. J Immunol 98: 923–934

108. Johnson JS, Vaughn JH, Swisher SN (1967) Canine immunoglobulins. II. Antibody activities in six immunoglobulin classes. J Immunol 98: 935–940

109. Keckwick RA (1940) The serum proteins in multiple myelomatosis. Biochem J 34: 1248–1257

110. Kehoe MJ (1978) In Good RA, Day SB (eds), Comprehensive Immunology, Vol 5. Plenum Medical Book, New York

111. Kckki M, Eisalo A (1964) Turnover of ^{35}S-labeled serum albumin and gamma globulin in the rat: Comparison of the resolution of plasma radioactivity curve by graphic means (manually) and by computer. Ann Med Exp Fenn 42: 196–208

112. Kelus AS, Gell PGH (1967) Immunoglobulin allotypes of experimental animals. Progr Allergy 11: 141–184

113. Kindt TJ (1975) Rabbit immunoglobulin allotypes: Structure, immunology and genetics. Adv Immunol 21: 35–86

114. Klein J (ed) (1982) Immunology, the Science of Self–Nonself Discrimination. J Wiley & Sons, New York, pp 195–210

115. Kulczycki A, Jr, Isersky C, Metzger H (1974) The interaction of IgE with rat basophilic leukemia cells. I. Evidence for specific binding of IgE. J Exp Med 139: 600–616

116. Lakin JD, Patterson R, Pruzansky JJ (1969) Immunoglobulins of the rhesus monkey (*Macaca mulatta*). III. Structure and activity of rhesus IgG and IgM antibodies synthesized in the primary response and in the hyperimmune state. J Immunol 102: 975–985

117. Lamm ME, Small PA, Jr (1966) Polypeptide chain structure of rabbit immunoglobulins. II. γM-Immunoglobulin. Biochemistry 5: 267–276

118. Landucci-Tosi S, Mage RG (1970) A method for typing rabbit sera for the A14 and A15 allotypes with cross-linked antisera. J Immunol 105: 1046–1048

119. Lang GM, Conrad DH, Kelly KA, Carter BG, Froese A, Sehon AH (1977) Murine and rat IgE: Relationships in terms of binding to cell receptors and to antibodies against rat epsilon chain. J Immunol 118: 749–755

120. Langone JJ (1978) ^{125}I Protein A: A tracer for general use in immunoassay. J Immunol Methods 24: 269–285

121. Lay WH, Nussenzweig V (1969) Ca^{++}-dependent binding of antigen-19S antibody complexes to macrophages. J Immunol 102: 1172–1178

122. Leissring JC, Anderson JW (1961) The transfer of serum proteins from mother to young in the guinea-pig. I. Prenatal rates and routes. Am J Anat 109: 149–155

123. Leslie RGQ, Cohen S (1970) Chemical properties of guinea-pig immunoglobulins γ_1G, γ_2G and γM. Biochem J 120: 787–795

124. Leslie GA, Armen RC (1974) Structure and biological functions of human IgD. III. Phylogenetic studies of IgD. Int Arch Allergy Appl Immunol 46: 191–197

125. Levine BB, Vez NM (1970) Effect of combinations of inbred strain, antigen, and antigen dose on immune responsiveness and reagin production in the mouse. Int Arch Allergy 39: 156–171

126. Levy HB, Sober HA (1960) A simple method for preparation of gammaglobulin. Proc Soc Exp Med Biol 103: 250–252

127. Lieberman R, Potter M (1969) Crossing over between genes in the immunoglobulin in heavy chain linkage group of the mouse. J Exp Med 130: 519–541

128. Lippincott SW, Korman T, Fong C, Stickley E, Wolins W, Hughes WL (1960) Turnover of labelled normal gamma globulin in multiple myeloma. J Clin Invest 39: 565–572

129. Mage RG, Lieberman R, Potter M, Terry WD (1973) In Sela M (ed), The Antigens, Vol 1. Academic Press, New York

130. Martin LN, Leslie GA, Hindes R (1976) Lymphocyte surface IgD and IgM in non-human primates. Int Arch Allergy Appl Immunol 51: 320–329

131. Mayers GL, Bankert RB, Pressman D (1978) Comparison of the homogeneous primary anti-dextran B1355 antibody raised in BALB/c mice with protein 104E. J Immunol 120: 1143–1148

132. McGhee JR, Michalek SM, Ghanta VK (1975) Rat immunoglobulins in serum and secretions: Purification of rat IgM, IgA and IgG and their quantitation in serum, colostrum, milk and saliva. Immunochemistry 12: 817–823

133. McGhee JR, Mestecky J (eds) (1983) The Secretory Immune System. New York Academy of Science, New York

134. Melcher U, Vitetta ES, McWilliams M, Lamm ME, Phillips-Quagliata JM, Uhr JW (1974) Cell surface immunoglobulin. X. Identification of an IgD-like molecule on the surface of murine splenocytes. J Exp Med 140: 1427–1431

135. Mescher MF, Pollock RR (1979) Murine cell surface immunoglobulin: Two forms of δ-heavy chain. J Immunol 123: 1155–1161

136. Mestecky J, Schrohenloher RE (1974) Site of attachment of J chain to human immunoglobulin M. Nature 249: 650–652

137. Mishell RI, Fahey JL (1964) Molecular and submolecular localization of two isoantigens of mouse immunoglobulins. Science 143: 1440–1442.

138. Morris IG (1964) The transmission of antibodies and normal—γ globulins across the young mouse gut. Proc Roy Soc B 160: 276–292

139. Mostov KE, Kraehenbuhl J-P, Blobel G (1980) Receptor-mediated transcellular transport of immunoglobulin: Synthesis of secretory component

as multiple and larger transmembrane forms. Proc Natl Acad Sci USA 77: 7257–7261

140. Mostov KE, Bloebel G (1982) A transmembrane precursor of secretory component. The receptor for transcellular transport of polymeric immunoglobulins. J Biol Chem 257: 11816–11821

141. Mostov KE, Friedlander M, Blobel G (1984) The receptor for transepithelial transport of IgA and IgM contains multiple immunoglobulin-like domains. Nature 308: 37–43

142. Mota I, Peixoto JM (1966) A skin-sensitizing and thermolabile antibody in the mouse. Life Sci 5: 1723–1728

143. Muller-Eberhard HJ (1975) Complement. Ann Rev Biochem 44: 697–724

144. Mullock BPM, Hinton RH, Dobrota M, Peppard J, Orlans E (1979) Endocytic vesicles in liver carry polymeric IgA from serum to bile. Biochim Biophys Acta 587: 381–391

145. Nagura H, Nakane P, Brown WRJ (1979) Translocation of dimeric IgA through neoplastic colon cells in vitro. J Immunol 123: 2359–2368

146. Natvig JB, Kunkel HG (1973) Human immunoglobulins: Classes, subclasses and genetic variants and idiotypes. Adv Immunol 16: 1–59

147. Neoh SN, Jahoda DM, Rowe DS, Voller A (1973) Immunoglobulin classes in mammalian species identified by cross-reactivity with antisera to human immunoglobulin. Immunochemistry 10: 805–813

148. Nisonoff A, Hopper JE, Spring SB (eds) (1975) The Antibody Molecule, Chap 5, 8. Academic Press, London

149. Nisonoff A, Wissler FC, Lipman LN, Woernley DC (1960) Separation of univalent fragments from the bivalent rabbit antibody molecule by reduction of disulfide bonds. Arch Biochem Biophys 89: 230–244

150. Nisonoff A, Wissler FC, Lipman LN (1960) Properties of the major component of a peptic digest of rabbit antibody. Science 132: 1770–1771

151. Nisonoff A, Hopper JE, Spring SB (eds) (1975) The Antibody Molecule. Academic Press, New York, p 94

152. Nisonoff A, Hopper JE, Spring SD (1975) In Dixon FJ, Kunkel HG (eds), The Antibody Molecule in Immunology. Academic Press, New York, pp 346–406

153. Nussenzweig V, Benacerraf B (1964) Studies on the properties of fragments of guinea pig γ_1 and γ_2 antibodies obtained by papain digestion and milk reduction. J Immunol 93: 1008–1014

154. Nussenzweig V, Benacerraf B (1967) Third Nobel Symposium on Gammaglobulins. Interscience, New York, p 233

155. Ogra PL, Dayton DH (eds) (1979) Immunology of Breast Milk. Raven Press, New York

156. Olson JC, Leslie GA (1982) IgD: A component of the secretory immune system. Ann NY Acad Sci 339: 97–104

157. Ouchterlony O, Nilsson LA (1978) In Weir D (ed), Handbook of Experimental Immunology, Vol I, Chap 19. Blackwell Scientific, London

158. Oudin J (1960) Allotype of rabbit serum proteins. I. Immunochemical analysis leading to the individualization of seven main allotypes. J Exp Med 112: 107–124

159. Oudin J (1956) Reaction de précipitation specifique entre des serums d'animaux de même espèce. Complex Rednus de l'Acad Sci (Paris) 242: 2489–2490

160. Oudin J (1974) In Sela M (ed), The Antigens, Vol 2. Academic Press, New York, pp 277–364

161. Oudin J, Cazenave PA (1971) Similar idiotypic specificites in immunoglobulin fractions with different antibody functions or even without detectable antibody function. Proc Natl Acad Sci, USA 68: 2616–2620

162. Ovary Z, Kaplan B, Kojima S (1976) Characteristics of guinea pig IgE. Int Arch Allergy Appl Immunol 51: 416–428

163. Ovary Z, Barth WF, Fahey JL (1965) The immunoglobulins of mice. III. Skin sensitizing activity of mouse immunoglobulins. J Immunol 94: 410–415

164. Ovary Z (1964) In Ackroyd JF (ed), Immunological Methods. Blackwell, Oxford, p 259

165. Patterson R, Pruzansky JJ, Change WWY (1963) Spontaneous canine hypersensitivity to ragweed. Characterization of the serum factor transferring skin, bronchial and anaphylactic sensitivity. J Immunol 90: 35–42

166. Patterson R (1969) Laboratory models of reaginic allergy. Progr Allergy 13: 332–407

167. Pearson T, Galfre G, Ziegler A, Milstein C (1977) A myeloma hybrid producing antibody specific for an allotypic determinant on "IgD-Like" molecules of the mouse. Eur J Immunol 7: 684–690

168. Peri BA, Theodore CM, Losonsky GA, Fishaut JM, Rothberg RM, Ogra PL (1982) Antibody content of rabbit milk and serum following inhalation or ingestion of respiratory syncytial virus and bovine serum albumin. Clin Exp Immunol 48: 91–101

169. Perlmutter RM, Hansburg D, Briles DE, Nicolotti RA, Davie JM (1978) Subclass restriction of murine anticarbohydrate antibodies. J Immunol 121: 566–572

170. Porter RR (1959) The hydrolysis of rabbit γ-globulin and antibodies with crystalline papain. Biochemistry J 73: 119–126

171. Portis JL, Coe JE (1975) The immune response in the hamster. VII. Studies on cytophilic immunoglobulin. J Immunol 115: 693–700

172. Prouvost-Danon A, Peixoto JM, Queiroz-Javierre M (1968) Antigen-induced histamine release from peritoneal mast cells of mice producing reagin-like antibody. Immunology 15: 271–286

173. Putnam FW, Takahashi N, Tetaert D, Lin L-C, Debuire B (1982) The last of the immunoglobulins: Complete amino acid sequence of human IgD. Ann NY Acad Sci 399: 41–68

174. Quinlivan LG (1967) Gamma globulin-^{131}I transfer between mother and offspring in the rhesus monkey. Am J Physiol 212: 324–328

175. Rabbitts TH, Bentley DL, Milstein CP (1981) Human antibody genes: V gene variability and CH gene switching strategies. Immunol Rev 59: 69–91

176. Renston RH, Jones AL, Christiansen WD, Hradek GT, Underdown BJ (1980) Evidence for a vesicular transport mechanism in hepatocytes for biliary secretion of immunoglobulin A. Science 208: 1276–1278

177. Revoltella R, Ovary Z (1969) Reaginic antibody production in different mouse strains. Immunology 17: 45–54

178. Revoltella R, Ovary Z (1969) Preferential production of rabbit reaginic antibodies. Int Arch Allergy Appl Immunol 36: 282–289

179. Richerson HB, Ching HF, Seebohm PM (1968) Heterogeneity of rabbit anti-ovalbumin antibodies sensitizing human, guinea pig and rabbit skin. J Immunol 101: 1291–1299

180. Riesen WF, Skvaril F, Braun DJ (1976) Natural infection of man with group A streptococci. Levels, restriction in class, subclass and type, and clonal appearance of polysaccharide group-specific antibodies. Scand J Immunol 5: 383–390

181. Rogentine GN, Jr, Rowe DS, Bradley J, Waldman TA, Fahey JL (1966) Metabolism of human immunoglobulin D (IgD). J Clin Invest 45: 1467–1478

182. Rowe DS (1969) Radioactive single radial diffusion: A method for increasing the sensitivity of immunochemical quantitation of protein in agar gel. Bull Wld Hlth Org 40: 613–621

183. Ruddick JH, Leslie GA (1977) Structure and biologic functions of human IgD. XI. Identification and ontogeny of a rat lymphocyte immunoglobulin having antigenic cross-rectivity with human IgD. J Immunol 118: 1025–1031

184. Sakano H, Huppi K, Heinrich G, Tonegawa S (1979) Sequences at the somatic recombination sites of immunoglobulin light chain genes. Nature 280: 288–294

185. Seidman JG, Max EE, Leder P (1979) A κ-immunoglobulin gene is formed by site-specific recombination without further somatic mutation. Nature 280: 370–375

186. Sell S (1964) Globulin metabolism in germ free guinea pigs. J Immunol 92: 559–564

187. Sell S (1964) Evidence for species of differences in the effect of serum γ-globulin concentration on γ-globulin catabolism. J Exp Med 120: 967–986

188. Sieber A, Becker W (1974) Quantitation determination of IgE by single radial immunodiffusion. A comparison of three different methods of intensification of the precipitates. Clin Chim Acta 50: 153–159

189. Simionescu N (1979) The microvascular endothelium: Segmental differentiations, transcytosis, selective distribution of anionic sites. Adv Inflammation Res Vol. 1: 61–70

190. Sire JA, Colle A, Bourgois A (1979) Identification of an IgD like surface immunoglobulin on rabbit lymphocytes. Eur J Immunol 9: 13–16

191. Sitia R, Corte G, Ferrarini M, Bargellesi A (1977) Lymphocyte membrane immunoglobulins: Similarities between human IgD and mouse IgD-like molecules. Eur J Immunol 7: 503–507

192. Solomon A, Waldman TA, Fahey J (1963) Metabolism of normal 6.6S γ-globulin in normal subjects and in patients with macroglobulinemia and multiple myeloma. J Lab Clin Med 62: 1–17

193. Solomon A, Tomasi TB Jr (1964) Metabolism of IgA (β_2A) globulin. Clin Res 12: 452

194. Spiegelberg HL (1972) γD Immunoglobulin. Cont Top Immunochem 1: 165–180

195. Spiegelberg HL (1974) Biological activities of immunoglobulins of different classes and subclasses. Adv Immunol 19: 259–294

196. Spiegelberg H, Fishkin B, Grey H (1968) Catabolism of γG myeloma proteins of different subclasses in man. Fed Proc 27: 731

197. Spring SB, Nisonoff (1974) Allotypic markers on Fab fragments of mouse immunoglobulins. J Immunol 113: 470–478

198. Strober W, Wochner RD, Barlow MH, McFarlin DE, Waldmann TA (1968) Immunoglobulin metabolism in ataxia telangiectasia. J Clin Invest 47: 1905–1915

199. Sztul ES, Howell K, Palada GE (1983) Intracellular and transcellular transport of secretory component and albumin in rat hepatocytes. J Cell Biol 97: 1582–1591

200. Tada T (1975) Regulation of reaginic antibody formation in animals. Progr Allergy 19: 122–194

201. Terry WD (1966) Skin-sensitizing activity related to γ-polypeptide chain characteristics of human IgG. J Immunol 95: 1041–1047

202. Thorbecke GJ, Benacerraf B, Ovary Z (1963) Antigenic relationship between two types of 7S guinea pig γ-globulins. J Immunol 91: 670–676

203. Thorbecke GJ, Leslie GA (eds) (1982) Immunoglobulin D: Structure and function. New York Academy of Science, New York

204. Tomasi TB Jr, Bienenstock J (1968) Secretory immunoglobulins. Adv Immunol 9: 1–96

205. Tucker PW, Cheng H-L, Richards JE, Fitzmaurice L, Mushinski JF, Blattner FR (1982) Genetic aspects of IgD expression. III. Functional implications of the sequence and organization of the C δ gene. Ann NY Acad Sci 399: 26–40

206. Uhr JW (1965) Passive sensitization of lymphocytes and macrophages by antigen-antibody complexes. Proc Natl Acad Sci, USA 54: 1599–1606

207. Vaerman JP, Heremans JF (1972) The IgA system of the guinea pig. J Immunol 108: 637–648

208. Vaerman J-P, Heremans JF (1969) The immunoglobulins of the dog II. The immunoglobulins of canine secretions. Immunochemistry 6: 779–786

209. Valbuena O, Marcu KB, Weigert M, Perry RP (1978) Multiplicity of germline genes specifying a group of related mouse κ-chains with implications for the generation of immunoglobulin diversity. Nature 276: 780–784

210. VanLogham E, Litwin SD (1972) Antigenic determinants on immunoglobulins of nonhuman primates. Transpl Proc 4: 129–135

211. VanLoghem E, Shuster J, Fudenberg HH (1968) Gm factors in non-human primates. Vox Sang 14: 81–94

212. Vaz EM, Vaz NM, Levine BB (1971) Persistent formation of reagins in mice injected with low doses of ovalbumin. Immunology 21: 11–15

213. Vice JL, Hunt WL, Dray S (1970) Contribution of the b and c light chain loci to the composition of rabbit γ-G-immunoglobulin. J Immunol 104: 38–44

214. Waldmann TA, Strober W (1969) Metabolism of immunoglobulins. Progr Allergy 13: 1–110

215. Wang A-C, Shuster J, Epstein A (1968) Evolution

of antigenic determinants of transferrin and other
serum proteins in primates. Biochem Genet 1: 347–
358

216. Warner NL, Marchalonis JJ (1972) Structural
differences in mouse IgA myeloma proteins of
different allotypes. J Immunol 109: 657–661

217. Whitacre C, Lang RW (1975) Characterization of
IgG-containing DEAE fractions of canine serum.
Transpl Proc 7: 531–536

218. Wiener AS (1951) The half-life of passively acquired

antibody globulin molecules in infants. J Exp Med
94: 213–221

219. Williams AF (1984) The immunoglobulin super
family takes shape. Nature 308: 12–13

220. Yount WJ, Dorner MM, Kunkel HG, Kabat EA
(1968) Studies on human antibodies. VI. Selective
variations in subgroup composition and genetic
markers. J Exp Med 127: 633–646

221. Zvaifler NJ, Becker EL (1966) Rabbit anaphylactic
antibody. J Exp Med 123: 935–950

Appendix A. Properties of Rat Immunoglobulins

	Immunoglobulin Class/Subclass							
	IgG1	IgG2a	IgG2b	IgG2c	IgA	IgM	IgE	IgD
Sedimentation coefficient	7S	7S	7S	7S	7S–19S[a]	19S	8S	8S
Molecular weight	150K	150K	150K	150K	$\geqslant$150K	900K	185K	190K
Electrophoretic mobility	Fast$_\gamma$	Slow$_\gamma^b$	Slow$_\gamma$	Slow$_\gamma$	β	...	...	...
Half-life in serum	———————— 5-days ————————[c]				...	...	...	...
Concentrations								
Serum (mg/ml)	0.5[d]	7	0.9	...	0.2	ND[e]	...	...
Colostrum (mg/ml)	...	0.7	0.3	...	1.2	ND	...	...
Saliva (mg/ml)	...	0.05	ND	...	0.1–0.2	ND	...	...
Placental transfer (prenatal)	+	+	+	...	ND	ND	...	...
Intestinal transfer (postnatal)	+	++	+	...	ND	ND	+	...
PCA reaction[f]								
Homologous	+[g]	————ND————[h]			...	...	+	...
Heterologous[i]	ND	———— + ————[h]			ND	ND	ND	...
Protein A binding[j]	———————— + ————————[]				ND	+	...	...

[a] The predominant form in serum is 7S, whereas polymeric forms of IgA can be found in the secretions.
[b] Electrophoretic mobility increases slightly from G2a to G2c.
[c] The half-life was determined for rat IgG only and therefore mainly reflects catabolism of the predominant IgG subclass (G2a).
[d] The serum concentration of this subclass is highly variable and may reach levels 10 times those reported after immunization or appear naturally in certain strains (ie, Wistar).
[e] ND means not detected by the assay procedure used.
[f] Passive cutaneous anaphylaxis.
[g] There appears to be a controversy as to the ability of this subclass to mediate a homologous PCA reaction, although it does compete with IgE for cellular binding.
[h] These three subclasses were not separated when assayed and were simply referred to as IgG2.
[i] The heterologous reaction was performed using guinea pigs as recipients.
[j] Rat IgG as a whole exhibits only weak binding, and no distinction is made between the subclasses. IgM binds more weakly than does IgG.

Appendix B. Properties of Rabbit Immunoglobulins

	Immunoglobulin Class/Subclass					
	IgG1	IgG2	IgA[a]	IgM	IgE	IgD
Sedimentation coefficient	7S	7S	...	19S	8S	8S
Molecular weight	150K	150K	>150K[b]	900K	180K	190K
Electrophoretic mobility	...	γ	...	...	...	...
Half-life in serum (days)	...	7–9	...	34	...	...
Concentration						
Serum (mg/ml)	Minor	9–12	<1	<1	<0.01	...
Complement fixation						
Classical	ND[c]	+	ND	+	ND	...
Alternate	+	ND	...	ND	...	...
Placental transfer (prenatal)	...	+	ND	+	ND	...
Cytophilic for						
Basophil	ND	ND	...	ND	+	...
Mast cells	ND	ND	...	ND	+	...
PCA reaction[d]						
Homologous	ND	ND	ND	ND	+	...
Heterologous[e]	ND	+	ND	ND	ND	...
Protein A binding	...	+	ND	+[f]	...	...

[a] Two subclasses of IgA have been described in the rabbit (IgA1 and IgA2) as in the human.
[b] Polymeric forms of IgA are found similar to those of other species.
[c] ND means not detected in the assay procedure used.
[d] Passive cutaneous anaphylaxis.
[e] The heterologous reaction was performed using guinea pigs as recipients.
[f] IgM binding is much weaker than IgG binding.

Appendix C. Properties of Guinea Pig Immunoglobulins

	Immunoglobulin Class/Subclass				
	IgG1	IgG2	IgA	IgM	IgE
Sedimentation coefficient	7s	7S	7S–11S[a]	19S	8S
Molecular weight	165K	161K	...	970K	185K
Electrophoretic mobility	Fast γ	γ	β	...	...
Half-life in serum (days)	7.1	5.1	...	...	...
Concentrations (mg/ml)					
Serum	2.6–7	7–10	0.07	0.43	...
Urine	0.001	0.02	0.001	0.002	...
Saliva	0.006	0.01	0.005	0.001	...
Bile	0.001	0.002	0.005	0.001	...
Colostrum	0.14	0.49	0.76	0.11	...
Tears	0.16	0.42	0.15	0.009	...
Placental transfer (prenatal)	+	+	ND[b]	ND	...
Complement fixation					
Classical	ND	+	...	+[c]	...
Alternate	+	+	...	...	...
Cytophilic for					
B-cells	...	...	...	+	...
Mast cells	...	...	...	...	+
Basophils	+	ND	...	...	...
Macrophages	ND	+	...	...	...
PCA reaction:[d]					
Homologous	+	ND	...	...	+
Protein A binding	+	+	ND	ND	...

[a] Polymeric forms of IgA are found in guinea pigs as in other species.
[b] ND means not detected by the assay procedure used.
[c] A noncomplement binding population of IgM has also been described.
[d] Passive cutaneous anaphylaxis.

Appendix D. Properties of Hamster Immunoglobulins

	Immunoglobulin Class/Subclass				
	IgG2	IgG1	IgA	IgM	IgE
Sedimentation coefficient	7S	7S	7S–13S[a]	20S	8S
Electrophoretic mobility	Slow γ	Fast γ	β	β	...
Half-life in serum (hr)	91.1	75.2	20	26.5	...
Concentrations					
Serum (mg/ml)	5.3	2.1	0.24	1.5	...
Complement fixation					
Classical	+	ND[b]	ND	+	...
Presence in fluids					
Saliva	+	ND	+	ND	...
Enteric fluids	ND	ND	+	ND	...
Colostrum/milk	+	+	+	ND	...
Urine	ND	ND	+	ND	...
Cytophilic for					
Macrophages	+	+	...	...	...
Mast cells	+	ND	...	ND	+
PCA reactions[c,d]					
Homologous	...	...	...	...	+
Heterologous	+	ND	...	...	ND

[a] Monomeric (7S) and dimeric (13S) forms of IgA can be found in hamster secretions.
[b] ND means not detected by the assay procedure used.
[c] Passive cutaneous anaphylaxis.
[d] The heterologous reaction was performed using guinea pigs as recipients.

Appendix E. Properties of Nonhuman Primate Immunoglobulins

	Immunoglobulin Class/Subclass				
	IgG	IgA	IgM	IgE	IgD
Sedimentation coefficient	7S	7S–13S[a]	19S	8S	8S
Number of subclasses	4[b]	...	2[c]	...	...
Half-life in serum (days)					
Rhesus monkey	6.6	...	...	...	...
Baboon	12	...	...	...	...
Serum concentration (mg/ml)					
Chimpanzee	8–13	0.8–2.9	0.2–0.8	...	...
Orangutan	11–13	0.9–1.9	0.2–0.9	...	...
Baboon	11–14	1.1–4.1	0.3–1.8	...	...
Rhesus monkey	12–30	0.3–0.9	0.8–2.0	...	...
Vervet monkey	10	4	1.5	...	...
Placental transfer (prenatal)	+	ND[d]	ND	...	...
Cytophilic for					
Basophils	ND	ND	ND	+	...
Mast cells	ND	ND	ND	+	...
PCA reaction[e]					
Homologous	ND	ND	ND	+	...
Heterologous[f]	+	ND	ND	+	...

[a] Polymeric forms of IgA can be found as in human serum and secretions.

[b] Four subclasses have been identified in apes using antihuman IgG subclass antiserum In the baboon, determinants cross-reactive with the antihuman antisera were not identified; however, four structural forms of IgG could be identified using antibaboon IgG antisera.

[c] Two subclasses have been defined in the rhesus monkey.

[d] ND means not detected by the assay procedure used.

[e] Passive cutaneous anaphylaxis.

[f] The heterologous reaction was performed using guinea pigs as recipients.

Appendix F. Properties of Dog Immunoglobulins

	Immunoglobulin Class/Subclass						
	IgG1	IgG2a	IgG2b	IgG2c	IgA	IgM	IgE
Sedimentation coefficient	7S	7S	7S	7S	11S[a]	19S	8S
Electrophoretic mobility	Fast	Slow	Slow	Slow	...	...	...
Half-life in serum	———— 8 days————			[b]	...	...	...
Concentrations (mg/ml)							
Serum	3–6	——— 5–8 ———[c]		1	0.8	1.5	...
Colostrum	6.9	——— 6.7 ———[c]		0.9	3.1	2.2	...
Intestine	3.5	——— 0.6 ———[c]		0.5	3.0	0.9	...
Saliva	———— 0.015 ————[b]				0.033	0.51	...
Placental transfer (prenatal)	———————— + ————————[b]				ND[d]	ND	...
Intestinal transfer (postnatal)	———————— ND ————————[b]				+	ND	...
Cytophilic for							
Mast cells	———————— ND ————————[b]				...	...	+
Basophils	———————— ND ————————[b]				...	...	+
PCA reaction[e]							
Homologous	———————— ND ————————[b]				ND	ND	+
Protein A binding	———————— + ————————[b]				...	ND	...

[a] Serum IgA has a slightly lower molecular weight than the secreted IgA although similar.

[b] The IgG subclasses were not differentiated in the study; therefore, the values given probably refer mainly to the predominant subclasses IgG1 and IgG2a,b.

[c] No distinction was made between IgG2a and IgG2b.

[d] ND means not detected by the assay procedure used.

[e] Passive cutaneous anaphylaxis.

Richard B. Bankert and Paul K. Mazzaferro

Appendix G. Properties of Mouse Immunoglobulins

	Immunoglobulin Class/Subclass							
	IgG1	IgG2a	IgG2b	IgG3	IgA	IgM	IgE	IgD
Sedimentation coefficient	7S	7S	7S	7S	7S–13S[a]	18S	8S	8S
Molecular weight	150K	150K	150K	150K	$\geqslant$150K	900K	190K	180K
Electrophoretic mobility	Fast γ	Slow γ	Slow γ	Slow γ	β	Mid γ	...	...
Half-life in serum (days)	4	5	2	4	1	1	...	...
Concentration								
Serum (mg/ml)[b]	6.5	4.2	1.2	0.1–0.2	0.7	1	<0.01	<0.01
Placental transfer (prenatal)	+	+	+	+ + +	ND[c]	ND	ND	ND
Complement fixation								
Classical	ND	...	+	ND	...	+	ND	...
Alternate	+	+	...	...	+	...	...	...
Cytophilic for								
Macrophages	ND	+	...	ND	...	...	...	...
Mast cells	+	ND	ND	ND	ND	ND	+	ND
PCA reaction[d]								
Homologous	+	ND	ND	ND	ND	ND	+	ND
Heterologous[e]	ND	+	ND	ND	ND	ND	+	ND

[a] Monomeric and polymeric forms of IgA exist in the secretions.

[b] Serum concentrations for a normal BALB/c mouse.

[c] ND means not detected by the assay procedure used.

[d] Passive cutaneous anaphylaxis.

[e] The heterologous reaction was performed using guinea pigs as recipients.

B. Complement

FRED QUIMBY, VMD, PhD, and LLOYD DILLINGHAM, DVM

The complement system is composed of 20 or more chemically and immunologically distinct plasma glycoproteins capable of interacting with each other, with antibody, with certain bacterial products, and with cell membranes. The ability of C1 (the first component of the complement system) to bind a specific site on certain immunoglobulin molecules (which are themselves bound to antigen) and activate a sequence of reactions leading to the production of a unit capable of lysing a target cell membrane has established the complement system as the primary mediator of the antigen-antibody reaction(177).

Each protein of the complement system is normally present in the circulation as a functionally inactive molecule. Together they make up approximately 15 per cent (wt/wt) of the plasma globulin fraction in man. The sequential activation of individual complement proteins from inactive to functionally active substances is a dynamic event called the complement cascade. As specific inactive complement proteins (designated by arabic numerals, eg, C-1, C-2, etc) become activated (designated with an overbar, ie, C-$\overline{1}$, and C-$\overline{2}$), they serve as enzymes that catalyze the activation of the next complement protein in the cascade. Biologically active, nonenzymatic proteins generated during

the cascade are also designated with an overbar (C$\overline{4b2a}$); however, biologically active split products that do not contribute to the cascade are designated by a letter following the term used for the component (eg, C4a and C4b). The five proteins unique to the alternative pathway are designated by letters, eg, B, D, P, H, and I. Their reaction products are also designated by a lower case letter preceded by the component symbol (eg, Bb).

In addition to their role as effectors of cell membrane lysis, many of the biologically active split products of complement proteins participate in the pathogenesis of inflammatory reactions (262). The physiology, biochemistry, and measurement of these split products, as well as the specific cellular receptors that bind them, have recently been reviewed and will not be covered extensively in this section (2,71,78, 140,277,285).

In man there are two parallel but independent pathways leading to the activation of the terminal, biologically important portion of the complement sequence, that is, membrane attack complex (MAC). These pathways are termed classic and alternative (or properdin) and are triggered by different substances (Figure 10.B.1). Both pathways converge at the midpoint of the complement cascade and thus share

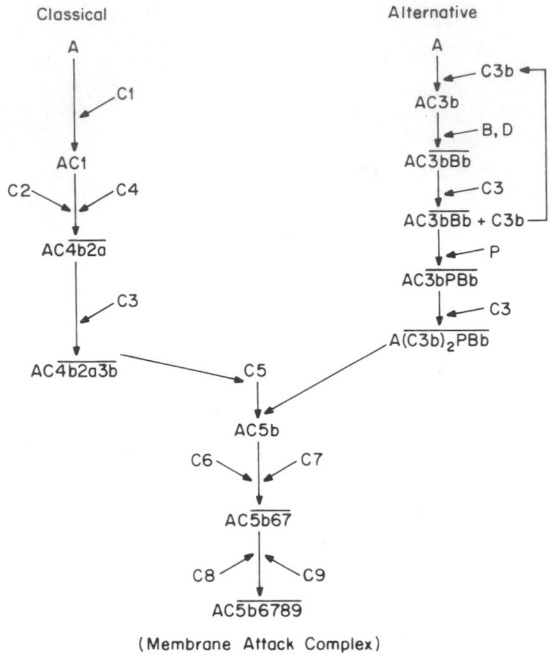

Figure 10.B.1. A schematic representation of the classical and alternative pathways for complement activation.

a common terminal activation sequence involving components C5 through C9. The classical pathway is activated by antibody-antigen complexes and has been demonstrated in man and all mammals in which it has been sought. Evidence exists for dual pathways in man, mouse, guinea pig, rabbit, rat, baboon, and rhesus monkey (103).

COMPLEMENT CASCADE

Classical Pathway

The classical pathway is initiated when C1 is activated to the active esterolytic enzyme $C\bar{1}$ (188). $C\bar{1}$, by limited proteolysis of C4 and C2, produces C3 convertase, $C\overline{4b2a}$. The potential for tremendous amplification of this sequence is demonstrated by the finding that $C\bar{1}$ can split several hundred C4 molecules. Activated $C\overline{4b2a}$ interacts with C3 to form $C\overline{4b2a3b}$ as well as several biologically active C3 split products such as C3a and C3b. The $C\overline{4b2a3b}$ complex (C5 convertase) has a functional counterpart in the alternative pathway $C\overline{3bPBb}$; both interact with C5, resulting in cleavage of the C5 molecule into C5a and C5b. $C\overline{5b}$ then attaches to the cell membrane through a C5b membrane-binding site. The interaction of $C\overline{5b}$ with C6 forming $C\overline{5b6}$ does not lead to cleavage of C6. The union of $C\overline{5b6}$ allows C7, C8, and C9 to combine, in sequence, without molecular cleavage. The $C\overline{5b6789}$ complex arranges itself on the target cell membrane so that the inner hydrophilic core is surrounded by a hydrophobic rim (188). The core or "hole" forms a transmembrane channel that allows water and ions to pass into the cell. This results in swelling; eventually the cell will burst (134). Recently it was shown that the MAC was composed of one molecule each of C5, C6, C7 and C8 with a variable number of C9 molecules. The $C\overline{5b678}$ attach to the cell surface, whereas C9 inserts into the membrane bilayer and polymerizes into a ring structure producing the channel. Depending on membrane fluidity, leaks may be caused by $C\overline{5b67}$ or $C\overline{5b678}$ as well as the totally assembled membrane attack complex (188). In fact, liposomal membranes, viral membranes, and bacterial cell walls may be disassembled by the MAC independent of the formation of transmembrane channels.

Both calcium and magnesium are essential cofactors in classical pathway activation (23). Substances shown to activate the classical pathway of complement include: immunoglobulin G and M, trypsin-like enzymes, staphylococcal protein A, teichoic acids and C-reactive protein, a number of polyanions, DNA precipitates, heparin, dextran sulfate, kallekrein, plasmin, and certain RNA tumor viruses (23,46,188,262).

Alternative Pathway

The alternative or properdin pathway is initiated by a number of nonimmunologic processes including lipopolysaccharides, staphylococcal peptidoglycans, cobra venom factor, zymosan, bacteria, viruses, parasites, and certain eukaryotic cells (116,190). In addition, heat-aggregated immunoglobulins and certain monomeric immunoglobulins can initiate alternative pathway activation (120) as can IgA immune precipitates in some species (233).

In plasma C3 has been shown to spontaneously and continuously break down, forming C3a and C3b. Factor C3b, thus formed, binds to cell surfaces where it complexes with factor B. Complex C3bB is split by the enzyme, factor D, in the presence of magnesium to form C3bBb which acts as a C3 convertase (190). C3 convertase ($\overline{C3bBb}$) is capable of cleaving C3 to C3a and C3b. Approximately 10 per cent of the C3b so released may bind activator surfaces, resulting in amplification of the sequence.

Stable complex $\overline{C3bPBb}$ acts as a C3 convertase which converts C3 to C3b and C3a. Some of the C3b formed here binds to the activator surface to produce the $(C3b)_2BbP$ complex called C5 convertase. This molecular complex recognizes and activates C5 as in the classical pathway.

Normal plasma contains two inhibitors of alternative pathway activation, factor H and factor I (Figure 10.B.2). Factor H splits the C3bPBb complex into C3b and PBb, allowing C3b to again bind cell surfaces. Factor I inactivates C3b in the presence of factor H by hydrolysis of its α-polypeptide, rendering it incapable of forming a C3 convertase. Thus, the products of the alternative pathway are nor-

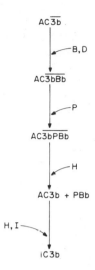

Figure 10.B.2. A schematic representation for the inactivation of the alternative complement pathway.

mally destroyed by circulating inhibitors soon after they are formed.

The current hypothesis for the activation of the alternative pathway is that certain substances, such as bacterial cell walls, fungi, helminth cuticles, and tumor cells, inhibit the activity of factor H (and possibly factor I), allowing the C3bPBb complex to develop into C5 convertase. The alternative pathway does not require specific antibody for its activation, yet it appears quite effective in inactivating a wide variety of infectious agents and it probably evolved earlier (82). A standard nomenclature for all inactive and active components of the alternative pathway has been published (144).

METHODS OF ANALYSIS

The various components of the complement system are quantitated by assays designed to measure the functional properties of these proteins or their antigenic properties. Although assays for individual components have unique benefits and disadvantages, tests designed to measure the antigenic properties of complement generally are simpler, less subject to error due to mishandling of serum, and less expensive; however, they have the disadvantage of measuring both active and inactive forms of these proteins and therefore may not necessarily correlate well with the functionally active protein concentration. Functional assays measure the ability of the entire classical or alternative pathway or individual components of pathways to lyse (hemolyze) antibody-coated (sensitized) or non-coated (for alternative pathway) red cells. Functional assays are both precise and sensitive (23).

The hemolytic assay is a useful screening test for complement activity of whole serum or plasma. However, for most complement component assays, serum rather than plasma is used because the anticoagulant may affect the assay. In addition, calcium and magnesium are required to measure early classical components; therefore, chelating agents strongly inhibit their activity. The hemolytic assay may be conducted on large volumes of serum in tubes or with smaller volumes in a microtiter test system. This assay, when used to measure classical pathway complement activity in human serum, uses sheep erythrocytes (E), rabbit antibody to sheep red cells (A), and fresh (or fresh frozen, $-70°C$) guinea pig serum as a source of complement (C). The degree of hemolysis is measured spectrophotometrically as the absorbance of released hemoglobin and can be directly related to the number of red blood cells lysed. The percentage of red cell lysis in a standardized system describes an S-shaped curve when plotted against increasing amounts of added complement. In the mid-region of the curve, there is nearly a linear relationship between the degree of hemolysis and the amount of complement added. The amount of complement required to achieve 50 per cent hemolysis is referred to as the CH_{50}. When human or animal serum is submitted to this procedure, a whole complement titer (CH_{50}) is measured. The titer is expressed as the reciprocal of the dilution of serum that lyses 50 per cent of a standard suspension of erythrocytes. If any single component of the classical pathway is missing, hemolysis will not occur; however, the total absence of a component is rare in most clinical situations, and often large reductions in individual components are necessary before the CH_{50} is reduced significantly (102). When testing animal serum, each individual species has optimum conditions for hemolysis. The target red cell, buffer pH, buffer ionic strength, and concentration of calcium ions must all be carefully selected (30). Serum for all animal species should be harvested within 60 minutes of blood collection and either tested immediately or stored at $-70°C$ until tested. Both swine and chicken complement are relatively unstable even at $-70°C$ (30). Care must be taken to sensitize red cells properly with a complement binding class or subclass of rabbit antibody, to standardize the population of target cells, and to include proper reference and internal standard sera. These techniques were thoroughly reviewed for both human (9,100,102) and animal assays (30,121). Using this basic technique, the total hemolytic complement of animals was measured in dogs (28,172,191,272,286), rats (243), mice (205), guinea pigs (270), nonhuman primates (84,234), rabbits (199), sheep (147,258), goat (213), swine (213), cat (33), hamster (287), horse (31), and chicken (29). Modifications to the hemolytic assay have been made to measure hemolytic complement in bovine milk (229). A test for measuring cytotoxic complement in rabbits using murine lymphocytes and mouse alloantisera in a microtiter system has been reported (97–99).

Fresh human serum is capable of lysing unsensitized rabbit erythrocytes in the presence of Mg-EDTA by the alternative pathway (23). However, the use of this assay to measure alternative pathway components in animals except cattle (180) has not been widely reported.

The functional (hemolytic) assay is also used to measure individual complement components. To accomplish this, cellular intermediates (target red cells with membrane-bound components) are used. All cellular intermediates are prepared by first producing antibody-sensitized sheep red cells (EA) and then incubating the cells in purified guinea pig or human Cl. This reaction mixture yields EAC1. Incubation of EAC1 with fresh human serum in EDTA yields EAC14 and EAC4. The application of EAC1 to test serum allows for the rapid binding of C4 which, in the presence of fresh guinea pig serum containing C3–9, will result in hemolysis limited only by the concentration of C4 in the test sample. Likewise, the application of the cellular intermediate EAC14 to test serum allows for the binding of C2 from the test serum which, in the presence of fresh guinea pig serum, allows for hemolysis limited only by the concentration of C2 in the test serum. The use of cellular intermediates and purified components for the measurement of all nine classical pathway components was reviewed for use in man (100) and other animals (30). Testing animal complement components using commercially available reagents for humans has produced acceptable results for the measurement of C1 and C5 through C9; however, the results obtained when measuring C4, C2, and C3 are generally much lower in domestic animals than in the human or the guinea pig (32). For this reason the purification of C4, C2, and C3 from each species and their use in a homologous assay is encouraged. The hemolytic assay for individual components using cellular intermediates was used to measure C1 through C7 in rats (21,243), C1 through C9 in rabbits (180), C1 through C9 and Factor B in nonhuman primates (178,227,248), C1 through C9 in guinea pigs (36,200), and C1 through C6 in the mouse (205).

Several modifications to the hemolytic assay have been made for the measurement of individual components in man and animals. In one modification EA cells are incubated with test serum in the presence of serum genetically deficient in one complement component. The most widely used assay employs sera from C4-deficient guinea pigs and has been used to measure C4 in man, mouse, and rat (21,24,100). Similarly, human C2-deficient sera and rabbit C6-deficient sera have been used to measure levels of these components in human and animal serum (24,36,100). In a second modification Pepys et al in 1974 (220) measured murine C3 by observing rosette formation where EAC142^{gp} (isolated components of guinea pig origin) bound to C3 on mouse mesenteric lymph node cells.

Antigenic assays including radial immunodiffusion, electroimmunodiffusion (rocket electrophoresis), automated immunoprecipitation (measured nephelometrically), and crossed immunoelectrophoresis (70,102,173) have all been used to measure complement components in man and other animals. Perhaps the simplest and most widely used is radial immunodiffusion which is based on the principle that a quantitative relationship exists between the amount of antigen placed in a well cut in the agar-antibody plate and the resulting ring of precipitation. The assay may be conducted using one of two methods. In the Mancini method specific antibody raised against the complement component to be measured is added to agar so that the antibody is in excess (relative to the concentration of the complement component in test sera). In this assay the incubation time is not critical. The Fahey (87) method employs antibody that is not in excess, and therefore, the time of incubation is critical. In both assays a standard curve is first generated using purified complement components and the diameter of the precipitin ring is directly related to antigen (complement) concentration through a logarithmic relationship. When universal reference standards or chemically pure components are unavailable, a standard reference serum may be used in which the exact concentration of the specific complement component is known. The radial immunodiffusion assay should be run on fresh or fresh frozen ($-70°C$) serum and, as in all complement assay methods, attempts should be made to avoid bacterial contamination of the test serum. Reference standards should be frozen as aliquots because repeated freeze-thawing may influence the results. The radial immunodiffusion assay has been used successfully to measure various complement components in guinea pigs (270), cattle (263), mouse (91,150), and nonhuman primates (139).

The electroimmunodiffusion (rocket electrophoresis) assay is based on the principle of electrophoresis of antigen (complement) into antiserum-containing agarose (102). In this assay the peak heights of rocket-shaped precipitin bands are measured and compared with those of standards for quantitation of antigen in the test sample. This method is both sensitive and rapid, but it requires some special equipment. Rocket electrophoresis has been used to quantitate complement components in nonhuman primates (12,178), dogs (90), mice (91,195,221), and guinea pigs (36).

A modification of rocket electrophoresis used for rapid qualitative assessment of complement components was described by Natsuume-Sakai et al (195). In this procedure wells are cut from agarose-coated glass slides, and antigen is first isolated by charge using constant voltage. After a period of time a trough is cut between two wells and specific antiserum is added. Precipitin bands occur when antigen and antiserum reach equivalence by double diffusion. This technique is useful to detect the presence or absence of a component and to observe charge variation in components. It has been used to evaluate complement in such divergent species as mouse (196) and cattle (263).

Crossed immunoelectrophoresis is a varient of immunoelectrophoresis and is more sensitive. It allows precise measurement of the amount of each antigen present in a mixture. Antigens placed in the sample slot are electrophoresed in agarose. A central strip of agarose, which contains all the isolated components, is then removed and placed on a second slab of agarose which contains the antisera (164). This assay has the advantage of providing quantitative estimations of complement component conversion, and therefore, it can assess complement activation which occurred in vivo (9). Crossed immunoelectrophoresis has been used successfully to quantitate complement components in dogs (117), cats (118), nonhuman primates (288), and mice (221).

Additional tests that are capable of detecting and quantitating complement activation have been developed. A sensitive radioimmumoassay was developed to measure the anaphylatoxins C3a, C4a, and C5a (276). This radioimmunoassay could be used to detect anaphylatoxins in rhesus monkey and baboon serum; however, the test appears to be no more than 10 per cent efficient in measuring C3a in nonhuman primate samples. Activation of the human classical and alternative pathway may be measured by enzyme-linked immunosorbant assay (ELISA); however, little information is available on its use in other animals (71).

As with most immunologic assays specificity and sensitivity are enhanced when specific antisera are employed. Table 10.B.1 lists the known sources of antibodies directed against the purified complement components of a particular species.

THE THIRD COMPONENT OF COMPLEMENT (C3)

Structure

The third component of complement (C3) is a secreted glycoprotein with the electrophoretic migration properties of a β-globulin (62). It is present in human serum in concentrations higher than those of any other complement component and was the first C component isolated in pure form. The molecules of C3, C4, and C5 have common structural and functional properties, and it has therefore been postulated that they may all have arisen from a common ances-

tral molecule (188). The molecular weight of secreted (extracellular) human C3 is 180,000 daltons (d) (45). It consists of two chains linked by disulfide bonds (203,266). The C3 α-chain weighs 110,000 d, and the C3 β-chain weighs 70,000 d. Both chains are part of a large intracellular polypeptide, pro-C3, which in mouse and guinea pig has the subunit arrangement NH_2-β-α-COOH (111). The pro-C3 subunits are linked by four arginine residues that must be cleaved to produce the native two-chain molecule (95). The secreted two-chain molecule undergoes extracellular enzymatic cleavage which selectively affects the larger α-chain. Cleavage of the chain leads to production of the C3a and C3b fragments, each with biologic activity. Further cleavage of the C3b fragment of the α-chain leads to production of C3c, C3d, and C3e (188). A similar two-chain protein has been described for feline C3. The intact protein has a molecular weight of 185,000 d. The C3 α-chain in cats weighs 128,000 d, whereas the C3 β-chain weighs 71,000 d (146). Rat C3 has a molecular weight of 187,000 d (74) and consists of two polypeptide chains weighing 125,000 and 73,000 d (122).

The amino acid sequence of the C3 chain is known for mouse and man (95). In addition, the sequence of C3a (anaphylatoxin) is also known for rat (145) and pig (72). Mouse C3a shares 92 per cent amino acid homology with rat C3a, 67 per cent homology with human C3a (141,150), and 65 per cent homology with swine C3a. All 10 amino acid residues common to the thioester bond region of human C2, C4, and α_2-macroglobulin (the thioester bond is considered essential for function) are also identical to those in mouse C3.

The C3 gene has been cloned in both mouse and man (134). C3 is coded by a single gene in both species, and strong homologies are seen in the primary structure of each C3 gene. The gene for human C3 is located on chromosome 19 unlinked to the major histocompatibility complex (MHC) (95). The murine C3 gene is linked to the MHC on chromosome 17 but maps outside the MHC, that is, a recombination distance of 12 centimorgans. Mouse C3 has three electrophoretic variants (219). Two variants, fast migrating (F) and slow migrating (S), are analogous to the two forms found in man (282). However, most mouse strains are homozygous for the S variant. The alleles responsible for

Table 10.B.1. Species Specific Antibodies to Purified Complement Components

Species	C2	C3	C4	C5	C6	Factor B
Mouse	...	196, 221, 92 CAP, NOR, RES, ACC, USB, MEB	196, 150, 216 ...	215, 86, 205, 55 ...	129 ...	196 ...
Rat	...	74 USB, ROC, CAP, NOR, RES, INV, ACC	21 ...	...	...	...
Guinea pig	110	CAP, NOR, RES, USB	35, 16, 110 MEB	...	...	35
Hamster	...	RES, USB	...	...	...	...
Rabbit	...	RES, SOC, USB, CAP, MEB, NOR	...	...	129, 113, 162	...
Dog	...	284, 118 NOR, RES, USB	...	...	...	...
Cat	...	146, 118	...	...	...	...
Cow	...	...	...	...	...	263
Human	248 CAI	248 ATL, INV, USB, CAP, MEB, NOR, RES, COR	248 ATL NOR, MBE, ACC, KEN, CAI, CAL, CAP	248 KEN, GEN, ATL, CAB, CAI, CAP, MEB, NOR, RES, ACC, CEN	248 CAB, CAI, CAP, RES	248 ATL, GEN, CAI, CAL, KEN, NOR, RES, MEB, ACC

ACC: Accurate Chemical & Scientific Corp., Westbury, NY 11590.
ATL: Atlantic Antibodies, Scarborough, ME 04074.
CAB: Calbiochem-Behring, San Diego, CA 92112.
CAI: California Immuno Diagnostics, Inc., San Marcos, CA 92069.
CAL: Cal-Med Corp., South San Francisco, CA 94083.
CAP: Cappel Laboratories, Division of Cooper Diagnostics, Malvern, PA 19355.
CEN: Central Laboratory of Netherlands Red Cross Blood Transfusion Service 1006 AD, Amsterdam, The Netherlands.
COR: Cordis Laboratories, Inc., Miami, FL 33152.
GEN: Genzyme Corp., Boston, MA 02111.
INV: In Vitro Research Sources, Inc., Benson, MD 21018.
KEN: Kent Laboratory, Redmond, WA 98052.
MEB: Medical and Biological Laboratories Co., LTD., Nagoya, Japan.
MEL: Meloy Laboratories, Inc., Springfield, VA 22151.
NOR: Nordic Immunological Laboratories, El Toro, CA; Britain, Tilburg, The Netherlands.
RES: Research Plus Inc., Bayonne, NJ 07002.
ROC: Rockland Inc., Gilbertsville, PA 19525.
USB: United States Biological Corp., Cleveland, OH 44128.

these variants in both species are codominantly expressed (195), and the allotypic determinants are located on the C3c fragment (as part of the primary structure). Antigenic variants in murine C3 have been demonstrated using specific alloantisera (197).

Three electrophoretic variants of C3 have been described in the rhesus monkey. The three alleles have been designated $C3^S$, $C3^F$, and $C3^{F1}$, with a gene frequency of 0.66, 0.33, and 0.01 among 81 rhesus monkeys (12). Using high voltage electrophoresis Gorman et al (118) described three allotypes of canine C3 designated F, FS, and S. Family studies in dogs demonstrated that the C3F and C3S alleles are codominantly expressed at a single autosomal locus. The canine C3 genetic locus was not linked to the MHC.

Human C3 α- and C3 β-chains are both glycosylated, whereas only the C3 β-chain is glycosylated in the mouse (95). It is also known that the mouse C3 β-chain is 9,000 d smaller than the human C3 β-chain because of a difference in the amino acid chain length. A number of rare variants of the S and F alleles have been described in man; however, they are all functionally identical (64,65).

Function

Because of its central position in both the alternative and classical pathways, C3 is of paramount importance in the generation of both the MAC and biologically active split products. The initial extracellular enzymatic cleavage of C3 occurs in the α-chain by C3 convertase (either classical or alternative), yielding a small molecular weight (9,000 d) C3a and the large C3b fragments. The C3b fragment has a binding site, allowing for its attachment to other acceptor molecules. Once bound, C3b has a second binding site, allowing it to react with the immune adherence receptor on a variety of cells (188). The binding of C3b to these receptors allows polymorphonuclear leukocytes and macrophages to engage in phagocytosis (104).

The C3b fragment is also subject to another enzymatic cleavage by C3 inactivator which also occurs on the α-chain (39). During this cleavage a small peptide, C3d, remains attached to the cell and a larger molecule, C3c, is released (241). The C3c fragment maintains an intact β-chain, but during fission from C3b it loses another small frgment (16,000 d), C3e (39).

The biologic activities of C3a include receptor binding and histamine release from mast cells (148), polymorphonuclear leukocyte chemotaxis (188), and contraction of smooth muscle (38).

The membrane-bound C3b combines with classical pathway C3 convertase to yield the trimolecular complex C4b2a3b which acts as a C5 convertase, cleaves C5, and initiates the assembly of the membrane attack complex, C5b–C9 (158). Likewise, the alternative pathway C3 convertase, C3bBb, may initiate a similar sequence, resulting in activation of C3–C9 (89).

Another interesting feature of C3 is that its blood concentrations increase during acute and chronic inflammation and after tissue injury (161,188). Although the acute phase reactants C-reactive protein and serum amyloid A protein rise rapidly after injury (within hours), C3 levels rise more slowly (2 to 10 days) and often parallel ceruloplasmin. The concentrations of C3 in the blood often increase by 50 per cent during this acute phase response, whereas other acute phase reactants, that is, C-reactive protein and serum amyloid A protein, have several hundredfold increases. Furthermore, although most acute phase reactants of hepatic origin are induced by interleukin-1 (see section D, on acute phase reactants), glucocorticoids are the only well-characterized C3 regulators (95).

Synthesis and Catabolism

Estimates of C3 synthetic rates in man range between 0.45 and 2.7 mg/kg/h (8,223,256). C3, like most of the C proteins, is synthesized early in fetal life (133). Gitlin and Biasucci (106) demonstrated fetal C3 synthesis in as early as the fourth week of gestation. In normal human adults, the liver was shown to be the principal, if not the only, site of C3 synthesis (13); however, small amounts of C3 have been produced in short-term culture of human monocytes, lymphoid cells, and certain epithelial cells (95).

The livers of adult rats and mice failed to synthesize C3 in vitro except after endotoxin stimulation; however, C3 synthesis was easily demonstrated in unstimulated liver from juvenile animals (269). In mice a locus that maps in the MHC controls the serum levels of C3 in the newborn; however, no significant differences in C3 are seen in adults (91,92).

Several investigators (259,261) have shown that hydrocortisone increases the synthesis of C3 in vitro; however, injection of cortisone acetate into experimental animals has yielded contradictory results (22). In one study periorbital abscesses secondary to bleeding procedures abolished the expected depression of the C3–C9 complex (62).

It has been shown that the placenta of man, rodents, and ungulates is an effective barrier in preventing the passage of complement either to or from the fetus (62).

C3a is inactivated in serum by carboxypeptidase B (an α-globulin) which removes the COOH-terminal arginine residue from C3a and neutralizes its activity. The trimolecular complex C4b2a3b decays with the dissociation of the C2 fragment. C3b inactivator splits cell-bound or soluble C3b into two fragments, C3c and C3d, and the function of C3b is thus abolished (189,267).

Deficiencies of C3

Genetic deficiencies in C3, although rare, have been described in man (14), dog (283,284), and guinea pig (47,184). Total (homozygous) C3 deficiency in man is characterized by the complete absence of C3 in the serum and it is usually associated with recurrent pyogenic infections. Many individuals with total deficiency have died in childhood. Transfusion with normal plasma gives patients transient relief from systemic infections. Sera from these patients lack the typical complement-mediated biologic functions, such as hemolytic activity, opsonization of endotoxin-coated particles, and chemotaxic and bactericidal activities (15,16). Dogs with total C3 deficiency display similar signs and a lack of normal complement-mediated functions. In both man and dog the defect is inherited as an autosomal recessive trait; heterozygotes have half the normal C3 concentrations. The first report of a complement defect in a laboratory animal was published in 1919 by Moore (184). He studied a guinea pig strain whose serum failed to lyse antibody-sensitized horse erythrocytes. This guinea pig serum showed reduced opsonization capacity, and affected guinea pigs were more susceptible to infection with *Bacillus cholerae suis* (*Salmonella cholerae suis*). This colony was decimated by an infectious disease; therefore, the true nature of the defect will never be known. The defect was transmitted as a simple Mendelian recessive trait. Burger et al (47) in 1986 described a colony of guinea pigs with C3 deficiency. Animals homozygous for the deficiency had markedly reduced lytic activity, reduced antigenic activity (6 per cent normal), reduced bacteriocidal activity, and impaired antibody responses (42,43,47). The defect in guinea pigs is inherited in a codominant autosomal fashion and is not linked to the MHC locus (47).

Partial deficiencies also have been described in man. These deficiencies may be due to either a partially inactive gene product or partially reduced synthesis of a normal product from at least one defective allele. Carriers of a partial deficiency are generally healthy (95).

Analysis of C3

A detailed description of the technical aspects of assays available for the measurement of C3

in man and animals appears in another section of this chapter (Methods of Analysis). C3 was measured by hemolytic assay using cellular intermediates in eight species of nonhuman primates. The hemolytic titers for C3 were equivalent to those in man for five species of Old World nonhuman primates; however, both antigenic and functional assays were inadequate in several New World primates (227,248). C3 was also measured by rocket electrophoresis in four species of Old World primates (12,178) and by radial immunodiffusion using human antiserum in nine nonhuman primates. In all these studies, Old World primates had strong cross-reactivity (rhesus monkey nearly identical to man) and prosimians had no detectable reactivity (139). The cellular intermediate $EAC1^{gp}4^{hu}2^{gp}$ has been used successfully to measure feline C3 (146).

In rabbits, rats, guinea pigs, and mice, C3 was measured by immunoelectrophoresis, double diffusion in agar, and immune adherence (58). Both rocket electrophoresis and crossed electrophoresis were used successfully to quantitate C3 in the mouse (195,221). C3 was also quantitated in rabbits using radial immunodiffusion (149,273). Canine C3 has been measured by rocket electrophoresis (90), and crossed immunoelectrophoresis has been used to measure C3 in the cat (118).

As with all other C-component assays, the lack of universal reference standards in animals makes comparison between laboratories impossible. These and other technical considerations are reviewed by Barta and Barta (30) as the tests are applied to domestic animal species.

Assays designed to measure antigenic determinants on the split products of C3 have been developed for man, but little use has been made of these assays in animals (255).

Interpretation

When measured by radial immunodiffusion, the adult levels of C3 in man are 1 to 2 mg/ml (95). Levels of serum C3 in women are known to increase during late pregnancy (230). Humans with obstructive jaundice have an increase in C3 (62), and patients with membranoproliferative glomerulonephritis have a decrease in serum C3 (11,223). Because liver samples from two patients with membranoproliferative glomerulonephritis failed to produce C3 in culture, it was postulated that the decrease in C3 seen in this condition is due to both decreased synthesis as well as increased catabolism (67). Decreased serum C3 due to increased catabolism is also seen in patients with diseases characterized by circulating immune complexes such as systemic lupus erythematosus.

The concentrations of total hemolytic complement (CH_{50}) and C3 were significantly depressed in dogs with acute necrotizing pancreatitis (90) and in rats fed a protein-deficient (0.5 per cent) diet (244). Rabbits developing disseminated intravascular coagulation had significantly depressed levels of C3 and CH_{50} (149). These studies documented a relationship between clotting and complement activation and demonstrated that platelets were responsible in part for the activation of complement.

Cobra venom factor (CoF) has been widely used in experimental animals to evaluate the role of complement in various biologic systems. CoF is composed of two anticomplementary factors: a low molecular weight factor (140,000 d), which activates both C3 and C5, and a high molecular weight factor (10^6 d), which is anticomplementary for the early complement components only (27). The effect of CoF has been studied in rats, rabbits, guinea pigs, and mice (58). In these studies C3, as measured by immunoelectrophoresis, double diffusion, and immune adherence, was depressed to less than 10 per cent normal in all animals after treatment with CoF. Furthermore, complement-depleted animals undergoing acute nephrotoxic nephritis had fewer neutrophils infiltrating the glomeruli. CoF was also shown to inhibit the Arthus reaction, thus demonstrating an important pathologic effect associated with C3 activation.

Mice depleted of C3 by CoF treatment had no change in the rate of clearance of pre-formed immune complexes in vivo (37), but had greatly prolonged survival of *Trypanosoma lewisi* (4). These investigators concluded that resistance to *T. lewisi* involved activation and binding of C3b by uncoated tyrpanosomes (76).

Rabbits treated with CoF and depleted of C3 (measured by radial immunodiffusion) had rapid C3-dependent depression of platelets and blood pressure. The hypotensive effects could be blocked by a histamine H2-receptor antagonist (272). Mathison and Ulevitch (174) also showed that thrombocytopenia associated with endotoxemia in rabbits could be abrogated if the

animals were depleted of C3. However, despite the abrogation of this early reaction, CoF had no effect on the final development of hypotension and disseminated intravascular coagulation in these animals.

Concentrations of C3 are depressed in the serum of baboons undergoing experimental toxic shock syndrome (227).

THE FOURTH COMPONENT OF COMPLEMENT (C4)

Structure

The fourth component of complement (C4) was first described in 1926 by Gordon et al (115) but was not isolated until 1963 (187). Human C4 is a glycoprotein weighing 209,000 d and containing 8 per cent carbohydrate. It migrates electrophoretically as a β-protein. Human C4 is composed of three unequal, covalently linked polypeptide chains designated as α, β, and γ with molecular weights of 93,000, 78,000 and 33,000 d, respectively (245). Guinea pig and mouse C4 have a similar molecular weight and three-chain structure (125). The mouse has two C4-like molecules, each coded by a separate gene in the S-region of the major histocompatibility complex (253); however, only one of these molecules (Ss protein) is the functional homologue of guinea pig and human C4 (93). Molecules having C4-like functional activity have also been described in the rat and hamster, but the proteins have not been isolated and characterized (21). Canine C4 containing three polypeptide subunit chains has also been described (211). The order of subunit composition in man, mouse, and guinea pig is β–α–γ (50,186,209). In mouse and man, the carbohydrate moiety is found on the α- and β-chains only (50).

There are two C4 structural gene loci in man, that is, C4A (acidic) and C4B (basic) (210), with allelic variants described for each locus (26). Complement 4 variants have been identified in the mouse and are linked to the S-region (93). The product of one locus, Slp, is hormone regulated (253). There is some evidence that the two C4 loci of man and mouse arose by gene duplication (253). Only a single C4 gene has been identified in guinea pigs, and it is linked to the MHC (249). Three variants of guinea pig C4, called C4-F, C4-S, and C4-S1, have been identified by electrophoresis (35). These varients are under the control of three codominant alleles at the single C4 locus (35). Despite duplication of the C4 gene in mice, only one gene product is hemolytically active (Ss protein). The product of the second C4 gene, Slp, contains a thioester site in a different portion of the molecule, preventing it from being cleaved by C1 (134). Five C4 variants have been described in dogs; they arise from the combination of two allelic products in both the α- and γ-chains (211). The two allelic products of the canine C4 α-chain also differ in molecular weight (in contrast to the human gene products which are of identical molecular weight). As in the mouse, the dog C4 γ-chain variant also shows molecular heterogeneity (94). The dog appears to have only a single C4 structural gene which is linked to the major histocompatibility complex (DLA). Two structural genes encoding C4 appear to be present in certain nonhuman primates (181).

The structural genes for C4, C2, and factor B have all been mapped to the MHC region in guinea pig, mouse, and man and are referred to as class III genes (36,159,214,235,252). The DNA sequence of the various murine and human complement component genes is 5'-C2-Bf—C4-3'. The Slp gene of mice is closer to Bf than to C4. Similarly the C4A gene of humans is closer to the Bf gene than it is to the C4B gene (134). The observation of frequent gene deletion and variations in the number of C4 genes in both mouse and man suggests that this class III region is not genetically stable and may still be undergoing gene expansion and contraction (251).

Function

During activation of the classical pathway, C4 is cleaved by C1 to produce two split products, C4a and C4b. In man C4a has a molecular weight of 10 kd and acts as a weak anaphylatoxin. The human C4b fragment is much larger, at 190 kd and covalently binds the biologic material. This bound C4b fragment combines with activated C2 to form a C3 convertase capable of completing the classical pathway of activation (188). A similar role has been proposed for functionally active C4 of all other species.

Synthesis and Catabolism

Using immunologic methods C4 biosynthesis has been demonstrated for macrophages and hepatocytes (62). In vitro production of functionally active guinea pig C4 has been demonstrated using cultures of bone marrow, spleen, and liver (254), and again the cell type responsible for production of C4 was a phagocytic cell (143,170). Using allogeneic bone marrow chimeras established in mice Geng et al (101) found that circulating C4 in the blood was not primarily synthesized by descendants of bone marrow cells. Recent studies using cell-free biosynthetic systems have shown that guinea pig (125), mouse (214), and human (105) C4 is synthesized from a single stranded precursor protein (pro-C4) (151) which undergoes intracellular processing including the cleavage of two proteolytic bonds, sulfation and glycosylation, subsequent to secretion as native C4 (281), known as $C4^s$ (s designates the secreted form). Approximately 8 per cent of the circulating C4 of mouse and man is $C4^s$ (49,150); the remaining C4 circulates as $C4^p$, a molecule produced by extracellular proteolytic cleavage. Both $C4^s$ and $C4^p$ are active in the fluid phase of blood and respond to regulatory enzymes. The combination of posttranslational intracellular processing, as well as extracellular cleavage, is responsible for as many as 20 structural variants of plasma C4 in a single human being (50). Each of the major intracellular and extracellular cleavage products has also been demonstrated in murine biosynthetic systems.

Control of C4 biosynthesis in guinea pigs has been shown to involve a specific feedback mechanism involving C4 itself (25). This feedback control of synthesis appears to be directed at the level of transcription or is a function of the stability of C4-specific mRNA. No similar feedback control of C4 biosynthesis, using similar systems, has been detected in mice (201). In vitro culture systems have also identified specific antibody and a lymphoid cell as suppressors of guinea pig macrophage C4 production (179).

In normal humans approximately 2 per cent of the plasma pool of C4 turns over each hour; therefore, 50 per cent of the plasma pool must be newly synthesized daily (23). When Ruddy et al (242) compared fractional catabolic or synthetic rates for C4 in normal humans with serum concentrations, they concluded that the primary determinant of serum concentrations was the synthetic rate. The turnover rate for other animal species is not known.

Deficiencies

A genetic deficiency of C4 has been described in guinea pigs, Wistar strain rats, and humans and a quantitative reduction in the hemolytic activity of C4 has been described in mice (150). In man, guinea pig, and rats, C4 deficiency is inherited as an autosomal recessive trait, with heterozygotes expressing intermediate levels of C4 (21,85, 206,244). Homozygotes in all three species can not activate complement through the classical pathway. Human patients with C4 deficiency have no detectable C4A or C4B gene products (236).

The deficiency in guinea pigs has been studied extensively. C4 deficiency is thought to have arisen from a mutation in the C4-F allele which is designated Co-4. Deficient guinea pig cells have no detectable intracellular pro-C4 (66); however, a C4 precursor RNA was detected using a cDNA probe for the fourth component of complement (281). These authors speculate that the basis for the C4 deficiency in guinea pigs is a posttranscriptional defect in the processing of C4 precursor RNA to mature C4 mRNA. Affected guinea pigs are more susceptible to experimental infection with *B. (S.) cholerae suis* or injection of endotoxin, had markedly impaired antibody responses to certain T-dependent antigens (176,184,207,208), and displayed characteristics of immune complex disease (42).

Mice expressing the H-2^{w7} haplotype (major histocompatibility complex) have C4 (Ss), which has only 30 per cent of the functional activity of other strains (24). In affected mice the C4 α-chain has a lower molecular weight because of a difference in its carbohydrate content (152). This genetic variation in glycosylation was shown to affect directly the hemolytic activity of the C4 molecule. Quantitative differences in the circulating levels of C4 have been demonstrated in certain strains of mice. The Ss locus is directly involved with 20-fold reduced levels of C4 being expressed in low (Ss-L) level mice. These quantitative differences in C4 are linked to the H-2k haplotype. Despite these low levels of C4, Ss-L mice do have an intact classical pathway for activation of complement and are not prone to infectious disease (252); however, they do have a greatly prolonged contact sensitivity reaction to picryl chloride (77).

Analysis of C4

The fourth component of complement may be measured using radial immunodiffusion, electroimmunodiffusion (rocket electrophoresis), automated immunoprecipitation, and sheep red cell hemolysis using C4-deficient guinea pig serum. Electroimmunodiffusion is an extremely sensitive assay for human C4 and requires less total time. Universal reference standards for human C4 are readily available for calibration of all immunologic methods. When C4-deficient guinea pig serum is available, the hemolytic assay is simple and accurate; however, care must be taken to use only fresh or fresh frozen guinea pig serum to prevent the loss of complement activity (71,100,102,173). One benefit of the hemolytic assay is that unlike immunologic assays, functionally active C4 is measured. Human C4 is measured in a hemolytic assay in which sheep erythrocytes are sensitized with antibody and C1; however, this cellular intermediate, while commercially available using purified guinea pig or human C1, is unreliable for testing many animal sera for C4, and therefore, purification of homologous C1 is usually necessary (30).

Rats have been successfully evaluated for C4 using the hemolytic assay and the cellular intermediate EAC1^{gp} and adding human C2. Hemolysis was expressed as a percentage of the maximum hemolysis obtained by substituting purified human C4 in the reaction mixture (21). Using a similar technique Sakamoto et al (243) expressed the results of C4 as the reciprocal of the end titer serum dilution giving 50 per cent hemolysis. The values for normal rats were 419 ± 93 (SD).

Mouse C4 has been successfully quantitated by a sensitive one-step hemolytic assay in which sensitized sheep red cells and C4-deficient guinea pig sera were present in the reaction mixture (24). Results of this assay were expressed in arbitrary hemolytic units in which B10.D2 mouse serum was used as the positive control. These investigators found that the addition of purified human C2 to the assay increased hemolytic titers twofold. They speculate that the human C2 helped to overcome a partial incompatibility between guinea pig C2 and mouse C4. Murine C4 also has been measured using agarose electrophoresis coupled with immunodiffusion (196). In this case alloantisera specific for each

C4 allotype were prepared by injecting mice that did not express the allotype with purified mouse C4. The method for purification of mouse C4 closely followed the method described for human C4 (40). Heterologous antimouse C4 has also been prepared for immunoprecipitation assays (216).

Immunoprecipitation procedures using heterologous goat antihuman C4 have been described for canine C4 (153).

Taking advantage of the absolute C4 deficiency of C4D guinea pigs (Co-4) Ellman et al (85) were able to develop an anti-guinea pig C4 antiserum that was effective in precipitating guinea pig C4 by gel diffusion. This principle of immunoprecipitation has been used by others to develop an effective radial immunodiffusion technique for guinea pigs (270). In addition, guinea pig C4 can be quantitated in a hemolytic assay using the cellular intermediate EAC1, with C1 of human origin (85).

Rabbit C4 has been measured in the hemolytic assay using the EAC1 cellular intermediate with C1 of guinea pig origin. After initial incubation of intermediate cells with rabbit test sera, normal guinea pig serum in EDTA is added to complete the reaction (199).

The sera of various nonhuman primates have been evaluated for detection of C4 by double immunodiffusion using goat antihuman C4. Although cross-reactivity was observed between rhesus, stumptail, and cynomolgus macaques, as well as Patas and African green monkeys, differences in migration distances, lengths of arcs, and spur formation suggested molecular differences in the proteins among species. Although this method may be useful in detecting genetic polymorphic forms of C4 among nonhuman primates, purified homologous C4 is necessary to quantitate this complement component (178). Baboon C4 was measured using cellular intermediates prepared with human purified complement components. The hemolytic activity of baboon C4 was found to be similar to that of human C4 (227).

In most studies performed to evaluate C4 in various animals, internal laboratory standards rather than commercially available reference standards were used; therefore, a direct comparison between laboratories is often difficult. A more complete discussion of the various methods is presented in the section on Methods of Analysis in this chapter, and the technical aspects of the hemolytic assays for various domestic species have previously been reviewed (30).

Analysis of C4 Activation

The fourth component of complement is activated by limited proteolysis to produce a large cleavage product (C4b) and a small product (C4a). Because the charge of C4b differs from that of the parent molecule, activation can be detected by immunoelectrophoresis (71). C4b is broken down in human serum to C4d, a smaller fragment that is antigenically different from C4. Immunoelectrophoresis in agarose allows for the simultaneous quantitation of C4 and C4d. This method has been particularly useful in the assessment of such clinical conditions as rheumatoid arthritis, hereditary angioedema, and systemic lupus erythematosus (182). Extremely sensitive radioimmunoassays have been developed to detect the smaller C4a fragment; however, although as little as 10 ng/ml of C4a can be detected in human plasma, the plasma must first be treated for selective precipitation of the native C4 molecule before application of the radioimmunoassay (119,276). Measurement of C4a has been a particularly sensitive marker of classical pathway activation in systemic lupus erythematosus (276). Although these methods could be adapted for the measurement of C4 activation in various animals, little information is currently available describing their use in species other than man.

Interpretation

In man serum C4 concentrations of 200 to 800 μg/ml (as measured by radial immunodiffusion) are considered normal (3); however, as previously mentioned, the use of different techniques and the lack of reference standards prevent a comparison of C4 concentrations (in animal species) among the various laboratories. As in man, the assays for native C4 have been particularly useful in the detection of genetic C4 deficiency in the guinea pig and rat as well as the quantitative deficiency in mice (21,85,160).

In man C4 acts as an acute phase reactant with levels increasing two- to threefold during acute inflammation. Elevations in C4 also parallel increases in corticosteroids. The serum C4 concentrations of man and animals increase from birth to sexual maturity, and levels in women increase during pregnancy (23,30).

Few attempts have been made to measure C4 during rheumatic and infectious disease in animals. In man marked depression of C4 is seen during exacerbations of systemic lupus erythematosus. Increased catabolism is the suspected cause of the lower C4 levels seen in hereditary angioedema, systemic lupus erythematosus, and complement-mediated anemias (9,23). Whereas total hemolytic complement activity is decreased during certain rheumatic diseases in dogs, the levels of specific components have not been measured (30,286).

In man C4 levels are decreased during infections associated with the development of antigen-antibody complexes such as malaria and poststreptococcal glomerulonephritis (23). In our own studies, baboons immune to staphylococcal toxic shock toxin (TSST-1) and injected with TSST-1 through the intravenous route have a rapid and prolonged decrease in C4 (227). Depression of C4 has been associated with acute aflatoxicosis in guinea pigs (270) and dietary protein restriction in rats (243). Sex-limited protein (Slp), the nonfunctional homologue of C4 in mice, has an androgen-dependent inducible synthesis in some strains (217) and constitutive (androgen-independent) synthesis in other strains (128). Recent studies suggest that hormonal regulation of the Slp gene product is associated with DNase I-hypersensitive sites in the 5′ regions of the Slp gene (130). Strains showing androgen-independent expression of Slp have C4-Slp recombinant genes with the 5′ region derived from the C4 gene (194). No other differences in circulating C4 have been described in animals of different gender, in association with natural cycles, or in response to specific drugs.

THE SECOND COMPONENT OF COMPLEMENT (C2)

Structure

In man the second component of complement is a single-chain glycoprotein with a molecular weight of 117,000 d (63). Human C2 migrates as a β_1-globulin with a sedimentation constant of 6S (62). In man the C2 molecule has two free reactive SH groups that are positioned in close proximity to form an intramolecular disulfide bond on oxidation with iodine. This reaction allows for an extraordinary increase in hemolytic activity (188,228). Guinea pig C2 has a molecular weight of 130,000 d (62).

Factor B, C2, and C4 are coded within the MHC in man, guinea pig, and mouse. In man C2 and Bf genes are very close and separated from C4 genes by 50 kilobases (134).

Genetic polymorphism of C2 has been described in man (6,135). In contrast to humans, who have one main C2 allotype and two rare allotypic variants, guinea pigs have six C2 phenotypes resulting from three alleles occurring with equal gene frequency. The three allotypic variants are known as $C2^B$ (basic), $C2^A$, and $C2^{A1}$, the latter two both being acidic variants. These variants of a single structural C2 gene behave as autosomal codominant traits (36).

Function

C2 is a serine protease found normally as a trace protein in serum and it is one of the two precursor molecules of the complex enzyme C3 convertase (188). C3 convertase (C4b,2a) is assembled by the enzyme C1s. The cleavage products of C2 are C2a (80,000 d) and C2b (37,000 d). C3 convertase is then capable of activating C3 and continuing the classical pathway.

Synthesis and Catabolism

A variety of studies have demonstrated that monocytes and tissue macrophages are the cellular sites of C2 synthesis in the human and the guinea pig (62). Human monocytes in culture generally require 3 days of incubation in vitro before C2 synthesis is detected. This delay in C2 secretion can be shortened by adding a lymphokine to the culture medium (171). Human bronchoalveolar macrophages incubated in vitro initiate C2 synthesis without this 3-day lag period (59). Likewise, differences are seen in the rate of C2 synthesis by guinea pig macrophages; however, in this species the proportion of tissue macrophages bound to synthesize C2 varies from 2 per cent for bronchoalveolar macrophages to 45 per cent for peritoneal or splenic macrophages (17). The plasma levels of C2 vary greatly between strains of mice, and genes outside the MHC are thought to be involved in the transcriptional control of C2 (88). In addition, exogenous IL-1 has been shown to increase specific C2 mRNA levels in murine kidney and lung (88,222).

In healthy humans, approximately 2 per cent of the plasma pool of C2 turns over each hour (23). The human C3 convertase $\overline{C4b2a}$ has a half-life at 37°C of 10 minutes (227).

Deficiencies

Deficiency of C2 occurs in 1 in 10,000 individuals, making it the most common human complement deficiency (107). Macrophages from deficient humans function normally but are incapable of secreting C2 (63).

Recently, Cole et al (60), using a combination of protein radiolabeling, immunoprecipitation, and Northern and Southern blot analyses, discovered that C2-deficient humans do not have a major gene deletion or rearrangement, but rather they have a specific and selective pretranslational regulatory defect in C2 gene expression. This leads to a lack of detectable C2 mRNA and a lack of C2 synthesis.

The C2 deficiency in guinea pigs is the first C2 deficiency described in an animal besides man (126). Homozygous deficient guinea pigs have no detectable hemolytic activity, whereas heterozygotes have 50 to 70 per cent hemolytic activity (36). These C2-deficient guinea pigs show no C1s-induced vascular permeability (260), have impaired humoral immunity (41), and demonstrate characteristics of immune complex disease (42). Guinea pigs homozygous for C2 deficiency synthesize a C2-like protein that can be detected immunologically within the cytoplasm of monocytes, but it is not secreted. Extracellular fluid from in vitro cultured C2-deficient macrophages contained reduced amounts of C2 antigen which consisted of small molecular weight molecules (14 to 15 kd). These studies suggested that C2-deficient guinea pig macrophages produce a structurally abnormal C2 protein, but they could not distinguish between a block in secretion or secretion of an instable C2 protein (111). The C2° allele of C2 deficient guinea pigs appears to be a silent $C2^B$ allele.

Analysis of C2

Guinea pig C2 may be quantitated using the cellular intermediate EAC14^{gp} and guinea pig serum diluted 1:10 in Veronal Buffered Saline-EDTA as a source of C3 to C9 (36). Similarly C2-deficient guinea pig serum may be used in a one-step hemolytic assay. Quantitative estimates for guinea pig C2 have also been conducted by rocket immunoelectrophoresis using homologous anti-guinea pig C2 antibody (36).

Mouse C2 has been quantitated by hemolytic assay using the cellular intermediate EAC1^{gp}4^{h} (112). Rat and rabbit C2 has similarly been quantitated with cellular intermediates made from purified guinea pig C1 and C4 (199,243).

Baboon C2 was quantitated employing intermediates prepared from human purified complement components. In this assay the hemolytic activities of baboon C2 were found to be approximately fivefold greater than those of human C2 (227). Likewise, Schur et al (248) quantitated the hemolytic activity for individual complement components in eight species of nonhuman primates using cellular intermediates prepared from purified human components. The C2 hemolytic titers of chimpanzees and gibbon ape were roughly the same as those of the human. The C2 hemolytic titers of *P. anubis* (baboon), *M. fuscicularis* (crab-eating macaque), *A. geoffrayi* (spider monkey), and *Cebus albifrins* (cebus monkey) were all greater than those of the human, and the titer of *Galago crassincaydatus* (greater bush baby), a prosimian, was approximately one tenth that of the human (248).

Interpretation

Humans have 25 μg/ml of C2 in serum as measured by radial immunodiffusion (188). The hemolytic titer of C2 measured in Old World nonhuman primates and Great Apes is similar to human titers when purified human components are used as intermediates. (See Analysis of C2.) The concentration of C2 in other species varies with methodology and the laboratory standard used.

Studies of 26 families with homozygous C2 deficiency (C2D) probands demonstrated that 23 of 38 C2D patients had diseases of the autoimmune type. Fourteen (37 per cent) had systemic lupus erythematosus or discoid lupus erythematosus (3). Only 2 of 38 patients had recurrent infections. As a primary clinical problem, however, an increased susceptibility to infections is thought to occur in all C2D homozygotes. The disease manifestations in C2D patients with systemic lupus erythematosus are different from those of "classic" systemic lupus erythematosus because C2D patients do not have anti-DNA antibodies and do have reduced immunoglobulins deposited in skin, a low incidence of renal disease, and an increased frequency of discoid lesions, suggesting that certain genes that control the disposition to this pathology may be missing in C2D patients. A similar systemic lupus erythematosus-like syndrome has not been described in the C2D guinea pig; however, circulating immune complexes are seen in these animals (42).

In several cases of C2D in humans there has also been a partial deficiency in factor B (202). These patients suffer from repeated *Streptococcus pneumoniae* infections. Because clearance of this organism is thought to depend on C3b-induced opsonization, an inability to activate C3 through the alternative pathway would predispose individuals to streptococcal infection.

Humans afflicted with autoimmune disorders characterized by antibody-antigen binding and activation of the classical pathway of complement, such as systemic lupus erythematosus, and autoimmune hemolytic anemia, characteristically have sharp depressions in serum C2 (and most other classical components). Although not specifically studied, it is assumed that C2 levels are depressed in animals that develop spontaneous systemic lupus erythematosus and autoimmune hemolytic anemia because dramatic decreases in total hemolytic complement are apparent during disease in susceptible strains of mice (19).

In humans afflicted with malaria there is rapid activation of the classical pathway and a resultant sharp decline in serum C1, C4, C2, and C3 levels concomitant with schizont rupture and intravascular release of malaria antigens (23). Patients afflicted with cutaneous necrotizing vasculitis and disseminated intravascular coagulation also have depressed serum C2 levels. A similar depression may be expected in animals with disseminated intravascular coagulation. (See the section on interpretation of C3.)

C2, like C1, C4, and C3, and factor B, acts as an acute phase reactant, increasing two- to fourfold during inflammation in man. C2 levels are also elevated in women during pregnancy; however, similar findings in animals have not been reported.

The functional levels of C2 were found to vary among inbred strains of mice (112). Serum C2 levels in mice appear to be controlled by genes closely linked to the Ss locus. Rats maintained on protein-deficient diets (0.5 vs 18 per cent) for 8 weeks had a 58 per cent depression in serum C2 activity (243). In addition, normal Sprague-Dawley pathogen-free rats challenged with an intradermal inoculation of 2×10^9 *Staphylococcus aureus* organisms had a 100 per cent elevation in serum C2, which remained elevated 14 days following inoculation (243).

Baboons subjected to intravenous injection of the TSST-1 toxin of *S. aureus* developed a 50 per cent depression of serum C2 within 2 hours which coincided with hypotension. This depression of serum C2 persisted for 3 days (227).

While evaluating total hemolytic complement in the sera of approximately 5,000 dogs, Neil Gorman (personal communication) discovered a complete absence of hemolytic activity in one animal which, on further evaluation, was a total deficiency of hemolytically active C2. Unfortunately this animal was not available for breeding; however, this large scale testing has demonstrated that C2 deficiency in dogs may not be rare.

Finally, there has been some speculation that the pathogenesis of the edema in hereditary angioedema (C1 esterase inhibitor deficiency) of man is mediated by a cleavage product of C2 with kinin-like activity (79). Serum C2 levels are also known to be very low during acute attacks of this disease. No equivalent deficiency has been described in animals.

THE FIFTH COMPONENT OF COMPLEMENT (C5)

Structure

Human C5 has a molecular weight of 180,000 d and is a β_1-globulin. The human C5 glycoprotein contains approximately 20 per cent carbohydrate. This C5 molecule is a two-chained structure with chains linked by disulfide bonds (203). The approximate molecular weights of alpha (α) and beta (β) chains are 110,000 and 70,000 d, respectively (188). A protein immunochemically defined as C5 in the mouse was previously called MuB1. In mice, plasma C5 consists of two chains of unequal size, an α-chain

(115,000 d) and a β-chain (82,000 d) structurally similar to those of both human and guinea pig C5 (218).

Function

When C5 is subjected to enzymatic attack by C5 convertase (C4b2a3b), the resulting product, C5b, serves as the focus for a self-assembling process leading to the stable C5b-9 complex (158). The entire membrane attack complex is composed of one molecule each of C5, C6, C7, and C8 and a variable number (8 to 18) of C9 molecules (134). This large molecular complex is assembled without the need for enzymatic activity following C5 convertase (188). One recent report (155) suggests that at least in some cases of human C3 deficiency, C5 may compensate for the lack of C3. These investigators provide evidence for the direct activation of C5 by the C3 convertase (C4b2a), resulting in the formation of the membrane attack complex C5b-9.

C5a biologically behaves very similar to C3a, causing the release of histamine from mast cells, chemotaxis of neutrophils, and contraction of smooth muscle. The C5a of pig, rat, and guinea pig differs from human C5a in that their COOH-terminus is susceptible to inactivation by serum carboxypeptidase B, which forces a conformational change on this molecule, resulting in reactivation and resistance to carboxypeptidase B (142,275,277). C5a and C3a bind to specific receptors on lymphocytes and macrophages and are potent regulators of the immune response (277). Human C5a triggers a wide variety of neutrophil responses after binding to the neutrophil receptor (140). Murine C5a binds to specific receptors on murine macrophages, but murine lymphocyte C5a receptors have not been identified. Purified C5a, given in physiologic doses, was shown to enhance the primary murine anti-SRBC response in vitro by induction of cytokine by macrophages (114). Furthermore, C5a stimulates the production of interleukin-1 by murine macrophages (277).

Synthesis and Catabolism

Evidence from several studies suggests that C5 may be synthesized in many human tissues including lung, liver, spleen, thymus, placenta, peritoneal cells, bone marrow, and fetal intestine (61,156). In the mouse, splenic macrophages were shown to be a site of C5 (MuB1) synthesis by one group (62), whereas another group found that circulating C5 was not synthesized by descendants of bone marrow cells (101). Studies of murine C5 synthesis in C5-deficient (C5D) strains have demonstrated the presence of a 200,000 d single polypeptide located intracellularly, but no extracellular C5 was detected. These authors suggested that C5D strains produce a nonglycosylated pro-C5 molecule intracellularly but that the product is not secreted (212). Studies conducted in mice have shown that C5 is synthesized in the fetus at 10 to 12 days of gestation, and that passive transfer of C5 from mother to fetus does not occur (264).

C5 convertase (C4b2a3b) cleaves a small fragment (molecular weight 17,000 d) from the α-chain, called C5a, leaving a slightly smaller biologically active C5b molecule (molecular weight 163,000 d). The C5b molecule is inactivated by a second enzymatic cleavage, also of the α-chain, which yields a small C5d fragment. The biologically active C5a, like C3a and C4b, binds to surface receptors on white blood cells. It has been shown that neutrophils and macrophages in both mouse and man are capable of degrading C5a following its specific receptor binding (277). The turnover rate of C5 in man has been approximated at 2 per cent of the plasma pool per hour (23).

Deficiencies

Humans with both total deficiency of C5 and C5 dysfunction have been described. The deficiency disease is rare and has been associated with absence of C5 (immunogenic and hemolytic) and increased susceptibility to infection, particularly pneumococcal pneumonia, and, in some, to systemic lupus erythematosus. One patient with C5D and systemic lupus erythematosus had typical serologic and dermal manifestations of systemic lupus erythematosus, but the renal disease was not progressive (238). In vitro studies with C5D serum demonstrated impaired cytolytic and bactericidal activities. Deficient sera could not generate chemotaxic factor, but they could provide normal opsonization of Baker's yeast (239). The disease is transmitted as an autosomal trait in which heterozygotes have half normal levels.

Several families have been reported on in which family members have normal antigenic and hemolytic C5 levels, yet are predisposed to infections. A functional defect in C5 is postulated because purified C5 corrects the opsonization defect but C5D serum does not. These patients have Leiner's disease characterized by eczema and secondary infections in infants (183). Because the defect in opsonization is not seen in homozygous C5-deficient serum, another factor may be responsible for this phenomenon.

Mice deficient in the fifth component of complement were first described by Rosenberg and Tachibana (237) who were able to show that two strains, DBA/2 and B10.D2 (old), were lacking in hemolytic activity. They also demonstrated that the defect was inherited as a single Mendelian recessive trait, the locus of which was designated as Hc (131,265). By immunizing DBA/2 mice with serum from other normal mice, two groups of investigators independently discovered a new serum beta globulin (also called MuB1) which was present only in mice with normal hemolytic activity (54,86). Homologous and heterologous antibody to MuB1 reacted with the serum of many mammalian species, demonstrating common antigenic specificities among them (55). Later a protein contaminant of murine β1c, β1F glycoprotein, was characterized as the fifth component of complement (204) and shown to be the same as MuB1 (205). Because purified human C5 was able to reconstitute mice bearing the homozygous Hc° (deficient) gene, it was concluded that the Hc locus controlled the production of C5 in mice. As in humans, there is no linkage between the Hc gene and the major histocompatibility complex (H-2) in mice. There is some evidence that the molecular basis for C5 deficiency in mice involves an abnormal primary transcript of the C5 gene, retarding the processing of C5 mRNA and resulting in an abnormal C5 protein (280).

The availability of two coisogenic lines of mice, one deficient in C5 (B10.D2/oSn) and the other (B10.D2/nSn) containing normal levels of C5, has allowed investigations concerning the role of C5 in a variety of experimental situations. The ability to reject large numbers of sarcoma I tumor cells was shown to require the presence of C5 (224). Two groups demonstrated that C5D strains of mice were not as capable of rejecting skin allografts after treatment with anti-lymphocyte serum (57,278). Lindberg and Rosenberg (169) found that C5-sufficient (B10.D2/nSn) strains were at risk of developing experimental nephritis; however, complement-deficient strains of mice were more susceptible to the development of experimental thyroiditis (193).

The importance of C5 in resistance to experimental bacterial infections has been studied extensively. Killing of *Escherichia coli* but not phagocytosis (109), in vivo and in vitro defense against *S. pneumoniae* (250), opsonization of *S. aureus* (81), and the early attraction of neutrophils against *Listeria monocytogenes* (165) all required C5 for maximum activity. Later studies showed that C5 yields important neutrophil chemotaxins during the early period after intrapulmonary inocuation with *S. pneumoniae* and that pulmonary clearance of the organism is impaired in C5D mice (271). Similar findings regarding pulmonary clearance of aerosolized *S. aureus* have also been reported (48).

Morelli and Rosenberg (185) demonstrated that normal mice survived longer than C5D mice when injected with *Candida albicans*. Moreover, infection of C5D mice with *Mycoplasma pulmonis* resulted in a more severe and persistent arthritis than that seen in normal mice (154). Furthermore, the incidence of pulmonary consolidation and mortality seen in mice inoculated with influenza virus was much higher in C5D mice (132).

Analysis of C5

The hemolytic assay for murine C5 is conducted using the EAC1a,4,^{oxy}2a3b intermediate constructed from purified human components. The use of oxidized C2 resulted in 10 times greater stability of the complex (205). The cellular intermediate can also be constructed using certain purified guinea pig components (268). Qualitative determination for the presence or absence of murine C5 has been assayed using immunodiffusion with antihuman C5 (215).

The hemolytic titers of C5 for cow, goat, pig, and chicken were very low when measured using cellular intermediates constructed from human components; therefore, the isolation of autologous components for accurate testing is required (32). Feline and canine hemolytic C5 titers are intermediate in activity when compared to large ruminant species. (For details see Methods of Analysis.)

Hemolytic titers for C5 can be measured accurately in guinea pigs using cellular intermediates constructed of either guinea pig or human purified components (162,199).

Interpretation

Humans average 80 $\mu g/ml$ of C5 in serum as measured by radial immunodiffusion (188). The mouse was once considered to have particularly low amounts of hemolytically active complement until it was realized that many inbred strains and outbred mice are deficient in the fifth component (131). An early attempt to develop a more sensitive assay using radioactive chromium-labeled sheep erythrocytes was described by Rosenberg and Tachibana (237). However, the development of cellular intermediates from purified components as well as specific antisera against C5 has rectified this situation. Many Hc° homozygous strains have been described (257).

Cinader et al (56) and Dubiski and Cinader (80) showed that adult female mice have only two thirds the concentration of MuB1 found in adult C5-sufficient males.

The kinin, coagulation, and fibrinolytic systems share important relationships with the complement system. In particular, the activation of these systems (as in experimental endotoxemia) may provide substances that activate certain complement proteins including C5 (262). Furthermore, those conditions that lead to the activation of C3 and the production of C5 convertase will result in decreased concentrations of C5 (and other late phase components) in the serum. Direct measurement of C5 activity during disease in animals has not been extensively reported; however, it is assumed that changes in C5 concentration in most mammalian species will parallel changes seen in similar human conditions (3,9,23).

THE SIXTH COMPONENT OF COMPLEMENT (C6) WITH COMMENTS ON THE SEVENTH COMPONENT (C7)

Structure

The sixth component of human complement is a β-globulin with a molecular weight of 111,000 d (225). Homogenous preparation of C6 from rabbit and guinea pig serum revealed proteins of similar molecular weight and structure (20).

Murine C6 is also a single peptide chain with a molecular weight slightly larger than that of human C6 (140,000 d); the PI range of murine C6 is more basic than that of human C6 (129). Purified C7 from humans has a molecular weight of 102,000 d and an electrophoretic mobility identical to that of C6. Both C6 and C7 are single polypeptide chains (225). Additional investigations showed similarities between C6 and C7 in both amino acid and carbohydrate content, and trypsinization studies suggest similar tertiary structures (226).

Both C6 and C7 in man show polymorphisms by isoelectric focusing (136). Polymorphisms have also been demonstrated for C6 of rhesus monkey (124), chimpanzee (231), rabbit (160), dog (18,83), and mouse (129). Canine C7, like human C7, is polymorphic (83).

Murine C6 occurs as two major protein bands by isoelectric focusing designated as C6A and C6M. Each protein band is also associated with one or more minor acidic bands. The major protein is controlled by a single codominant autosomal locus with alleles C6ᵃ and C6ᵐ which encode for C6A and C6M, respectively (129). Two common variants of human C6 were also described by isoelectric focusing, and they are designated as the A and B variants. Individuals may express any of three phenotypes, C6A, C6B, and C6AB, which occur with frequencies of 37 per cent, 14 per cent, and 45 per cent respectively (136).

Studies by Hobart, Cook, and Lachmann (138) showed that the gene responsible for C6 deficiency in man is not linked to HLA but is closely linked to the gene for C7.

Function

Regardless of which pathway is activated, C5 convertase cleaves C5, producing C5b which attacks the membrane at a third topologically distinct site (188). The final membrane attack complex C5-9 is constructed when one molecule each of C5, C6, C7 and C8 attaches to the cell surface, and a variable number of C9 molecules insert themselves into the membrane bilayer and polymerize into a ring containing a central channel (134). The attachment of late-acting complement components (C6 through C9) takes place spontaneously without the necessity for enzymatic cleavage (188). The soluble C5-9 complex circulates in the fluid phase following cytolysis and has a molecular weight of 1,040,000 d (157).

Synthesis and Catabolism

Following liver transplantation in one human who expressed the C6B phenotype, there was total conversion from C6B to C6A phenotype by day 10 (137). Thus, the liver must be the major if not the only site of C6 synthesis in man.

The half-life ($t\frac{1}{2}$) of rabbit C6, calculated by infusion of plasma from normal into C6D rabbits, is 30 hours (34).

Deficiency of C6

Deficiency of C6 (C6D) has been described in humans who lack antigenic and functional levels of C6 in their plasma. The disease is transmitted in families with an autosomal codominant pattern of inheritance (3). Heterozygotes for the C6D gene have half-normal antigenic levels of C6 but normal CH_{50} levels. Although some C6D patients appear to be normal, others have been described with Raynaud's syndrome, recurrent gonococcal septicemia, and recurrent meningococcal meningitis (23).

A biologically normal individual was found who had a partial genetic deficiency of both C6 and C7. Plasma levels of C6 were low and the molecular size of the C6 was smaller than normal. A structural mutation in the C6 gene causing hyposynthesis of C6 and C7 was hypothesized (108,163). In most instances, however, human C6 deficiency is not associated with reduced C7 (166,168). In addition, C6D rabbits have normal levels of C7 (199). A simultaneous deficiency of C6 and C2 occurred in three members of a single family; however, the deficient genes segregated independently, indicating separate genetic events (75).

At least three separate instances of spontaneous C6 deficiency have occurred among different strains of rabbits. In each instance C6D rabbits had little or no hemolytic C6 in their serum. The hemolytic activity of serum was reconstituted in one C6D strain by adding purified human or rabbit C6 (240) and by adding purified guinea pig C6 in another C6D strain (199). Lachmann (162) showed that C6D rabbits had no circulating antigenic C6. Given the fact that these deficiencies occurred in different strains of rabbits in England, Mexico, and Ger-

many, it is assumed that the defect in C6 synthesis in this breed is fairly common. The defect in C6 synthesis in rabbits was shown to be transmitted as a single autosomal recessive trait with heterozygotes containing half-normal serum levels of C6 (162).

C6D rabbits appear to withstand common infections well and have normal antibody production. Abnormal coagulation, as measured by prolonged whole blood clotting time and reduced prothrombin consumption, was observed in C6D rabbits and corrected by adding purified C6 to deficient blood (290).

C6 deficiency has been reported in the Syrian hamster (287). Serum from C6D hamsters could not reconstitute C6D serum from humans or rabbits; however, normal hamster serum could. Although no differences between C6D and normal hamster sera were noted in induction of immune adherence or phagocytosis, this colony was extremely susceptible to proliferative enteritis and was subsequently lost.

Analysis of C6 and C7

Hemolytic assays designed to measure C6 in various animals have taken advantage of the availability of C6D human and rabbit serum, thus allowing for simple one-step assays to quantitate C6 activity in the hamster (287), dog (83), rabbit (113), and mouse (205). The quantitation of both rabbit (199) and mouse (205) C6 and C7 using cellular intermediates and purified components has been documented. The details for measuring C6 and C7 in man and nine animal species using purified components on cellular intermediates were given by Barta and Hubbert (32) in 1978. The hemolytic titers for both C6 and C7 for seven nonhuman primate species were published by Schur et al (248). Immunologic techniques have been employed for measurement of C6 in mouse (129) and rabbit (113).

Interpretation

The levels of antigenic C6 and C7 in human serum average 60 μg/ml (23).

Quantitation of murine C6 in plasma revealed that females had much lower levels of antigenic and functional C6 than did males (53,205). In addition, levels of antigenic C7 in female mice were lower than male C7 levels (205).

As with most complement components, the measurement of C6 and C7 in animals varies between laboratories according to the methodology used. The lack of species-specific reference standards makes direct comparisons between laboratories difficult.

ALTERNATIVE PATHWAY COMPONENT FACTOR B

Structure

In man factor B is a single chain glycoprotein with a molecular weight of 95,000 d (52) and migrates as a β-globulin (190). This thermolabile glycoprotein is composed of 7.3 per cent carbohydrate (73), and its amino acid composition is known (167). Murine factor B has a molecular weight of approximately 100,000 d (198,235).

The intact human factor B is cleaved into Ba and Bb fragments of 30,000 d and 61,000 d molecular weight, respectively (188). The Ba and Bb fragments of murine factor B have similar molecular weights (235).

Multiple alleles of Bf (the factor B structural gene) have been described in man (10), mouse (198,235), guinea pig (35), and rhesus monkey (289). Multiple alleles in all species are codominantly expressed. Four allelic variants have been found in mice (198), two variants in guinea pigs (35), and six in the rhesus monkey (289).

The gene for human factor B is closely linked to the gene for C2 (7,35), C4 (26), and the major histocompatibility locus (5,232). Linkage between Bf, C2, C4, and the MHC has also been demonstrated for the rhesus monkey (288), guinea pig (159), and mouse (198,235). Restriction map analysis of the genomic clone and total genomic DNA have elucidated a single Bf gene (per haploid) spanning more than 5.5 kilobases. Using a human factor B cDNA probe, a murine cDNA clone that has 85 per cent homology with the human cDNA was isolated (63). Restriction enzyme analysis of multiple human and murine cDNA clones failed to reveal differences in the DNA sequence among members of the same species.

Function

When factor B (bound to C3b) is cleaved by factor D (in the presence of Mg^{2+}), it generates C3bBb, an unstable C3 cleaving enzyme. This cleaving enzyme is stabilized by the addition of properdin (P) to form C3 and C5 convertases (see Figure 10.B.2) (63). Because Bb can hydrolyze the synthetic ester, acetyl-glycyl-lysine methyl ester, in a form unassociated with C3b, it is classified as a serine protease (68).

Schreiber et al (246) have found that the mixture of isolated alternative pathway proteins and the isolated membrane attack pathway proteins constitutes an intact cytolytic pathway capable of killing bacteria in the absence of antibody. The activated alternative pathway appears to be effective in the lysis of some virus-infected cells (247), inactivation of viruses (69), killing of certain parasites (96), and influencing many host cellular functions. Guinea pig Ba has neutrophil chemotaxic activity (127); however, human Ba does not (167).

Synthesis and Catabolism

Human factor B is synthesized by macrophages (44,279) and lymphocytes (123) and accounts for 0.1 per cent of the total protein synthesized by the liver (135). Similarities between factor B and C2 have been seen in biosynthesis, post-synthetic processing, and secretion (175).

Factor B is activated by enzymatic cleavage into fragments Ba (the N-terminal component that behaves electrophoretically as an α-globulin) and Bb (which behaves as a γ-globulin). Under physiologic activation, Bb remains complexed to C3b (forming alternative pathway C3 convertase) and Ba is released. The maintenance of stable $\overline{C3bBb}$ and the formation of C3/C5 convertase requires an activator that prevents the interaction of C3b with factor H. Many such activators are known including lipopolysaccharide, viruses, fungi, bacteria, parasites, and some animal cells; however, the critical feature of their structure that inhibits the C3b-factor H interaction is not known. Increased catabolism of factor B has been observed in patients with immune complex-mediated diseases (51).

Analysis of Factor B (and Activation of the Alternative Pathway)

In man factor B is routinely measured using the radial immunodiffusion assay (100). Erythrocytes of some animal species are sensitive to alternative complement pathway-mediated lysis by fresh heterologous sera in the presence of magnesium and ethyleneglycol-bis-(2-amino-ethyl)-tetra-acetic acid (EGTA). The proper target red cell for 12 animal species has been reported (274). Antigenic analysis using specific anti-factor B antisera has been published for guinea pigs (35) and mice (198).

Factor B has been measured in cattle using a hemolytic diffusion plate assay and radial immunodiffusion, with poor concordance between these assays (263). The investigators suggest that because hemolytic activity depends on the concentration of other complement components, it is not as reliable as radial immunodiffusion. Rocket immunoelectrophoresis has been developed for measuring consumption of factor B after activation with zymosan (263).

Schur et al (248) demonstrated lines of identity between factor B of six nonhuman primate species and anti-human factor B. This observation was confirmed by McMahan (178) and used as a basis for crossed electrophoresis to measure rhesus monkey factor B (289). A hemolytic assay was used to measure factor B in baboon serum; however, activation of the alternative pathway yielded significantly less lysis of guinea pig or rabbit red cells (in Mg^{2+}, EGTA) than did human sera. Preliminary studies indicate that baboon factor B is as hemolytically active with these cells as is human factor B. Studies are currently underway to determine which other component of the alternative pathway in baboon sera is responsible for this reduced activity (227).

Interpretation

The serum concentrations of factor B in healthy humans average 200 μg/ml (190) and range from 180 to 230 μg/ml (1,192). In cattle, mean factor B levels in serum were 34 mg/dl (263). In mice, sexual dimorphism is seen in the expression of factor B variants, with female mice lacking several anodal bands present in males; however, no differences in total factor B were seen using radial immunodiffusion or rocket immunoelectrophoresis (235). Strain-specific differences in plasma levels of factor B have been documented, with 10-fold differences seen between B10.WR and B10.SM strains (88). Factor B levels are commonly elevated in inflammatory disorders, leaving some to classify factor B as an acute phase reactant (23). In both man

and mouse interleukin-1 has been shown to modulate factor B gene expression, resulting in increased mRNA levels in tissues and increased factor B in plasma (88,222).

Inherited deficiencies in complement components of the alternative pathway have not been described in animals.

REFERENCES

1. Adinolfi M, Beck S (1975) Human complement C7 and C9 in fetal and newborn. Sera Arch Dis Childhood 50: 562–564
2. Aegerter-Shaw M, Cole JL, Klickstein LB, Wong WW, Fearon DT, Lalley PA, Weis JH (1987) Expansion of the Complement Receptor Gene Family. J. Immunol 138: 3488–3494
3. Agnello V (1978) Complement deficiency states. Medicine 57: 1–23
4. Albright JW, Albright JF (1985) Murine natural resistance to *Trypanosoma lewisi* involves complement component C3 and radiation-resistant, silica dust-sensitive effector cells. Infect Immunol 47: 176–182
5. Allen FH (1974) Linkage of HLA and GBG. Vox Sang 27: 382–384
6. Alper CA (1976) Inherited structural polymorphism in human C2: Evidence of genetic linkage between C2 and Bf. J Exp Med 144: 1111–1115
7. Alper CA, Beonisch T, Watson L (1972) Genetic polymorphism in human glycine-rich beta-glycoprotein. J Exp Med 135: 68–80
8. Alper CA, Rosen FS (1967) Studies of the *in vivo* behavior of human C3 in normal subjects and patients. J Clin Invest 46: 2021–2034
9. Alper CA, Rosen FS (1975) Complement in laboratory medicine. In: Laboratory Diagnosis of Immunologic Disorders. Vyas GN, Stites DP, Brecher G (eds), Grune & Stratton, New York, pp 47–68
10. Alper CA, Goodofsky I, Lepow IH (1972) The relationship of glycine rich B glycoprotein to factor B in the properdin system and to cobra factor binding protein of human serum. J Exp Med 137: 424–437
11. Alper CA, Levin AS, Rosen FS (1966) Beta-IC-Globulin: Metabolism in glomerulonephritis. Science 153: 180–182
12. Alper CA, Robin NI, Refetoff S (1971) Genetic polymorphism in rhesus C3 and Gc globulin. J Immunol 107: 96–98
13. Alper CA, Johnson AM, Birtch AG, Moore FD (1969) Human C3: Evidence for the liver as the primary site of synthesis. Science 163: 286–288
14. Alper CA, Propp RP, Klemperer MR, Rosen FS (1969) Inherited deficiency of the third component of human complement (C3). J Clin Invest 48: 553–557
15. Alper CA, Colten HR, Gear JJS, Rabson AR, Rosen FS (1976) Homozygous human C3 deficiency. J Clin Invest 57: 222–229
16. Alper CA, Colten HR, Rosen FS, Rabson AR,

MacNab GM, Gear JSS (1972) Homozygous deficiency of C3 in a patient with repeated infections. Lancet II: 1179–1181

17. Alpert SE, Auerbach HS, Cole FS, Colten HR (1983) Macrophage maturation: Differences in complement secretion by marrow, monocyte, and tissue macrophages detected with an improved hemolytic plaque assay. J Immunol 130: 102–107

18. Anderson JE, Ladiges WC, Giblett ER, Weiden P, Storb R (1983) Polymorphism of the sixth component of complement (C6) in the dog. Biochem Genet 21: 155–160

19. Andrews BS, Eisenberg RA, Theofilopoulos AN, Izui S, Wilson CB, McConahey PJ, Murphy ED, Roths JB, Dixon FJ (1978) Spontaneous murine lupus-like syndromes. Clinical immunopathological manifestations in several strains. J Exp Med 148: 1198–1215

20. Arroyave CM, Muller-Eberhard JH (1971) Isolation of the sixth component of complement from human serum. Immunochemistry 8: 995–1006

21. Arroyave CM, Levy RN, Johnson JS (1977) Genetic deficiency of the fourth component of complement (C4) in wistar rats. Immunology 33: 453–459

22. Atkinson JP, Frank MM (1973) Effects of cortisone therapy on serum complement components. J Immunol 111: 1061–1070

23. Atkinson JP, Frank MM (1980) Complement. In Parker CW (ed), Clinical Immunology, Vol 1. W. B. Saunders, Philadelphia, Chap 8, pp 219–271

24. Atkinson JP, McGinnis K, Brown L, Peterein J, Shreffler D (1980) A murine C4 molecule with reduced hemolytic efficiency. J Exp Med 151: 492–497

25. Auerbach IIS, Lalande ME, Latts S, Colten HR (1983) Isolation of guinea pig macrophages bearing surface C4 by fluroescence activated cell sorting: Correlation between surface C4 antigen and C4 protein secretions. J Immunol 131: 2420–2426

26. Awdeh ZL, Alper CA (1980) Inherited structural polymorphism of the fourth component of complement (C4). Proc Natl Acad Sci USA 77: 3576–3580

27. Ballow M, Cochrane CG (1969) Two anticomplementary factors in cobra venom: Hemolysis of guinea pig erythrocytes by one of them. J Immunol 103: 944–952

28. Barta O, Barta V (1973) Canine hemolytic complement: Optimal conditions for its titration. Am J Vet Res 34: 653–657

29. Barta O, Barta V (1975) Chicken (Gallus gallus) hemolytic complement: Optimal conditions for its titration. Immunol Commun 4: 337–351

30. Barta O, Barta V (1984) Laboratory Techniques of Veterinary Clinical Immunology. Barta O (ed), Charles C Thomas, Springfield, IL, pp 138–155

31. Barta O, Barta V, Williams EI (1973) A method for titrating equine haemolytic complement. A Immunitaetsforsch Immunobiol 146: 114–122

32. Barta O, Hubbert NL (1978) Testing of hemolytic complement components in domestic animals. Am J Vet Res 39: 1303–1308

33. Barta O, Oyekan PP (1981) Feline (cat) hemolytic complement optimal testing conditions. Am J Vet Res 42: 378–381

34. Biro CE, Ortega ML (1966) Algunas caracteristicas del sexto componente del complemento. Arch Inst Cardiol Mex 36: 166–168

35. Bitter-Suermann D, Kronke M, Brade V, Hadding U (1977) Inherited polymorphism of guinea pig factor B and C4: Evidence for genetic linkage between the C4 and Bf loci. J Immunol 118: 1822–1826

36. Bitter-Suermann D, Hoffmann T, Burger R, Hadding U (1981) Linkage of total deficiency of the second component (C2) of the complement system and the genetic C2-polymorphism to the major histocompatibility complex of the guinea pig. J Immunol 127(2): 608–612

37. Bockow B, Mannik M (1981) Clearance and tissue uptake of immune complexes in complement-depleted and control mice. Immunology 42: 497–604

38. Bokisch VA, Muller-Eberhard HJ (1970) Anaphylatoxin inactivator of human plasma: Its isolation and characterization as a carboxypeptidase. J Clin Invest 49: 2427–2436

39. Bokisch VA, Muller-Eberhard HJ, Dierich MP (1975) Third component of complement (C3): Structural properties in relation to functions. Proc Natl Acad Sci USA 72: 1989–1993

40. Bolotin CG, Morris S, Tack B, Prahl J (1977) Purification and structural analysis of the fourth component of human complement. Biochemistry 16: 2008–2015

41. Bottger EC, Hoffmann T, Hadding U, Bitter-Suermann D (1985) Influence of genetically inherited complement deficiencies on humoral immune response in guinea pigs. J Immunol 135: 4100–4107

42. Bottger EC, Hoffmann T, Hadding U, Bitter-Suermann D (1986) Guinea pigs with inherited deficiencies of complement components C2 or C4 have characteristics of immune complex disease. J Clin Invest 78: 689–695

43. Bottger EC, Metzger S, Bitter-Suermann D, Stevenson G, Kleindienst S, Burger R (1986) Impaired humoral immune response in complement C3-deficient guinea pigs: Absence of secondary antibody response. Eur J Immunol 16: 1231–1235

44. Brade V, Fries W, Bentley C (1978) Identification of properdin B, D, and C3 as biosynthetic products of guinea pig peritoneal macrophages and influence of culture conditions on their secretion (abstr). J Immunol 120: 1766

45. Budzko DB, Bokisch VA, Muller-Eberhard HJ (1971) A fragment of the third component of human complement with anaphylatoxin activity. Biochemistry 10: 1166–1172

46. Burger R, Bitter-Suermann D, Loos M, Hadding U (1977) Insoluble polyanions as activators of both pathways of complement. Immunology 33: 827–837

47. Burger R, Gordon J, Stevenson G, Ramadori G, Zanker B, Hadding U, Bitter-Suermann D (1986) An inherited deficiency of the third component of complement, C3, in guinea pigs. Eur J Immunol 16: 7–11

48. Cerquetti MC, Sordelli DO, Ortegon RA, Bellanti JA (1983) Impaired lung defenses against Staphylococcus aureus in mice with hereditary deficiency of the fifth component of complement. Infect Immun 41: 1071–1076

49. Chan AC, Atkinson JP (1983) Identification and structural characterization of two incompletely processed forms of the fourth component of human complement. J Clin Invest 72: 1639–1649

50. Chan AC, Karp DR, Shreffler DC, Atkinson JP (1984) The 20 faces of the fourth component of complement. Immunology Today 5: 200–203

51. Charlesworth JA, Williams DG, Sherington E, Lachmann PJ, Peters DK (1974) Metabolic studies of the third component of complement and the glycine rich beta glycoprotein in patients with hypocomplementemia. J Clin Invest 53: 1578–1587

52. Christie DL, Gagnon J, Porter RR (1980) Partial sequence of human complement component factor B: Novel type of serine esterase. Proc Natl Acad Sci USA 77: 4923–4927

53. Churchill WH Jr, Weintraub RM, Borsos T, Rapp HJ (1967) Mouse complement: The effect of sex hormones and castration on two of the late-acting components. J Exp Med 125: 637–671

54. Cinader B, Dubiski S (1963) An alpha-globulin allotype in the mouse (MuB1). Nature 200: 781

55. Cinader B, Dubiski S (1964) Effects of autologous protein on the specificity of the antibody response: Mouse and rabbit antibody to MuB1. Nature 202: 102–103

56. Cinader B, Dubiski S, Wardlow AC (1964) Distribution, inheritance and properties of an antigen, MuB1, and its relation to hemolytic complement. J Exp Med 120: 879–924

57. Cinader B, Jeejeebhoy HF, Koh SW, Rabbat AG (1971) Immunosuppressive and graft-rejecting antibodies in heterologous antilymphocyte serum. J Exp Med 133: 81–99

58. Cochrane CG, Muller-Eberhard HJ, Aikin BS (1970) Depletion of plasma complement in vivo by a protein of cobra venom: Its effect on various immunologic reactions. J Immunol 105: 55–69

59. Cole FS, Schneeberger EE, Lichtenberg NA, Colten HR (1982) Complement biosynthesis in human breast-milk macrophages and blood monocytes. Immunology 46: 429–441

60. Cole FS, Whitehead AS, Auerbach HS, Phil D, Lint T, Zeitz HJ, Kilbridge P, Colten HR (1985) The molecular basis for genetic deficiency of the second component of human complement. N Engl J Med 313: 11–16

61. Colten HR (1974) Synthesis and metabolism of complement proteins. Transpl Proc 6: 33–38

62. Colten HR (1976) Biosynthesis of complement. Adv Immunol 22: 67–118

63. Colten HR (1983) Molecular biology and biosynthesis of the complement proteins. In Yamamura Y, Tada T (eds), Progress in Immunology, Vol 5. Academic Press, Tokyo, pp 397–406

64. Colten HR (1983) Molecular genetics of the major histocompatibility linked complement genes. Springer Sem Immunopathol 6: 149–158

65. Colten HR, Alper CA (1972) Hemolytic efficiencies of genetic variants of human C3. J Immunol 108: 1184–1198

66. Colten HR, Frank MM (1972) Biosynthesis of the second (C2) and fourth (C4) components of complement in vitro by tissues isolated from guinea

pigs with genetically determined C4 deficiency. Immunology 22: 991–999

67. Colten HR, Levy RH, Rosen FS, Alper CA (1973) Decreased synthesis of C3 in membranoproliferative glomerulonephritis (abstr). J Clin Invest 52: 20

68. Cooper NR (1971) Enzymes of the complement system. Prog Immunol 1: 567–577

69. Cooper NR (1979) Humoral immunity to viruses. Comprehensive Virol 15: 123–170

70. Cooper NR (1982) The complement system. In Stites DP, Stobe JD, Fudenberg HH, Wells JV (eds) Basic and Clinical Immunology, 4th ed. Lange Medical Publications, Los Altos, CA

71. Cooper NR, Nemerow GR, Mayes JT (1983) Methods to detect and quantitate complement activation. Springer Sem Immunopathol 6: 195–212

72. Corbin NC, Hugli TE (1976) The primary structure of porcine C3a anaphylatoxin. J Immunol 117: 990–995

73. Curman B, Sandberg-Tragardh K, Peterson PA (1977) Chemical characterization of human factor B of the alternate pathway of complement activation. Biochemistry 16: 5368–5375

74. Daha MR, Stuffers-Heiman M, Kijlstra A, vanEst LA (1979) Isolation and characterization of third component of rat complement. Immunology 36: 63–70

75. Delage JM, Lehner-Netsch G, LaFleur R, Simard J (1979) Simultaneous occurrence of hereditary C6 and C2 deficiency in a French-Canadian family. Immunology 37: 419–428

76. Desai BB, Albright JW, Albright JF (1987) Cooperative action of complement component C3 and phagocytic effector cells in innate murine resistance to Trypanosoma lewisi. Infect Immun 55: 358–363

77. Dieli F, Salerno A (1986) Role of the fourth complement component (C4) in the regulation of contact sensitivity. Cell Immunol 105: 386–396

78. Dierich MP, Schultz T (1983) The nature and function of complement receptors. Prog Immunol 5: 407–418

79. Donaldson VH, Rafnoff OD, Dias da Silva W (1969) Permeability-increasing activity in hereditary angioneurotic edema plasma II. Mechanism of formation and partial characterization. J Clin Invest 48: 642–653

80. Dubiski S, Cinader B (1966) Gene dosage effect of serum concentration of a complement component, MuB1. Proc Soc Exp Biol Med 122: 775–778

81. Easmon CS, Glynn AA (1976) Comparison of subcutaneous and intraperitoneal staphylococcal infections in normal and complement deficient mice. Infect Immunity 13: 399–406

82. Egwang TG, Befus AD (1984) The role of complement in the induction and regulation of immune responses. Immunology 51: 207–224

83. Eldridge PR, Hobart MJ, Lachmann PJ (1983) The genetics of the sixth and seventh components of complement in the dog: Polymorphism, linkage, locus duplication and silent alleles. Biochem Genet 21: 81–91

84. Ellingsworth LR, Holmberg CA, Osburn BI (1983) Hemolytic complement measurement in eleven

species of nonhuman primates. Vet Immunol Immunopathol 5: 141–149

85. Ellman L, Green I, Frank M (1970) Genetically controlled total deficiency of the fourth component of complement in the guinea pig. Science 170: 74–75

86. Erickson RP, Tachibana DK, Herzenberg LA, Rosenberg LT (1964) A single gene controlling hemolytic complement and a serum antigen in the mouse. J Immunol 92: 611–615

87. Fahey JL, McKelvey EM (1965) Quantitative determination of serum immunoglobulins in antibody agar plates. J Immunol 94: 84–90

88. Falus A, Beuscher HU, Auerbach HS, Colten HR (1987) Constitutive and IL 1-regulated murine complement gene expression is strain and tissue specific. J Immunol 138: 856–860

89. Fearon DT, Austen KF, Ruddy S (1973) Formation of a haemolytically active cellular intermediate by the interaction between properdin factors B and D and the activated third component of complement. J Exp Med 138: 1305–1313

90. Feldman BF, Attix EA, Strombeck DR, O'Neill S (1981) Biochemical and coagulation changes in a canine model of acute necrotising pancreatitis. Am J Vet Res 42: 805–809

91. Ferreira A, Nussenzweig V (1975) Genetic linkage between serum levels of the third component of complement and the H-2 complex. J Exp Med 141: 513–517

92. Ferreira A, Nussenzweig V (1976) Control of C3 levels in mice during ontogeny by a gene in the central region of the H-2 complex. Nature 260: 613–614

93. Ferreira A, Takahashi M, Nussenzweig V (1977) Purification and characterization of mouse serum protein with specific binding affinity for C4 (Ss protein). J Exp Med 146: 1001–1018

94. Ferreira A, Michaelson J, Nussenzweig V (1980) A polymorphism of the γ-chain of mouse C4 controlled by the S region of the major histocompatibility complex. J Immunol 125: 1178–1182

95. Fey G, Domdey H, Wiebauer K, Whitehead AS, Odink K (1983) Structure and expression of the C3 gene. Springer Sem Immunopathol 6: 119–147

96. Flemmings B, Diggs C (1978) Antibody-dependent cytotoxicity against *Trypanosoma rhodesiense* mediated through an alternate complement pathway. Infect Immun 19: 928–933

97. Fox RR, Cherry M (1978) Effect of rabbit strain on activity level and cytotoxicity of serum complement. II. Comparison of 5 murine target cells. J Hered 69: 331–336

98. Fox RR, Cherry M, Schultz KL (1978) Effect of rabbit strain on activity level and cytotoxicity of serum complement. J Hered 69: 107–112

99. Fox RR, Cherry M, Shultz KL, Salvatore KJ (1979) Effect of rabbit strain on activity level and cytotoxicity of serum complement. III. Comparison of 4 tumor target cells. J Hered 70: 109–114

100. Gaither TA, Frank MM (1979) Complement. In Henry JB (ed), Clinical Diagnosis and Management by Laboratory Methods, Vol 2. WB Saunders, Philadelphia, pp 1245–1261

101. Geng L, Iwabuchi K, Sakai S, Ogasawara M, Fujita M, Ogasawara K, Kakinuma M, Good RA, Morikawa K, Onoe K (1986) Analysis of synthetic sites of fourth and fifth components of serum complement system in allogenic bone marrow chimaeras. Immunology 58:453–457

102. Gewurz H, Suyehira LA (1976) in Rose N and Friedman H (eds), Manual of Clinical Immunology. American Society of Microbiology, Washington, D.C. pp 36–47

103. Gigli I, Austen KF (1971) Phylogeny and function of the complement system. Ann Rev Microbiology 25: 309–332

104. Gigli I, Nelson RA (1968) Complement dependent immune phagocytosis I. Requirements for C1, C4, C2, C3. Exp Cell Res 51: 45–67

105. Gigli I (1978) A single chain precursor of C4 in human serum. Nature (London) 272: 836–837

106. Gitlin D, Biasucci A (1969) Development of γG, γA, γM, BIC/BIA, C1 esterase inhibitor, ceruloplasmin, transferrin, hemopexin, haptoglobin, fibrinogen, plasminogen, α_1-antitrypsin, orosomucoid, β-lipoprotein, macroglobulin, and prealbumin in the human conceptus. J Clin Invest 48: 1433–1446

107. Glass D, Raum D, Gibson D, Stillman JS, Schur PH (1976) Inherited deficiency of the second component of complement. Rheumatic disease associations. J Clin Invest 58: 853–861

108. Glass D, Raum D, Balavitch D, Kagan E, Rabson A, Schur PH, Alper CA (1978) Inherited deficiency of the sixth component of complement: A silent or null gene. J Immunol 120: 538–541

109. Glynn AA, Medhurst FA (1967) Possible extracellular and intracellular bactericidal actions of mouse complement. Nature 213: 608–610

110. Goldberger G, Cole SF, Einstein LP, Auerbach HS, Bitter-Suermann D, Colten HR (1982) Biosynthesis of a structurally abnormal C2 complement protein by macrophages from C2-deficient guinea pigs. J Immunol 129: 2061–2065

111. Goldberger G, Thomas ML, Tack BF, Williams J, Colten HR, Abraham GN (1981) NH2-terminal structure and cleavage of guinea pig pro C3, the precursor of the third component of complement. J Biol Chem 256: 12617–12619

112. Goldman MB, Goldman JN (1976) Relationship of functional levels of early components of complement to the H-2 complex of mice. J Immunol 117: 1584–1588

113. Goldman MB, Cohen C, Stronski K, Banaglore S, Goldman JN (1982) Genetic control of C6 polymorphism and C6 deficiency in rabbits. J Immunol 128: 43–48

114. Goodman MG, Chenoweth DE, Weigle WO (1982) Potentiation of the primary humoral immune response *in vitro* by C5a anaphlatoxin. J Immunol 129: 70–75

115. Gordon J, Whitehead HR, Wormall A (1926) The action of ammonia on complement. The fourth component. Biochem J 20: 1028–1035

116. Gorman NT (1984) Activation of the alternative complement pathway by lymphoblasts isolated from canine thymic lymphomas. Vet Immunol Immunopathol 7: 213–225

117. Gorman NT, Hobart MJ, Lachmann PJ (1981) Polymorphism of the third component of canine complement. Vet Immunol Immunopathol 2: 301–307

118. Gorman NT, McConnell I, Lachmann PJ (1981) Characterization of the third component of canine and feline complement. Vet Immunol Immunopathol 2: 309–320

119. Gorski JP (1981) Quantitation of human complement fragment C4ai in physiological fluids by competitive inhibition of radioimmune assay. J Immunol Methods 47: 61–62

120. Gotze O, Muller-Eberhard HS (1976) The alternative pathway of complement activation. Adv Immunol 24: 1–35

121. Grant CK (1977) Complement "specificity" and interchangeability: Measurement of hemolytic complement levels and use of the complement-fixation test with sera from common domesticated animals. Am J Vet Res 38: 1611–1617

122. Guiguet M, Dethieux MC, Exilie-Frigere MF, Bidan Y, Lautissier JL, Mack G (1987) Third component of rat complement. Purification from plasma and radioimmunoassay in culture media from cell lines. J Immunol Methods 96: 157–164

123. Halbwachs L, Lachmann PJ (1976) Factor B of the alternative complement pathway on human lymphocytes. Scand J Immunol 5: 697–704

124. Hall JR Jr, Alper CA (1977) Genetic polymorphism of the sixth component of complement (C6) in the rhesus monkey. J Immunol 119: 253–255

125. Hall RE, Colten HR (1977) Cell-free synthesis of the fourth component of guinea pig complement (C4): Identification of a precursor of serum C4 (pro-C4). Proc Natl Acad Sci USA 74: 1707–1710

126. Hammer CH, Gaither T, Frank MM (1981) Complement Deficiencies in Laboratory Animals. In Gershaw ME, Merchant B (eds), Immunologic Defects in Laboratory Animals, Vol 2. Plenum Press, New York, pp 207–240

127. Hamuro J, Hadding U, Bitter-Suermann D (1978) Fragments Ba and Bb derived from guinea pig factor B of the properdin system: Purification, characterization and biologic activities. J Immunol 120: 438–444

128. Hansen TH, Shreffler DC (1976) Characterization of a constitutive variant of the murine serum protein allotype, Slp. J Immunol 117: 1507–1513

129. Hayakawa J, Nikaido H, Koizumi T (1984) Genetic polymorphism of the sixth component of complement (C6) in mice. Immunogenetics 20: 633–638

130. Hemenway C, Robins DM (1987) DNase I-hypersensitive sites associated with expression and hormonal regulation of mouse C4 and Slp genes. Proc Natl Acad Sci 84: 4816–4820

131. Herzenberg LA, Tachibana DK, Herzenberg LA, Rosenberg LT (1963) A gene locus concerned with hemolytic complement in *Mus musculus*. Genetics 48: 711–715

132. Hicks JT, Ennis FA, Kim E, Verbonita M (1978) The importance of an intact complement pathway in recovery from a primary viral infection: Influenza in decomplemented and C5-deficient mice. J Immunol 121: 1437–1445

133. Hirschfeld J, Lunell NO (1962) Serum protein synthesis in foetus. Haptoglobins and group-specific components. Nature 196: 1220

134. Hobart M (1984) The biochemistry and genetics of complement component: Agreement now the norm. Immunol Today 5: 121–125

135. Hobart MJ, Lachmann PJ (1976) Allotypes of complement components in man. Transpl Rev 32: 26–42

136. Hobart MJ, Lachmann PJ, Alper CA (1975) Polymorphism of human C6. In Peeters H (ed), Protides of the Biological Fluids. Pergamon Press, Oxford, pp 575–580

137. Hobart MJ, Lachmann PJ, Calne RY (1977) C6: Synthesis by the liver *in vivo*. J Exp Med 146: 629–630

138. Hobart MJ, Cook PJL, Lachmann PJ (1977) Linkage studies with C6. J Immunogenet 4: 423–428

139. Holmberg CA, Ellingsworth L, Osburn BI, Grant CK (1977) Measurement of hemolytic complement and the third component of complement in non-human primates. Lab An Sci 27: 993–998

140. Hugli TE (1981) The structural basis for anaphylatoxin and chemotaxic functions of C3a, C4a and C5a. CRC Crit Rev Immunol 2: 321–366

141. Hugli TE (1975) Human anaphylatoxin (C3a) from the third component of complement: Primary structure. J Biol Chem 250: 8293–8301

142. Hugli TE, Callota EH, Muller-Eberhard (1975) Purification and partial characterization of human and porcine $C3_a$ anaphylatoxin. J Biol Chem 250: 1472

143. Ilgen CL, Burkholder PM (1974) Isolation of C4 synthesizing cells from guinea pig liver by ficoll density gradient centrifugation. Immunology 26: 197–203

144. International Union of Immunological Societies (1981) Nomenclature of the alternative activating pathway of complement. J Immunol 127: 1261–1262

145. Jacobs JW, Rubin JS, Hugli TE, Bogardt RA, Mariz IK, Davis JS, Daughaday WH, Bradshaw RA (1978) Purification, characterization, and amino acid sequence of rat anaphylatoxin (C3a). Biochemistry 17: 5031–5038

146. Jacobse-Geels HEL, Daha MR, Horzinek MC (1980) Isolation and characterization of feline C3 and evidence for the immune complex pathogenesis of feline infectious peritonitis. J Immunol 125: 1606–1610

147. Jonas W, Stankiewicz M (1981) Haemolytic activity of sheep complement for two assay systems. Vet Immunol Immunopathol 2: 393–400

148. Johnson AR, Hugli TE, Muller-Eberhard HJ (1975) Release of histamine from fat mast cells by the complement peptides C3a and C5a. Immunology 28: 1069–1080

149. Kalowski S, Howes EL, Margaretten W, McKay DG (1975) Effects of intravascular clotting on the activation of the complement system. Am J Pathol 78: 525–536

150. Karp DR, Atkinson JP, Shreffler DC (1982) Genetic variation in glycosylation of the fourth component of murine complement. J Biol Chem 257: 7330–7335

151. Karp DR, Parker KL, Shreffler DC, Capra JD

(1981) Characterization of the murine C4 precursor (Pro-C4): Evidence that the carboxy-terminal subunit is the C4 γ-chain. J Immunol 126: 2060–2061

152. Karp DR, Parker KL, Shreffler DC, Slaughter C, Capra JD (1982) Amino acid sequence homologies and glycosylation differences between the fourth component of murine complement and sex-limited protein. Proc Natl Acad Sci USA 79: 6347–6349

153. Kay PII, Dawkins RL (1984) Genetic polymorphism of complement C4 in the dog. Tissue Antigens 23: 151–155

154. Keystone E, Taylor-Robinson D, Pope C, Taylor G, Furr P (1978) Effect of inherited deficiency of the fifth component of complement on arthritis induced in mice by *Mycoplasma pulmonis*. Arth Rheum 21: 792–797

155. Kitamura H, Matsumoto M, Nagaki K (1984) C3-independent immune hemolysis: Hemolysis of EAC14^{oxy}2 cells by C5-C9 without participation of C3. Immunology 53: 575–582

156. Kohler PF (1973) Maturation of the human complement system. 1. Onset time and sites of fetal C1q, C4, C3 and C5 synthesis. J Clin Invest 52: 671–677

157. Kolb WP, Muller-Eberhard HJ (1973) The membrane attack mechanism of complement verification of a stable C5-9 complex in free solution, J Exp Med 138: 438–451

158. Kolb WP, Haxby JA, Arroyave CM, Muller-Eberhard HJ (1972) Molecular analysis of the membrane attack mechanism of complement. J Exp Med 135: 549–566

159. Kronke M, Hadding U, Geczy AF, DeWeck AL, Bitter-Suermann D (1977) Linkage of guinea pig Bf and C4 to the GPLA. J Immunol 119: 2016–2018

160. Kunstmann G, Mauff G (1980) Genetic polymorphism of rabbit C6. Immunology 158: 30–33

161. Kusher I (1982) The phenomenon of the acute phase response. Ann NY Acad Sci 389: 39–48

162. Lachmann PJ (1970) C6-deficiency in rabbits. In Peeters H (ed), Protides of the Biological Fluids. Pergamon Press, Oxford, pp 301–309

163. Lachmann PJ, Hobart MJ, Woo P (1978) Combined genetic deficiency of C6 and C7 in man. Clin Exp Immunol 33: 193–203

164. Laurell CB (1972) Electroimmunoassay. (Scand) J Clin Lab Invest 29 (Supple 124): 21–37

165. Lawrence DA, Schell RF (1978) Susceptibility of C5-deficient mice to listeriosis: Modulation by concanavalin A. Cell Immunol 39: 336–344

166. Leddy JP, Frank MM, Gaither T, Baum J, Klemperer MR (1974) Hereditary deficiency of the sixth component of complement in man. I. Immunochemical, biologic and family studies. J Clin Invest 53: 544–553

167. Lesavre P, Hugli TE, Esser AF, Muller-Eberhard HJ (1979) The alternative pathway of C3/C5 convertase: Chemical basis of factor B activation. J Immunol 123: 529–534

168. Lim D, Gewurz A, Lint TF, Chaze M, Sephein B, Gewurz H (1976) Absence of the sixth component of complement in a patient with repeated episodes of meningococcal meningitis. J Pediatr 89: 42–47

169. Lindberg LH, Rosenberg LT (1968) Nephrotoxic serum nephritis in mice with a genetic deficiency in complement. J Immunol 100: 34–38

170. Littleton C, Keisler D, Burkholder PM (1970) Cellular basis for the synthesis of the fourth component of guinea pig complement and determined by a hemolytic plaque technique. Immunology 18: 693–704

171. Littman BH, Ruddy S (1977) Production of the second component of complement by human monocytes: Stimulation by antigen-activated lymphocytes or lymphokines. J Exp Med 145: 1344–1352

172. Madewell BR (1978) Serum complement level in dogs with neoplastic disease. Am J Vet Res 39: 1373–1376

173. Mancini G, Carbonara AO, Heremans JF (1965) Immunochemical quantitation of antigens by single radial immunodiffusion. Immunochemistry 2: 235–254

174. Mathison JC, Ulevitch RJ (1981) *In vivo* interaction of bacterial lipopolysaccharide (LPS) with rabbit platelets: Modulation by C3 and high density lipoproteins. J Immunol 126: 1575–1580

175. Matthews WJ Jr, Goldberger G, Marino JT, Einstein LP, Gasj DJ, Colten HR (1982) The major histocompatibility complex linked complement protein C2, C4 and factor B: Effect of glycosylation on their secretion and catabolism. Biochem J 204: 839–846

176. May JE, Kane MA, Frank MM (1972) Host defense against bacterial endotoxemia. Contribution of the early and late components of complement to detoxification. J Immunol 109: 893–895

177. Mayer MM (1973) The complement system. Sci Am 229: 1–14

178. McMahan MR (1982) Complement components C3, C4 and Bf in six nonhuman primate species. Lab An Sci 32: 57–59

179. McMannis JD, Goldman MB, Goldman JN (1987) The role of lymphoid cells in antibody-induced suppression of the fourth component of guinea pig complement. Cell Immunol 106: 22–32

180. Menger M, Aston WP (1984) Factor D of the alternative pathway of bovine complement. Isolation and characterization. Vet Immunol Immunopathol 7: 325–336

181. Mevag B, Olaisen B, Teisberg P, Smith DG (1983) Two C4 loci in macaca monkeys (abstr). Immunobiology 164: 276–277

182. Milgrom H, Curd JG, Kaplan RA, Muller-Eberhard HJ, Vaughan JH (1980) Activation of the fourth component of complement (C4): Assessment by rocket immunoelectrophoresis in correlation with the metabolism of C4. J Immunol 124: 2780–2785

183. Miller ME, Nilsson UR (1970) A familial deficiency of the phagocytosis-enhancing activity of serum related to a dysfunction of the fifth component of complement (C5). N Engl J Med 282: 354–358

184. Moore HD (1919) Complementary and opsonic functions in their relation to immunity. A study of the serum of guinea pigs naturally deficient in complement. J Immunol 4: 425–432

185. Morelli R, Rosenberg LT (1971) Role of com-

plement during experimental *Candida* infection in mice. Infect Immun 3: 521–529

186. Morris KM, Aden DP, Knowles JF, Strominger JL (1982) Complement biosynthesis by the human hepatoma-derived cell line HepG2. J Clin Invest 70: 906–913

187. Muller-Eberhard HJ, Biro CE (1963) Isolation and description of the fourth component of human complement. J Exp Med 118: 447–466

188. Muller-Eberhard HJ (1975) Complement. Am Rev Biochem 44: 697–724

189. Muller-Eberhard HJ, Gotze O (1972) C3 pro-activator convertase and its mode of action. J Exp Med 135: 1003–1008

190. Muller-Eberhard HJ, Schreiber RD (1980) Molecular biology and chemistry of the alternative pathway of complement advances in immunology. Adv Immunol 29: 1–53

191. Muller-Peddinghaas R, Schwartz-Porsche D (1983) Klinische Bedeutung des Serumkomplements bei Hunden. Zbl Vet Med A 30: 698–711

192. Nagaki K, Hiramatsu S, Inai S, Saski A (1980) The effect of aging on complement activity (CH_{50}) and complement protein levels. J Clin Lab Immunol 3: 45–50

193. Nakamura RM, Weigle WO (1968) Experimental thyroiditis in complement intact and deficient mice following injections of heterologous thyroglobulins without adjuvant. Proc Soc Exp Biol Med 129: 412–416

194. Nakayama K, Nonaka M, Yokoyama S, Yeul YD, Pattanakitsakul SN, Takahashi M (1987) Recombination of two homologous MHC class III genes of the mouse (C4 and Slp) that accounts for the loss of testosterone dependence of sex-limited protein expression. J Immunol 138: 620–627

195. Natsuume-Sakai S, Hayakawa J, Takahashi M (1978) Genetic polymorphism of murine C3 controlled by a single co-dominant locus on chromosome 17. J Immunol 121: 491–498

196. Natsuume-Sakai S, Kaidoh T, Nonaka M, Takahashi M (1980) Structural polymorphism of murine C4 and its linkage to H-2. J Immunol 124: 2714–2720

197. Natsuume-Sakai S, Moriwaki K, Amano S, Hayakawa J, Kaidoh T, Takahashi M (1979) Allotypes of C3 in laboratory and wild mouse distinguished by alloantisera. J Immunol 123: 216–221

198. Natsuume-Sakai S, Moriwaki K, Migita S, Sudo K, Suzuki K, Lu D-Y, Wang C, Takahashi M (1983) Structural polymorphism of murine factor B controlled by a locus closely linked to the H-2 complex and demonstration of multiple alleles. Immunogenetics 18: 117–124

199. Nelson RA Jr, Biro CE (1968) Complement components of a haemolytically deficient strain of rabbits. Immunology 14: 525–540

200. Nelson RA Jr, Jensen J, Gigli I, Tamuro N (1966) Methods for the separation and measurement of nine components of hemolytic complement in guinea pig serum. Immunochemistry 3: 111–135

201. Newell SL, Atkinson JP (1983) Biosynthesis of C4 by mouse peritoneal macrophages: II. Comparison of C4 synthesis by resident and elicited cell populations. J Immunol 130: 834–838

202. Newman SL, Vogler LB, Feigin RD, Johnston RB (1978) Recurrent septicemia associated with congenital deficiency of C2 and partial deficiency of B and the alternative complement pathway. N Engl J Med 299: 290–292

203. Nilsson U, Mapes J (1973) Polyacrylamide gel electrophoresis (PAGE) of reduced and dissociated C3 and C5: Studies of polypeptide chain (PPC) subunits and their modifications by trypsin (TRY) and C42–C423 (abstr). J Immunol 111: 293–294

204. Nilsson UR, Muller-Eberhard HJ (1965) Isolation of B1F-globulin from human serum and its characterization as the fifth component of complement. J Exp Med 122: 277–298

205. Nilsson UR, Muller-Eberhard HJ (1967) Deficiency of the fifth component of complement in mice with inherited complement defect. J Exp Med 124: 1–16

206. Ochs HD, Rosenfeld SI, Thomas ED, Giblett ER, Alper CA, Dupont B, Schaller JG, Gilliland BC, Hansen JA (1977) Linkage between the fourth component of complement and the major histocompatibility complex. N Engl J Med 296: 470–475

207. Ochs HD, Jackson CG, Heller SR, Wedgewood RJ (1978) Defective antibody response to a T-dependent antigen in C4 deficient guinea pigs and its correction by addition of C4. Fed Proc 37: 1477

208. Ochs HD, Wedgewood RJ, Frank MM, Heller SR, Hosea SW (1983) The role of complement in the induction of antibody responses. Clin Exp Immunol 53: 208–216

209. Odink KG, Fey G, Wiebauer K, Digglemann H (1981) Mouse complement components C3 and C4. Characterization of their messenger RNA and molecular cloning of complementary DNA for C3. J Biol Chem 256: 1453–1458

210. O'Neill GJ, Yang SY, Dupont B (1978) Two HLA-linked loci controlling the fourth component of human complement. Proc Natl Acad Sci USA 75: 5165–5169

211. O'Neill GJ, Lang M, Nerl C, Deeg HJ (1984) C4 polymorphism in the dog: Molecular heterogeneity of the C4α and C4γ subunit chains. Immunogenetics 20: 649–654

212. Ooi YM, Colten HR (1979) Genetic defect in secretion of complement C5 in mice. Nature 282: 207–208

213. Oyekan PP, Barta O (1980) Hemolytic assay for goat (caprine) and swine (porcine) complement. Vet Immunol Immunopathol 2: 393–400

214. Parker KL, Roos MH, Shreffler DC (1979) Structural characterization of the murine fourth component of complement and sex-limited protein and their precursors: Evidence for two loci in the S region of the H-2 complex. Proc Natl Acad Sci USA 76: 5853–5857

215. Parrish DA, Mitchell BC, Henson PM, Larsen GL (1984) Pulmonary response of fifth component of complement-sufficient and deficient mice to hyperoxia. J Clin Invest 74: 956–965

216. Passmore HC, Beisel KW (1977) Preparation of antisera for the detection of the Ss protein and Slp alloantigen. Immunogenetics 4: 393–399

217. Passmore HC, Shreffler DC (1970) A sex-limited

serum protein variant in the mouse: Inheritance and association with the H-2 region. Biochem Genet 4: 351–365

218. Patel F, Minta JO (1979) Biosynthesis of a single chain pro-C5 by normal mouse liver mRNA: Analysis of the molecular basis of C5 deficiency in AKR/J mice. J Immunol 123: 2408–2414

219. Penalva da Silva F, Hoecker GF, Day NK, Vienne K, Rubinstein P (1978) Murine complement component 3: Genetic variation and linkage to H-2. Proc Natl Acad Sci USA 75: 963–965

220. Pepys MB (1974) Complement mediated mixed aggregation of murine spleen cells. Nature 249: 51–53

221. Pepys MB, Dash AC, Fielder AHL, Mirjah DD (1977) Isolation and study of murine C3. Immunology 33: 491–499

222. Perlmutter DH, Goldberger G, Dinarello CA, Mizel SB, Colten HR (1986) Regulation of class III major histocompatibility complex gene products by interleukin-1. Science 232: 850–852

223. Peters DK, Martin A, Weinstein A, Cameron JS, Barrett T, Ogg CS, Lachmann PJ (1972) Complement studies in membranoproliferative glomerulonephritis. Clin Exp Immunol 11: 311–320

224. Phillips ME, Rother V, Rother K (1968) Serum complement in the rejection of sarcoma I ascites tumor grafts. J Immunol 100: 493–500

225. Podack ER, Kolb WP, Muller-Eberhard HJ (1976) Purification of the sixth and seventh component of human complement without loss of hemolytic activity. J Immunol 116: 263–269

226. Podack ER, Kolb WP, Esser AF, Muller-Eberhard HJ (1979) Structural similarities between C6 and C7 of human complement. J Immunol 123: 1071–1078

227. Polley MJ, Quimby F (1987) Personal communication

228. Polley MJ, Muller-Eberhard HJ (1967) Enhancement of the hemolytic activity of the second component of human complement by oxidation. J Exp Med 126: 1013–1025

229. Poutrel B, Caffin JP (1984) Determination of hemolytic complement activity in bovine milk. Vet Immunol Immunopathol 5: 177–184

230. Propp RP, Alper CA (1968) C3 synthesis in the human fetus and lack of transplacental passasge. Science 162: 672–673

231. Raum D, Balner H, Peterson BH, Alper CA (1980) Genetic polymorphism of serum complement components in the chimpanzee. Immunogenetics 10: 455–468

232. Raum DP, Awdeh ZL, Glass D, Yunis E, Alper CA (1981) The location of C2, C4 and Bf relative to HLA-B and HLA-D. Immunogenetics 12: 473–483

233. Rits M, Kints JP, Bazin H, Vaerman JP (1987) Rat C3 conversion by rat anti-2,4, dinitrophenyl (DNP) hapten IgA immune precipitates. Scand J Immunol 25: 359–366

234. Rommel FA, Bendure DW, Kalter SS (1980) Hemolytic complement in nonhuman primates. Lab An Sci 30: 1026–1029

235. Roos MH, Demant P (1982) Murine complement factor B (Bf): Sexual dimorphism and H-2 linked polymorphism. Immunogenetics 15: 23–30

236. Rosen FS (1981) In Nathan DG, Oski FA (eds), Hematology of Infancy and Childhood, Vol 2. Saunders, Philadelphia, pp 866–886

237. Rosenberg LT, Tachibana DK (1962) Activity of mouse complement. J Immunol 89: 861–867

238. Rosenfeld SE, Kelly ME, Leddy JP (1976) Hereditary deficiency in the fifth component of complement in man. I. Clinical, immunochemical and family studies. J Clin Invest 57: 1626–1634

239. Rosenfeld SE, Baum J, Steigbigel RT, Leddy JP (1976) Hereditary deficiency of the fifth component of complement in man. II. Biological properties of C5 deficient human serum. J Clin Invest 57: 1635–1643

240. Rother K, Rother U, Muller-Eberhard HJ, Nilsson UR (1966) Deficiency of the sixth component of complement in rabbits with an inherited complement defect. J Exp Med 124: 773–785

241. Ruddy S, Austen KF (1971) C3b inactivator of man. II. Fragments produced by C3b inactivator cleavage of cell-bound or fluid phase C3b. J Immunol 107: 742–750

242. Ruddy S, Carpenter GB, Chin KW, Knostman JN, Soter NA, Goetz O, Muller-Eberhard HJ, Austen KF (1975) Human complement metabolism: An analysis of 144 studies. Medicine 54: 165–178

243. Sakamoto M, Ishii S, Nisheoka K, Shimasa K (1981) Level of complement activity and components C1, C4, C2 and C3 in complement response to bacterial challenge in malnourished rats. Infect Immun 32: 553–556

244. Schaller JG, Gilliland BG, Ochs HD, Leddy JP, Agodoa LCY, Rosenfeld SI (1977) Severe systemic lupus erythematosus with nephritis in a boy with deficiency of the fourth component of complement. Arth Rheum 20: 1519–1525

245. Schreiber RD, Muller-Eberhard HJ (1974) Fourth component of human complement: Description of three polypeptide chain structure. J Exp Med 140: 1324–1335

246. Schreiber RD, Morrison DC, Podack ER, Muller-Eberhard HJ (1979) Bactericidal activity of the alternative complement pathway generated from 11 isolated plasma proteins. J Exp Med 149: 870–882

247. Schreiber RD, Pangburn MK, Medicus RG, Muller-Eberhard HJ (1980) Raji cell injury and subsequent lysis by the purified cytolytic alternative pathway of human complement. Clin Immunol Immunopathol 15: 384–396

248. Schur PH, Connelly A, Jones TC (1975) Phylogeny of complement components in non-human primates. J Immunol 114: 270–273

249. Shevach E, Green I, Frank MM (1976) Linkage of C4 deficiency to the major histocompatibility locus in the guinea pig. J Immunol 116: 1750

250. Shin HS, Smith MR, Wood WB Jr (1969) Heat labile opsonins to pneumococcus. II. Involvement of C3 and C5. J Exp Med 130: 1229–1241

251. Shiroishi T, Sagai T, Natsuume-Sakai S, Moriwaki K (1987) Lethal deletion of the complement component C4 and steroid 21-hydroxylase genes in the mouse H-2 class III region, caused by meiotic recombination. Proc Natl Acad Sci 84: 2819–2823

252. Shreffler DC, Owen RD (1963) A serologically

detected variant in mouse serum: Inheritance and association with the histocompatibility-2 locus. Genetics 48: 9–25

253. Shreffler DC (1982) In Parham P, Strominger J (eds), Receptors and Recognition, Ser B, Vol 14. Chapman and Hall, London

254. Siboo R, Vas SI (1965) Studies on *in vitro* antibody production. III. Production of complement. Can J Microbiol 11: 415–425

255. Sinosich MJ, Best N, Teisner B, Grudzinskas JG (1982) Demonstration of antigen determinants specific for the split products of the third complement factor, C3. J Immunol Methods 51: 355–358

256. Sliwinski AJ, Zvaifler NH (1972) Decreased synthesis of the third component of complement (C3) in hypocomplementemic systemic lupus erythematosus. Clin Exp Immunol 11: 21–29

257. Staats A (1985) Standardized nomenclature for inbred species of mice 8th listing. Cancer Res 45: 945–977

258. Stankiewicz M, Jonas W (1981) Haemolysis of human erythrocytes heavily sensitized with sheep amboceptor by sheep complement chelated with EGTA or Mg^{+2}-EGTA. Vet Immunol Immunopathol 2: 253–264

259. Stecher VJ, Thorbecke GJ (1967) Sites of synthesis of serum proteins. II. Medium requirements for serum protein production by rat macrophages. J Immunol 99: 653–659

260. Strang CJ, Auerbach HS, Rosen FS (1986) C1s-induced vascular permeability in C2-deficient guinea pigs. J Immunol 137: 631–635

261. Strunk RS, Tashjian AH, Colten HR (1975) Complement biosynthesis *in vitro* by rat hepatoma cell strains. J Immunol 114: 331–335

262. Sundsmo JS, Fair DS (1983) Relationships among the complement, kinin, coagulation and fibrinolytic systems. Springer Sem Immunopathol 6: 231–258

263. Tabel H, Menger M, Aston WP, Cochran M (1983) Alternative pathway of bovine complement: Concentration of factor B, hemolytic activity and heritability. Vet Immunol Immunopathol 5: 389–398

264. Tachibana DK, Rosenberg LT (1966) Fetal synthesis of HC, a component of mouse complement. J Immunol 97: 213–215

265. Tachibana DK, Ulrich M, Rosenberg LT (1963) The inheritance of hemolytic complement activity on CF-1 mice. J Immunol 91: 230–232

266. Tack BF, Prahl JW (1976) Third component of human complement. Purification from plasma and physico-chemical characterization. Biochemistry 15: 4513–4521

267. Tamura N, Nelson RA (1967) Three naturally-occurring inhibitors of components of complement in guinea pig and rabbit serum. J Immunol 99: 582–589

268. Terry WD, Borsos T, Rapp H (1964) Differences in serum complement activity among inbred strains of mice. J Immunol 92: 576–578

269. Thorbecke GJ, Hochwald GM, vanFurth F, Muller-Eberhard HJ, Jacobson EB (1965) Complement: In: Ciba Foundation Symposium, p 99

270. Thurston JR, Baetz AL, Cheville NF, Richard JL (1980) Acute aflatoxicosis in guinea pigs: Sequential changes in serum proteins, complement, C4, and live enzymes and histopathologic changes. Am J Vet Res 41: 1272–1276

271. Toews GB, Vial WC (1984) The role of C5 polymorphonuclear leukocyte recruitment in response to *Streptococcus pneumoniae* Am Rev Resp Dis 129: 82–86

272. Trail PA, Yang TJ, Cameron JA (1984) Increase in the haemolytic complement activity of dogs affected with cyclic haematopoiesis. Vet Immunol Immunopathol 7: 359–368

273. Ulevitch RJ, Cochrane CG (1977) Complement dependent hemodynamic and hematologic changes in the rabbit. Inflammation 2: 199–216

274. Van Dijk H, Heezius E, Van Kooten PJS, Rademaker PM, Van Dam R, Willers JMN (1983) A study of the sensitivity of erythrocytes to lysis by heterologous sera via the alternative complement pathway. Vet Immunol Immunopath 4: 469–477

275. Vogt W, Lieflander M, Stalder KH, Lufft E, Schmidt G (1971) Functional identity of anaphylatoxin preparations obtained from different species and by different activation procedures. II. Immunological identity. Eur J Immunol 1: 139–140

276. Wagner JL, Hugli TE (1984) Radioimmunoassay for anaphylatoxins: A sensitive method for determining complement activation products in biological fluids. Analytical Biochem 136: 75–88

277. Weigle WO, Goodman MG, Morgan EL, Hugli TE (1983) Regulation of immune response by components of the complement cascade and their activated fragments. Springer Sem Immunopathol 6: 173–194

278. Weitzel HK, Rother K (1970) Studies on the role of serum complement in allograft rejection and in immunosuppression by antithymocyte serum. Eur Surg Res 2: 310–317

279. Whaley K (1980) Biosynthesis of the complement components and the regulatory proteins of the alternative complement pathway by human peripheral blood monocytes. J Exp Med 151: 501–516

280. Wheat WH, Wetsel R, Falus A, Tack BF, Strunk RC (1987) The fifth component of complement (C5) in the mouse. J Exp Med 165: 1442–1447

281. Whitehead AS, Goldberger G, Woods DE, Markham AF, Colten HR (1983) Use of a cDNA clone for the fourth component of human complement (C4) for analysis of a genetic deficiency of C4 in guinea pig. Proc Natl Acad Sci USA 80: 5387–5391

282. Wieme RJ, Demulenaare B (1967) Genetically determined electrophoretic variant of the human complement component C3. Nature 214: 1042–1043

283. Winkelstein JA, Cork LC, Griffin DE, Griffin JW, Adams RJ, Price DL (1981) Genetically determined deficiency of the third component of complement in the dog. Science 212: 1169–1170

284. Winkelstein JA, Johnson JP, Swift AJ, Ferry F, Yolken R, Cork LC (1982) Genetically determined deficiency of the third component of complement in the dog: *In vivo* studies on the complement system and complement mediated serum activities. J Immunol 129: 2598–2602

285. Wissler JH (1972) Chemistry and biology of anaphylatoxin related peptide system. I. Purification crystalization and properties of classical anaphylatoxin from rat serum. Eur J Immunol 2: 73–83

286. Wolfe JH, Halliwell REW (1980) Total hemolytic complement values in normal and diseased dog populations. Vet Immunol Immunopathol 1: 287–298

287. Yang SY, Jensen R, Folke L, Good RA, Day NK (1974) Complement deficiency in hamsters. Fed Proc 33: 795

288. Ziegler JB, Alper CA, Balner H (1975) Properdin factor B and histocompatibility loci linked in the rhesus monkey. Nature 254: 609–611

289. Ziegler JB, Watson L, Alper CA (1975) Genetic polymorphism of properdin factor B in the rhesus: Evidence for single subunit structure in primates. J Immunol 114: 1649–1653

290. Zimmerman TS, Arroyave CM, Muller-Eberhard HJ (1971) A blood coagulation abnormality in rabbits deficient in the sixth component of complement (C6) and its correction by purified C6. J Exp Med 134: 1591–1600

C. Transport Proteins

HAI T. NGUYEN, VMD, MS

Plasma proteins in most animal species make up approximately 7 per cent of the total plasma. These nitrogenous compounds are often unique and specific for individual species. Most plasma proteins have specific functions as, for example, enzymes, blood coagulation factors, hormones, antibodies, or transport compounds. This chapter deals with the last group of plasma proteins. Most transport proteins in humans have been well characterized. However, information on the animal counterparts is often scanty or lacking, as in the case of group-specific components and hemopexin. The major transport proteins covered in this chapter include prealbumin, thryoid hormone binding proteins, albumin, haptoglobin, group-specific components, hemopexin, transferrin, and corticosteroid-binding globulin. Ceruloplasmin is discussed elsewhere.

PREALBUMIN (TRANSTHYRETIN)

Biochemistry and Function

Prealbumin (PA) is a plasma protein of high negative charge when compared with other plasma proteins. Its electrophoretic mobility is greater than that of serum albumin. The PA band is usually visible only by transmitted light on an electrophoretogram (118). The name transthyretin was recently recommended for prealbumin to avoid confusion with albumin precursors and to indicate its function as a serum transport protein for both thyroxin and retinol-binding protein (217). The structure and physicochemical properties of PA in man have been well described (161,204,250). Human PA has a molecular weight of approximately 55,000 daltons (d) and is a stable tetramer of four identical polypeptide subunits. It is high in acidic protein but contains no sialic acid or carbohydrate groups. The complete amino acid sequence has been determined.

Prealbumin has not been as well characterized in animals as in man, and it may not even exist as such in some domestic animals (162). However, it has been reported in the nonhuman primate, horse, rabbit, rat, chicken, pigeon, and quail (89,131,242,271). Among all these species, only rat and monkey PA has been well studied. The rat PA is slightly smaller than human PA. It has a molecular weight of approximately 51,000 d as determined by sedimentation equilibrium analysis (215,233). There is evidence that rat PA also contains four identical subunits. Although rat and human PAs are immunologically distinct, their amino acid compositions are quite similar. Analysis of the

NH$_2$-terminal 30 amino acid residues of the rat PA subunit showed only four substitutions from that of the human PA subunit (225). Rhesus and cynomolgus monkey PAs have molecular weights of approximately 65,000 and 58,000 d, respectively, and are believed to be a tetramer similar to that of rat and man (37, 302). Rabbit PA contained the same number of amino acid residues and showed 80 per cent homology with rat and human PA by sequence analysis (290).

Prealbumin plays an important role in the plasma transport of thyroid hormones and is also involved in the transport of vitamin A (160,220). In man thyroxine-binding pre-albumin (TBPA) has been shown to have two binding sites for T$_4$, and although the binding sites are identical, the binding of T$_4$ to one site inhibits the binding to the other (250). Thus, one molecule of TBPA only binds one molecule of thyroxine. In contrast to human TBPA, which plays a minor role in transporting thyroid hormones compared to thyroxine-binding globulin (61), TBPA in the rat appears to be the major thyroid hormone transport protein (76,233, 271). T$_4$ binding to TBPA has also been reported in the rabbit, rhesus monkey, horse, pigeon, and chicken (242,271). T$_3$ binding to PA has been demonstrated in the pigeon (241). The electrophoretic mobility of TBPA differs considerably among animal species. In the monkey, horse, and chicken, the protein was found anodal to albumin, but in cattle, swine, dog, cat, rabbit, and frog it was cathodal to albumin, making the term "prealbumin" less suitable in these species (177).

Vitamin A normally circulates in plasma as retinol which is bound to retinol-binding protein (RPB). In turn, RPB strongly interacts with PA and circulates together with PA in plasma as a protein-protein complex. In man, purified RPB has α$_1$ mobility on electrophoresis and has a molecular weight of approximately 21,000 to 22,000 d (160). The RPB-PA interactions of rat and monkey are similar to those in man (233,302).

Experiments using rat liver perfusion and hepatocyte culture techniques as well as metabolic studies indicate that the liver is the site of PA synthesis (81,90,216). Hepatic secretion of PA and that of RPB are believed to be independently regulated processes and the PA-RPB complex is formed in the plasma after the independent secretion of the two proteins from liver cells (216). The rate of PA synthesis in the rat was estimated at 3.6 mg/100 g of body weight per day and the half-life of PA in the blood stream was 29 hours (81). Prealbumin also was reported to be synthesized and secreted by the choroid plexus in the rat, and the synthesis of PA by the liver and the choroid plexus appears to be independently regulated during the acute phase response (80,82).

Genetic polymorphism of PA has only been described for the nonhuman primate. *Macaca mulatta* (rhesus monkey) TBPA exists in three forms and is under the control of two autosomal codominant alleles: the fast PA, designated Pt^1, and the slow PA, designated Pt^2. The homozygous type Pt 1–1 migrates similar to human TBPA. The two homozygous types Pt 1–1 and Pt 2–2 migrate as single bands on 8.5 per cent polyacrylamide gel electrophoresis at pH 8.9. The heterozygote Pt 1–2 is seen as three bands between the two Pt 1–1 and Pt 2–2 bands. No polymorphism like that seen in macaques has been found in baboons, chimpanzees, or organutans but drills and mandrills have PA polymorphism. There is no evidence that the PA polymorphism affects thyroxine transport or RPB-PA complexing (11,37,40,249,312).

Measurement

Isolation and purification of PA is facilitated by the relative abundance of PA and especially by its high negative charge. For bulk preparation, precipitation methods have been used; however, ion-exchange chromatography, gel filtration, and preparative electrophoresis (250) are more commonly employed for purification. At high ionic strength, PA complexes with RPB which has a characteristic green flurescence; therefore, affinity chromatography on sepharose with covalently bound RPB has also been widely used for PA purification (92,215).

Serum levels of PA can be measured directly by radioimmunoassay (35,216) and radial immunodiffusion (81). Prealbumin concentrations can also be determined indirectly and expressed in terms of thyroxine-binding capacity (27). Serum PA is relatively stable under various storage conditions (56). The serum levels in selected animals are listed in Table 10.C.1.

Serum PA concentrations in man are

Table 10.C.1. Prealbumin Serum Levels of Various Animal Species

	Serum levels of Prealbumin	
Animal Species	μg/ml (refs)	μg of T4 bound/100 ml (refs)
Rat	400–500 (81)	140 (76)
	398 $\pm$ 50 (215,216)	
Rhesus monkey (*Macaca mulatta*)	291 (250)	
Green monkey (*Cercopithecus aethiops*)		203 $\pm$ 9 (25, 26)
Quail		
1 day old	220 (131)	
14 days old	430 (131)	

decreased in liver disease, hyperthyroidism, cystic fibrosis, and protein calorie malnutrition. They are unchanged in chronic renal disease (250). Acute inflammation induced by turpentine in rats was shown to decrease the serum PA level considerably (81). Therefore, PA is considered as a "negative" acute-phase protein. Androgenic steroids markedly increase serum PA concentrations, whereas estrogenic compounds have much less effect (25–27). Seasonal changes in TBPA concentrations have been described in quail, being lowest during the summer and highest during mid-winter (131).

THYROID HORMONE-BINDING PROTEINS

Biochemistry and Function

In plasma there are three proteins that regulate the circulation of thyroid hormones: (1) thyroxine-binding globulin (TBG), which is the most important and transports the major part of T_4 in most animals, except the rat; (2) thyroxine-binding prealbumin, which probably does not exist in all animals (see prealbumin); and (3) serum albumin, which usually plays a minor role in thyroid hormone transport (see albumin). In addition, lipoproteins also carry minor quantities of thyroxine, but their importance is unknown. These serum proteins may store thyroxine in a nondiffusible form in the extrathyroidal space, and they may serve to carry thyroxine from the circulation to target cells (61,141,250). In man TBG is responsible for the transport of 75 per cent of the thyroxine, TBPA transports 15 per cent, and albumin, despite its abundance in plasma, transports only about 10 per cent of the plasma thyroxine.

Thyroxine-binding globulin has the highest affinity for T_4 and binds most of the circulating T_4, with over one third of the binding sites on the protein occupied. Human TBG is a single polypeptide chain with a molecular weight of 54,000 to 63,000 d (141,250). It is an acidic inter-α-globulin rich in sialic acid. Bovine TBG has a molecular weight of 54,000 d and a carbohydrate content similar to that of human TBG (306). Thyroxine-binding globulin is synthesized by the liver (109,111).

With the use of agarose gel electrophoresis, rhesus monkey T_4 may be found bound to the inter-alpha, PA, and albumin zones; T_3 is bound to the inter-alpha and albumin zones only. The inter-alpha protein in rhesus monkey migrates slightly slower than does human TBG. Baboon and chimpanzee have thyroxine-binding patterns similar to those of rhesus monkey, but TBPA and its polymorphic variations have only been seen in mandrills and macaques (89, 242,312). In the dog and cat T_4 is bound to the inter-alpha and albumin zones and there is no binding to a prealbumin area. In the mouse T_4 is bound to albumin and α-globulin; however, there appears to be some interstrain variation in the electrophoretic mobility of these proteins. Mouse prealbumin does not bind T_4. In the rat T_4 is bound to PA and albumin. Postalbumin TBG was reported by some investigators (76) but not confirmed by others (89,242,271). Prealbumin in the rat was found to be the major T_4 transport protein, carrying 55 per cent of the total T_4 compared to 15 per cent and 18 per cent by albumin and TBG, respectively (76). Rabbit T_4 binds similarly to albumin and postalbumin and a small amount is also bound to PA (271). In the guinea pig thyroxine seems to be associated only with albumin. In cattle, sheep, and goat T_3 and T_4 are bound in postalbumin and albumin zones. In the horse and chicken a PA zone in addition to the albumin and post-

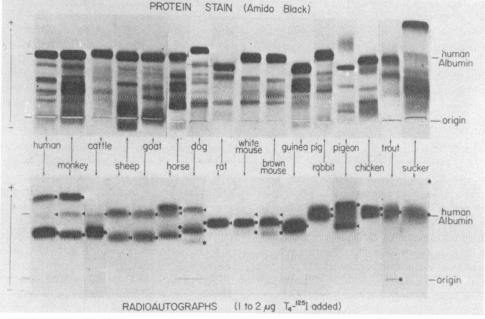

Figure 10.C.1. L-thyroxine binding patterns of serum proteins. Amido-Black protein stain (*top*) and corresponding radioautographic patterns (*bottom*) of agarose gel electrophoreses of sera from various vertebrate species enriched with a "tracer" of ^{125}I-labeled L-thyroxine. Dotted marks on the right of each pattern indicate the location of a radioautographic band distinctly visible on the original developed x-ray film. Triangles indicate the location of the albumin of each individual species. All photographic prints were copied on scale with the albumin band of the human control serum (present in each individual electrophoretic run) 5.5 cm from the origin, as indicated on the right. Reprinted by permission of J. B. Lippincott Co (242).

albumin zones is also found to bind T_4 (89,242). The ^{125}I-labeled L-thyroxine binding patterns for serum proteins of various species is shown in Figure 10.C.1. Apparently in many animal species the thyroxine carrier proteins reported in the literature are unspecific and poorly characterized, and TBG probably does not exist in a number of species including cat, rat, rabbit, frog, and chicken (177).

Measurement

Thyroxine-binding globulin may be isolated and purified using immunoprecipitation, affinity chromatography (throxine-coupled agarose), anion-exchange chromatography, and gel filtration. Serum TBG concentrations can be measured using radioimmunoassay methodology (110,112,141). In the rhesus monkey the serum TBG concentration is approximately 20 μg/ml and the synthesis rate of TBG in the rat is approximately 2 mg per day per 3 kg of body weight (112,194). The biologic significance of a

given serum TBG concentration is not completely understood. In humans with normal thyroid function the T_4/TBG ratio remains constant. Elevation in the T_4/TBG ratio is found in hyperthyroidism and a decreased T_4/TBG ratio is seen in hypothyroidism (141).

ALBUMIN

Biochemistry and Function

Serum albumin is the most abundant protein in the circulation and the most prominent component on electrophesis. Albumin is a single peptide chain of over 580 amino acid residues. The amino acid composition and sequence of albumin have been studied in many domestic and laboratory animals (49,50,228,231). The complete amino acid sequence of human and bovine albumin has been described (33,48,92, 197). The molecular weights of human and bovine albumin calculated from the sequences are 66,500 and 66,210 d, respectively. The proposed structure for both human and bovine albumin consists of three repeating units or domains. Each domain is composed of two large double loops and one small double loop (33,48). The double loops are formed by disulfide bonds between the 34 half-cystine residues. The structure of bovine albumin deduced by Brown (49) is shown in Figure 10.C.2. Only 20 per cent of the amino acid residues differed between human and bovine albumin.

Albumin serves many functions. It binds and transports large organic anions that are normally insoluble in aqueous fluid, particularly bilirubin and long-chain fatty acids, poorly soluble hormones such as steroid and thyroid hormones, and virtually all constituents of plasma not bound and transported by specific proteins. Albumin is a major contributor to the plasma osmotic pressure and accounts for 75 per cent of total osmotic activity. Albumin plays a minor nutritive role acting as reservoir and contributing approximately 5 per cent of amino acids used in peripheral tissues. It is also involved in the binding of heavy metals (118,162,228). The ligand-binding locations for several substances have been reported (228,241). Copper and nickel bind at the amino terminus. Cystine and glutathione bind near the first thiol group, and normally two fatty acids bind on loops 4–6 and 7.

Albumin synthesis takes place in the liver and is closely dependent on the amino acid supply. The synthesis of albumin involves an intracellular precursor form, proalbumin. Studies in the rat have shown that proalbumin, formed by the microsomes, contains a basic hexapeptide extension at the amino terminus. Proalbumin binds bilirubin and palminate as effectively as does albumin. Although the role of proalbumin is unknown, it has been suggested that the hexapeptide extension on proalbumin serves to channel the nascent albumin through the liver cell and to regulate albumin synthesis (228,229,231,232). The overall rates of albumin catabolism have been determined for various animal species by conventional protein tracer techniques such as radioiodination (9,83,192). The rate of catabolism varies with the species and is frequently measured as the time in which one half the serum concentration disappears ($T_{1/2}$). There appears to be a direct correlation between albumin turnover and body size. The $T_{1/2}$ for albumin in various species is listed in Table 10.C.2 (162).

The tissue sites for albumin catabolism have been studied using nondegradable radioactive tracers that accumulate in tissues following protein degradation. Studies in the rabbit using (^{14}C) sucrose-labeled albumin suggested that all tissues catabolized albumin with no tissue of predominant importance. The most active tissues were those with fenestrated or discontinuous capillary beds, suggesting that exposure to high concentrations of albumin was an important determinant in albumin degradation (318). Similar studies in rats showed that the major fraction of albumin catabolism occurs in muscle and hide (31).

Genetic polymorphism has been observed in many species, including domestic fowl, pig,

---

Figure 10.C.2. Structural organization of mammalian albumin. The layout of the sequence is based on the vertical alignment of the CYS-CYS sequences that occur in the large double loops. This results in vertical sequence alignment of similar structural features. The enclosed areas formed by disulfide bridges are black. The loops and connecting segments form a pattern that repeats three times. These three basic repeat units are proposed structural domains, as indicated in the figure. The junctions between domains occur at 190–191 and 382–383. Each domain can be divided into a subdomain that includes a "type C" loop and a fused subdomain that includes "type A and B" loops. The junctions between subdomains occur at 115–116, 306–307, and 503–504. The locations of CYS residues appear to be invariant in the sequences of all mammalian albumins analyzed. Because the pattern of loops and connecting segments is a consequence of the location and disulfide bridge pairing of CYS residues, all mammalian albumins probably have similar domain and subdomain structures. Several laboratories have prepared fragments of bovine and human albumin by specific cleavage with cyanogen bromide or limited proteolysis. The sites of these cleavages are indicated by a black triangle.

Partial amino acid sequences of sperm whale myoglobin and human alpha hemoglobin at the bottom of the figure are arranged so that the PRO residues (120 and 114) that occur at the ends of the G-helixes are aligned with PRO residues (146,222,337,413, and 534) that occur at the ends of the large loops of albumin. In myoglobin, PRO at position 100 starts the G-helix, and a similar PRO occurs at 514 in albumin. In hemoglobin, PRO-119 starts the H-helix; similar PRO residues occur in albumin at 151 and 418. The similarities in sequence between the globins and the various albumin loops are equal to or greater than the similarity between myoglobin and hemoglobin. Reprinted by permission of the Federation of American Societies for Experimental Biology (49).

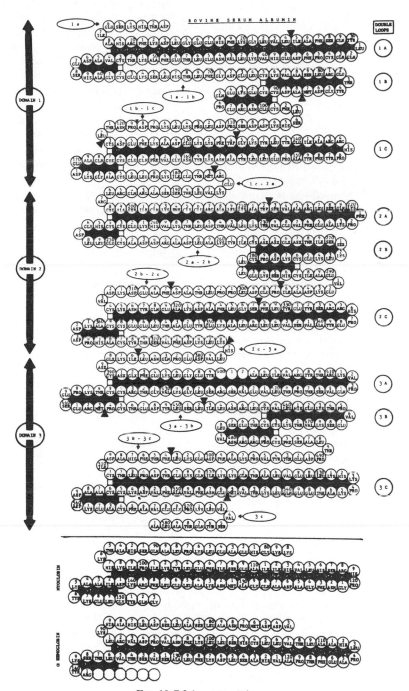

FIG. 10.C.2 (*see opposite*).

Table 10.C.2. Albumin Turnover in Animals

Species	$T_{1/2}$ (days)	Reference
Mouse	1.9	9
Rat	2.5	9
Guinea pig	2.8	9
Rabbit	5.7	83
Dog	8.2	83
Man	15	83
Baboon	16	64

cattle, horse, and toad (295). Breeding experiments with inbred lines of Brown Leghorns, White Leghorns, and Rhode Island Red chickens have shown three phenotypes of albumin controlled by two codominant autosomal alleles: a homozygous fast, a homozygous slow, and a heterozygous fast-slow combination type (195). Patterns of albumin polymorphism similar to those of chickens are also observed in turkeys (238) and horses (284). In pigs the genetic control of albumin phenotypes appears to involve three codominant alleles (170). Eleven albumin alleles present in 29 phenotypes were found in the American toad (*Bufo Americanus*) (66). Genetic variants have also been described in cattle (279). Immunologic cross-reactivity between serum albumin from various species has been studied and correlated with the phylogenetic relatedness between species. Cross-reactivity between human serum albumin and those of several primate species, as well as cross-reactivity among serum albumins of various domestic and laboratory animals, has been reported (158,239,255,257,311). In these studies, rabbit anti-bovine serum albumin antibodies will cross-react most strongly with sheep and goat albumin and less so with pig, horse, rodent, and chicken albumin in decreasing order.

Measurement

Currently used procedures for estimation of serum albumin are based on one of the following principles: (1) salt precipitation, (2) dye binding, (3) electrophoretic mobility, and (4) antigenicity (118,162,228). The most commonly used salts for precipitation are sodium and ammonium sulfate. Serum globulins can be removed selectively by salt precipitation and the remaining albumin assayed by the biuret method. Because the globulin concentrations differ in animals, the salt concentrations must be adjusted accordingly (162). Albumin has the tendency to bind certain dyes such as bromcresol green (BCG), methyl orange, and 2-(4′-hydroxyazobenzene)-benzoic acid (HABA). This characteristic has been used to measure albumin directly. HABA binds very poorly to albumin of domestic animals and is susceptible to bilirubin interference. The use of BCG appears to be quite accurate when compared to electrophoresis and is less affected by pigment interference. The assay of albumin using electrophoresis and protein staining has frequently been used as the reference against which other procedures are judged. However, there is no convincing evidence that the staining intensity is linear to protein concentration. Immunochemical techniques for albumin determination such as radial immunodiffusion and immunonephelometry are gaining popularity (228).

Measurement of serum albumin is of considerable diagnostic value as it relates to (a) general nutritional status, (b) the integrity of the vascular system, and (c) liver function. Serum albumin concentrations for most laboratory animal species are between 2.42 and 4.19 g/dl, and reference values for each laboratory animal species have been reported (200). In man the rate of albumin synthesis by the liver is approximately 14 g per day (237). In 5- to 7-week-old rats, it is 3.13 mg/100 g of body weight per hour (230).

Fasting rats for 18 hours caused a 40 per cent reduction in the rate of albumin synthesis (230). Circadian fluctuation of plasma protein and albumin levels in rats maintained on a 12-hour light-dark cycle has been reported, with highest levels observed at 0100 and 0800 hours and lowest levels observed at 1800 (260). The formation of albumin decreases with increasing age (155); however, the properties and composition of serum albumin from adult and aging mice are identical (261). Increased albumin production, in the true sense, has not been known to occur in animals. An increase in the serum albumin concentration is usually interpreted as consistent with dehydration (162). Hypoalbuminemia may result from: (a) impaired synthesis, as in malnutrition or chronic liver disease; (b) loss through urine and feces, as in renal and intestinal disease; (c) increased catabolism, as in neoplastic conditions and acute phase reaction (in this sense, albumin is a "negative" acute

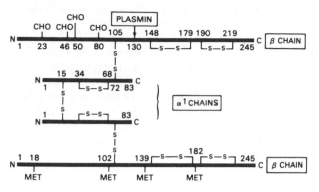

Figure 10.C.3. Summary representation of the major features of the human Hp 1-1 tetrachain structure. CHO indicates carbohydrate attachment to Asn. Plasmin cleaved at Lys-130 of both β chains. Reprinted by permission of the National Academy of Sciences (173).

phase reactant); and (d) changes in distribution between intra- and extravascular compartments (53,67,79,118,137,157,162,173,198).

HAPTOGLOBIN (SEROMUCOID α_2)

Biochemistry and Function

Haptoglobin (Hp) was first identified in 1939 as a serum component responsible for enhancing the peroxidase activity associated with hemoglobin (235). It is a serum α_2-glycoprotein present in man and animal that can bind free hemoglobin (Hb), forming a stable complex. This complex has a pink color and can be visualized after electrophoresis or chromatography. One known function of Hp is to protect the kidneys from tissue destruction by binding free Hb after hemolysis (43). The formation of Hp-Hb complexes may also be beneficial by decreasing the availability of Hb iron to support bacterial growth at sites of septic inflammation (87). In vitro studies on the inhibition of cathepsin B and cathepsin L by rat Hp suggest that haptoglobin inhibits lysosomal thiol proteinases specifically and therefore may have a regulatory role in tissue proteolysis associated with the inflammatory reaction (222). However, this characteristic of Hp has only been observed in rat Hp. Haptoglobin is one of the major acute-phase reactants (166). Its concentration in serum increases during inflammation and decreases after hemolysis.

Human Hp has a tetrachain structure with two α chains and two β chains (Figure 10.C.3). The α and β chains are covalently linked by disulfide bonds (173). Genetic studies showed that Hp polymorphism in man is controlled by three codominant alleles coding for the α chain, namely, Hp αIF (fast), Hp αIS (slow), and Hp α2. These three major alleles are responsible for the six common phenotypes observed (277). Other rare variants of human Hp have also been reported (43). The simplest phenotypic form, Hp 1-1, is monomeric (Figure 10.C.3) whereas phenotypes Hp 2–1 and Hp 2–2 are polymeric and appear as several bands on electrophoresis. Complete amino acid sequences of the α- and β-chains of human haptoglobin type 1–1 have been determined (173). Amino acid compositions of dog, rat, and rabbit Hps have also been reported (127,172,183,184). The carbohydrate moiety of human Hp is approximately 19.8 per cent (43), and of those of rabbit and rat, 17.9 and 14.1 per cent, respectively (184). The Hp β-subunit shows substantial homology to the chymotrypsinogen family of serine proteases. Evolution from a common ancestral molecule is suggested; however, no proteolytic activity remains in the case of Hp (28,173).

The dissociation of Hb tetramers into dimers is a prerequisite for binding to Hp. This suggests that the $\alpha_1\beta_2$ contact region between Hb dimers is the binding site for Hp (34,190). Evidence has also been presented that Hb binds to Hp as intact $\alpha_1\beta_1$ dimers and that the primary region of Hb involved in the intermolecular contact is the $\alpha_1\beta_2$ interface (149). Binding sites on the Hb α- and β-subunit interacting surfaces have been localized (164,319).

Concerning Hp binding sites for Hb, studies show that Hb binds to the β chain of Hp and the α chain does not directly participate in the binding (43,115). There is some evidence that tyrosyl or tryptophanyl residues are involved in the binding (236). The stable Hp-Hb complex, once formed in the blood stream following hemolysis, is rapidly cleared from the plasma and accumulates in the liver. When cats were injected intravenously with Hb in quantities sufficient to bind all circulating Hp, unbound Hp was not present after 3 hours and the Hp-Hb complexes were cleared in as little as 6 hours (128). Studies using solubilization and assay of the hepatic receptor for the Hp-Hb complex suggest that the carbohydrate moiety of haptoglobin did not appear to participate in the binding of the Hp-Hb complex to its receptors (186).

Haptoglobin has been found in the sera of all vertebrates studied (153,236). Haptoglobin isolated from most nonhuman species resembles human Hp 1 on gel electrophoresis and appears as a single component. Polymeric forms similar to human Hp 2 and Hp 2–1, however, have been observed in members of the Bovidae and Cervidae families such as goat, sheep, cattle, antelopes, giraffe, elephant, and hyrax (39,52, 248,297–299). Despite an extensive search in several species of nonhuman primates (39,52, 248,269), dogs (268), rabbits (121), and swine (168), there is no convincing evidence that polymorphism exists in any animals other than man (43,51). Other variations in the Hp structure have been observed in the chicken and dog. Chicken Hp is composed of only two chains with a molecular weight of 3,000 and 54,000 d (185). Dog Hp under standard gel electrophoretic conditions appears similar to human Hp 1 in both charge and size, with a molecular weight of approximately 100,000 d. However, under denaturing conditions employing 6M urea or 0.1 per cent sodium lauryl sulfate the molecular weight is that of an Hp $\alpha\beta$ subunit, which is 48,500 d (172).

Results of sequence analysis on the amino-terminal 40 residues of rat, rabbit, and dog Hp β chain indicated that the Hp β chain has been fairly well conserved during evolution. Both human and dog have carbohydrate moieties on β Asn-23, but rat and rabbit do not (171).

Haptoglobin appears to exhibit little species specificity in binding to Hb. Human Hp can bind Hb from numerous animals; however, very distantly related Hbs only bind weakly (63,85,190,234). Chicken Hp has a narrow specificity and binds only avian and reptilian Hb (214).

Haptoglobin is synthesized in the liver (166) and more precisely by the hepatocytes (91). It has a plasma half-life of about 3 days (10,166). Various hormones (30,116,156,183), endotoxins (116,140), and prostaglandins (140,270) have been studied regarding their influence on Hp synthesis. Injection of cortisone acetate in rats increased plasma Hp by 54 per cent (116). Prednisone-induced increases in serum Hp have also been reported in dogs (130). Leukocytic endogenous mediator appears to be an important factor in triggering the accelerated Hp synthesis associated with the acute phase response (41,140,159,296,301,310).

Measurement

Several methods for purifying (7,78) and quantitating serum Hp have been described (19,69,234). Methods for the isolation of Hp from plasma may need to be altered for use in different animal species. Modifications for the isolation of rat (7,183), rabbit (183), and canine (84) haptoglobins have been described.

The quantitating procedures include measuring enhancement of peroxidase activity, changes in electrophoretic mobility and rivanol precipitation, and immunochemical techniques. In most methods an excess of Hb is added to the serum to saturate the Hp. The amount of Hp-Hb complex is then estimated by peroxidase activity. The complex can also be separated from free hemoglobin by electrophoresis or gel filtration and the proportion of Hb bound to Hp is then calculated. Immunotechniques may be complicated, depending on the heterogeneity and the degree of polymerization of Hp. Immunochemical methods that have been used to measure Hp in animals include rocket electroimmunoassay (103,223,307), two-dimensional immunoelectrophoresis (1), immunonephelometry (69), ELISA (19), and radial immunodiffusion (19). Some degree of interspecies cross-reactivity does occur. Antiserum against human Hp was found to produce clear rockets when used in electroimmunoassay to measure rabbit (307) and mouse (309) haptoglobins. Hemolysis in samples does not affect Hp estimation, but hyperlipidemia may give high results (43,118,234). Normal Hp levels of some animal species are listed in Table 10.C.3.

Table 10.C.3. Normal Haptoglobin Levels of Some Animal Species

| Species | Serum Haptoglobin | | |
	mg/100 ml of Serum	mg Hb Bound/ 100 ml of Serum	Reference
Green monkey			
(*Cercopithecus aethiops*)	...	21–105	26
Cattle	...	0–50	46
Rabbit	10–30	...	183
Rat			
Unspecified	10–30	...	183
Unspecified	30–60	...	7
Unspecified	50	...	69
Sprague-Dawley	100	...	19
Mouse—DBA/2	...	50–150	226
Dog	...	14–252	129
Cat	...	31–216	129
Horse	...	19 177	129

Baseline Hp levels in human serum are influenced by genetic factors, gender, and age (236,291). Levels tended to be higher in men than in women (104). Pregnancy did not affect Hp levels (104), but contraceptive medications caused a 25 per cent decrease (178). Anhaptoglobinemia is common in human infants less than 3 months old (236).

Disease-related changes in human Hp concentrations include both increased and decreased levels (93,102,236,278,314). Raised levels are noted with acute or chronic inflammatory conditions and with neoplastic disease. Decreased levels are associated with hemolytic processes and with severe liver diseases.

Reported normal and acute phase concentrations for several species are shown in Table 10.C.4. Strain-dependent variation in Hp concentration was reported among 11 strains of mice examined (226). The DBA/2 and AKR strains represent the extremes of this variation, with serum Hp levels of 50 to 150 and 5 to 10

mg of hemoglobin binding capacity (HbBC) per 100 ml, respectively. No reports were found regarding gender-related differences in Hp levels in animals. In contrast to the unchanged concentration reported in pregnant women, Hp was increased in pregnant C57BL/10 mice (309). The increase was of greater degree and duration in allogeneic than in syngeneic pregnancy. Levels returned to normal by 8 days postpartum (309). Age also has an effect on baseline levels in mice. In newborn DBA/2 mice, serum Hp was about 50 per cent of the adult levels (223). The levels then dropped quickly and remained at only 10 to 30 per cent of the adult range during the first 2 weeks of life.

Changes associated with various pathologic processes are similar to those seen in humans. Decreased Hp levels were documented in cats with experimental and spontaneous hemolytic anemias (128) and in some rats with induced hepatic cirrhosis (68). Increased concentrations in response to various inflammatory stimuli

Table 10.C.4. Haptoglobin (Hp) in Several Species

| Species | Molecular Weight (dalton) | Serum Hp (mg/dl HbBC)[a] | | References |
		Normal (adult)	Acute Phase	
Human (1-1)	100,000	75–175	650	236
Rabbit	70,000	10–30	300	183
Rat	90,000	10–30	300	126, 183
Dog	81,000	15–250	500	103, 129
Mouse (DBA/2)	...	45–55	500	223

[a] HbBC = hemoglobin binding capacity.

have been observed in mice (223,226), rats (69,116,193), rabbits (29,117,183,213), cats (128), and dogs (103). Neoplasia-associated increases in serum Hp have been reported in rabbits (307), mice (224,226), and rats (1). In C3H mice with mammary tumor, however, the serum Hp remains low (226). Absence or a low level of Hp indicates hemolysis or acute hepatocellular damage (118).

GROUP-SPECIFIC COMPONENT

Biochemistry and Function

Group-specific component (Gc) was first discovered in human serum by Hischfeld (138) in 1959. It is an α_2-globulin with an electrophoretic mobility similar to but distinct from that of haptoglobin. The protein was later isolated and characterized and its amino acid composition was determined by various investigators (60,134,272). Variants of human Gc are controlled by some 30 different alleles (65), but the three most common phenotypes are the Gc 1–1, Gc 2–1, and Gc 2–2 controlled by codominant alleles Gc 1 and Gc 2. Gc 1 consists of two suballeles, Gc 1F (fast) and Gc 1S (slow) (59). The total amino acid composition and molecular weight of the major Gc phenotypes are very similar. They have a molecular weight of about 50,800 d and a low carbohydrate content (3.3 per cent) and appear to be a single polypepide chain (60). The Gc system has been used for individual identification and parentage exclusion, but the biologic function of Gc has been largely unknown until recently when it was found to be similar, if not identical, to the serum protein that binds vitamin D and its metabolites (42,73,74,292). Therefore, Gc may have a function in vitamin D transport and may also act as a buffer to prevent the toxic effects of vitamin D at the tissue level (73).

Measurement

Demonstration and quantitation of Gc components can be conducted using various methods such as electrophoresis, isoelectrofocusing, and immunoprecipitation (65,245). High doses of vitamin D, hemolysis, and bacterial contamination may induce modification of the Gc electrophoretic pattern (65).

Group-specific component in various animal species including primates, cattle, pig, horse, rodent, and rabbit has been reported (13,58,59,245,313). Antiserum specific to human Gc was found to cross-react with serum from horse, cow, rhesus monkey, chimpanzee, goat, sheep, rat, and mouse (73,245), but not with rabbit and guinea pig serum (73). In many species, Gc appears as single-band components on electrophoresis. However, genetic polymorphism of Gc has been observed in cattle (13), mouse (58), horse (313), and primate (59). In the horse, Gc polymorphism is apparently under the control of two autosomal codominant alleles, with three different phenotypes found in standard bred, thoroughbred, and Arabian horses as well as the Shetland pony (313). Kitchin and Bearn (165) studied Gc polymorphism in chimpanzees, orangutans, rhesus monkeys and a gorilla and found genetic variations only in orangutans. Cleve and Patutschnick (59), however, observed two phenotypes in a group of 78 chimpanzees and postulated that two alleles controlled the genetic variation in chimpanzee Gc. Two phenotypes, Gc pan 1–1 and Gc pan 2–1, were found, but the third phenotype, Gc pan 2–2, was not observed.

HEMOPEXIN

Biochemistry and Function

During intravascular hemolysis, hemoglobin is released into the circulation and cleared by glomerular filtration or hepatocellular uptake. Haptoglobin, albumin, and hemopexin (Hx) are the three plasma proteins associated with the transport of circulating hemoglobin and heme (heme in this discussion is defined as ferriprotoporphyrin IX). In man, haptoglobin binds hemoglobin but not heme, and Hx and albumin bind heme but not hemoglobin (136,210). Mouse Hx has been reported to bind both heme and hemoglobin (316).

Hemopexin is a β-glycoprotein. Human and rabbit Hx have been found to be very similar (144,267). They both have a molecular weight of approximately $57,000 \pm 3,000$ d and appear to consist of a single polypeptide chain. The carbohydrate content is about 20 per cent and consists of sialic acid, mannose, galactose, and glucosamine. The amino acid composition of both human and rabbit Hx has been determined (144,308), and recently complete amino acid sequence of human Hx has been reported (294). Pig Hx has been isolated in pure form by affinity chromatography and ion-exchange chromatography and has a molecular weight of approximately 57,000 d (189). Mouse Hx was reported as a β-2-III globulin with a molecular weight of approximately 65,000 d (316). Bovine Hx migrates as a β_1-globulin (46). Rat and guinea pig heme-Hx complexes have also been reported to migrate with β-globulins (148). Rhesus monkey Hx purified by the wheat-germ lectin-sepharose method has a molecular weight of 60,000 d (95). The chemical composition and molecular weight (56,000 d) of sheep Hx have also been reported (286).

Studies on the immunologic cross-reactivity of serum Hx from 64 vertebrates representing many different phylogenetic orders revealed that many antigenic determinants are shared by the Eutherian mammals but not by the non-Eutherian mammals and lower animals. The Hx of apes and man appears to be identical (70).

Genetic polymorphism of Hx has been described in rabbits, pigs, and sheep. Studies in rabbits (122,125) suggest that rabbit Hx is controlled by four-codominant autosomal alleles and that the Hx locus is located between the color locus (c) and the Hq blood group locus (Linkage Group I). American and European pigs are reported to have a Hx system under the control of seven alleles (Hpx^0, Hpx^1, Hpx^{1F}, Hpx^2, Hpx^3, Hpx^{3F}, and Hpx^4) (22,23). A new allele Hpx^5 was recently described in East Asian pigs (Ohmini miniature pigs) (219). The Hpx locus in pigs appears to be linked to the K blood group system (12,124). In sheep and probably goats, Hx is genetically controlled from a single locus by two codominant alleles, and three phenotypes, Hpx A, Hpx AB, and Hpx B, have been described (286).

Hemopexin is synthesized by the liver. It binds heme specifically and carries circulating heme to the liver for uptake and breakdown (212). Radiolabeled heme-Hx complex given intravenously was found exclusively in the liver parenchymal cells, whereas spleen, kidney, lung, and bone marrow cells remained free of radiolabeled material, suggesting that plasma heme is eliminated as a heme-Hx complex by the hepatocyte (176,211). Evidence supports a rapid receptor-mediated interaction between heme-Hx complexes and cells of the liver, followed by the uptake of heme into the cells

and the release of Hx intact into the circulation (273,274).

Measurement

Several methods for Hx purification and serum level determination including preparative electrophoresis, affinity and ion-exchange chromatography, rivanol precipitation, immunoelectrophoresis, and immunodiffusion have been described (95,144,189,293,308,316). The normal plasma concentration of Hx in New Zealand white rabbits is 31 to 52 mg/100 ml (176). As in humans, neonatal rabbits have much lower levels of Hx than adults, and adult rabbit Hx values are reached at about 30 to 60 days of age (210). Rhesus monkeys have serum Hx levels of 53.3 ± 2.8 units/100 ml (1 unit represents the amount of monkey Hx equivalent to 1.0 mg of Hx per milliliter of human serum) (95).

In man, decreased serum levels of Hx are associated with severe hemolytic diseases or fulminant rhabdomyolysis (4,208,266). Increased Hx levels have been observed in certain heme deficiency diseases and chronic neuromuscular diseases in which small amounts of heme are released from increased circulating myoglobin (3,175). However, the most important factor controlling the plasma level of Hx is heme (208,266). Unlike haptoglobin and other acute phase reactants, Hx levels are rarely and only minimally affected by nonspecific stimuli such as acute inflammation, connective tissue disease, surgical procedures, and fractures. Serum Hx is probably a more reliable measurement of the severity of hemolysis (174).

Experiments in calves, however, have shown that turpentine injection produced a marked increase in plasma Hx (46). The same investigator also reported a transient elevation of serum Hp in calves infected experimentally with the nematode *Oesophagostomum radiatum* and the disappearance of Hx from the plasma of calves during the hemolytic crisis of babesiosis. In rabbits receiving varying amounts of heme, the level of Hx was lowest 4 to 6 hours after injection. Thereafter, plasma Hx concentration rose slowly in rabbits injected with large amounts of heme. These observations suggest that the administration of heme may stimulate Hx synthesis or mobilize it from the extravascular site, or both (209). Heterologous Hxs from rabbits and man maintains the heme transport function when injected into rats (180). In the rhesus monkey, small doses of heme administered intravenously elevated serum Hx to 150 per cent of control levels with a 76 per cent increase in the net rate of Hx synthesis, whereas large doses of heme caused a 60 per cent decrease in the serum Hx level; and intermediate doses of heme produced no change in the circulating Hx levels (95). The changes observed following heme administration appeared to be specific for Hx because serum haptoglobin and transferrin levels were unaffected by heme administration.

TRANSFERRIN

Biochemistry and Function

Transferrin (formerly called siderophilin), the major component of β-globulin, is the iron-transporting protein of plasma. The molecular weight of human transferrin ranges from 75,000 to 80,000 d as estimated by sedimentation equilibrium and diffusion (191,251). The molecular weight of most animal transferrins also falls within this range, whereas turtle and hagfish transferrins have molecular weights of 92,000 and 44,000 d respectively (145,225,262,282).

The structure and composition of transferrin have been studied in several species. Generally, it is a glycoprotein consisting of a single peptide chain with a varying number of heteropoly-saccharide units attached to it (5,119, 145,225,247). Rabbit transferrin was reported to contain two heterosaccharide units per molecule by some investigators (145), and only one unit by others (132,179). Most serum transferrin molecules in the rabbit contain two sialic acid residues. Transferrin isolated from rabbit milk appears to be identical to serum transferrin except that most milk transferrin molecules contain only one sialic acid residue (20). Analysis of pooled plasma from 116 rats revealed that one third of the total transferrin contains 3 moles of sialic acid and two thirds contain 2 moles of sialic acid per mole of transferrin (262). The N-terminal sequences of rabbit and rat transferrins show clear homology with human transferrin (132,187,262).

Bovine transferrin exhibits a very complex heterogeneity on starch-gel electrophoresis. In addition to genetic polymorphism, which will be described herein, each homozygous variant of bovine transferrin may exhibit multiple bands which are due, in part, to differing numbers of sialic acid residues (247,281,283,287). With high resolution chromatographic and electrophoretic techniques, 12 components (six pairs) can be visualized in the TfA homozygous variant of bovine transferrin (287). These components have been designated as 0a, 0b, 1a, 1b, 2a, 2b, 3a, 3b, 4a, 4b, and 5a, 5b (in increasing order of mobility). The numeral in each designation reflects the number of residues of sialic acid per mole of transferrin. After complete removal of sialic acid by neuraminidase treatment, all the a bands have the same mobility and all the b bands have the same mobility. However, the b bands have greater mobility than do the a bands. Because the a and b components of a single genetic variant have the same molecular weight, same amino acid composition, and identical peptide maps (247), it is suggested that the difference in mobility is due to scission of the b component peptide chain (188).

Sheep transferrin has an amino acid composition similar to that of cattle. Individual components of two variants of sheep transferrin containing 3 to 4 sialic acid residues have been isolated. However, there is no evidence for pairs of bands with the same number of sialic acid residues, as seen in cattle (282). Transferrin in carp (*Cyprinus carpio L.*) contains no sialic acid (303). The sialic acid content may be of importance in transferrin catabolism. The catabolic rate of asialotransferrin in rabbits was found to be higher than the corresponding value for normal transferrin (243).

Each transferrin molecule has two active sites for iron binding with the exception of hagfish transferrin, which has only one (225). Sequence studies of human and rabbit transferrin polypeptide chains revealed two regions of internal homology (187,289). This internal homology reflects a doubling of an ancestral structural gene responsible for the production of a transferrin with 2 metal binding sites from a precursor with a single metal-binding site (187). There are definite physicochemical differences between the two iron-binding sites (6,77); however, it is unclear whether functional differences exist. Several investigators have observed functional heterogeneity of the two iron-binding sites (16–18,75,94), whereas others have not (77,120,133, 145,320).

Transferrin polymorphism has been observed

in man as well as many animal species (51,106,107). In man at least 18 genetic variants have been described; however, only 28 phenotypes have been observed (107). All genetic variants appear to be compatible with good health. In animals, transferrin polymorphism has been observed in many species including nonhuman primates, cattle, sheep, swine, fish, and toad. Of the nonhuman primates, the chimpanzee has the greatest variation of transferrin phenotpyes. A remarkable number of variants are observed in baboons and macaques. The genus *Macaca* has at least 11 variants; of the 66 possible phenotypes, 34 have been described (113). The transferrins of prosimians are extremely complex, particularly in lemurs where 22 alleles are described. Some monkeys, such as the *C. patas*, appear to have no transferrin variants (51). Certain transferrin variants such as Tf-D and Tf-G in rhesus monkeys may be responsible for or associated with lower infant growth rates and decreased fertility (275).

In cattle, transferrin polymorphism is under the control of four alleles: Tf^A, Tf^{D1}, Tf^{D2}, and Tf^E (14,169,276,280). In addition, polymorphic variation in the amount of sialic acid attached to bovine transferrin is believed to be controlled by a recessive epistatic gene with two alleles: Tfs A and Tfs a. Thus, Tfs a/a cattle are lacking the two faster transferrin bands from the four bands normally observed in any Tf allele. Tfs A/a and Tfs A/A animals have a full complement of phenotypes (283). The Tf and Tfs loci are apparently not linked.

There are 10 known transferrin variants in horses (D, F1, F2, F3, G, H, J, M, O, and R) of which the F variant is the most common. As in cattle, equine transferrins are highly heterogeneous (57,285,288). Transferrin polymorphism has also been observed in Duroc and Hampshire pigs (23), the American toad (*Bufo americanus*) (123), and carp (*Cyprinus carpio*) (303). In the toad, 13 transferrin alleles are present, and 36 phenotypes have been described. Seven variants (A, B, C, D, E, F, and G) are found in the carp. Shifrine and Stormont studied variants of transferrin in 100 samples of plasma from beagles and found a single phenotype with a three-band pattern (268). Other transferrin variants in the dog have been reported (45).

Although transferrin may be synthesized by tissues other than the liver, such as testes, lung, brain, hematopoietic and mammary tissues, the liver is the major site of transferrin synthesis in adult animals (44,151,167,196,203). In the rat and rabbit, the rate of transferrin production is about 95 and 27 mg/kg of body weight per day, respectively. In the rat, the rate of transferrin syntheisis is one fifth the rate of albumin synthesis (202). In mouse embryos, transferrin can be detected by immunoperoxidase staining in the egg cylinders from the seventh day of gestation onwards and in the visceral yolk sac at all gestational stages (2). Thus, transferrin can be produced by both mature and immature hepatocytes. Fasting decreases and reduced ambient temperature increases transferrin synthesis (105).

Precise information about the site of transferrin catabolism is unavailable. It is probably taken up by the cells of many tissues and enzymatically degraded intracellularly (5). Studies of transferrin turnover in 11 mammalian species showed that the turnover rate closely correlated with species size (244).

Transferrin carries iron from cells involved with absorption or storage of iron to cells that utilize iron, as in hemoglobin synthesis (erythroblasts and reticulocytes), incorporation into cytochromes involved with electron transfer, or as a component of an enzyme system. Transferrin may also play a role in the regulation of iron absorption in the intestine (96,146,147). More recently it has been suggested that transferrin may serve as a physiologic regulator of granulocyte maturation (88). It is now generally accepted that transferrin is transported across the cell membrane by receptor-mediated endocytosis. Transferrin receptors on reticulocyte and hepatocyte membranes in rat, rabbit, and mouse have been studied extensively (108,150,182,300,305,321). Transferrin receptors of rabbit mammary gland cells and placenta have also been described (21,206).

Measurement

Several methods for isolation and purification of transferrin have been described. Most commonly, methods involve precipitation or fractionation with rivanol or ammonium sulfate followed by ion-exchange chromatography (181,225,259,282). Serum transferrin may be estimated directly by immunochemical methods such as radial immunodiffusion or electrodiffusion or indirectly by measuring the maximum amount of iron the serum can bind. This total iron-binding capacity (TIBC) includes both bound iron and the unbound or latent iron-binding capacity; therefore, it represents the total amount of apotransferrin in the serum. The indirect method overestimates transferrin by 10 to 20 per cent because the metal attaches to proteins other than transferrin when the latter is more than half saturated (118,162). The average concentration of transferrin in human plasma is about 290 mg/100 ml (about 30 μmol/1) or, in terms of TIBC, about 300 μg/100 ml (60 μmol/l) (118). There are no sex differences or diurnal variation, but there is a tendency for the transferrin level to fall with age (36). Serum transferrin concentrations of many animal species, such as baboon, goat, mouse, rabbit, and sheep, fall within a broad range of 250 to 350 mg/100 ml. The pig and rat have higher mean concentrations, that is, 593 and 458 mg/100 ml, respectively, whereas the dog and guinea pig have somewhat lower mean levels, that is, 192 and 187 mg/100 ml, respectively (244). Adult male hamsters have a TIBC level of 104.5 μmol/1 with 44 per cent transferrin saturation (246). Increased serum transferrin levels have been observed in pregnancy (118,139), iron deficiency anemia (205), and cortisol and estrogen administration (142,154). Low levels, usually accompanied by low albumin, are found in many diseases and are due either to impaired synthesis, as in cirrhosis, starvation, and chronic infection, or to increased excretion as in the nephrotic syndrome (118,152,201).

CORTICOSTEROID BINDING GLOBULIN

Biochemistry and Function

Corticosteroid binding globulin (CBG) or transcortin is a plasma carrier protein of obscure biologic function. It is generally accepted that CBG protects the corticosteroids from peripheral metabolism and loss through the kidney, and therefore helps maintain relatively constant plasma corticosteroid levels; however, firm evidence supporting this hypothesis is lacking. Corticosteroid binding globulin has been found in all vertebrate species examined. The CBG binding capacities of 131 vertebrate species have been determined by Seal and Doe (263–265). A comprehensive review of the CBG of various animal species was made by Westphal (315).

Table 10.C.5. Characteristics of Corticosteroid Binding Globulin from Several Animals

Species	Molecular Weight (daltons)	Percentage of Carbohydrates	References
Human	52,000	14–26	207, 265
Rat	53,000	27.8	54, 253
Rabbit	40,700	29.2	55
Guinea pig	43,300	29.0	199

Human CBG was recently reviewed by Brien (47).

Human and animal CBGs are α-globulins of similar size. The amino acid composition and carbohydrate content of CBG in rats, rabbits, and guinea pigs have been reported (54,55, 199,253). Table 10.C.5 compares the molecular weight and carbohydrate composition of CBG in several animal species and man. Rat and rabbit CBG has more half cystine than does human CBG. Because cystine is involved in the maintenance of the conformational structure of CBG, the higher cystine content found in rat CBG may be related to its greater tendency to form polymeric structures after removal of corticosterone (315). The number of corticosteroid-binding sites per molecule of CBG is one in all species tested (199,253,254). The amino acid sequence of CBG has not been established.

CBG, like other glycoproteins, is synthesized in the liver. Indirect evidence for this includes the low levels of CBG observed in rats submitted to subtotal hepatectomy (100) and in some human patients with liver disease (86). Recently, immunocytochemical localization studies demonstrating CBG in guinea pig hepatocytes (227), and in vitro synthesis of CBG by fetal rat hepatocytes (8) and by translation of rat liver m RNA in the *Xenopus laevis* oocyte system (317) provide more direct evidence in support of the liver as the site of CBG synthesis. Some evidence suggests that the liver also plays a major role in the degradation and plasma clearance of CBG. The clearance of CBG is greatly enhanced by removal of its sialic acid (143).

Measurement

Plasma CBG can be measured indirectly by determining the cortisol or corticosterone-binding capacity, and is expressed as micrograms of cortisol or of corticosterone per 100 ml of plasma. The most commonly used methods for indirect measurement are equilibrium dialysis, competitive binding analysis, and gel filtration (315). The CBG can be measured directly using radial immunodiffusion (304) and radioimmunoassay (38). The results obtained by homologous radioimmunoassay for rat CBG were consistently 0.25 μM lower than those obtained by the steroid-binding method (240). Chemical alteration of the protein and radioisotope decay are inherent problems in the radioimmunoassay for guinea pig CBG (252). The CBG concentrations calculated by radial immunodiffusion are in good agreement with estimates made by equilibrium dialysis (114). Normal CBG reference values for practically all vertebrate species have been compiled by Westphal (315).

The female rat has a higher CBG level than does the male; however, there is no change in CBG concentration during estrus or pregnancy (98,99). The CBG activity of female mice is three times that of the male. In contrast to that in rats, pregnancy in mice results in a 13-fold increase in CBG activity (101). This increase during pregnancy is also observed in rabbits and guinea pigs (101). The rise in guinea pig plasma CBG during gestation is as dramatic as that seen in the mouse with peak values of 900 μg of CBG per milliliter of plasma (compared to 75 to 155 μg per milliliter in nonpregnant animals) (114). Pregnant baboons have only a moderate increase in CBG during pregnancy (59 ± 6.4 μg of cortisol/100 ml of plasma in pregnant animals compared to 33.4 ± 5.5 μg/100 ml in nonpregnant animals) (218). The CBG levels in fetuses are higher than those in neonates, and newborn animals have much lower levels of CBG than do adults (24,32,72,135). The development and synthesis of CBG are probably regulated through the pituitary-adrenal-thyroid axis (24,72,97,252,256). Estrogen administration caused a marked increase in CBG activity in rats and monkeys (25,62,100). This effect was not observed in hypophysectomized rats, suggesting that thyroid-stimulating hormone is involved in the estrogen effect because it is the only pituitary hormone that influences CBG activity. Conversely, testosterone administration depresses CBG activity in the rat. Testosterone also depresses CBG activity in monkeys, but not significantly (27). Testosterone did not seem to

have a depressive effect on CBG in badgers (15); in Peking ducks, in which males have higher CBG levels than do females, testosterone was found to stimulate CBG production without altering thyroxine levels (75).

Diurnal variations in CBG levels have been observed in the guinea pig, rat, and mouse. The guinea pig has a maximum CBG binding capacity at 1600 hours (9 hours of light per day cycle and lights on at 0800 hours) and the lowest binding capacity at 1200 and 2400 hours (97). Biphasic circadian rhythm for CBG has been observed in the rat. D'Agnostino et al (71) observed two distinct peaks, one during the light phase and the other during the dark phase, which were sustained for almost the entire dark period. Other investigators (221) found both peaks in the light period. The CBG rhythm in the mouse is monophasic, with peak levels found during the dark phase (221).

Pathologic variations in CBG levels in man have been reviewed (47). Altered values have been reported in liver disease, nephrosis, and other protein-losing conditions, thyroid disease, adrenal diseases (including Cushing's syndrome and Addison's disease), mental illness, and stress. Sows and gilts subjected to stress (heat and crowding) during midgestation had lower CBG levels (163). Acute inflammation induced by subcutaneous injection of turpentine produced an average threefold decrease in serum corticosterone and CBG levels in both pregnant and nonpregnant rats (258). Like transferrin and albumin, CBG may represent one of the "negative" acute phase proteins.

REFERENCES

1. Abd-el Fattah, Reiner M, Scherer, Fouad FM, Ruhenstroth, Bauer G (1981) Kinetics of the acute-phase reaction in rats after tumor transplantation. Cancer Res 41: 2548–2555
2. Adamson ED (1982) The location and synthesis of transferrin in mouse embryos and terato carcinoma cells. Devel Biol 91: 227–234
3. Adornato BT, Engel WK, Foidart-Desalle M (1978) Elevations of hemopexin levels in neuromuscular disease. Arch Neurol 35: 577–580
4. Adornato BT, Kagen LJ, Garver FA, Engel WK (1978) Depletion of serum hemopexin in fulminant rhabdomyolysis. Arch Neurol 35: 547–548
5. Aisen P, Brown EB (1977) The iron-binding function of transferrin in iron metabolism. Sem Hematol 14: 31–53
6. Aisen P, Liebman A, Zweier J (1978) Stoichiometric

and site characteristics of the binding of iron to human transferrin. J Biol Chem 253: 1930–1937

7. Akaiwa S (1982) Purification of haptoglobin from rat serum. Anal Biochem 123: 178–182

8. Ali M, Vranckx, Nunez EA (1986) Origin of corticosteroid-binding globulin in fetal rat. J Biol Chem 261: 9915–9921

9. Allison AC (1960) Turnovers of erythrocytes and plasma proteins in mammals. Nature (London) 188: 37–40

10. Alper CA, Peters JH, Birtch AG, Gardner FH (1965) Haptoglobin synthesis. In vivo studies of the production of haptoglobin, fibrinogen, and γ-globulin by the canine liver. J Clin Invest 44: 574–581

11. Alper CA, Robin NI, Refetoff S (1969) Genetic polymorphism of Rhesus thyroxine-binding prealbumin: Evidence for tetrameric structure in primates. Proc Nat Acad Sci USA 63: 775–781

12. Andersen E (1966) Linkage between the K blood group locus and the Hp locus for hematin-binding globulins in pigs. Genetics 54: 805–812

13. Ashton GC (1963) Polymorphism in the serum post-albumins of cattle. Nature 198: 1117–1118

14. Ashton GC (1963) Cattle serum transferrins: A balanced polymorphism? Genetics 52: 983–997

15. Audy MC, Marin B, Charron G, Bonnin M (1982) Steroid-binding proteins and testosterone level in the badger plasma during the animal cycle. Gen Comp Endocrinol 48: 239–246

16. Awai M, Chipman B, Brown EB (1979) In vivo evidence for the functional heterogeneity of transferrin-bound iron. I. Studies in normal rats. J Lab Clin Med 85: 769–784

17. Awai M, Chipman B, Brown EB (1979) In vivo evidence for the functional heterogeneity of transferrin-bound iron. II. Studies in pregnant rats. J Lab Chem Med 85: 785–796

18. Baarlen JV, Brouwer JT, Liebman A, Aisen P (1980) Evidence for the functional heterogeneity of the two sites of transferrin in vitro. Br J Haematol 46: 417–426

19. Baglia FA, Kwan SW, Fuller GM (1981) Haptoglobin biosynthesis in rats. Biochim Biophys Acta 696: 107–113

20. Baker E, Shaw DC, Morgan EH (1968) Isolation and characterization of rabbit serum and milk transferrin. Evidence for difference in sialic acid contentiony. Biochemistry 7: 1371–1378

21. Baker E, VanBockxmeer FM, Morgan EH (1983) Distribution of transferrin and transferrin receptors in the rabbit placenta. Quart J Exp Physiol 69: 359–372

22. Baker LN (1967) A new allele, Hp⁴, in the hemopexin system in pigs. Vox Sang 12: 397–400

23. Baker LN (1968) Serum protein variation in Duroc and Hampshire pigs. Vox Sang 15: 154–158

24. Ballard PL, Kitterman JA, Bland RD, Clyman RI, Gluckman PD, Platzker ACG, Kaplan SL, Grunbach MM (1982) Ontogeny and regulation of corticosteroid-binding globulin in plasma of fetal and newborn lambs. Endocrinology 110: 359–366

25. Barbosa J, Doe, RP, Seal US (1970) Effects of Clomiphene on estrogen induced changes in plasma proteins in monkeys. J Clin Endrocinol 31: 654–658

26. Barbosa J, Seal US, Doe RP (1973) Anti-estrogens and plasma proteins. I. Clomiphene and isomers, ethamoxytriphetol, U-11, 100A and U-11, 555A. J Clin Endocrinol Metab 36: 666–678

27. Barbosa J, Seal US, Doe RP (1971) Effects of anabolic steroids on hormone-binding proteins, serum cortisol and serum non-protein bound cortisol. J Clin Endocrinol Metab 32: 232–240

28. Barnett DR, Lee TH, Bowman BH (1972) Amino acid sequence of the human haptoglobin B chain. I. Amino- and carboxy-terminal sequences. Biochemistry NY 11: 1189–1194

29. Baseler MW, Burrell R (1981) Acute-phase reactants in experimental inhalation lung disease. Proc Soc Exp Biol Med 168: 49–55

30. Baumann H, Jahreis GP (1983) Regulation of mouse haptoglobin synthesis. J Cell Biol 97: 728–736

31. Baynes JW, Thorpe SR (1981) Identification of the sites of albumin-catabolism in the rat. Arch Biochem Biophys 206: 372–379

32. Beamer N, Hagemenas FC, Kittinger GW (1973) Development of cortisol-binding in the rhesus monkey. Endocrinology 93: 363–368

33. Behrens PQ, Spikerman AM, Brown JR (1975) Structure of human serum albumin. Fed Proc 34: 591

34. Benesch RE, Ikeda S, Benesch R. (1976) Reaction of haptoglobin with hemoglobin covalently cross-linked between the αβ dimers. J Biol Chem 251: 465–470

35. Benvenga S, Bartalena L, Antonelli A, Calzi LL, Pasquale GD, Trimarchi F, Pinchera A (1986) Radioiummonoassay for human thyroxine-binding prealbumin. Ann Clin Lab Sci 16: 231–240

36. Bernat I (1983) Iron Metabolism. Plenum Press, New York, p 82

37. Bernstein RS, Robbin J, Rall JE (1970) Polymorphism of monkey thyroxine-binding prealbumin (TBPA). Mode of inheritance and hybridization. Endocrinology 86: 383–390

38. Bernutz C, Horn K, Pickardt CR (1977) Corticosteroid-binding globulin (CBG) isolation and radio-immunological determination in serum. Acta Endoc (Kbh) 87 (Suppl 215): 25–26

39. Blumberg BS (1960) Biochemical polymorphisms in animals. Haptoglobin and transferrins. Proc Soc Exp Biol Med 104: 25–28

40. Blumberg BS, Robbins J (1960) Thyroxine-serum protein complexes. Single dimension gel and paper electrophoresis studies. Endocrinology 60: 368–378

41. Bornstein DL, Walsh EC (1978) Endogenous mediators of the acute-phase reaction. I. Rabbit granulocyte pyrogen and its chromatographic subfractions. J Lab Clin Med 91: 236–245

42. Bouillon R, Baelen HV, Rombauts W, DeMoor P (1976) The purification and characterization of the human-serum protein for the 25-hydroxy-cholecalciferol (transcalciferin). J Biochem 66: 285–291

43. Bowman BH, Kurosky A (1982) Haptoglobin: The evolutionary product of duplication, unequal crossing over, and point mutation. Adv Hum Genet 12: 189–261

44. Bradshaw JP, Hatton J, White DA (1985) The hor-

monal control of protein N-glycosylation in the developing rabbit mammary gland and its effect upon transferrin synthesis and secretion. Biochim Biophys Acta 847: 344–352

45. Braend M (1966) Serum transferrin in dog. In 10th European conference on animal blood groups and biochemical polymorphism. Paris, Institut National de la Recherche Agronomique, pp 319–322

46. Bremner KC (1966) Studies on haptoglobin and haemopexin in the plasma of cattle. Aust J Exp Biol Med Sci 42: 643–656

47. Brien TG (1981) Human corticosteroid binding globulin. Clin Endocrinol 14: 193–212

48. Brown JR (1975) Structure of bovine serum albumin. Fed Proc 34: 591

49. Brown JR (1976) Structural origins of mammalian albumin. Fed Proc 35: 2141–2144

50. Brown JR, Lou T, Behrens P, Sepulveda M, Parker M, Blakeney E (1971) Amino acid sequence of bovine and porcine serum albumin. Fed Proc 30: 1241

51. Buettner-Janusch J (1970) Evolution of serum polymorphisms. Ann Rev Genet 4: 47–68

52. Buettner-Janusch J, Buettner-Janusch V, Sale JB (1964) Plasma proteins and hemoglobin of the African elephant and the hyrax. Nature 210: 510–511

53. Campbell RM, Cuthbertson DP, Mackie E, McFarlane AS, Phillipson AT, Sudaneh S (1961) Passage of plasma albumin into the intestine of the sheep. J Physiol (London) 158: 113–131

54. Chader GJ, Westphal U (1968) Steroid-protein interactions. XVIII. Isolation and observations on the polymertic nature of the corticosteroid-binding globulin of the rat. Biochemistry 7: 4272–4282

55. Chader GJ, Westphal U (1968) Steroid-protein interactions. XVI. Isolation and characterization of the corticosteroid-binding globulin of the rabbit. J Biol Chem 243: 928–939

56. Chen BH, Turley CP, Brewster MA, Arnold WA (1986) Storage stability of serum transthyretin. Clin Chem 32: 1231–1232

57. Chung MCM, McKenzie HA (1985) Studies on equine transferrin I. The isolation and partial characterization of the D and R variants. Comp Biochem Physiol 80B: 287–297

58. Cinader B, Dubinski S (1963) An alpha-globulin allo-type in the mouse (MuBI). Nature 200: 781

59. Cleve H, Patutschnick W (1979) Different phenotypes of the group-specific component (Gc) in chimpanzees. Hum Genet 50: 217–220

60. Cleve H, Prunier JH, Bearn AG (1963) Isolation and partial characterization of the two principal inherited group-specific components of human serum. J Exp Med 118: 711–726

61. Cody V (1980) Thyroid hormone interactions: Molecular conformation, protein binding, and hormone action. Endocrinol Rev 1: 140–166

62. Coe CL, Murai JT, Wiener SG, Levine S, Siiteri PK (1986) Rapid cortisol and corticosteroid-binding globulin responses during pregnancy and after estrogen administration in the squirrel monkey. Endocrinology 118: 435–440

63. Cohen-Dix P, Noble RW, Reichlin M (1973) Comparative binding studies of the hemoglobin-haptoglobin and hemoglobin-antihemoglobin reactions. Biochemistry 12: 3744–3751

64. Cohen S (1956) Plasma protein distribution and turnover in the female baboon. J Biochem 64: 286–296

65. Constans J (1976) Group-specific component. Report on the first International Workshop. Human Genet 48: 143–149

66. Constans J, Viau M (1977) Group-specific component. Evidence for two subtypes of the Gc^1 gene. Science 198: 1070–1071

67. Cornelius CE, Baker NF, Kaneko JJ, Douglas JR (1962) Distribution and turnover of iodine-131-tagged bovine albumin in normal and parasitized cattle. Am J Vet Res 23: 837–842

68. Courtoy PJ, Feldman G, Rogier E, Moguilevsky N (1981) Plasma protein synthesis in experimental cirrhosis. Lab Invest 45: 67–76

69. Courtoy PJ, Lombart C, Feldman G, Moguilevsky N, Rogier E (1981) Synchronous increase of four acute phase proteins synthesized by the same hepatocytes during the inflammatory reaction. Lab Invest 44: 105–115

70. Cox KH, Wormley S, Northway NA, Creighton L, Muller-Eberhard U (1978) Immunological cross-reactions between heterologous hemopexin. Comp Biochem Physiol 60(B): 473–479

71. D'Agostino J, Vaeth GF, Henning SJ (1982) Diurnal rhythm of total and free concentrations of serum corticosterone in the rat. Acta Endocrinol 100: 85–90

72. D'Agostino J, Henning SJ (1982) Postnatal development of corticosteroid-binding globulin. Effect of thyroxine. Endocrinology 111: 1476–1482

73. Daiger SP, Schanfield MS, Cavalli-Sforza LL (1975) Human group specific component (Gc) proteins bind vitamin D and 25—hydroxy-vitamin D. Proc Nat Acad Sci USA 72: 2076–2080

74. Daiger SP, Cavalli-Sforza LL (1977) Detection of genetic variation with radioactive ligands. II. Genetic variants of vitamin D-labelled group specific component (Gc) proteins. Am J Hum Genet 29: 593–604

75. Daniel JY, Malaval F, Assenmacher I (1981) Evidence of a sex-related difference of transcortin level in adult ducks. Steroids 38: 29–34

76. Davis PJ, Spaulding SW, Gregerman RI (1970) The three thyroxine-binding proteins in rat serum. Binding capacities and effect of binding inhibitors. Endocrinology 87: 978–986

77. Delaney TA, Morgan WH, Morgan EH (1982) Chemical, but not functional, differences between the iron-binding sites of rabbit transferrin. Biochim Biophys Acta 701: 295–304

78. Delers F, Lombart C, Domingo M, Musquera S (1981) A novel and specific method for the purification of hemoglobin-binding proteins. Anal Biochem 118: 353–357

79. Dick J, Nielson K (1963) Metabolism and distribution of 131 I-labelled albumin in the pig. Canad J Comp Med Vet Sci 27: 269–273

80. Dickson PW, Aldred AR, Marley PD, Bamister D, Schreiber G (1986) Rat choroid plexus specializes

in the synthesis and the secretion of transthyretin (prealbumin). J Biol Chem 261: 3475–3478

81. Dickson PW, Howlett GJ, Schreiber G (1982) Metabolism of prealbumin in rats and changes induced by acute inflammation. Eur J Biochem 129: 289–293

82. Dickson PW, Howlett GJ, Schreiber G (1985) Rat transthyretin (prealbumin). J Biol Chem 260: 8214–8219

83. Dixon FJ, Maurer PH, Deichmiller MP (1953) Half-lives of homologous serum albumin in several species. Proc Soc Exp Biol Med 83: 287–288

84. Dobryszycka W, Elwyn DH, Kukral JC (1969) Isolation and chemical composition of canine haptoglobin. Biochim Biophys Acta 175: 220–222

85. Dobryszycka W, Osada J (1977) Hybridization of human and porcine haptoglobins. Int J Biochem 8: 511–515

86. Doe RP, Fernandez R, Seal US (1964) Measurement of corticosteroid-binding globulin in man. J Clin Endocrinol 24: 1029–1039

87. Eaton JW, Brandt P, Mahoney JR, Lee JT (1982) Haptoglobin: A natural bacteriostat. Science 215: 691–692

88. Evans WE, Wilson SM, Mage MG (1986) Transferrin induces maturation of neutrophil granulocyte precursors in vitro. Leuk Res 10: 429–436

89. Farer LS, Robbins J, Blumberg BS, Rall JE (1962) Thyroxine-serum protein complexes in various animals. Endocrinology 70: 686–696

90. Felding P, Fex G (1982) Cellular origin of prealbumin in the rat. Biochim Biophys Acta 716: 446–449

91. Feldman G (1979) Morphologic aspects of hepatic synthesis and secretion of plasma proteins. In Progress in Liver Disease, Popper H and Schaffner F (eds) Grune & Stratton, New York, p 23

92. Fex G, Laurell CB, Thulin E (1977) Purification of prealbumin from human and canine serum using a two-step affinity chromatographic procedure. Eur J Biochem 75: 181–186

93. Fischer CL, Gill C, Forrester MG, Nakamura R (1976) Quantitation of "Acute-phase Proteins" postoperatively. Am J Clin Pathol 66: 840–846

94. Fletcher J, Huehns ER (1968) Function of transferrin. Nature 218: 1211–1218

95. Foidart M, Eisman J, Engel WK, Adornato BT, Liem HH (1982) Effect of heme administration on hemopexin metabolism in Rhesus monkey. J Lab Clin Med 100: 451–460

96. Forth W, Rummel W (1973) Iron absorption. Physiol Rev 53: 724–792

97. Fujieda K, Goff AK, Pugeat M, Strott CA (1982) Regulation of the pituitary-adrenal axis and corticosteroid-binding globulin-cortisol interaction in the guinea pig. Endocrinology 111: 1944–1950

98. Gala RR, Westphal U (1965) Corticosteroid-binding globulin in the rat. Studies on the sex difference. Endocrinology 77: 841–851

99. Gala RR, Westphal U (1965) Corticosteroid-binding globulin in the rat. Possible role in the initiation of lactation. Endocrinology 76: 1079–1088

100. Gala RR, Westphal U (1966) Further studies on the corticosteroid-binding globulin in the rat. Proposed endocrine control. Endocrinology 79: 67–76

101. Gala RR, Westphal U (1967) Corticosteroid-binding activity in serum of mouse, rabbit, guinea pig during pregnancy and lactation. Possible involvement in the initiation of lactation. Acta Endocrinology 55: 47–61

102. Ganrot K (1974) Plasma protein pattern in acute infectious diseases. Scand J Clin Lab Invest 34: 75–81

103. Ganrot K (1973) Plasma protein response in experimental inflammation in the dog. Res Exp Med 161: 251–161

104. Ganrot PO (1972) Variation of the concentrations of some plasma proteins in normal adults, in pregnant women and in newborns. Scand J Clin Lab Invest 29 (Suppl 124): 83–88

105. Gardiner ME, Morgan EH (1981) Effect of reduced atmospheric pressure and fasting on transferrin synthesis in the rat. Life Sci 29: 1641–1648

106. Giblett ER, Hickman CG, Smithies O (1959) Serum transferrins. Nature 183: 1589–1590

107. Giblett ER (1969) Genetic Markers in Human Blood. Oxford, Blackwell Scientific Publications pp 126–159

108. Glass J, Nunez M, Robinson SH (1980) Transferrin-binding and iron-binding proteins of rabbit reticulocytic plasma membrane. Biochim Biophys Acta 598: 293–304

109. Glinoer D, Gershengorn MC, Robbins J (1970) Thyroxine-binding globulin biosynthesis in isolated monkey hepatocytes. Biochim Biophys Acta 418: 232–244

110. Glinoer D, McGuire RA, Gershengorn MC, Robbins J, Berman M (1977) Effects of estrogen on thyroxine-binding globulin metabolism in rhesus monkeys. Endocrinology 100; 9–17

111. Glinoer D, Gershengorn MC, Dubois A, Robbins J (1977) Stimulation of thyroxine-binding globulin synthesis by isolated rhesus monkey hepatocytes after in vivo B-estradiol administration. Endocrinology 100: 807–813

112. Glinoer D, McGuire RA, Cogen JP, Robbins J, Berman M (1979) Thyroxine-binding globulin metabolism in rhesus monkeys. Effects of hyper- and hypothyroidism. Endocrinology 104: 175–183

113. Goodman M, Kulkarni A, Poulik E, Reklys E (1965) Species and geographic differences in the transferrin polymorphism of Macaques. Science 147: 884–886

114. Goodman WC, Mickelson KE, Westphal U (1981) Immunochemical determination of corticosteroid-binding globulin in the guinea pig during gestation. J Steroid Biochem 14: 1293–1296

115. Gordon S, Bearn AG (1966) Hemoglobin binding capacity of isolated haptoglobin polypeptide chains. Proc Soc Exp Biol Med 121: 846–850

116. Gordon AH, Limaos EA (1979) Effects of bacterial endotoxin and corticosteroids on plasma concentrations of α_2 macroglobulin, haptoglobin and fibrinogen in rats. Br J Exp Pathol 60: 343–440

117. Got R, Cheftel RI, Font J, Moretti J (1967) Etude de l α_1—macroglobuline du serum de lapin. III. Biochimie de la copule glucidique. Biochim Biophys Acta 136: 320–330

118. Grant GH, Kachmar JF (1976) The proteins of

body fluids. In Tietz NW (ed), Fundamentals of Clinical Chemistry. W. B. Sanders, Philadelphia pp 298–376

119. Greene FC, Feeney RE (1968) Physical evidence for transferrin as single polypeptide chains. Biochemistry 7: 1366–1371

120. Greene R, Hendrickson P, Young S, Leibman A, Aisen P (1982) Molecular ferrokinetics in the rabbit. Br J Haematol 50: 43–53

121. Grunder AA (1966) Inheritance of a heme-binding protein in rabbits. Genetics 54: 1085–1093

122. Grunder AA (1968) Hemopexin of rabbits. Vox Sang 14: 218–223

123. Guttman SI, Wilson KG (1973) Genetic variation in the genus Bufo. I. An extreme degree of transferrin and albumin polymorphism in a population of American toad (*Bufo americanus*). Biochem Genet 8: 329–340

124. Hagen K, Rasmusen BA, Mittal KK (1968) Further investigations on linkage between the loci for heme-binding globulins and K blood groups in pig. Vox Sang 15: 147–151

125. Hagen KL, Suzuki Y, Tissot R, Cohen C (1978) The hemopexin locus. Its assignment to linkage group I in the laboratory rabbit (*Oryctolagus cuniculus*) and evidence for a forth allele. Anim Blood Grps Biochem Genet 9: 151–159

126. Hangen TH, Hanley JM, Heath EC (1981) Haptoglobin. A novel mode of biosynthesis of a liver secretory glycoprotein. J Biol Chem 256: 1055–1057

127. Hanley JM, Haugen TH, Heath EC (1983) Biosynthesis and processing of rat haptoglobin. J Biol Chem 258: 7858–7869

128. Harvey JW, Gaskin JM (1978) Feline haptoglobin. Am J Vet Res 39:549–553

129. Harvey JW (1976) Quantitative determinations of normal horse, cat and dog haptoglobins. Theriogenology 6: 133–138

130. Harvey JW, West CL (1987) Prednisone-induced increases in serum alpha-2-globulin and haptoglobin concentration in dogs. Vet Pathol 24: 90–92

131. Heaf DJ, El-Sayed M, Glover J (1980) Changes in plasma concentrations of thyroxine-binding prealbumin and retinol binding protein in Japanese quail after hatching. Br J Nutr 44: 287–293

132. Heaphy S, Williams J (1978) The preparation and partial characterization of N-terminal and C-terminal iron-binding fragments from rabbit serum transferrin. Biochem J 205: 611–617

133. Heaphy S, Williams J (1982) Removal of iron from differic rabbit serum transferrin by rabbit reticulocytes. Biochemistry 205: 619–621

134. Heimburger N, Heide K, Haupt H, Schultze HE (1964) Bausteinanalysen von human serum proteinen. Clin Chim Acta 10: 292–307

135. Henning S (1978) Plasma concentrations of total and free corticosterone during development in the rat. Am J Physiol: Endocr Metab Gastrointest Physiol 4: E451–E456

136. Hershko C (1975) The fate of circulating haemoglobin. Br J Haematol 29: 199–204

137. Hickman DM, Miller RA, Rombeau JL, Twomey PL, Frey CF (1980) Serum albumin and body weight as predictions of postoperative course in colorectal cancer. J Parenteral Enteral Nutr 4: 314–316

138. Hirschfeld J (1959) Immune-electrophoretic demonstration of qualitative differences in human sera and their relation to the haptoglobins. Acta Path Microbiol Scand 47: 160–168

139. Hofvander Y (1968) Hematological investigation in Ethiopia. Acta Med Scand 185 (Suppl 494): 1–74

140. Hooper DC, Steer CJ, Dinarello CA, Peacock AC (1981) Haptoglobin and albumin synthesis in isolated rat hepatocytes. Response to potential mediators of the acute-phase reaction. Biochim Biophys Acta 653:118–129

141. Horn K, Gartner R (1979) Thyroxine-binding globulin-structure, assay and function. Acta Endocrinal 225: 447–448

142. Horne CHW, Mallison AC, Ferguson J, Goudie RB (1971) Effects of estrogen and progestogen on serum levels of α2-macroglobulin, transferrin, albumin and IgG. J Clin Pathol 24: 464–466

143. Hossner KL, Billiar RB (1981) Plasma clearance and organ distribution of native and desialylated rat and human trancortin—species specificity. Endocrinology 108: 1780–1786

144. Hrkal Z, Muller-Eberhard U (1971) Partial characterization of the heme-binding serum glycoproteins—rabbit and human hemopexin. Biochemistry 10: 1746–1750

145. Hudson BG, Ohno M, Brodeway WJ, Castellino FJ (1973) Chemical and physical properties of serum transferrin from several species. Biochemistry 12: 1047–1053

146. Huebers H, Urelli D, Celada A, Josephson B, Finch C (1982) Basis of plasma iron exchange in the rabbit. J Clin Invest 70: 769–779

147. Huebers HA, Huebers E, Csiba E, Rummel W, Finch CA (1983) The significance of transferrin for intestinal iron absorption. Blood 61: 283–290

148. Hughes-Jones NC, Gardner B, Helps R (1961) Observation on the binding of haemoglobin and hematin by serum proteins of the rabbit, rat and guinea pig. Biochem J 79: 220–223

149. Hwang PK, Greer J (1980) Interaction between hemoglobin subunits in the hemoglobin-haptoglobin complex. J Biol Chem 255: 3038–3041

150. Iacopatta BJ, Morgan EH, Yeoh GCT (1983) Receptor-mediated endocytosis of transferrin by developing erythroid cells from the fetal rat liver. J Histochem Cytochem 31: 336–344

151. Idzerda RL, Huebers H, Finch CA, McKnight GS (1986) Rat transferrin gene expression: Tissue-specific regulation by ion deficiency. Proc Natl Acad Sci 83: 3723–3727

152. Jarnum S, Lassen NA (1961) Albumin and transferrin metabolism in infectious and toxic disease. Scand J Clin Lab Invest 13: 357–368

153. Javid J (1978) Human haptoglobins. Current Topic in Hematol 1: 151–192

154. Jeejeebhoy KN, Bruce-Robertson A, Ho J, Sodtke U (1972) The effect of cortisol on the synthesis of rat plasma albumin, fibrinogen, and transferrin. Biochemistry J 130: 533–538

155. Jeffrey H (1960) The metabolism of serum proteins. J Biol Chem 235: 2352–2356

156. John DW, Miller LL (1969) Regulation of net biosynthesis of serum albumin and acute phase plasma proteins. J Biol Chem 244: 6134–6142

157. Kalberg HI, Hern KA, Fischer JE (1983) Albumin turnover in sarcoma-bearing rats in relation to cancer anorexia. Am J Surg 145: 95–101

158. Kamiyama T (1976) Immunological cross reactions and species specificities of cyanogen bromide cleaved fragments of bovine, goat and sheep serum albumins. Immunochemistry 14: 91–98

159. Kampschmidt RF, Upchurch HF (1974) Effects of leukocytic endogenous mediator on plasma fibrinogen and haptoglobin. Proc Soc Exp Biol Med 146: 904–907

160. Kanai M, Raz A, Goodman DeWS (1968) Retinol-binding protein. The transport protein for vitamin A in human plasma. J Clin Invest 47: 2025–2044

161. Kanda Y, Goodman DeWS, Canfield RE, Morgan FJ (1974) The amino acid sequence of human plasma prealbumin. J Biol Chem 249: 6796–6805

162. Kaneko JJ (1980) Serum proteins and dysproteinemias. In Kaneko JJ (ed), Clinical Biochemistry of Domestic Animals. Academic Press, New York, pp 97–118

163. Kattesh HG, Kornegay ET, Knight JW, Gwazdauskas, FG, Thomas HR, Notter DR (1980) Glucocorticoid concentrations, corticosteriod-binding protein characteristics and reproduction performance of sows and gilts subjected to applied stress during midgestation. J An Sci 50: 897–905

164. Kazim AL, Atassi MZ (1981) Hemoglobin binding with haptoglobin. Biochem J 197: 507–510

165. Kitchin FD, Bearn AG (1965) The serum group specific component in non-human primates. Am J Human Genet 17: 42–50

166. Koj A (1974) Acute phase reactants. In Allison AC (ed), Structure and Functions of Plasma Proteins. Plenum Press, New York, pp 73–133

167. Kraemer M, Vassey J, Foucrier J, Chalumeau MT (1981) Ultrastructural localization of transferrin synthesis in rat hepatocytes during prenatal and postnatal development. Cell Differentiation 10: 211–217

168. Kristjansson FK (1961) Genetic control of three haptoglobins in pigs. Genetics 46; 907–910

169. Kristjansson FK, Hickman CG (1965) Subdivision of the alleles TfD for transferrin in Holstein and Ayrshire cattle. Genetics 52: 627–630

170. Kristjansson FK (1966) Fractionation of serum albumin and genetic control of two albumin fractions in pigs. Genetics 53: 675–679

171. Kurosky A, Kim KH, Touchstone B (1976) Comparative sequence analysis of the N-terminal region of rat, rabbit and dog haptoglobin β-chains. Comp Biochem Physiol 55B: 453–459

172. Kurosky A, Hay RE, Bowman BH (1979) Canine haptoglobin, a unique haptoglobin subunit arrangement. Comp Biochem Physiol 62B: 339–344

173. Kurosky A, Barnett DR, Lee TH, Touchstone B, Hay RE, Arnott MS, Bowman BH, Fitch WM (1980) Covalent structure of human haptoglobin—serine protease homolog. Proc Natl Acad Sci USA 77: 3388–3392

174. Kusher I, Edington TS, Trimble C, Leim HH, Muller-Eberhard U (1972) Plasma hemopexin homeostasis during the acute phase response. J Lab Clin Med 80: 18–25

175. Lamon JM, Sach J, Zavazal V, Nozlckova M, Mateja F (1978) Hematine therapy in acute prophyria and observation on hemopexin. In Doss M (ed), Diagnosis and Therapy of Porphyrias and Lead Intoxication. Berlin, Springer Verlag, p 285

176. Lane RS, Rangeley DM, Liem HH, Womsley S, Muller-Eberhard U (1973) Plasma clearance of 125 I-labelled haemopexin in normal and heme loaded rabbits. Br J Haematol 25: 533–540

177. Larsson M, Pettersson T, Carlstrom A (1985) Thyroid hormone binding in serum of 15 vertebrate species: Isolation of thyroid-binding globulin and prealbumin analogs. Gener Comp Endocrinol 58: 360–375

178. Laurell CB, Kullander S, Thorell J (1969) Plasma protein changes induced by sequential type of contraceptive steroid pills. Clin Chim Acta 25: 294–296

179. Leger D, Tordera V, Spik G (1978) Structure determination of the single glycan of rabbit serotransferrin by methylation analysis and 360 MH$_z$ ^{1}H NMR spectroscopy. FEBS-Lett 93: 255–260

180. Leim HH (1976) Catabolism of homologous and heterologous hemopexin in the rat and uptake of hemopexin by isolated perfused rat liver. Ann Clin Res 8 (Suppl 17): 233–238

181. Letendre ED, Holbein BE (1981) A sensitive and convenient assay procedure for transferrin and its application to the purification of mouse transferrin. Can J Biochem 59: 906–910

182. Loh TT (1983) Studies on the forms of iron-transferrin released from rabbit reticulocytes. Life Sci 32: 915–920

183. Lombart C, Moretti J, Jayle MF (1965) Préparation et propriétés physiques des haptoglobines de lapin et de rat. Biochim Biophys Acta 97: 262–269

184. Lombart C, Dautrevaux M, Moretti J (1965) Compostion chimique des haptoglobines de lapin et de rat. Biochim Biophys Acta 97: 270–274

185. Lombart C, Musquera S, Delers F (1979) Characterization and specific properties of chicken haptoglobin. In XIth International Congress of Biochemistry. N.R.C.C., Toronto, Canada, p 178

186. Lowe ME, Ashwell G (1982) Solubilization and assay of an hepatic receptor for the haptoglobin-hemoglobin complex. Arch Biochem Biophys 216: 704–710

187. MacGillivray RTA, Mendez E, Brew K (1977) Structure and evolution of serum transferrin. In Brown EB, Aisen P, Feilding J, Crichton RR (eds), Proteins of Iron Metabolism. Grune & Stratton, New York pp 133–141

188. Maeda K, McKenzie HA, Shaw DC (1980) Nature of the heterogeneity within genetic variants of bovine serum transferrin. An Blood Grps Biochem Genet 11: 63–75

189. Majuri R (1982) Purification of pig serum haemopexin by haemin-sepharose affinity chromatography. Biochim Biophys Acta 719: 53–57

190. Makinen MW, Milstein JB, Kon H (1972) Specificity of interaction of haptoglobin with mammalian hemoglobin. Biochemistry 11: 3851–3860

191. Mann KG, Fis WW, Cox AC, Tanford C (1970) Single chain nature of human serum transferrin. Biochemistry 9: 1348–1354

192. Mattheeuws DRG, Kaneko JJ, Loy RG, Cornelius CE, Wheat JD (1966) Compartmentalization and turnover of 131 I-labelled albumin and gamma globulin in horses. Am J Vet Res 27: 699–705

193. Maung M, Baker DG, Murray RK (1968) Studies on the nature of the seromucoid and haptoglobin responses to experimental inflammation. Can J Biochem 46: 477–481

194. McGuire RA, Glinoer D, Albert MA, Robbins J (1982) Comparative effects of thyroxine (T_4) and triiodothyronine on T_4-binding globulin metabolism in rhesus monkeys. Endocrinology 110: 1340–1346

195. McIndoe WM (1962) Occurrence of two plasma albumins in the domestic fowl. Nature 195: 353–354

196. Meek J, Adamson E (1985) Transferrin in foetal and adult mouse tissues: Synthesis, storage and secretion. J Embryol Exp Morph 86. 205–218

197. Meloun B, Moravek L, Kostka V (1975) Complete amino acid sequence of human serum albumin. FEBS Lett 58: 134–137

198. Meuten DJ, Butler DG, Thompson GW, Lumsden JH (1978) Chronic enteritis associated with malabsorption and protein-losing enteropathy in the horse. J Am Vet Med Assoc 172: 326–333

199. Mickelson KE, Westphal U (1979) Purification and characterization of the corticosteroid-binding globulin of pregnant guinea pig serum. Biochemistry 18: 2685–2690

200. Mitruka BM, Rawnsley HM (1977) Clinical, Biochemical and Haematological Reference Values in Normal Experimental Animals. Masson Publishing USA, New York, pp 117–181

201. Morgan EH, Peters T (1971) The biosynthesis of rat serum albumin. V. Effects of protein depletion and refeeding on albumin and transferrin synthesis. J Biol Chem 246: 3500–3507

202. Morgan EH, Peters T (1971) Intracellular aspects of transferrin synthesis and secretion in the rat. J Biol Chem 246: 3508–3511

203. Morgan EH (1974) Transferrin and transferrin iron. In Jacobs A, Worwood M, (eds), Iron in Biochemistry and Medicine. Academic Press, London, pp 29–71

204. Morgan FJ, Canfield RE, Goodman DeWS (1971) The partial structure of human plasma prealbumin and retinol-binding protein. Biochim Biophys Acta 236: 798–801

205. Morton AG, Tavill AS (1975) Studies on the mechanism of iron supply in the regulation of hepatic transferrin synthesis. In Crichton RR (ed), Proteins of Iron Storage and Transport in Biochemistry and Medicine. Amsterdam, North-Holland, pp 167–172

206. Moutafchiev DA, Shisheva AC, Sirakov M (1983) Binding of transferrin-iron to the plasma membrane of a lactating rabbit mammary gland cell. Int J Biochem 15: 755–758

207. Muldoon TG, Westphal U (1967) Steroid-protein interactions. XV. Isolation and characterization of corticosteroid-binding globulin from human plasma. J Biol Chem 242: 5636–5643

208. Muller-Eberhard U, Javid J, Liem HH, Hamstein A, Hanna M (1968) Plasma concentration of hemopexin, haptoglobin and heme in patients with various hemolytic disease. Blood 32: 811–815

209. Muller-Eberhard U, Liem HH, Hamstein A, Saarinen PA (1969) Studies on the disposal of intravascular heme in the rabbit. J Lab Clin Med 73: 210–218

210. Muller-Eberhard U (1970) Hemopexin. New Engl J Med 283: 1090–1094

211. Muller-Eberhard U, Bosman C, Leim HH (1970) Tissue localization of the heme-hemopexin complex in the rabbit and the rat as studied by light microscopy with the use of radiosotopes. J Lab Clin Med 76: 426–431

212. Muller-Eberhard U (1978) Heme transport and properties of hemopexin. In Blauer G, Sund H (eds), Transport by Proteins. Walter de Gruyter & Co., Berlin, p 295

213. Murray RK, Connel GE (1960) Elevation of serum haptoglobin in rabbits in response to experimental inflammation. Nature 186: 86

214. Musquera S, Lombart C, Jayle MF, Rogard M, Waks M (1979) Identification of haptoglobin in chicken serum and specificity of the chicken haptoglobin-hemoglobin complex formation. Comp Biochem Physiol 62B: 241–244

215. Navab M, Mallia AK, Kanda Y, Goodman DeWS (1977) Rat plasma prealbumin: Isolation and partial characterization. J Biol Chem 252: 5100–5106

216. Navab M, Smith JE, Goodman DeWS (1977) Rat plama prealbumin. J Biol Chem 252: 5107–5114

217. Nomenclature Committee of IUB (NC-IUB) IUB-IUPAC Joint Commission on Biochemical Nomenclature (1981) Newsletter. J Biol Chem 256: 12–14

218. Oakey RE (1975) Serum cortisol binding capacity and cortisol concentration in the pregnant baboon and its fetus during gestation. Endocrinology 97: 1024–1029

219. Oishi T, Tomita T, Komatsu M (1980) New genetic varients detected in the haemopexin and ceruloplasmin systems of Ohmini miniature pigs. An Blood Grps Biochem Genet 11: 59–62

220. Oppenheimer JH, Surks MI, Smith JC, Squef R (1965) Isolation and characterization of human throxine-binding prealbumin. J Biol Chem 240: 173–180

221. Ottenweller JE, Meier AH, Russo AC, Frenske ME (1979) Circadian rhythms of plasma corticosteroid binding activity in the rat and the mouse. Acta Endocrinol (Kbh) 91: 150–157

222. Pagano M, Nicola MA, Engler P (1982) Inhibition of Cathepsin L and B by haptoglobin, the haptoglobin-hemoglobin complex and asialohaptoglobin. "In vitro" studies in the rat. Can J Biochem 60: 631–637

223. Palmer WG (1976) The serum haptoglobin response to inflammation in neonatal mice and its relationship to phagocytosis. J Reticuloendothel Soc 19: 301–309

224. Palmer WC, Costlow RD (1981) Reproducibility of serum haptoglobin profiles in mice with transplanted tumors. Oncology 38: 116–120

225. Palmour RM, Sutton HE (1971) Vertebrate transferrins. Molecular weights, chemical compositions and iron-binding studies. Biochemistry 10: 4026–4032

226. Peacock AC, Gelderman AH, Ragland RH, Hoffman HA (1967) Haptoglobin levels in serum of various strains of mice. Science 158: 1703–1704

227. Perrot-Applanat M, David-Ferreira JF, David-Ferreira KL (1981) Immunocytochemical localization of corticosteroid-binding globulin (CBG) in guinea pig hepatocytes. Endocrinology 109: 1625–1633

228. Peters T Jr (1977) Serum albumin: Recent progress in the understanding of its structure and biosynthesis. Clin Chem 23: 5–12

229. Peters T Jr, Davidson LK (1986) The biosynthesis of rat serum albumin. J Biol Chem 261: 7242–7246

230. Peters T Jr, Peters JC (1972) The biosynthesis of rat serum albumin. VI. Intracellular transport of albumin and rates of albumin and liver protein synthesis in vivo under various physiological conditions. J Biol Chem 247: 3858–3863

231. Peters T Jr, Reed RG (1980) The biosynthesis of rat serum albumin. J Biol Chem 255: 3156–3163

232. Peters T Jr, Davidson LK (1982) The biosynthesis of rat serum albumin. J Biol Chem 257: 8847–8853

233. Peterson PA, Rask L, Ostberg L, Anderson L, Kamwendo F, Pertoft H (1973) Studies on the transport and cellular distribution of vitamin A in normal and vitamin A-deficient rats with special reference to the vitamin A-binding plasma protein. J Biol Chem 248: 4009–4022

234. Pintera J (1971) The biochemical, genetic and clinicopathological aspects of haptoglobin. Jenson KG, Killman SA (eds), Series Hematologica. Vol IV. Munksgaard, Copenhagen

235. Polonovski M, Jayle MF (1939) Peroxidases animales. Leur specificities at leur role biologiques. Bull Soc Chim Biol Paris 21: 66–91

236. Putman FW (1975) Haptoglobin. In Putman FW (ed), The Plasma Proteins, Structure, Function and Genetic Control, Vol 2. Academic Press, New York, pp 1–50

237. Putman FW (1975) Serum albumin. In Putman FW (ed), The Plasma Protein. Academic Press, New York, pp 133–181

238. Quinteros IR, Stevens SC, Stormont C, Asmundson VS (1964) Albumin phenotypes in turkeys. Genetics 50: 579–582

239. Rangel H (1965) Study of the cross-reaction between rabbit and anti-bovine serum albumin and equine serum albumin. Immunology 8: 88–94

240. Ramoure WJ, Kuhn RW (1983) A homologous radioimmunoassay for rat corticosteroid-binding globulin. Endocrinology 112: 1091–1097

241. Reed RG, Feldhoff RC, Clute OL, Peters T Jr (1975) Fragments of bovine serum albumin produced by limited proteolysis. Conformation and ligand binding. Biochemistry 14: 4578–4583

242. Refetoff S, Robin N, Fang VS (1970) Parameters of thyroid function in serum of 16 selected vertebrate species: A study of PBI, serum T_4, free T_4 and the pattern of T_4 and T_3 binding to serum proteins. Endocrinology 86: 793–805

243. Regoeczi E, Hatton MWC, Wong KL (1974) Studies of the metabolism of asialotransferrins: Potentiation of the catabolism of human sialotransferrin in the rabbit. Can J Biochem 52: 155–161

244. Regoeczi E, Hatton WC (1980) Transferrin catabolism in mammalian species of different body sizes. Am J Physiol 238: R306–R310

245. Reinskou T (1968) The Gc system. Ser Haematol 1: 21–37

246. Rennie JS, MacDonald DG, Douglas TA (1981) Haemoglobin, serum iron and transferrin values of adult male Syrian hamsters (*Mesocricetus auratus*). Lab An 15: 35–36

247. Richardson NE, Buttress N, Feinstein A, Stratil A, Spooner RL (1973) Structural studies on individual components of bovine transferrin. Biochem J 135: 87–92

248. Ritter H, Smith J (1971) Hp 2-2 like phenotypes in mammals. Humangen 12: 351–353

249. Robbins J (1973) Inherited variations in thyroxine transport. Mt Sinai J Med, New York 40: 511–519

250. Robbins JR, Cheng SY, Gershengorn MC, Glinoer D, Chanman HJ, Edelnoch H (1978) Thyroxine transport proteins of plasma. Molecular properties and biosynthesis. Recent Progress Horm Res 34: 477–519

251. Roberts RC, Makey DG, Seal US (1966) Human transferrin molecular weight and sedimentation properties. J Biol Chem 241: 4907–4913

252. Rosenthal HE, Paul MA, Sandberg AA (1974) Transcortin. A corticosteroid-binding protein of plasma. XII. Immunologic studies on transcortin in guinea pig tissues. J Steroid Biochem 5: 219–225

253. Rosner W, Hochberg R (1972) Corticosteroid-binding globulin in the rat: Isolation and studies of its influence on cortisol action in vivo. Endocrinology 91: 626–632

254. Rosner W (1972) Recent studies on the binding of cortisol in serum. J Steroid Biochem 3: 531–542

255. Sakata S, Atassi MZ (1979) Immunochemistry of serum albumin. VI. A dynamic approach to the immunochemical cross-reactions of proteins using serum albumins from various species as models. Biochim Biophys Acta 579: 322–332

256. Sakly M, Koch B (1983) Ontogenetical variation of transferrin modulate glucocorticoid receptor function and corticotropic activity in the pituitary gland. Horm Metabol Res 15: 92–96

257. Sarich VM, Wilson AC (1966) Quantitative immunochemistry and the evolution of primate albumins: Micro-complement fixation. Science 154: 1563–1566

258. Savu L, Lombart C, Nunez EA (1980) Corticosteroid-binding globulin: An acute-phase "negative" protein in the rat. FEBS Lett 113: 102–106

259. Sawatzki G, Anselstetter V, Kubanek B (1981) Isolation of mouse transferrin using salting-out chromatography on sepharose CL-6B. Biochim Biophys Acta 667: 132–138

260. Scheving LE, Pauly JE, Tsai TH (1968) Circadian fluctation in plasma proteins of the rat. Am J Physiol 215: 1096–1101

261. Schofield JD (1980) Altered proteins in ageing

organisms: Purification and properties of serum albumin from adult and ageing C57B1 mice. Exp Geront 15: 433–455

262. Schreiber G, Doryburgh H, Millership A, Matsuda Y, Inglis A, Phillips J, Edwards K, Maggs J (1979) The synthesis and secretion of rat transferrin. J Biol Chem 254: 12012–12019

263. Seal US, Doe RP (1963) Corticosteroid-binding globulin: Species distribution and small scale purification. Endocrinology 73: 371–376

264. Seal US, Doe RP (1965) Vertebrate distribution of corticosteroid-binding globulin and some endocrine effects on concentration. Steroids 5: 827–841

265. Seal US, Doe RP (1966) Corticosteroid-binding globulin: Biochemistry, physiology, and phylogeny. In Pincus G, Nakao T, Tait JF (eds), Steroid Dynamics. Academic Press, New York, p 63

266. Sears DA (1968) Plasma heme-binding in patient with hemolytic disorders. J Lab Clin Med 71: 484–494

267. Seery VL, Hathaway G, Muller-Eberhard U (1972) Hemopexin of human and rabbit: Molecular weight and extinction coefficient. Arch Biochem Biophys 150: 269–272

268. Shifrine M, Stortmont C (1973) Hemoglobins, haptoglobins and transferrins in beagles. Lab An Sci 23: 704–706

269. Shim BS, Bearn AG (1965) The distribution of haptoglobin subtypes in various populations, including subtype patterns in some non-human primates. Am J Hum Genet 16: 477–483

270. Shim BS (1976) Increase in serum haptoglobin stimulated by prostaglandins. Nature 259: 326–327

271. Shutherland RL, Brandon MR (1976) The thyroxine-binding properties of rat and rabbit serum proteins. Endocrinology 98: 91–98

272. Simons K, Bearn AG (1967) The use of preparative polyacrylamide-column electrophoresis in isolation of electrophoretically distinguishable components of the serum group-specific proteins. Biochim Biophys Acta 133: 499–505

273. Smith A, Morgan WT (1979) Heme transport to the liver by haemopexin receptor-mediated uptake with recycling of the protein. Biochem J 182: 47–54

274. Smith A, Morgan WT (1985) Hemopexin-mediated heme transport to the liver. J Biol Chem 260: 8325–8329

275. Smith DG (1982) Iron binding and transferrin polymorphism in rhesus monkey (*Macaca mulatta*). Lab An Sci 32: 153–156

276. Smithies O, Hickman CG (1958) Inherited variations in the serum proteins of cattle. Genetics 43: 374–385

277. Smithies D, Connel GE, Dixon GH (1962) Inheritance of haptoglobins subtypes. Am J Hum Genet 14: 14–21

278. Snyder S, Ashwell G (1971) Quantitation of specific serum glycoproteins in malignancy. Clin Chim Acta 34: 449–455

279. Soos P (1971) Genetic variants of serum albumin in two Hungarian cattle breeds. Acta Vet Acad Sci Hung 24: 341–343

280. Spooner RL, Baxter G (1969) Abnormal expression of normal transferrin alleles. Biochem Genet 2: 371–382

281. Spooner RL, Land RB, Oliver RA, Stratil A (1970) Fetal and neonatal transferrin in cattle. An Blood Grps Biochem Genet 1: 241–246

282. Spooner RL, Oliver RA, Richardson N, Buttress N, Feinstein A, Maddy AH, Stratil A (1974) Isolation and partial characterization of sheep transferrin. Comp Biochem Physiol 52B: 515–522

283. Spooner RL, Oliver RA, Williams G (1977) Polymorphic variation in the amount of sialic acid attached to bovine transferrin. An Blood Grps Biochem Genet 8: 21–24

284. Stormont C, Suzuki Y (1963) Genetic control of albumin phenotypes in horses. Proc Soc Exp Biol 114: 673–675

285. Stratil A, Glasnak V (1981) Partial characterization of horse transferrin heterogeneity with respect to the atypical type, Tfc. An Blood Grps Biochem Genet 12: 113–122

286. Stratil A, Glasnak V, Tomasek V, Williams J, Clamp JR (1984) Haemopexin of sheep, mouflon and goat: Genetic polymorphism, heterogeneity and partial characterization. An Blood Grps Biochem Genet 15: 285 297

287. Stratil A, Spooner RL (1971) Isolation and properties of individual components of cattle transferrin: The role of sialic acid. Biochem Genet 5: 347–365

288. Stratil A, Tomasek V, Bobak P, Glasnak V (1984) Heterogeneity of horse transferrin: The role of carbohydrate moiety. An Blood Grps Biochem Genet 15: 89–101

289. Strickland DK, Hudson BG (1978) Structural studies on rabbit transferrin: Isolation and characterization of the glycopeptides. Biochemistry 17: 3411–3418

290. Sundelin J, Melhus H, Das S, Erikson U, Lind P, Tragardh L, Peterson PA, Rask L (1985) The primary structure of rabbit and rat prealbumin and a comparison with the tertiary structure of human prealbumin. J Biol Chem 260: 6481–6487

291. Sutton HE (1970) In Steinburg AG, Bearn AG (eds), Progress in Medical Genetics, Vol VII. Grune & Stratton, New York and London

292. Svasti J, Bowman BH (1978) Human group-specific component: Changes in electrophoretic mobility resulting from vitamin D binding and from neuraminidase digestion. J Biol Chem 253: 4188–4194

293. Takahashi N, Takahashi Y, Heiny ME, Putnam FW (1985) Purification of hemopexin and its domain fragments by affinity chromatography and high performance liquid chromatography. J Chromatography 326: 373–385

294. Takahashi N, Takahashi Y, Putnam FW (1985) Complete amino acid sequence of human hemopexin, the heme-binding protein of serum. Proc Natl Acad Sci USA 82: 73–77

295. Tarnoky AL (1980) Genetic and drug induced variations in serum albumin. Adv Clin Chem 21: 101–146

296. Thompson WL, Abeles FB, Ball FA, Dinterman RE, Wannemacher RW (1976) Influence of the adrenal glucocorticoids on the stimulation of synthesis of hepatic ribonucleic acid and plasma acute-phase globulins by leucocytic endogenous mediator. Biochem J 156: 25–32

297. Travis TC, Brown SO, Sanders BG (1970) A polymeric form of haptoglobin in the gamma irradiated Spanish goat. Biochem Genet 4: 639–649

298. Travis JC, Sanders BG (1972) Haptoglobin evolution: Polymeric forms of Hp in the bovidal and cervidal families. J Exp Zool 180: 141–148

299. Tranz JC, Garza T, Sanders BG (1975) Structural characterization of polymeric haptoglobin from goats. Comp Biochem Physiol 51B: 93–97

300. Trowbridge IS, Lesley J, Schulte R (1982) Murine cell surface transferrin receptor: Studies with an anti-receptor monoclonal antibody. J Cell Physiol 112: 403–410

301. Turchik JB, Bornstein DL (1980) Role of the central nervous system in acute-phase response to leukocytic pyrogen. Infect Immun 30: 439–444

302. Vahlquist A, Petersone PA (1972) Comparative studies on the vitamin A transporting protein complex in human and cynomolous plasma. Biochemistry 11: 4526–4532

303. Valenta M, Stratil A, Slechtova V, Kalal L, Slechta V (1976) Polymorphism of transferrin in carp (*Cyprinus carpio L*). Genetic determination, isolation, and partial characterization. Biochem Genet 14: 27–45

304. Van Baelan H, De Moor P (1974) Immunochemical quantitation of human transcortin. J Clin Endocrinol Metab 39: 160–163

305. Van Der Heul C, Froos MJ, Van Eijk HC (1982) Characterization and localization of the transferrin receptor or rat reticulocytes. Int J Biochem 14: 467–476

306. Van Der Walt BJ, Van Jaarsveld (1978) Bovine thyroxine-binding globulin. Biochim Biophys Acta 535: 44–53

307. Voelkel EF, Levine L, Alper CA, Tashjian AH (1978) Acute-phase reactants ceruloplasmin and haptoglobin and their relationship to plasma prostaglandins in rabbits bearing the VX$_2$ carcinoma. J Exp Med 147: 1078–1088

308. Vretblad P, Hjort R (1977) The use of wheat-germ lectin sepharose for the purification of human haemopexin. Biochem J 167: 759–764

309. Waites GT, Bell AM, Bell SG (1983) Acute phase serum proteins in syngeneic and allogeneic mouse pregnancy. Clin Exp Immunol 53: 225–232

310. Wannemacher RW, Pekarek RS, Thompson WL, Curnon RT, Beall FA, Zenser TV, DeRubertis FR, Beisel WR (1975) A protein from polymorphonuclear leukocytes (LEM) which affects the rate of hepatic amino acid transport and synthesis of acute phase globulins. Endocrinology 96: 651–661

311. Weigle WO (1961) Immunochemical properties of the cross-reactions between anti-BAS and heterologous albumins. J Immunol 87: 599–607

312. Weiss ML, Goodman M, Prychodko W, Tanaka T (1971) Species and geographic distribution patterns of the Macaque prealbumin polymorphism Primates 12: 75–80

313. Weitkamp LR (1978) Equine markers genes: Polymorphism for group-specific components (Gc). An Blood Grps Biochem Genet 9: 123–126

314. Werner M (1969) Serum protein changes during the acute phase reaction. Clin Chim Acta 25: 299–305

315. Westphal U (1971) Steroid Protein Interactions. Springer-Verlag, Berlin, pp 164–350

316. Witz I, Gross J (1965) Purification and partial characterization of mouse hemopexin (beta 2-III globulin). Proc Soc Exp Med 118: 1003–1006

317. Wolf G, Armstrong EG, Rossner W (1981) Synthesis in vitro of corticosteroid-binding globulin from rat liver messenger ribonucleic acid. Endocrinology 108: 805–811

318. Yedgar S, Carew TE, Pittman RC, Beltz W, Steinberg D (1983) Tissue sites of catabolism of albumin in rabbits. Am J Physiol 244: E101–E107

319. Yoshioka N, Atassi MZ (1986) Hemoglobin binding with haptoglobin. Biochem J 234: 453–456

320. Young S (1982) Evidence for the functional equivalence of the iron-binding sites of rat transferrin. Biochim Biophys Acta 718: 35–41

321. Young SP, Bomford A, Williams R (1983) Dual pathways for the uptake of rat asialotransferrin by rat hepatocytes. J Biol Chem 258: 4972–4976

D. Acute Phase Proteins

TRACY FRENCH, DVM

The host response to tissue injury involves, in addition to local inflammation, a wide range of systemic alterations known collectively as the acute phase response. Fever and leukocytosis have long been recognized as components of this reaction, but only more recently have the endocrine, metabolic, and immunologic manifestations been appreciated (245). The acute phase proteins (acute phase reactants) are a diverse group whose plasma levels rise, as part of this systemic response, during the first hours to days following tissue injury. Though termed "acute" because the prototype of this group (C-reactive protein) was first noted in sera from human patients with acute bacterial infection, the response may be initiated by a variety of conditions that need not be acute (or primarily inflammatory) in nature. Tissue damage associated with surgery, infarction, burns, or trauma can elicit the response. Neoplasms of many types, localized or disseminated, have been associated with increased plasma levels of various acute phase proteins. Bacterial, viral, immune-mediated, and idiopathic inflammatory conditions are all capable of inducing this response. Endotoxin is a particularly potent acute phase stimulus.

Although no precise criteria can be given, certain common denominators apply to most of the proteins commonly categorized under this heading. Designation as an acute phase reactant has generally been restricted to those plasma proteins whose levels increase by at least 25 per cent during the first few days after injury (245). The primary site of production for most acute phase proteins is the liver, and the observed increases are the result of accelerated hepatic synthesis (231). Most acute phase proteins contain a significant amount of carbohydrate and display alpha or beta electrophoretic mobility on paper. The functions of the individual proteins in this group, when known, vary widely and will be discussed in more detail in the following sections. In many cases, however, they are involved in modulating various aspects of the host response to the tissue injury that induced their increased concentrations.

Numerous potential mediators have been studied to explain how this hepatic synthetic response is triggered by tissue damage at distant sites. Various hormones (cortisol, epinephrine, sex hormones, and others), prostaglandins, biogenic amines, fibrinogen degradation products, and central nervous system effects, to name but a few, have all been reported to play roles in controlling the synthesis of various acute phase

201

proteins. Undoubtedly, a complex interaction of many factors is involved, and the dominant elements likely vary depending on the protein in question and the nature of the inciting stimulus. However, leukocytic pyrogen (interleukin-1) appears to be emerging as a major mediator that is able to induce, whether directly or indirectly, the characteristic protein changes as well as other systemic features of the acute phase response such as fever, granulocytosis, and hypoferremia (reviewed in reference 56).

The patterns of acute phase protein alterations in human sera have been studied in various clinical conditions including infectious diseases (154), myocardial infarction (215), liver disease (183, 336), rheumatic diseases (226, 244), and the postoperative period (98,147). As a rule, such profiles do not give specific diagnostic information. However, they are often helpful in monitoring the activity of, and the response to therapy for, various inflammatory and neoplastic diseases. The two-dimensional immunoelectrophoretograms in Figure 10.D.1a,b depict the effect of tumor implantation on the numerous proteins in rat serum. The pattern returned toward normal 3 days after removal of the tumor (1).

The plasma levels of the various acute phase reactants are influenced by physiologic as well as pathologic factors. Age, sex, and reproductive status affect the basal levels for some of the specific proteins. Circadian fluctuations have been reported in some instances. For some proteins, the species and strain of animal influence both the basal levels and the acute phase behavior observed. C-reactive protein, for example, increases after tissue injury in most species but is relatively unchanged in mice. Conversely, serum amyloid P-component displays convincing acute phase increases in mice but not in other species studied (329).

The following sections will present information on some of the major acute phase proteins in animals in comparison to the homologous human proteins. The proteins selected are those that appeared best studied in animals. Plasminogen, antithrombin III, and α_1-antichymotrypsin, among others, are sometimes classified as acute phase reactants but will not be covered here. The complement component C3, also often considered with this group, is covered with the rest of the complement system in this text.

C-REACTIVE PROTEIN

C-reactive protein (CRP) is the prototype of the acute phase proteins in humans (423) and also has been described in many animal species (16,112,326,331,357,358,364). The homologous protein in rabbits is sometimes termed C_x-reactive protein (8). Comprehensive reviews, which include discussion of the biology of CRP, have been published (248,327,335).

Biochemistry and Physiology

The CRP molecule of human origin is composed of five identical polypeptide subunits, each with a molecular weight of about 21,000 daltons (d) (263), which associate in a noncovalent manner to form an annular disk with cyclic pentameric symmetry (pentraxin) (315). The same basic structure with some variations was also reported for CRP isolated from several animal species (16,74,112,331). Glycosylation of polypeptide subunits has been reported for dog (74) and rat (112) molecules in contrast to those of other mammals. This distinctive pentraxin configuration is shared by the closely related proteins serum amyloid P-component (315) and hamster female protein (92). These three proteins also share an important functional characteristic, the capacity for calcium-dependent ligand binding (16,92). Differences in the binding specificities are used to identify and selectively isolate these proteins from serum. C-reactive protein was classically defined by, and named for, its calcium-dependent reactivity with the C-polysaccharide of pneumococcal bacteria. This interaction reflects the binding of CRP to phosphorylcholine residues (441), which is a consistent feature of CRP from different species. Many other ligand specificities, including binding to lipids and lipoproteins, have been reported and recently were reviewed (335). Binding of fibronectin (374) and of chromatin and nucleosome core particles (363) by CRP also has been demonstrated.

The major site of synthesis of CRP is the hepatocyte (246,266,409); however, recent reports indicate that some human lymphocyte populations also are capable of synthesizing the protein (205,249). The rate of production can increase rapidly following tissue injury, and leukocytic pyrogen (IL-1) is an important mediator of this response (57). Rabbit CRP mRNA syn-

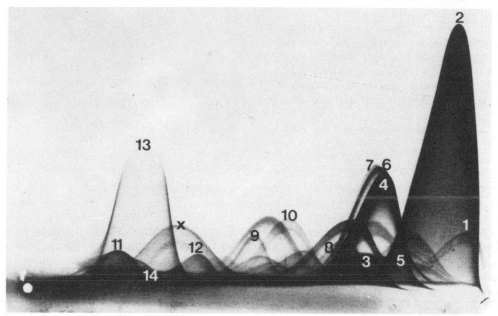

A

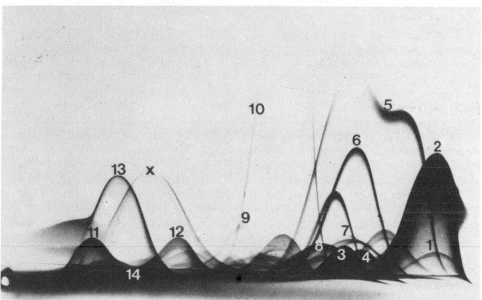

B

Figure 10.D.1 Crossed two-dimensional immunoelectrophoresis using antiserum to whole rat serum proteins. Proteins identified are: 1, Prealbumin; 2, albumin; 3, α-lipoprotein; 4, α-1-macroglobulin; 5, α-1-acid glycoprotein; 6, α-1-antitrypsin; 7, cholinesterase; 8, ceruloplasmin; 9, hemopexin; 10, haptoglobin; 11, C_3; 12, C_3c; 13, transferrin; 14, β-lipoprotein; X, unidentified peak. (A) Control rat serum; (B) Rat serum 6 days after transplantation of Yoshida sarcoma. Reproduced with permission from Cancer Research, Inc. (ref.1).

thesis and concentration increase in hepatocytes during the acute phase response (375,409). The plasma half-life of CRP is short, ranging from 3 to 4.5 hours in normal rabbits, rats, and mice, but is somewhat longer (6.5 hours) in rabbits undergoing an acute phase response (20,81,371). Consequently, plasma levels can decrease rapidly once the stimulus for enhanced production is removed.

The exact function of CRP remains unclear;

however, a variety of in vitro and in vivo biologic activities have been described which suggest an important role in initiating and modulating inflammatory and immune responses (reviewed in references 161 and 335). Reported effects of CRP include activation or regulation of the classical and alternative complement cascades following binding to various ligands (44,220,285,316,344,394), opsonin-like enhancement of phagocytosis (284,286), modulation of platelet function (59,143,146,229), interactions with lymphoid cells (208,453,455), induction of macrophage tumoricidal activity (467), regulation of bone-marrow monocyte progenitor cells (293), enhancement of cell-mediated cytotoxicity (26,438), and modulation of blood coagulation (144) and of monocyte chemotaxis and procoagulant activity (454). The recent demonstration of high affinity binding of CRP to chromatin and nucleosome core particles (363) has led to the finding that CRP can mediate the complement-dependent solubilization of DNA (362,391). Hence, CRP may be important as a scavenger for chromatin released from damaged cells.

Analysis

Early methods for detecting CRP, based on precipitation reactions with the pneumococcal C-polysaccharide (423) or with monospecific rabbit antisera (7), were relatively insensitive and failed to detect the low levels present in normal sera. Newer methods include electroimmunoassay (252), latex slide agglutination tests (443), radial immunodiffusion (304), ELISA (22), luminometry (60), immunoturbidimetry (279, 341), and immunonephelometry (142). The most sensitive methods, which are able to detect CRP in all human sera, include radioimmunoassay (88), quantitative latex immunoagglutination (387), and particle counting immunoassay (97) which can detect CRP in the range of 1 to 10 ng/ml. Application of these methods to CRP in a given species will generally require the appropriate species-specific antiserum; however, some cross-reactivity does occur (16,326). A simple, nonimmunologic, qualitative test for detecting high CRP concentration in human sera has been described (200). This test involves agglutination of a fat emulsion and is based on the calcium-dependent interaction of CRP and liposomes.

Table 10.D.1. C-reactive Protein (CRP) in Various Species

| Species | CRP (mg/l) | | References |
	Normal Sera	Acute Phase Sera	
Human[a]	0.07–8.0	300–500	88,161
Mouse	2.0	2.0	326
Rat[a]	300–600	700–900	112
Rabbit	2.0	100–200	246
Dog	10.0	100–400	152

[a] Adult levels. Range is known to be lower for the young of these species. (See text.)

C-reactive protein can be isolated from the sera of many species by calcium-dependent affinity chromatography on phosphorylcholine or C-polysaccharide-substituted agarose beads (16,331).

Concentration

The normal concentration of CRP varies markedly in the serum of different species (Table 10.D.1). The rat is noteworthy in that baseline levels in this species may exceed even the maximal acute phase levels in other species (112). Normal levels in other species are generally very low. Some investigators studying rabbit CRP have accepted higher baseline levels (20 to 100 mg/l) than those indicated for that species in Table 10.D.1 (57,67). This variation may reflect differences in the measurement techniques or the presence of subclinical inflammatory processes.

Normal values for CRP in human neonates are considerably lower than those in adults (88). Similarly, young August rats (3 weeks old) were found to have much lower levels (70 to 200 mg/l) than did mature animals (112). In the same study, no differences in the level of CRP were noted between adult rats of different strains or sexes. Increased levels of CRP have been associated with pregnancy and the use of contraceptive medications in women (100), but reports regarding similar effects in animals were not found. Lactation in women had no effect on plasma CRP content (119).

Causes of pathologic increases in serum CRP levels in humans are numerous, including most diseases with associated inflammation or tissue destruction. Consequently, elevations are of little specific diagnostic value. However, serial

Table 10.D.2. Serum Amyloid P-Component (SAP) in Various Species

Species	SAP (mg/l)		
	Normal Sera	Acute Phase Sera	References
Human	30–40	Little change[a]	332
Rat	20–50	Little change	112
Mouse strains:			
C57BL/10SN	20–30	170–200	291
BALB/c	90–110	190–210	291
DBA/2	150–180	210–230	291

[a] May increase slightly in chronic inflammatory or neoplastic diseases.

determinations have been useful in monitoring disease activity, progression, and response to therapy in inflammatory and neoplastic conditions in humans (24,161,175,244,288,333). Repeated measurement of CRP has also been valuable in detecting infections in patients with neutropenic leukemia and in gauging their response to antibiotic therapy (367). Measurement of CRP in cerebrospinal fluid has been of value in the diagnosis of bacterial meningitis (417).

In animals with various, mostly experimentally induced, inflammatory conditions, CRP levels have been shown to respond in a species-dependent manner (Table 10.D.1). In the rabbit CRP has long been known to show dramatic acute phase increases (8). Following subcutaneous injection of croton oil or turpentine in rabbits, elevations in CRP were noted as early as 6 hours and peak levels were reached by 40 to 48 hours (67,246). Turpentine-induced pleurisy in rabbits resulted in raised CRP levels in serum by 12 hours, which peaked at 50-fold normal by 36 hours; however, none was detected in the inflammatory exudate (162). Dogs (118, 152,358) and monkeys (2) also were reported to show acute phase increases in CRP levels. In a recent study, high serum CRP concentrations were detected in dogs with various naturally occurring and experimental conditions (75). Rats injected with croton oil showed only moderate increases relative to the high basal levels reported (112), and mice given similar treatment showed barely detectable increases (326).

SERUM AMYLOID P-COMPONENT

Serum amyloid P-component (SAP) is a normal plasma glycoprotein of man and many species of animals (112,271,326,331). The overall biology of SAP was recently reviewed (328). It is a major acute phase reactant in the mouse (329), but remains relatively constant during disease in other species (16,112,271).

Biochemistry and Physiology

Serum amyloid P-component is closely related to CRP and hamster female protein. All three display a similar molecular configuration (pentraxins), amino acid sequence, and capacity for calcium-dependent ligand binding (16,93,315). Despite these similarities, SAP is antigenically distinct. No cross-reactivity has been noted between SAP and CRP in any species. Also SAP differs in that its calcium-dependent binding activity is strongest for plain agarose, rather than the C-polysaccharide or phosphorylcholine substituted agarose that binds CRP most effectively (16). This specificity is due to the pyruvate acetal of galactose contained in agarose (192) and also present in the cell wall of some bacteria (191).

Serum amyloid P-component appears to be identical to the amyloid P-component that can be isolated from amyloid deposits of all types. It was first identified as a protein in normal serum that cross-reacted with antisera produced against soluble extracts of secondary amyloid deposits from affected livers (77). Synthesis of SAP is believed to occur mainly in the liver (17,18,328). The rate of synthesis is likely constant in most species as evidenced by the stability of serum concentrations. In mice however, serum levels increase following induction of acute phase responses with various stimuli (329). Because the normal murine SAP turnover rate of 7.0 to 8.25 hours has been reported to remain unchanged during such responses, the observed serum increases are likely due to enhanced hepatic synthesis (18,328). The nature of the signal that triggers this increase is not yet clear. Interleukin-1 (IL-1) has been studied as a possible mediator of the response (256,291,398,418), with somewhat variable results. A recent report indicated that although purified mouse IL-1 increases production by individual SAP-secreting hepatocytes, other monokines are important in the induction of nonsynthesizing cells into new SAP synthesis (255). Complement activation alone did not induce elevation of SAP in mice, and an intact complement system was not required for the acute phase increases to occur following tissue injury (334). T-cell deprivation had little effect on the SAP response in mice infected with *Schistosoma mansoni* (330).

The function of SAP is not known. It may be the precursor of the glycoprotein amyloid P-component consistently found in all types of amyloid deposits; however, its significance, if any, in the pathogenesis of amyloidosis has yet to be proven. A SAP-related material, identified by immunofluorescent staining with anti-SAP antibodies, has been demonstrated in normal human renal glomerular basement membranes and elastic fibers in blood vessels and various other tissues (61,126). Reported activities that may relate to its biologic function include modulation of blood coagulation (144), regulation of platelet reactivity (145), enhancement of bactericidal activity (395) and complement-mediated phagocytosis (460) in monocyte/macrophage populations, enhancement of IL-1 production by elicited monocytes/macrophages (378), elastase inhibition (259), and modulation of lymphocyte function (258,261). It has also been shown that fibronectin and C4-binding protein are selectively bound in a calcium-dependent fashion by aggregated SAP immobilized on agarose beads (111). Such findings have opened new avenues for investigating possible roles of SAP in physiologic as well as pathologic processes.

Analysis

Measurement of SAP in plasma has been accomplished by the use of antisera raised against either SAP isolated from serum (112,326) or amyloid P-component extracted from amyloid deposits (398). Such antisera have been employed in electroimmunoassay (112,252,326), ELISA (388), rate nephelometry (160), quantitative Western blot (180), and radioimmunoassay procedures (398). The antisera to SAP from different mammals appear to be species specific and also fail to react with CRP from the same or other species (16).

Concentration

Reported normal SAP levels for humans, rats, and several strains of mice are shown in Table 10.D.2. Mice are unique among the species studied in that baseline levels show marked strain-dependent variation (291,329). The strains shown in Table 10.D.2 demonstrate the range of this variation, which is reportedly influenced more by the non-H-2 background genes than by the H-2 complex (291). It recently was shown that endogenous murine SAP concentration is controlled by a major locus on chromosome 1 (292). This locus has been designated *Sap*, and it is linked to the Ly-9 lymphocyte differentiation antigen locus. No significant variation in baseline levels was noted among several strains of rats examined (112).

Normal SAP levels in humans are influenced by gender, males having slightly higher levels than females (332). No significant variation between sexes has been found in mice or rats (112,291). Age has an effect on SAP levels in humans. Neonates have low levels which rise to the adult range at a few weeks of age (328). In contrast, neonatal mice had levels in or above the adult range (444). Three-week-old rats had SAP values in the adult range, but levels in neonatal rats were not determined (112).

The effect of syngeneic and allogeneic pregnancy on SAP levels in C57BL/10 mice has been studied (444). Levels increased slightly during the final 3 days of syngeneic pregnancy and returned to baseline by 8 days postpartum. Allogeneic pregnancy (CBA/Ca males) resulted in a marked triphasic response with a peak on day 4 (twofold increase), a plateau from days 8 to 12 (threefold increase), followed by a climb to maximum levels (five- to sixfold increase) on day 18 of gestation. As with syngeneic pregnancy, SAP levels returned to baseline by day 8 postpartum.

In mice, SAP increases in a variety of pathologic states. Elevated levels were induced by local inflammation, endotoxin (in responsive strains), tumor implantation, and infection with *Schistosoma mansoni* (329). The SAP concentration was elevated in mice within the first 2 days after their infection with the nematode parasite *Nippostrongylus brasiliensis* (250). The SAP response is very sensitive to bacterial endotoxin (338), but mice infected with *Mycobacterium leprae* maintained normal SAP concentrations (421). The magnitude of the acute phase SAP response in mice is strain dependent, and in some experimental situations, it is inversely related to baseline levels (Table 10.D.2). At 24 hours after intraperitoneal thioglycollate administration, strains with low baseline levels showed a proportionally greater increase (up to 10-fold) compared to the 35 to 50 per cent increase seen in strains with high baseline levels (291). Differences in SAP response are also evident between amyloid-resistant and amyloid-susceptible strains of mice given daily injections of casein (19). Resistant strains showed only a transient increase in SAP, whereas susceptible strains sustained high levels as long as the injections continued. The SAP response also displays specificity with regard to the levels attained in different mouse models of autoimmune disease (366). Mice which develop a spontaneous systemic lupus erythematosus-like syndrome (NZBxW), failed to show SAP increases related to the progression of their underlying chronic inflammatory disease. However, they were able to respond with increased SAP when challenged with superimposed stimuli such as injection of casein or endotoxin. In contrast MRL/1 mice, which develop a more aggressive lupus-like disease with polyarthritis and circulating rheumatoid factors, showed a marked SAP response which correlated well with the activity of their disease (365,366).

HAMSTER FEMALE PROTEIN

Female protein (FP) is the hamster homolog of CRP/SAP in other species, but it is unique in the sex-dependent expression implied by its name. It is a prominent plasma protein (1 to 2 g/l) in female hamsters, but it is present in only 1/100th that concentration in normal adult males. Female protein has been demonstrated in Syrian hamsters and the closely related Kurdistan hamster, but not in several other species examined (91).

Biochemistry and Physiology

Female protein was first noted on immunoelectrophoretic patterns as a fast gamma globulin present in sera from normal female hamsters but not detectable in sera from normal adult male hamsters (90). It is similar to CRP and SAP in other species in terms of its calcium-dependent ligand binding, pentraxin structure, amino acid composition, and sequence (93). The derived amino acid sequence of FP is 69 per cent identical to that of human SAP and 50 per cent identical to that of human CRP (124). Female protein will bind to plain agarose and to

phosphorylcholine-substituted agarose, but it appears to have greater affinity for the latter (93). Female protein is synthesized by hepatocytes, the relative FP-specific mRNA content of which corresponds to the relative concentration of FP in the serum of the animal of origin (124). Studies of FP catabolism using ^{125}I-FP suggest that the differences in serum levels between normal males and females, as well as the changes observed in inflammatory states, are primarily due to variation in the rate of synthesis (94). In hamsters with amyloidosis, however, the serum metabolism of FP is altered in that the terminal ^{125}I-FP half-life is prolonged (124). The function of FP is not known. Female protein has been shown capable of activating the classical complement cascade following binding to phosphorylcholine-coupled sheep red blood cells, and it resembles CRP in this regard (131). Female protein also has been reported to be a constituent of Syrian hamster amyloid, the deposition of which is directly associated with high serum levels of FP (95). These findings correlate with the observed earlier onset and higher incidence of amyloidosis in female Syrian hamsters compared to males.

Analysis

Radial immunodiffusion with appropriate dilution of antiserum is sufficiently sensitive to quantify low levels of FP (10 to 15 mg/l) such as those found in adult males (90,94). Specific antiserum can be prepared by absorption of anti-whole normal hamster (male and female) serum with normal male hamster serum or by inoculating rabbits with purified FP preparations emulsified in complete Freund's adjuvant (90,93). Pure FP can be isolated from serum by affinity chromatography using phosphorylcholine-agarose or rabbt anti-FP-agarose (93).

Concentration

Normal FP levels in serum are influenced by age as well as gender (90,92). First detected at 10 days of age in hamsters of both sexes, FP then increased to higher levels with different patterns depending on gender. In males, FP levels were noted to peak at 21 days of age (400 to 500 mg/l) and then decline to the low levels typical of adult males (10 to 20 mg/l) by 60 to 90 days of age.

Female hamsters had a rapid increase in FP and reached levels typical of adult females (1 to 2 g/l) by 30 to 35 days of age. After this peak, levels in females tended to decrease as aging continued. Individual female hamsters showed considerable, apparently random variation in FP levels when examined daily over periods of 1 to 3 weeks (94). Fluctuations of 600 to 800 mg/l were observed and did not appear to correlate to the estrus cycle or time of day.

The lower levels of FP in sera from adult males are due to suppression of synthesis by testosterone (90). Castration or the administration of estrogens to males resulted in increased FP levels (up to 500 mg/l) within 14 days. Administration of testosterone to females reduced FP levels to the same range as that of intact males, whereas ovariectomy caused no significant change (90).

Following induction of acute inflammation, FP shows a unique dichotomous response which depends more on the initial level than on gender per se (94). Hamsters with high initial FP levels (females and castrated or estrogen-treated males) had a transient decrease (50 per cent) within 24 hours following turpentine injection. Hamsters with low initial FP levels (males and testosterone-treated females) had up to fivefold increases by 48 hours after the same inflammatory stimulus. Daily administration of exogenous corticosteroids to female hamsters caused a relatively slow progressive decline in FP to levels of about 70 mg/l by day 11 of treatment, but it did not match the rapid drop seen in the first 24 hours after turpentine injection (94). The persistence of very low FP levels (100 mg/l or 10 per cent of normal) in injured or diseased female hamsters (turpentine injection, "wet tail" disease) indicated a poor prognosis and was often associated with subsequent fatality (92).

SERUM AMYLOID A

Serum amyloid A (SAA) is an α_1-globulin that displays marked acute phase increases in response to a wide variety of tissue injuries. It has been studied in humans and several species of animals. It is believed to be the precursor of the AA fibrils present in secondary amyloid deposits in tissues.

Biochemistry and Physiology

Serum amyloid A is a single polypeptide chain with a molecular weight of about 12,000 daltons. This same molecule has also been termed apo SAA because in serum it associates with high-density lipoproteins to yield a 180,000-dalton complex (34). Heterogeneity of SAA has been reported in several species including the human (30,128), rabbit (424), mouse (5,172), monkey (325), and mink (5). In mice, SAA is encoded by at least three genes, designated SAA_{1-3} (265,462). The hepatocyte is likely the major site of SAA synthesis during the acute phase response (37,272,386,415); however, detection of SAA-specific mRNA has been reported in various extrahepatic sites in mice treated with endotoxin or IL-1 (346). Serum levels of SAA can increase very rapidly following tissue injury. Mice injected with casein may show a 100- to 200-fold increase by 12 to 18 hours, with detectable elevations as early as 3 hours after injection (42). Interleukin-1 (IL-1) is an important mediator of the acute phase synthesis of SAA (398), and it has been shown to cause a dose-dependent increase in SAA-specific hepatic mRNA (347). Clearance of SAA in mice is rapid, with an estimated plasma half-life of 75 to 80 minutes (194). The turnover of Vervet monkey SAA from plasma was biphasic, with a half-life of 0.39 to 0.48 days during the initial phase and 2.5 to 4.3 days during the second phase (325). Human apo SAA-rich high-density lipoproteins injected into rats had a half-life of 11 hours (127).

The function of SAA is not well defined. A role in regulation of the immune response has been suggested on the basis of experiments that demonstrate SAA-mediated suppression of the in vitro antibody response of mouse spleen cells to sheep red blood cells (40). This suppression is not due to any direct effect of SAA on B-lymphocytes, but it may instead result from an influence on macrophage/T-cell interactions (38,39). Suppression of human peripheral blood lymphocyte function has also been shown to occur after treatment with SAA (39,260). A recent study indicated that association with apo SAA causes remodeling of high-density lipoprotein particles with regard to size, density, and apo-A-I-content; however, the metabolic consequences of such alterations remain unknown (96).

Though its function remains obscure, the role of SAA in amyloidogenesis is being clarified. Acute phase mice given human high-density lipoprotein-SAA developed amyloid deposits that contained both mouse and human AA protein, evidence supporting a precursor/product relationship (202). The murine isotype SAA_2 appears to be the sole precursor of amyloid fibril protein AA, because of the apparent selective removal of this isotype from the circulation in this species (276). Acute phase SAA_2 gene expression is minimal in SJL mice, perhaps accounting for the resistance to azocasein-induced amyloidosis (462).

Analysis

Many immunologic assays have been described for the quantitation of SAA in various species. In addition to differences in analytic methods per se (ELISA, radioimmunoassay, etc.), these assays vary with regard to the source of protein standard (protein AA or SAA), the antisera used (anti-SAA or cross-reacting anti-protein AA), units used to express results (AA equivalents or SAA concentration), and the pre-assay sample treatment (untreated or denatured with acid, alkali, or heat). Consequently, interlaboratory variation hinders comparison of results (129, 270).

Interspecies cross-reactivity for SAA generally has not been found (5,247,272). In a study using a sensitive enzyme-linked immunosorbent assay (ELISA), however, cross-reactivity between rhesus protein AA and SAA and xenotypic (mouse and human) protein AA was demonstrated (120). Other ELISA methods for murine SAA, using monoclonal (458) and polyclonal (469) antibodies, have been described. These methods avoid the need to denature the protein as is required for optimal reactivity in some assays (396). A quantitative radial immunodiffusion assay for SAA, also using untreated serum, has been described (78). Determination of SAA concentration in serum also has been accomplished by radioimmunoassay (42,129, 270,396).

Concentration

Reported SAA concentrations in normal human sera vary from mean values as low as 94 μg AA equivalent per liter (246) or 2.0 mg AA equivalent per liter (49), to a derived reference range of 5 to 30 mg/l (78). (See comments under Analysis.) Relatively higher levels have been reported for pregnant women and individuals of advanced age (369). In mice, values from 200 μg AA equivalent per liter (273) to 40 mg/l (250) have been reported for normal sera. Thymus-deficient nude mice were found to have high baseline SAA concentrations compared to 11 other strains of mice (273).

Levels of SAA increase rapidly following tissue damage and may remain elevated while the stimulus persists. Increases of up to 1000-fold may occur. Levels return to normal quickly when the stimulus is removed (273). Various acute and chronic inflammatory diseases and neoplasms have been associated with increased SAA in humans (350,369). Serum amyloid A has been evaluated as a biochemical marker to detect dissemination of neoplasms and to monitor response to therapy (41,49,370). The extreme sensitivity of the SAA response in humans mandates cautious interpretation, because its concentration may be raised by both trivial and asymptomatic viral infections (452).

Most studies in animals have involved the induction of inflammation to examine the mechanisms controlling SAA synthesis and its role in amyloid formation. Marked strain-dependent variation in SAA response was reported in mice given endotoxin (273). At 24 hours post-injection, SAA levels ranged from 200 to 750 mg/l for 11 strains examined. Endotoxin-resistant C3H/HeJ mice required much larger doses to induce a significant SAA increase, yet their response to casein injection was similar to that of other strains (273). Latent phase serum from endotoxin-sensitive strains given endotoxin contained an SAA inducer (probably IL-1) capable of stimulating SAA synthesis in endotoxin-resistant strains (397,410). A biphasic SAA response was observed in mice infected with the nematode parasite *N. brasiliensis*, with peak increases of 13- and 8-fold normal occurring on postinfection days 1 to 1.5 and 12, respectively (250).

Hamsters injected with casein had high SAA levels during the pre-amyloid period, but a significant decline occurred during the development of amyloidosis. This decline was followed by a later increase in some individuals when amyloid was deposited in large amounts (195).

A study involving strains of mice differing in their propensity for amyloid deposition subsequent to repeated injections of casein showed similar SAA responses among the strains examined (42). This finding is consistent with the observation that elevated SAA levels occur in many human disorders not usually associated with amyloid deposition (171). Consequently, the presence of an increased level of SAA is of no value in the diagnosis of amyloidosis. A normal level of SAA generally argues against the presence of secondary amyloidosis (247).

α_2-MACROGLOBULIN

The α-macroglobulins (αM) are large, tetrameric, glycoproteins that possess an unusual broad-spectrum antiprotease activity (reviewed in reference 138). Proteins of this type have been identified in the plasma of many species including humans, rats (446), guinea pigs (407), rabbits (174), dogs (309), mice (177,465), hamsters (403), and others (402). The α-macroglobulins from the various mammals are generally of similar size and antiprotease activity (402). Immunologic relationships have been identified between the αM of several species (45,407,451). Results of amino acid sequence comparisons indicate the likelihood of a common evolutionary origin of α_2-macroglobulin and the complement components C3 and C4 (399). In human plasma, there is only a single αM, which is designated α_2-macroglobulin. Several animal species (including rats, rabbits, and dogs) possess two forms termed α_1- and α_2-macroglobulins (α_1M and α_2M). In some species, such as humans, mice, and dogs, the α-macroglobulins fail to increase in most diseases and therefore are not typical acute phase reactants in these species (152,309,361,465). In contrast, rabbit α_1M (173,257,294,437) and rat α_2M (446) do increase following tissue injury. Rat α_2M is the best studied of the α-macroglobulins in animals, and it is often considered to be the prototype acute phase reactant in this species. The following discussion will therefore center on rat α_2M. Numerous synonyms including α_2-macrofetoprotein, α_2 acute-phase globulin, fetal globulin, abnormal serum globulin, and reproduction-associated globulin have been used for this protein in the rat. These names reflect the finding of increased levels in the plasma of pregnant, fetal, neonatal, and injured rats.

Biochemistry and Physiology

Rat α_2M has a molecular weight of about 700,000 d and a carbohydrate content of 9 to 10 per cent (157). It consists of four identical subunits with a molecular weight of 170,000 d (187), and DNA sequence analysis has revealed 80 per cent homology to human α_2M (305). Synthesis in the rat occurs mainly in the liver in adult, fetal, and neonatal animals (35,376,377). Additional sites in pregnant rats are the decidual tissue and metrial gland of the uterus (31,32,323), spleen, thymus, and blood lymphocytes (323). Following injury, such as turpentine or endotoxin injection, α_2M levels in plasma increase quickly as a result of increased hepatic synthesis (105,169,211) which reportedly is regulated mainly at the level of gene transcription (50,187,305). Synthesis in acute-phase male rats also has been reported to occur in kidney, spleen, thymus, and blood lymphocytes (323). Leukocytic endogenous mediator (or IL-1) has been shown to play an important role in triggering this response (12,25,170,445). Several hormones including glucocorticoids (169,216,422), adrenaline (165), estrogen, and progesterone (33,380) are also involved in facilitating and/or regulating synthesis of α_2M.

α_2M is unique as an antiproteinase in terms of both the broad spectrum of enzymes inhibited and the nature of its inhibitory activity. α_2M is able to bind a number of serine proteases (e.g., trypsin, chymotrypsin, thrombin, and plasmin) as well as other types of endopeptidases (23, 442). This binding results in substantial inhibition of the enzyme's activity against large proteins, but the complex retains significant esterolytic or amidase activity against low molecular weight substances. The complexed enzyme, designated as trypsin-protein esterase in the case of trypsin, is immune to further inactivation by high molecular weight inhibitors (e.g., soybean trypsin inhibitor) that would immediately inactivate the unbound enzyme (186). These characteristics are believed to result from a "trapping" mechanism whereby, once bound, the active site of the enzyme is free to react with small molecules, whereas steric hindrance limits interaction with larger substrates or inhibitors (23,140). α_2M-enzyme complexes are quickly cleared from the circulation (167,303,308). The half-life of ^{125}I-labeled human α_2M-trypsin in rats was 2 minutes (110). Cellular uptake is receptor mediated, and hepatocytes account for most of the plasma clearance in both rats and mice (110,141). Macrophages, fibroblasts, and adipocytes also bear the receptor for the α_2M recognition site, which is exposed on reaction with active protease or methylamine (141,164). Therefore, by removing, inhibiting, and altering the specificity of various enzymes, α_2M may play a role in controlling coagulation, fibrinolysis, and kinin formation as well as limiting proteolytic tissue damage at sites of inflammation (150,167,359). The injection of purified α_2M into rats has been reported to reduce the inflammatory edema and subsequent development of granulation tissue induced by the administration of carragccncn (300,431), and to inhibit thc hepatotoxicity induced by galactosamine (429). α_2M also has been reported to mitigate the hemodynamic effects of early endotoxic shock in rats, possibly by inhibition of prostaglandin E_2 activity (435). However, other studies involving rat models for counter-irritation (14) and experimentally induced arthritis (193) have not supported a role for α_2M as an endogenous antiinflammatory protein. Enhanced development of post-CCl_4 cirrhosis was observed in rats with elevated α_2M levels as part of an induced acute-phase response, and it possibly was based on the increased anticollagenase activity (432).

α_2M may also affect the proliferation and activities of various cell types. Purified protein has been reported to inhibit the in vitro mitogen-induced stimulation of lymphocytes in humans (348), rats (283), and hamsters (185). Residual enzymatic activity of human α_2M-protease complexes appears to play a role in the inhibition of natural killing, antibody-dependent cell-mediated cytotoxicity (117), and the modulation of antigen-induced T-cell proliferation (268), the latter possibly a result of α_2M-protease inactivation of interleukin-2 (58). Growth inhibitory activity against several types of tumor cells has been attributed to mouse (238) and rat (442) α_2M or to small biomediators carried by the mouse protein (239). Polymorphonuclear leukocyte chemotactic activity was reported to be inhibited, both in vitro and in vivo, by rat α_2M (430).

Analysis

Immunochemical methods that have been used to determine α_2M concentrations in the plasma of rats include rocket electroimmunoassay (15,151,321), radioimmunoassay (199,322), immunonephelometry (105), and radial immunodiffusion (168). Though species-specific antisera generally have been employed, cross-reactivity between rat α_2M and some antihuman α_2M antisera does occur (15). α_2M has been isolated from serum by many methods including gel filtration followed by either negative affinity chromatography (321) or ultracentrifugation and DEAE-cellulose chromatography (168).

α_2M has also been measured as the trypsin-protein esterase (155). This spectrophotometric method involves the addition of trypsin in sufficient quantity to saturate the α_2M present in the specimen, followed by the addition of soybean trypsin inhibitor in cxccss. A synthctic low molecular weight substrate is then used to measure the activity of the α_2M-trypsin complex, which is unaffected by the soybean trypsin inhibitor. This method correlates well with immunochemical methods for measuring α_2M in normal human plasma, which contains only a single α-macroglobulin. However, it is not specific, and in animals with two α-macroglobulins both may contribute to the observed trypsin-protein esterase activity (153). Storage-associated in vitro inactivation of α_2M and the abnormal presence of α_2M-protease complexes formed in vivo are possible causes of lowered functional, compared to immunoreactive, estimations of α_2M concentration (155,179).

Concentration

The levels reported for α_2M in normal adult rats vary somewhat but are generally less than 50 mg/l (168,199,320,429). Much higher concentrations are found in pregnant, fetal, and neonatal rats (199,320,379,429,446). In pregnant rats, there is a biphasic increase (320). The normal range is first exceeded around day 7 of gestation and levels continue to increase through day 12. This early elevation has been attributed to synthesis of α_2M in the metrial gland. The second phase increase begins about day 17 and peaks during labor. Much of this late rise may be due to transplacental passage of α_2M produced in fetal liver (320). Reported concentrations for pregnant rats at or near term are roughly 50- to 100-fold normal (199,320). Maternal levels decrease after parturition but remain somewhat elevated during the lactation period before returning to baseline by day 48 postpartum. In fetal rats, $\alpha_2 M$ increases during gestation and reaches maximum levels at delivery. The neonatal levels (150- to 300-fold normal) decrease to the nonpregnant adult range by 7 to 8 weeks of age (320,379). Induction of inflammation in 4-day-old rats caused an acute-phase $\alpha_2 M$ response despite the already high concentration present at this age (420). At 1.5 to 2.0 years of age, levels begin to increase somewhat (379).

$\alpha_2 M$ in the rat shows a marked increase in response to tissue injury of various causes. Increased levels can be detected as soon as 12 hours after injury, and peak levels may be reached by 40 hours (105,310,429). Concentrations as great as 10 g/l may be attained in acute inflammatory conditions (199,429). The response is generally greater (3- to 10-fold) in male rats than in females (15,33). Strain-dependent differences in response have been reported as well (15,429,447). At 48 hours after turpentine injection, for example, $\alpha_2 M$ levels in August and Lewis rats are about 9,500 mg/l compared to only 3,500 mg/l in Fullindorf rats (15).

Antiinflammatory agents of the nonsteroidal type (e.g., aspirin and indomethacin) have been shown to inhibit the acute phase increase of $\alpha_2 M$ following turpentine injection, suggesting the possible use of the $\alpha_2 M$ response as an aid in screening for new classes of antiinflammatory compounds (13,15).

α_1-ANTITRYPSIN

α_1-Antitrypsin ($\alpha_1 AT$) also termed α_1-trypsin inhibitor and α_1-protease inhibitor ($\alpha 1 PI$), is a glycoprotein of hepatic origin and a major inhibitor of serine proteases in plasma. The recognition that early onset pulmonary emphysema and childhood cirrhosis were often associated with abnormally low levels of $\alpha_1 AT$ prompted extensive investigation of the human protein and the genetically determined deficiency (reviewed in references 73,109,289,290). Corresponding proteins have been isolated from the plasma of several animal species including rats (204,412,425), mice (297,413), rabbits (233), rhesus monkeys (46), guinea pigs (227), and dogs (3,309). Moderate acute phase increases (two- to fourfold) of $\alpha_1 AT$ occur in most species.

Biochemistry and Physiology

The human $\alpha_1 AT$ molecule is a single polypeptide chain with three carbohydrate side chains (277). The homologous proteins in those animal species studied are relatively similar to the human molecule in carbohydrate content and molecular weight (Table 10.D.3). Human $\alpha_1 AT$ displays microheterogeneity (multiple bands) when examined by acid electrophoresis (137) or electrofocusing (64,214). Variation in sialic acid content accounts for much of the observed banding. Microheterogeneity has also been demonstrated by similar techniques for $\alpha_1 AT$ isolated from mice (251,297,413), monkeys (46), rabbits (233), and rats (204,412,425). The human protein is controlled by a single genetic locus with numerous independent alleles, a few of which are associated with abnormally low levels of $\alpha_1 AT$ in plasma. Single amino acid substitutions have been identified in the deficient proteins encoded by two alleles (73). In mice, two α_1-protease inhibitors have been isolated and were termed α_1-PI(E) and α_1-PI(T) to indicate the observed preferential inhibition of elastase and trypsin (302). The same proteins have been designated by other workers as α_1-antitrypsin and contrapsin, respectively (413, 414). Though similar in many respects, the two are antigenically distinct and are thought to be products of different genes (301,413). Rat serum was reported to contain at least two major α_1-protease inhibitors, also immunologically distinct and of differing inhibitory spectra (240, 368). A third rat α_1-PI, resembling mouse contrapsin, has been identified by some investigators (240). Three genetically determined electrophoretic phenotypes of $\alpha_1 AT$ have been reported to occur among rabbits of various strains, and they appear to be controlled by codominant alleles at a single autosomal locus (241).

Synthesis of $\alpha_1 AT$ occurs mainly in the liver (71,436), but also has been reported to occur in human leukocytes (6). In a single mouse species, the wild-derived *Mus caroli*, the kidneys also synthesize an $\alpha_1 AT$ which is detectable in urine but not in serum (43). The plasma half-life of 6 days for human $\alpha_1 AT$ (73) is long compared to those reported for the homologous protein in several animals. Values from 4 to 15.5 hours have been reported for the $T\frac{1}{2}$ of mouse $\alpha_1 AT$ (251,301) and 14 hours for the rat counterpart

Table 10.D.3. α_1-Antitrypsin in Various Species

Species	Molecular Weight (daltons)	Carbohydrate Content (%)	Plasma Concentration		References
			Normal (g/l)	Acute Phase (times normal)	
Human	50,000–55,000	12.0	1.0–1.6	2–4x	73,253,361
Rat[a]	50,000	10.3	1.10 ± 0.09	1.3–3x	1,232,310,412
Mouse[b]	53,000	9.6	Male 5.2 ± 0.6	1.5x	149,413
			Female 3.5 ± 0.2		
Rabbit[c]	57,000–59,000	11.4–11.8	1.03 ± 0.15	1.75x	233,235
Rhesus	60,000	11.7	2.5–3.7	ND[d]	46

[a] Normal plasma concentration given is from adult male Buffalo rats.

[b] Plasma levels given are for adults ICR albino mice. See text regarding values in young mice.

[c] Plasma levels given are for adult male New Zealand White Rabbits. See text regarding strain- and sex-related variation.

[d] ND = not determined in references cited.

(425). Rabbit α_1AT is cleared somewhat more slowly, with half-lives of 68.1 and 55.3 hours reported for the F- and S-forms, respectively (352).

The main function of α_1AT is thought to be to limit the activity of proteolytic enzymes released at sites of tissue damage. Studies in rats with experimentally induced granulomatous and neoplastic lesions showed that α_1AT accumulated in the abnormal tissues (207). Human α_1AT inhibits a number of enzymes in vitro including leukocyte elastase, chymotrypsin, cathepsin G, trypsin, plasmin, and thrombin. Evidence suggests that the inhibition of leukocyte elastase, an enzyme important in the development of pulmonary emphysema, is most significant in vivo (73). The spectra of enzymes inhibited by the various α_1-proteinase inhibitors isolated from several animals have been studied and, despite some differences, they were consistent with this proposed main function (236,240,282,302,368,414). Supporting this view, rats artificially rendered deficient in α_1AT were shown to have increased susceptibility to endotoxin-induced emphysema compared to similarly treated rats with normal α_1AT (52).

Human α_1AT is reported to reduce natural killer cell activity by decreasing the binding of natural killer cells to their specific target cells. This effect is apparently mediated by the carbohydrate moieties, rather than the antiprotease activity, of the α_1AT molecule (311).

Analysis

Immunochemical methods provide the most specific means of quantitating α_1AT in plasma.

These methods generally require specific antisera and, to obtain results in absolute terms, purified α_1AT to use in calibrating the assays. Rhesus monkey α_1AT was measured using commercially prepared radial immunodiffusion plates containing antihuman α_1AT, but incomplete cross-reactivity caused falsely high results if read from the calibration curve prepared using human standards (46). Lower values were obtained when calibrated with purified monkey α_1AT. Other immunochemical procedures applied to animal samples include electroimmunoassay (235,251,413), immunonephelometry, and ELISA (251). More recently described immunoassays for human α_1AT include luminometric and turbidimetric procedures (60,439). The need for monospecific antiserum and purified protein can be avoided with quantitative two-dimensional immunoelectrophoresis (1,87). Polyvalent antiserum to whole serum is used, and results can be expressed as a percentage relative to the concentration in pooled normal serum.

Functional assays measure spectrophotometrically the residual activity of trypsin solutions following incubation with dilutions of the serum being tested (130), and automated procedures have been described (296). The decrease in activity is a measure of the trypsin inhibitory capacity (TIC) of the serum, with results usually expressed in milligrams of trypsin inhibited per milliliter of serum. The specificity of this method is less than that of the immunochemical methods, and it is influenced by the substrate used to measure the residual activity. The use of low molecular weight substrates (e.g., benzoyl-arginine-*p*-nitroanilide) rather than proteins such as casein prevents α-macroglobulins from contributing to the trypsin inhibitory capacity, because αM-trypsin complexes remain active against the smaller synthetic compounds (253). The source of the trypsin employed also is important. Mouse α_1AT, for example, inhibited bovine, but not murine, trypsin, though its bovine-trypsin–inhibiting capacity was much weaker than that of the homologous human protein (413,414). Variation in the activity of the trypsin used can influence the assay as well. Standardization of the trypsin used (80), or reporting results relative to a pooled normal serum standard (289), will minimize this problem. A good correlation between trypsin inhibitory capacity and several immunochemical methods was found in a study involving murine α_1AT (251). Correlation between results of functional and immunologic assays was lower in human sera from diseased individuals as compared to healthy ones, possibly because of endogenous complex formation between the inhibitor protein and proteinases in serum (179).

Concentration

Normal plasma levels for α_1AT as determined by immunoassay methods in several species are given in Table 10.D.3. α_1AT levels in a number of other species were studied using functional assay methods, and considerable variation was shown (203,411). The levels in rats, mice, and guinea pigs were roughly twice the normal human range (411). Strain-related variation in α_1AT and contrapsin levels of mice has been reported (251,282,463). For example, as measured by nephelometry, pooled plasma from mature mice of strains CBA/J, C3H, and C3D2 contained 3.0 ± 0.7, 3.5 ± 0.6, and 4.6 ± 1.0 g/l of α_1AT, respectively (251).

In addition to the genetic influence mentioned before, the concentration of α_1AT in human plasma is affected by age and reproductive status. α_1AT levels in human newborns are slightly below the normal adult range, but they rise rapidly after a few days (156,361). Pregnant women at term have levels as much as twice normal (156), and contraceptive steroids may raise levels by about 50 per cent (254). Lactation in women has no effect on α_1AT levels (119), and gender per se does not appear to influence the concentration of α_1AT in adult humans (156).

Studies have shown that the behavior of α_1AT in mice differs markedly from the pattern in humans. Mice were born with levels only 15 to 20 per cent of the normal adult range and required roughly 25 to 40 days to reach adult levels (251,464). Though initially reported to remain unchanged throughout the gestation period (251,464), maternal α_1AT levels were found in a later study to undergo a sharp, transient increase associated with parturition (465). Lastly, male mice showed significantly higher levels than did females (Table 10.D.3) (282,413,464). Orchiectomy reduced α_1AT levels, whereas the administration of testosterone to female mice caused increased levels (463,465).

Mouse contrapsin levels also are low (<0.5 g/l) in newborns, but rise sharply at 2 to 3 weeks, and reach adult values (2 to 3 g/l) by 4 to 6 weeks of age (464). Maternal contrapsin levels are half normal (1 g/l) at term, show a transient increase with parturition, then gradually return to nonpregnant adult concentrations by 6 weeks postpartum (465). As with murine α_1AT, serum contrapsin concentration is greater (30 to 50 per cent) in males than in females (413,464). Contrapsin levels decrease with orchiectomy and increase with testosterone administration in females (463,465).

Rabbits also exhibit sexual dimorphism with regard to α_1AT, as females had concentrations 16 per cent lower than those of males. In addition, the genetically determined electrophoretic phenotypes are associated with quantitative differences in α_1AT concentration. The P phenotype α_1AT level was about 56 per cent of that associated with the M phenotype, whereas levels in the heterozygous MP phenotype were intermediate between those in the M and P types (241).

Human α_1AT increases in inflammatory and neoplastic disorders (73,147,154,289,450). In comparison to CRP and SAA, however, the increase is slow (days rather than hours) and of low magnitude (2- to 4-fold rather than 100- to 1,000-fold).

Reports on the α_1AT response to disease in rats show considerable variation. In one study, no increases were found following injection of turpentine, endotoxin, or diethylstilbestrol (425). In another experiment, slight (1.3-fold) increases were observed during acute inflammation and hepatoma growth, but they were considered insufficient to qualify α_1AT as a true acute phase reactant in the rat (232). However, other workers have reported more vigorous responses (1.8-fold normal) after induction of sterile inflammation (310). Furthermore, transplantation of tumors in rats resulted in a biphasic response involving α_1AT and several other acute phase reactants (1). In the first phase, attributed largely to trauma associated with the implantation, levels increased to about 2.5 times normal within 2 days. The second phase, attributed to effects of tumor growth, began on the fourth day and was characterized by a slow steady increase. Removal of the solid tumor led to a gradual return to normal levels (1).

Reports also vary regarding the behavior of mouse α_1AT (α_1PI-E) in response to inflammation. Some investigators found plasma levels to decrease slightly (465), whereas others reported a threefold increase in specific hepatic mRNA and an associated 35 to 50 per cent elevation in plasma levels after induction of the acute phase response (149). Plasma contrapsin (α_1PI-T) levels apparently remain unchanged in the acute phase response, despite reported increases in specific hepatic mRNA similar to those for α_1PI-E (149,465).

Induction of inflammation by injection of turpentine in rabbits caused a doubling of α_1AT levels by the third day after injection (235). In contrast, α_1AT in dogs is reported to show little to no change in a variety of experimentally induced inflammatory conditions (152).

α_1-ACID GLYCOPROTEIN

α_1-Acid glycoprotein (α_1AGP, orosomucoid) is a constituent of normal plasma that increases in concentration in the acute phase response. Human α_1AGP has been studied extensively (382). Corresponding proteins have been isolated from the plasma of several animal species, and it is best studied in rats and mice.

Biochemistry and Physiology

Human α_1AGP consists of a monomeric polypeptide with five carbohydrate side chains and an overall molecular weight of about 40,000 d. The carbohydrate chains account for 45 per cent of the molecular weight, and this protein alone comprises about 10 per cent of the total protein-bound carbohydrate of normal plasma (382).

Rat α_1AGP is similar in size (mol wt 43,000 d) and carbohydrate content (34 per cent) (212), as are the homologous proteins isolated from the plasma of rabbits, pigs, and chickens (79). The complete amino acid sequence of human α_1AGP, isolated from pooled plasma, has been determined (383). Many amino acid substitutions and a significant homology to portions of human immunoglobulin G were noted. The amino acid sequence of the rat homolog, inferred from the mRNA nucleotide sequence, has also been determined and is notably similar to that of the human protein (356). Comparison of the amino acid sequences derived from α_1AGP cDNA sequences of rats and mice showed still greater homology between the rodent proteins (101).

Human α_1AGP exists in several genetically determined variants, demonstrated by starch gel electrophoresis or isoelectric focusing, which differ in either amino acid sequence or composition of the carbohydrate side chains (382). Microheterogeneity also has been noted on acid electrophoresis of α_1AGP derived from the serum of rats, nonhuman primates, dogs, horses, cows, and chickens (47). Crossed immunoaffinoelectrophoresis using concanavalin A has been employed to study the carbohydrate variations in human (389) and rat (116,232,287) proteins, the latter of which is resolved into three to four peaks by this method.

Based on studies of specific hepatic mRNA and its cell-free translation products, α_1AGP is polymorphic in its expression in different strains and species of mice. Inbred strains of *Mus musculus* typically expressed two forms, termed AGP-1 and AGP-2 (28), whereas wild-derived species expressed up to six different polypeptide forms (27). It is thought likely that multiple genes are involved in encoding for murine α_1AGP (27,101). However, studies in the rat indicate there is but a single α_1AGP gene (262,353).

α_1AGP is synthesized in the liver, and the elevated serum levels observed during acute phase responses are due to increased production (105,209). The hepatic biosynthesis of α_1AGP and the kinetics of its induction have been studied (210,298,354,355). The increased α_1AGP synthesis associated with acute inflammation is due to accumulation of specific mRNA (116,354) which results largely from increased gene transcription (50,242). Monocyte-derived cytokines injected into rats mimicked the acute phase increase in plasma levels (457). Gluco-corticoids also are involved either directly by stimulating gene transcription and/or indirectly by inducing another protein which subsequently enhances α_1AGP gene transcription or mRNA stability (242,353,433). The serum half-life of α_1AGP is 5.5 days in humans (449), about 1 day in rats (243), and 3.7 days in dogs (468). Studies of α_1AGP catabolism in rats indicate that several tissues, including kidney, liver, muscle, and hide, may be active in degrading the protein (243).

The function of α_1AGP is not known; however, many roles have been postulated (summary in references 382 and 393). The iodinated protein was shown to accumulate in granulo-matous and neoplastic lesions in rats, suggesting a possible role in modulating inflammatory or cell proliferative processes (393). Human α_1AGP inhibited neutrophil activation by a variety of stimuli in vitro (103). The human protein, and especially the agalacto/asialo derivative, suppressed a number of immune functions of mouse spleen cells (36), and similar effects of the native protein on human peripheral blood lymphocytes were demonstrated (83,84). Natural killer cell activity was inhibited by α_1AGP, possibly as a result of its interaction with a cytotoxic factor secreted from natural killer cells following effector-target interaction (311). Human α_1AGP was also shown to exert an inhibitory influence on platelet aggregation induced by ADP, collagen, or thrombin (102). Once again, the desialyzed protein was more potent than the native form. This finding may be important because the sialic acid content of α_1AGP in humans with some chronic diseases was found to be lower than normal (382,389). Platelet activating factor appears to bind to α_1AGP, an interaction that may serve to stabilize, transport, and regulate the activity of platelet activating factor (275). Many drugs bind to α_1AGP in plasma, an interaction with potentially important pharmacokinetic and pharmacodynamic consequences when the concentration of this protein is altered in disease conditions (459,466).

Analysis

Methods for specific determination of α_1AGP concentration which have been applied to animal samples include radial immunodiffusion (298,392), rocket immunoelectrophoresis (152, 354), immunonephelometry (105), quantitative precipitation (211), immunoturbidimetric assay (113), zone immunoelectrophoresis (9), and two-dimensional immunoelectrophoresis (1). In addition, ELISA (125) and luminometric assays (60) have been described for quantitating the human protein.

Isolation of α_1AGP is facilitated by its low isoionic point which gives the molecule a strong negative net charge at pH above 4.0 and by its marked solubility near neutrality. Several isolation procedures were reviewed by Schmid (382). A relatively rapid and simple two-step purification procedure applied to rat serum was described by Shibata et al (392). High-performance liquid chromatography was used to isolate purified human α_1AGP from small volumes of plasma (188).

Concentration

Reported levels of α_1AGP in normal human serum vary somewhat but generally range from 0.5 to 1.0 mg/ml (147,382,450). Levels are not affected by gender. An approximately 20 per cent reduction was reported in pregnant women at term (156). Administration of oral contraceptives caused a similar lowering of α_1AGP concentration in women (254). Newborn infants had levels roughly one third those of adults (156).

The reported normal levels for rat α_1AGP vary widely, ranging from as low as 0.064 mg/ml (354) to as high as 2.3 mg/ml (211). In several other studies, intermediate levels were reported, ranging from 0.13 to 0.77 mg/ml (105,298,392). These studies employed several different assays and various strains of rats, and so the source of this variation cannot be determined. No reports documenting gender-related variation in α_1AGP concentration in rats were found. However, administration of pharmacologic doses of estrogen to male rats both increased the serum levels of the protein (14-fold) and changed its glycosylation as evidenced by increased relative proportions of the concanavalin A reactive peaks on crossed immunoaffinoelectrophoresis (116). Phenobarbital treatment in rats also increased serum α_1AGP levels and effected changes in the oligosaccharide structure of the protein (287). α_1-Acid glycoprotein levels in neonatal rats remained very low until the time of weaning (about 2 week of age), at which time its concentration increased rapidly, reaching 80 per cent of the adult level at 36 days of age (420). Normal dog serum contained 0.2 to 1.0 mg/ml of α_1AGP as determined by electroimmunoassay (152) or single radial immunodiffusion (468).

Acute phase increases in human α_1AGP generally range 2 to 4 times normal levels (245). Several studies have documented such changes in infectious diseases (154), in the postoperative period (147), and in other conditions including autoimmune and neoplastic disorders (450).

The magnitude of the α_1AGP response in rats is greater than that in humans. Increases of 5- to 20-fold following induction of inflammation were reported (105,116,298,392). This response was fairly rapid in rats. Elevations were detectable at 12 to 16 hours and peak levels were reached by 24 to 72 hours (105,116,211,232). In addition to elevating serum α_1AGP levels in rats, inflammation also altered the concanavalin A immunoaffinoelectrophoretic pattern of the protein in favor of the reactive forms (116,232). Neonatal rats, despite their naturally low endogenous α_1AGP levels, are capable of responding with marked increases when challenged with inflammatory stimuli. Injection of turpentine into 4-day-old rats caused a two-stage increase in α_1AGP levels. The concentration climbed slowly for the first 24 hours, then rose more rapidly to peak at better than 10-fold normal by 3 days after injection (420).

In dogs with turpentine-induced inflammation, increased levels of α_1AGP were detected at 6 to 9 hours and peak levels, ranging from 2.6 to 3.7 mg/ml, were reached at 3 to 8 days after injection (468). Increases as great as 17-fold have been reported in dogs with inflammatory conditions (152).

Genetic analysis of the α_1AGP acute phase response in mice indicates variation among different strains and species. In most inbred strains of *M. musculus*, the two forms (AGP-1 and AGP-2) are equally inducible by acute inflammation; however, the predominant expression switches to AGP-2 in chronic inflammation (163). However, mice of strain CE/J lack detectable mRNA for AGP-2, apparently because of a deletion of the coding elements (27). Polymorphism of α_1AGP expression is great among wild-derived species of mice, as exemplified by *Mus spretus*. Mice of this species possess an electrophoretic variant of

AGP-2 that is more basic and smaller than that of inbred strains. In addition, although all *M. spretus* mice carry an AGP-1 allele, not all individuals respond with increased levels of the corresponding protein when challenged with inflammation, a finding that suggests the presence of regulatory variation within the population (28).

Neoplasia also is associated with increased α_1AGP in animals. Sarcoma implantation in rats resulted in a five- to sixfold increase in serum levels by 2 weeks after implantation (392). Morris hepatoma implantation in rats caused a biphasic α_1AGP response. The initial rapid increase, which reached ninefold normal on day 4 after implantation, likely reflected inflammation associated with the implantation procedure. Subsequently, levels decreased to about fivefold normal on day 14, at which time a slower, secondary increase began which was related to tumor growth (232).

CERULOPLASMIN

Ceruloplasmin (Cp) (ferroxidase and copper oxidase) is a metalloprotein with intense blue color that is found in the plasma of all mammals. About 90 per cent of the copper present in plasma is bound to this protein, yet copper transport is but one of its several possible functions.

Biochemistry and Physiology

Ceruloplasmin is a glycoprotein (8 to 9 per cent carbohydrate) that migrates as an α_2-globulin. Human Cp is a monomeric protein with a molecular weight of 128,000 to 135,000 d (65,306) and 6 to 7 copper atoms per molecule (340,373). The amino acid sequence for the entire human protein has been determined (416). It is structurally related to coagulation factors V and VIII, possibly indicating a common evolutionary origin for the group (85). Rat Cp was purified and found to have a similar molecular weight (124,000 d) but somewhat different amino acid composition (267). Ceruloplasmins of pig, horse, and rabbit are reported to be single peptides with a molecular size similar to that of the human (372). Bovine Cp has a molecular weight of 125,000 d and contains approximately 4 copper atoms per molecule (68). Chicken Cp has a molecular weight of 158,000 d with 5 copper atoms per molecule. It has amino acid composition and electrophoretic mobility similar to those of human protein, but appears to be more labile than mammalian Cp (401).

Genetically determined variants were demonstrated by starch gel electrophoresis in humans (reviewed in reference 340), pigs (206), and rats (404,405). The porcine variants were noted in sera from the Landrace breed. Three phenotypes were seen, which appeared to be controlled by two allelic genes at a single locus. No polymorphism was found in a study of numerous chimpanzee sera (339). Another study analyzed small numbers of samples from 10 primate species by polyacrylamide gel electrophoresis (274). Variation in Cp migration between different species was evident, but no variants within a species could be proven. Ceruloplasmin migrated as a single band except in the one spider monkey tested, which displayed two bands of equal concentration.

Ceruloplasmin is synthesized in the liver and its production is reported to be affected by several factors including copper (133) and various hormones (132,135,448 reviewed in 106). The incorporation of copper into Cp takes place in the liver (66,197). Rats fed a copper-deficient diet were found to have little or no Cp oxidase activity and the apoceruloplasmin concentration was approximately 25 per cent that of normal rats (196). Removal of sialic acid with resulting exposure of galactosyl residues caused rapid clearance of Cp from the circulation (178,190,428). Hepatic uptake of native Cp appears to be mediated by liver endothelial cells, which bind, internalize, desialate, and then release the protein for subsequent galactosyl receptor-mediated uptake by hepatocytes (419). In vitro experiments have shown that dexamethasone increased both synthesis and secretion of Cp by cultured hepatocytes and that adrenaline increased the incorporation of copper into newly synthesized Cp (448). Interleukin-1 increases plasma Cp and is likely important in acute phase responses caused by inflammation (57,445).

Several potential functions, a few of which follow, have been proposed for Cp. It may in fact be a protein of multiple functions. Because it contains most of the copper present in plasma, Cp has been studied for its role in the transport of this element (70,198,312,317). Ceruloplasmin has significant oxidase activity, which may be involved in its physiologic function in several ways. It is likely involved in the mobilization of stored iron by oxidizing it to permit incorporation into circulating transferrin (313,314, 345). Ceruloplasmin may also be involved in limiting autoxidation by abolishing the catalytic action of free iron in this process (4,123) and by acting as a scavenger of superoxide anion radicals (166,181). Administration of zinc or 13-cis-retinoic acid to rats with adjuvant arthritis augmented the increase in serum Cp levels and was associated with a reduction in inflammation (107). One study aimed at identifying anti-inflammatory activity by injecting Cp together with an experimental irritant in copper-deficient rats was interpreted as yielding positive results (i.e., reduced swelling compared to irritant alone). However, a similar experiment found no such effect in rats consuming a normal diet (299). Mouse Cp recently was reported to potentiate immune function in vitro, enhancing antibody formation and macrophase activation and restoring the depressed immune responses of tumor-bearing mice (237).

Analysis

Ceruloplasmin concentration has been measured by both functional and immunologic assays. Human Cp oxidase activity in serum and synovial fluid deteriorates in storage even when frozen, whereas the immunoreactive levels are much more stable (182). Fresh specimens are therefore important for accurate results.

Several functional methods for quantitation of Cp, based on its oxidase activity, use p-phenylenediamine as a substrate (108,189). Care must be taken to avoid contamination of samples or reagents with traces of copper or iron because this can result in nonenzymatic degradation of p-phenylenediamine (108). Serum or heparinized plasma may be used, but EDTA should be avoided because it inhibits the oxidase activity of Cp (48,189). The optimum pH for the reaction varies with the species and it should be adjusted accordingly (48).

Immunologic assays that have been applied to the quantitation of Cp include radial immunodiffusion, electroimmunoassay, immunonephelometry, radioimmunoassay, and two-dimensional immunoelectrophoresis. Antisera to Cp show some cross-reactivity between species. Rabbit antihuman Cp cross-reacted with

Cp from dogs and rhesus monkeys (152,340). Several immunologic methods have been evaluated and compared as applied to measurement of human Cp (63,337).

Concentration

The normal Cp level in serum from human adults is 30.4±0.5 mg/dl (108). Ceruloplasmin in newborns is low (about 14 mg/dl) compared to that in adults (156). Levels increase to 40 to 45 mg/dl at 2 to 3 years of age before declining to the normal adult range by 12 years of age (108). The menstrual cycle has no effect (108), but pregnancy (156), lactation (119), and contraceptive drugs (254) cause increases of about two- to threefold. Genetic factors may influence Cp levels in humans (108).

Normal Cp levels were determined for a number of animal species and were found to vary considerably (48). Female rats of the Lewis and Brown Norway strains had higher Cp levels than did males (404). Age influenced Cp concentration in normal Sprague-Dawley and Wistar rats (134,135). Ceruloplasmin was low at birth (1.4±0.83 mg/dl), but increased quickly to about 20 mg/dl by 20 days of age. Thereafter, the rate of increase slowed, and adult levels of about 30 to 35 mg/dl were reached by 1 year of age (134). Guinea pigs at birth had serum Cp levels 21 per cent those of adults; concentrations neared the adult range by 30 days of age (400). Pregnancy in rabbits resulted in consistent increases in Cp levels (up to threefold) during the second half of gestation (426). Administration of estradiol increased Cp levels by about 75 per cent in female rats (132). Quantitative differences in serum Cp were demonstrated in a study involving 27 inbred strains of mice (278). Differences between strains were statistically significant and the degree of heritability was considerable. Reduced Cp levels were reported in mice of the X-linked mottled locus, particularly the tortoiseshell (Mo^{to}) and brindled (Mo^{br}) mutants (69,201,390). The mottled mutant mice are animal models for Menkes kinky hair disease in man which is also sex linked. Lewis rats had Cp levels two- to threefold those of Brown Norway rats. This strain difference was reported to be regulated by two alleles at an autosomal locus (404).

Humans respond with elevated Cp levels in various inflammatory and neoplastic conditions (108,147,154,340,450). In comparison to several other acute phase reactants however, the increase is relatively low in magnitude (1.5- to 2-fold) and slow to develop.

Similar conditions result in elevated Cp levels in animals. In rats with carrageenan-induced inflammation, serum Cp increased roughly twofold by 22 hours after injection of the irritant (99). Elevated levels have also been reported in rats intoxicated by orally administered pyrrolizidine alkaloids (408). Treatment with oxyphenylbutazone and hydrocortisone failed to inhibit the acute phase increase of serum Cp in rats with induced inflammatory conditions (115). Dogs with bacterial arthritis or turpentine-induced inflammation showed similar moderate increases (152). Chicks, which normally have low plasma Cp levels, showed marked elevation when subjected to salmonella infection (401). Ceruloplasmin levels in rabbits with turpentine-induced pleurisy had increased by 12 hours and peaked at two to threefold normal by 48 to 72 hours after induction (162). Ceruloplasmin has been reported to be a marker of neoplastic activity in rabbits bearing the VX-2 carcinoma (426). In this model Cp increased four- to eightfold, often before the tumor could be detected by palpation. Ceruloplasmin levels returned to normal if tumors regressed, but remained high if metastasis developed. However, control rabbits with induced subcutaneous abscesses showed no significant change in Cp levels in this study. Further investigation of this model showed that the tumor cells produced an unidentified factor which, when injected into normal rabbits, caused Cp levels to rise (427). Because the tumor also produced a 20-fold increase in plasma prostaglandin E$_2$ and because indomethacin given at the time of tumor implantation largely inhibited the increase in Cp, the increase in Cp may be related to arachidonic acid metabolism (440). In another study, rats with transplanted tumors showed much less pronounced elevations (50 per cent increase) in serum Cp levels (1).

FIBRINOGEN

Fibrinogen is a large, poorly soluble β-globulin present in the plasma of all vertebrates. The conversion of fibrinogen (factor I) to insoluble fibrin is the central event in blood coagulation. Fibrinogen qualifies as an acute phase reactant because its plasma concentration increases in response to tissue injury of various types. The synthesis, structure, and function of fibrinogen were the topic of a comprehensive review (122).

Biochemistry and Physiology

The fibrinogen molecule is composed of three pairs of covalently linked, nonidentical polypeptide chains (termed A_α, B_β, and γ) with a relatively low (4 per cent) carbohydrate content. The overall molecular weight of rat fibrinogen was determined to be 340,000 d (434). Fibrinogens from various vertebrates are fairly constant in their physical properties (121), and binding studies suggest homology of the functionally important polymerization domains (86).

Plasma fibrinogen is synthesized by hepatocytes and has a relatively short half-life ranging from 1.3 to 3.4 days in various species (231). Platelets also contain fibrinogen which, though apparently the product of the same gene, is thought to be synthesized in megakaryocytes (221,456). Numerous studies have been aimed at identifying factors involved in the regulation of normal and acute phase synthesis of fibrinogen by the liver. Substances that have been investigated in this regard include leukocytic endogenous mediator (218,219), glucocorticoids (169,213,216,342), corticotropin (10,82), endotoxin (169,234,461), sex hormones (159,318, 319), fibrinogen and fibrin/fibrinogen degradation products (11,148,224,225,343), hepatocyte-stimulating factor (29,360), prostaglandins (72,158), and biogenic amines (406). A complex interaction of many factors is likely responsible for controlling synthesis in various physiologic and pathologic states.

The main function of fibrinogen is to provide substrate for the formation of fibrin. The essential assembly events have been outlined as follows (122,184). Initial activation results from the action of thrombin which cleaves a small polar peptide (fibrinopeptide A) from the amino-terminus of the $A\alpha$ chain. This trimming results in the formation of fibrin monomers which then undergo spontaneous polymerization to form long thin protofibrils. Fibrinopeptide B is released, and lateral association of the protofibrils leads to the formation of thick, highly interconnected fibers. These are eventually stabilized further by the factor $XIIIa/Ca^{2+}$-catalyzed addition of several interchain covalent bonds. Fibrinogen also contributes to hemostasis by acting as a cofactor for platelet aggregation induced by ADP and other stimuli (269). Defective platelet-fibrinogen interaction appears to be the cause of platelet dysfunction in hereditary canine thrombopathia (76).

Congenital abnormalities of fibrinogen documented in humans include both quantitative defects (afibrinogenemia and hypofibrinogenemia) and qualitative defects (dysfibrinogenemia). These rare conditions have been well summarized in recent articles (51,280). Documentation of similar problems in animals is scarce. Afibrinogenemia in goats (62) and hypofibrinogenemia in dogs (217) have been reported.

Analysis

Methods for quantitation of plasma fibrinogen fall into three main categories: biologic (clottable protein), physicochemical (precipitable protein), and immunologic. The strengths and weaknesses of a number of methods have been studied and compared (136,176,228).

In the clottable protein methods, fibrinogen in the plasma is converted to fibrin by the addition of thrombin (or Ca^{2+} in some methods). The separated clot may then be rinsed, dried, and weighed, with the weight being taken as an estimation of the initial fibrinogen content of the plasma (21). Alternatively, the rinsed, separated clot may be dissolved in NaOH or alkaline urea solutions in which the protein is then measured spectrophotometrically (54,231,349). Another variation that has gained widespread acceptance for clinical use is the thrombin clotting time (89). With this method, the time required for clot formation to occur following the addition of thrombin to the diluted plasma sample is inversely proportional to the concentration of fibrinogen in the plasma. The clotting time obtained is then compared with that of a standardized fibrinogen preparation. High concentrations of heparin or fibrinolytic degradation products may interfere with these methods. In addition, fibrinogens with abnormal function (dysfibrinogenemia) may not be quantitated accurately.

Physicochemical methods take advantage of the relatively poor solubility of fibrinogen to more or less selectively precipitate it from the plasma. Ammonium sulfate (324) and glycine (222) have been used to precipitate fibrinogen, which may then be measued by turbidometry or spectrophotometry. Fibrinogen can also be precipitated by heating the plasma to 56°C for 3 minutes. The fibrinogen content can then be quantitated by microscopic measurement of the precipitate column obtained by centrifugation (53,281).

Immunologic assays that have been applied to the quantitation of fibrinogen include electroimmunoassay, immunoturbidometry, and immunonephelometry. These methods measure immunoreactive fibrinogen but do not correlate with the functionality of the molecules. They are useful in the detection of dysfibrinogenemias, which are recognized by the discrepancy between apparently low fibrinogen levels measured by thrombin clotting time and normal to high levels measured by immunologic methods.

Concentration

Fibrinogen concentration in normal human plasma ranges from about 200 to 400 mg/dl (121) and is not influenced by age or gender. Levels increase during normal pregnancy and with the administration of contraceptive medications (156,361).

The reported normal fibrinogen levels in plasma from various animal species also range from 200 to 400 mg/dl (264,385). Circadian fluctuation in plasma fibrinogen concentration has been reported in normal rats (55). Pregnancy was associated with a two- to threefold increase in fibrinogen in the bitch, and administration of progesterone resulted in a smaller but still significant increase (159). Both increased (406) and unchanged (295) fibrinogen levels have been reported in pregnant rabbits. Slight (25 per cent) increases were noted in a group of pregnant rhesus monkeys (351).

Pathologic processes in humans may result in increased or decreased fibrinogen levels. Increases are seen with many conditions associated with tissue damage including surgery (98), myocardial infarction (215), and various infectious diseases (154). Marked increases have also been noted in cases of membranoproliferative glomerulonephritis (361). Decreased fibrinogen may be seen in some phases of chronic liver disease (176) and disseminated intravascular

coagulation as well as in the previously mentioned congenital disorders.

Disease-related variations in plasma fibrinogen concentration in animal species parallel those described in humans. Increases are seen with various inflammatory conditions. Acute phase increases in hepatic synthesis appear to be controlled at the mRNA level (384). Injection of turpentine, for example, results in two- to fivefold increases in plasma fibrinogen by 40 to 50 hours after injection in dogs, rats, and rabbits (105,152,223,230,235). Increased levels have also been reported in dogs with various naturally occurring inflammatory and neoplastic conditions (307,381). Glomerulonephritis in dogs has sometimes been associated with marked increases (up to 1,300 mg/dl) in dogs (381). Decreased fibrinogen has been reported in some dogs with advanced liver disease (381) and in dogs with disseminated intravascular coagulation (139).

REFERENCES

1. Abd-el-Fattah M, Reiner, Scherer, Fouad FM, Ruhenstroth-Bauer G (1981) Kinetics of the acute-phase reaction in rats after tumor transplantation. Cancer Res 41: 2548–2555
2. Abernathy TJ (1937) Studies on the somatic C polysaccharide of pneumococcus. II. The precipitation reaction in animals with experimentally induced pneumococcic infection. J Exp Med 65: 75–89
3. Abrams WR, Kimbel P, Weinbaum G (1978) Purification and characterization of canine α_1-antiproteinase. Biochemistry 17: 3556–3561
4. Al-Timimi D, Dormandy TL (1977) The inhibition of lipid autoxidation by human caeruloplasmin. Biochem J 168: 283–288
5. Anders RF, Natvig JB, Sletten K, Husby G, Nordstoga K (1977) Amyloid-related serum protein SAA from three animal species: Comparison with human SAA. J Immunol 118: 229–234
6. Andersen MM (1983) Leukocyte-associated plasma proteins. Scand J Clin Lab Invest 43: 49–59
7. Anderson HC, McCarty M (1950) Determination of C-reactive protein in the blood as a measure of the activity of the disease process in acute rheumatic fever. Am J Med 8: 445
8. Anderson HC, McCarty M (1951) The occurrence in the rabbit of an acute phase protein analogous to human C-reactive protein. J Exp Med 93: 25–36
9. Appel M, Davy J, Duvand G, Biou D, Feger J, Agneray J (1984) Zone immunoelectrophoresis assay applied to α_1-acid glycoprotein secretion by isolated rat hepatocytes. Experientia 40: 1443–1445
10. Atencio AC, Chao P-Y, Chen AY, Reeve EB (1969) Fibrinogen response to corticotropin preparations in rabbits. Am J Phys 216: 773–780
11. Atencio AC, Joiner K, Reeve EB (1969) Exper-

imental and control systems studies of plasma fibrinogen regulation in rabbits. Am J Physiol 216: 764–772

12. Bailey PT, Abeles FB, Hauer EC, Mapes CA (1976) Intracerebroventricular administration of leukocytic endogenous mediators (LEM) in the rat. Proc Soc Exp Biol Med 153: 419–423

13. Baldo BA (1982) Additional inhibitors of rat serum acute phase α_2-macroglobulin levels. Effect of 6-mercaptopurine and some lipoxygenase and cyclooxygenase inhibitors. Agents Actions 12: 340–343

14. Baldo BA (1982) Inflammation, counter irritation and rat serum acute phase α_2-macroglobulin levels. Agents Actions 12: 333–339

15. Baldo BA, Chow SC, Evers C (1981) A new screen for anti-inflammatory agents. Estimation of rat serum acute phase α_2-macroglobulin levels using an electroimmunoassay. Agents Actions 11: 482–489

16. Baltz ML, deBeer FC, Feinstein A, Munn EA, Milstein CP, Fletcher TC, March JF, Taylor J, Bruton C, Clamp JR, Davies AJS, Pepys MB (1982) Phylogenetic aspects of C-reactive protein and related proteins. Ann NY Acad Sci 389: 49–73

17. Baltz ML, Dyck RF, Pepys MB (1980) Amyloid P-component in mice injected with casein: Identification in amyloid deposits and in the cytoplasm of hepatocytes. Immunology 41: 59–65

18. Baltz ML, Dyck RF, Pepys MB (1985) Studies of the *in vivo* synthesis and catabolism of serum amyloid P component (SAP) in the mouse. Clin Exp Immunol 59: 235–242

19. Baltz ML, Gomer K, Davies AJS, Evans DJ, Klaus GGB, Pepys MB (1980) Differences in the acute phase responses of serum amyloid P-component (SAP) and C3 to injections of casein or bovine serum albumin in amyloid-susceptible and -resistant mouse strains. Clin Exp Immunol 39: 355–360

20. Baltz ML, Rowe IF, Pepys MB (1985) *In vivo* turnover studies of C-reactive protein. Clin Exp Immunol 59: 243–250

21. Bang HO (1957) Quantitative determination of fibrinogen in plasma. Gram's method modified. Scand J Clin Lab Invest 9: 205–207

22. Barka N, Tomasi J-P, Stadtbaeder S (1985) Use of whole *Streptococcus pneumoniae* cells as a solid phase sorbent for C-reactive protein measurement by ELISA. J Immunol Methods 82: 57–63

23. Barrett AJ, Starkey PM (1973) The interaction of α_2-macroglobulin with proteinases. Characteristics and specificity of the reaction, and a hypothesis concerning its molecular mechanism. Biochem J 133: 709–724

24. Bartoloni C, Guidi L, Baroni R, Wieser A, Barone C, Gambassi G (1985) Immune complexes and acute phase proteins in human cancer: preliminary evaluation by laser nephelometric techniques. Oncology 42: 150–156

25. Bauer J, Weber W, Tran-Thi T-A, Northoff G-H, Decker K, Gerok W, Heinrich PC (1985) Murine interleukin-1 stimulates α_2-macroglobulin synthesis in rat hepatocyte primary cultures. FEBS Letters 190: 271–274

26. Baum LL, James KK, Glaviano RR, Gewurz H (1986) Possible role for C-reactive protein in the human natural killer cell response. J Exp Med 157: 301–311

27. Baumann H, Berger FG (1985) Genetics and evolution of the acute phase proteins in mice. Mol Gen Genet 201: 505–512

28. Baumann H, Held WA, Berger FG (1984) The acute phase response of mouse liver. J Biol Chem 259: 566–573

29. Baumann H, Hill RE, Sander DN, Jahreis GP (1986) Regulation of major acute-phase plasma proteins by hepatocyte-stimulating factors of human squamous carcinoma cells. J Cell Biol 102: 370–383

30. Bausserman LL, Herbert PN, McAdams KPWJ (1980) Heterogeneity of human serum amyloid A proteins. J Exp Med 152: 641–656

31. Bell SC (1979) Immunochemical identity of "decidualization-associated protein" and α_2 acute-phase macroglobulin in the pregnant rat. J Reprod Immunol 1: 193–206

32. Bell SC (1979) Synthesis of "decidualization-associated protein" in tissues of the rat uterus and placenta during pregnancy. J Reprod Fert 56: 255–262

33. Bell SC (1980) Effects of oestradiol and progesterone on the concentration of α_2-macroglobulin in the sera of injured male and female rats. J Endocrinol 86: 189–191

34. Benditt EP, Hoffman JS, Eriksen N (1982) SAA, an apoprotein of HDL: Its structure and function. Ann NY Acad Sci 389: 183–189

35. Benjamin DC, Weimer HE (1966) Synthesis of α_2-AP (acute phase) globulin of rat serum by the liver. Nature 209: 1032–1033

36. Bennett M, Schmid K (1980) Immunosuppression by human plasma α_1-acid glycoprotein: Importance of the carbohydrate moiety. Proc Natl Acad Sci USA 77: 6109–6113

37. Benson MD (1982) In vitro synthesis of the acute phase reactant SAA by hepatocyes. Ann NY Acad Sci 389: 116–119

38. Benson MD, Aldo-Benson M (1979) Effect of purified protein SAA on immune response *in vitro*: Mechanisms of suppression. J Immunol 122: 2077–2082

39. Benson MD, Aldo-Benson MA (1982) SAA suppression of in vitro antibody response. Ann NY Acad Sci 389: 121–125

40. Benson MD, Aldo-Benson MA, Shirahama T, Borel Y, Cohen AS (1975) Suppression of *in vitro* antibody response by a serum factor (SAA) in experimentally induced amyloidosis. J Exp Med 142: 236–241

41. Benson MD, Eyanson S, Fineberg NS (1986) Serum amyloid A in carcinoma of the lung. Cancer 57: 1783–1787

42. Benson MD, Scheinberg MA, Shirahama T, Cathcart ES, Skinner M (1977) Kinetics of serum amyloid protein A in casein-induced murine amyloidosis. J Clin Invest 59: 412–417

43. Berger FG, Baumann H (1985) An evolutionary switch in tissue-specific gene expression. Abundant expression of α_1-antitrypsin in the kidney of a wild mouse species. J Biol Chem 260: 1160–1165

44. Berman S, Gewurz H, Mold C (1986) Binding of C-reactive protein to nucleated cells leads to comp-

lement activation without cytolysis. J Immunol 136: 1354–1359

45. Berne BH, Dray S, Knight KL (1971) Immunological relationships of serum α-macroglobulins in the human, rat, and rabbit. Proc Soc Exp Biol Med 138: 531–535

46. Berninger RW, Mathis RK (1976) Isolation and characterization of α1-antitrypsin from rhesus-monkey serum. Biochem J 159: 95–104

47. Binette JP (1968) Patterns of polymorphism of α_1-acid glycoprotein in different species. Biochim Biophys Acta 154: 234–235

48. Bingley JB, Dick AT (1969) The pH optimum for ceruloplasmin oxidase activity in the plasma of several species of animal. Clin Chim Acta 25: 480–482

49. Biran H, Friedman N, Neumann L, Pras M, Shainkin-Kestenbaum R (1986) Serum amyloid A (SAA) variations in patients with cancer: Correlation with disease activity, stage, primary site, and prognosis. J Clin Pathol 39: 794–797

50. Birch HE, Schreiber G (1986) Transcriptional regulation of plasma protein synthesis during inflammation. J Biol Chem 261: 8077–8080

51. Bithell TC (1985) Hereditary dysfibrinogenemia. Clin Chem 31: 509–516

52. Blackwood RA, Moret J, Mandl I, Turino GM (1984) Emphysema induced by intravenously administered endotoxin in an α_1-antitrypsin-deficient rat model. Am Rev Resp Dis 130: 231–236

53. Blaisdell FS, Dodds WJ (1977) Evaluation of two microhematocrit methods for quantitating plasma fibrinogen. J Am Vet Med Assoc 171: 340–342

54. Blomback B (1958) On the properties of fibrinogen and fibrin. Arkiv Kemi 12: 99

55. Bocci V, Viti A (1971) Factors regulating plasma protein synthesis. I. Circadian fluctuations of plasma fibrinogen mass in the rat. Am J Physiol 221: 719–725

56. Bornstein DL (1982) Leukocytic pyrogen: a major mediator of the acute phase reaction. Ann NY Acad Sci 389: 322–337

57. Bornstein DL, Walsh EC (1978) Endogenous mediators of the acute-phase reaction. I. Rabbit granulocytic pyrogen and its chromatographic subfractions. J Lab Clin Med 91: 236–245

58. Borth W, Teodorescu M (1986) Inactivation of human interluekin-2 (IL-2) by α_2-macroglobulin-trypsin complexes. Immunology 57: 367–371

59. Bout D, Joseph M, Pontet M, Vorng H, Deslee D, Capron A (1986) Rat resistance to Schistosmiasis: Platelet-mediated cytotoxicity induced by C-reactive protein. Science 231: 153–156

60. Braun J, Schultek T, Tegtmeier K-F, Florenz A, Rhode C, Wood WG (1986) Luminometric assays of seven acute-phase proteins in minimal volumes of serum, plasma, sputum, and bronchoalveolar lavage. Clin Chem 32: 743–747

61. Breathnach SM, Mekose SM, Bhogal B, deBeer FC, Dyck RF, Tennant G, Black MM, Pepys MB (1981) Amyloid P component is located on elastic fibre microfibrils in normal human tissue. Nature 293: 652–654

62. Breukink HJ, Hart HC, Arkel C, Veldon NA, Watering CC (1972) Congenital afibrinogenemia in goats. Zentralbl Veterinaermed Reihe A 19: 661–676

63. Buffone GJ, Brett EM, Lewis SA, Losefsohn M, Hicks JM (1979) Limitations of immunochemical measurement of ceruloplasmin. Clin Chem 25: 749–751

64. Buffone GJ, Stennis BJ, Schimbor CM (1983) Isoelectric focusing in agarose: Classification of genetic variants of α_1-antitrypsin. Clin Chem 29: 328–331

65. Burnett D, Chandy KG (1983) Evidence for a single-chain structure of native human ceruloplasmin using sodium dodecyl sulfate-polyacrylamide-crossed immunoelectrophoresis. Anal Biochem 128: 317–322

66. Bush JA, Mahoney JP, Markowitz H, Gubler CF, Cartwright GE, Wintrobe MN (1955) Studies on copper metabolism. XVI. Radioactive copper studies in normal subjects and in patients with hepatocellular degeneration. J Clin Invest 34: 1766–1778

67. Cabana VG, Gewurz H, Siegel JN (1983) Inflammation-induced changes in rabbit CRP and plasma lipoproteins. J Immunol 130: 1736–1742

68. Calabrese L, Malatesta F, Barra D (1981) Purification and properties of bovine ceruloplasmin. Biochem J 199: 667–673

69. Camakaris J, Danks DM, Mann JR (1979) Copper metabolism in mottled mutants. Biochem J 180: 597–604

70. Campbell CH, Brown R, Linder MC (1981) Circulating ceruloplasmin is an important source of copper for normal and malignant animal cells. Biochim Biophys Acta 678: 27–38

71. Carlson J, Stenflo J (1982) The biosynthesis of rat α_1-antitrypsin. J. Biol Chem 257: 12987–12994

72. Carlson TH, Fradl DC, Leonard BD, Wentland SH, Reeve EB (1977) Fibrinogen synthesis stimulation by prostaglandin in E_1 and some other vasodilators. Am J Physiol 233: 1–9

73. Carrell RW, Jeppsson J-O, Laurell C-B, Brennan SO, Owen MC, Vaughan L, Boswell DR (1982) Structure and variation of human α_1-antitrypsin. Nature 298: 329–334.

74. Caspi D, Baltz ML, Snel F, Gruys E, Niv D, Batt RM, Munn EA, Buttress N, Pepys MB (1984) Isolation and characterization of C-reactive protein from the dog. Immunology 53: 307–313

75. Caspi D, Snel FWJJ, Batt RM, Bennett D, Rutteman GR, Hartman EG, Baltz ML, Gruys E, Pepys MB (1987) C-reactive protein in dogs. Am J Vet Res 48: 919–921

76. Catalfamo JL, Raymond SL, White JG, Dodds WJ (1986) Defective platelet-fibrinogen interaction in hereditary canine thrombopathia. Blood 67: 1568–1577

77. Cathcart ES, Comerford FR, Cohen AS (1965) Immunologic studies on a protein extracted from human secondary amyloid. New Engl J Med 273: 143–146

78. Chambers RE, Whicher JT (1983) Quantitative radial immunodiffusion assay for serum amyloid A protein. J Immunol Methods 59: 95–103

79. Charlwood PA, Hatton MWC, Regoeczi E (1976) On the physicochemical and chemical properties of α_1-acid glycoproteins from mammalian and avian plasmas. Biochem Biophys Acta 453: 81–92

80. Chase T, Shaw E (1967) p-nitrophenyl-p^1-guanidinobenzoate HC1: A new active site titrant for trypsin. Biochem Biophys Res Commun 29: 508–514

81. Chelladurai M, MacIntyre SS, Kushner I (1983) In vivo studies of serum C-reactive protein turnover in rabbits. J Clin Invest 71: 604–610

82. Chen Y, Briese F, Reeve EB (1974) Relation of fibrinogen secretion (synthesis) to ACTH dose. Am J Physiol 227: 932–939

83. Cheresh DA, Haynes DH, Distasio JA (1984) Interaction of an acute phase reactant, α_1-acid glycoprotein (orosomucoid), with the lymphoid cell surface: A model for non-specific immune suppression. Immunology 51: 541–548

84. Chiu KM, Mortensen RF, Osmand AP, Gewurz H (1977) Interactions of alpha 1 -acid glycoprotein with the immune system. Immunology 32: 997–1005

85. Church WR, Jernigan RL, Toole J, Hewick RM, Knopf J, Knutson GJ, Nesheim ME, Mann KG, Fass DN (1984) Coagulation factors V and VIII and ceruloplasmin constitute a family of structurally related proteins. Proc Natl Acad Sci USA 81: 6934–6937

86. Cierniewski CS, Krajewski T, Janiak A (1980) Homology of polymerization domains in vertebrate fibrinogens. Throm Res 19: 599–607

87. Clark MHG, Freeman T (1968) Quantitative immunoelectrophoresis of human serum proteins. Clin Sci (Oxf) 35: 403–413

88. Claus DR, Osmand AP, Gerwurz H (1976) Radioimmunoassay of human C-reactive protein and levels in normal sera. J Lab Clin Med 87: 120–128

89. Clauss A (1957) Gerinnungs physiologische schnell methode zur Bestimmung des Fibrinogens. Acta Haematol 17: 237–246

90. Coe JE (1977) A sex-limited serum protein of Syrian hamsters: Definition of female protein and regulation by testosterone. Proc Natl Acad Sci USA 74: 730–733

91. Coe JE (1981) Comparative immunology of old world hamsters—*Cricetinae*. Adv Exp Med Biol 134: 95–101

92. Coe JE (1982) Female protein of the Syrian hamster: A homolog of C-reactive protein. Ann NY Acad Sci 389: 299–305

93. Coe JE, Margossian SS, Slayter HS, Sogn JA (1981) Hamster female protein. A new pentraxin structurally and functionally similar to C-reactive protein and amyloid P component. J Exp Med 153: 977–991

94. Coe JE, Ross MJ (1983) Hamster female protein. A divergent acute phase protein in male and female Syrian hamsters. J Exp Med 157: 1421–1433

95. Coe JE, Ross MJ (1985) Hamster female protein, a sex-limited pentraxin, is a constituent of Syrian hamster amyloid. J Clin Invest 76: 66–74

96. Coetzee GA, Strachan AF, van der Westhuyzen DR, Hoppe HC, Jeenah MS, de Beer FC (1986) Serum amyloid A-containing human high density lipoprotein 3. Density, size, and apolipoprotein composition. J Biol Chem 261: 9644–9651

97. Collet-Cassart D, Mareschal JC, Sindic CJM, Tomasi JP, Masson PL (1983) Automated particle-counting immunoassay of C-reactive protein and its application to serum, cord serum, and cerebrospinal fluid samples. Clin Chem 29: 1127–1131

98. Colley CM, Fleck A, Goode AW, Muller BR, Myers MA (1983) Early time course of the acute phase protein response in man. J Clin Pathol 36: 203–207

99. Conforti A, Franco L, Milanino R, Velo GP (1982) Copper and ceruloplasmin (Cp) concentrations during the acute inflammatory process in the rat. Agents Actions 12: 303–307

100. Connell EB, Connell JT (1971) C-reactive protein in pregnancy and contraception. Am J Obstet Gynecol 110: 633–639

101. Cooper R, Papaconstantinou J (1986) Evidence for the existence of multiple α_1-acid glycoprotein genes in the mouse. J Biol Chem 261: 1849–1853

102. Costello M, Fiedel BA, Gewurz H (1979) Inhibition of platelet aggregation by native and desialised alpha-1 acid glycoprotein. Nature 281: 677–678

103. Costello MJ, Gewurz H, Siegel JN (1984) Inhibition of neutrophil activation by α_1-acid glycoprotein. Clin Exp Immunol 55: 465–472

104. Courtoy PJ, Feldmann G, Rogier E, Moguilevsky N (1981) Plasma protein synthesis in experimental cirrhosis. Lab Invest 45: 67–76

105. Courtoy PJ, Lombart C, Feldmann G, Moguilevsky N, Rogier E (1981) Synchronous increase of four acute phase proteins synthesized by the same hepatocytes during the inflammatory reaction. Lab Invest 44: 105–115

106. Cousins RJ (1985) Absorption, transport, and hepatic metabolism of copper and zinc: Special reference to metallothionein and ceruloplasmin. Physiol Rev 65: 238–309

107. Cousins RJ, Swerdel MR (1985) Ceruloplasmin and metallothionein induction by zinc and 13-cis-retinoic acid in rats with adjuvant inflammation. Proc Soc Exp Biol Med 179: 168–172

108. Cox DW (1966) Factors influencing serum ceruloplasmin levels in normal individuals. J Lab Clin Med 68: 893–904

109. Cox DW (1986) Clinical and molecular studies of alpha 1-antitrypsin deficiency. Prog Clin Biol Res 214: 373–384

110. Davidsen O, Christensen EI, Gliemann J (1985) The plasma clearance of human α_2-macroglobulin-trypsin complex in the rat is mainly accounted for by uptake into hepatocytes. Biochim Biophys Acta 846: 85–92

111. deBeer FC, Baltz ML, Holford S, Feinstein A, Pepys MB (1981) Fibronectin and C4-binding protein are selectively bound by aggregated amyloid P component. J Exp Med 154: 1134–1149

112. deBeer FC, Baltz ML, Munn EA, Feinstein A, Taylor J, Bruton C, Clamp JR, Pepys MB (1982) Isolation and characterization of C-reactive protein and serum amyloid P component in the rat. Immunlogy 45: 55–70

113. Delcroix C, Fraeyman N, Belpaire F (1984) A method for the assay of α_1-acid glycoprotein in dog serum and its application to the plasma binding of propranolol and oxprenolol in animals receiving rifampicin. J Pharmacol Methods 12: 97–105

114. Denko CW (1979) Protective role of ceruloplasmin in inflammation. Agents Actions 9: 333–336

115. Deshmukh VK, Raman PH, Dhuley JN, Naik SR (1985) Role of ceruloplasmin in inflammation: Increased serum ceruloplasmin levels during inflammatory conditions and its possible relationship wth anti-inflammatory agents. Pharmacol Res Commun 17: 633–642

116. Diarra-Mehrpour M, Bourguignon J, Leroux-Nicollet I, Marko-Vercaigne D, Biou D, Hiron M, Lebreton J-P (1985) The effects of 17 α-ethynyloestradiol and of acute inflammation on the plasma concentration of rat α_1-acid glycoprotein and on the induction of its hepatic mRNA. Biochem J 225: 681–687

117. Dickinson AM, Shenton BK, Alomran AH, Donnelly PK, Proctor SJ (1985) Inhibition of natural killing and antibody-dependent cell-mediated cytotoxicity by the plasma protease inhibitor α_2-macroglobulin (α_2M) and (α_2M protease complexes. Clin Immunol Immunopathol 36: 259–265

118. Dillman RC, Coles EH (1966) A canine serum fraction analogous to human C-reactive protein. Am J Vet Res 27: 1769–1775

119. DiSilvestro RA (1986) Plasma levels of immunoreactive ceruloplasmin and other acute phase proteins during lactation. Proc Soc Exp Biol Med 183: 257–261

120. Doepel FM, Glorioso JC, Newcomer CE, Skinner M, Abrams GD (1981) Enzyme-linked immunosorbent assay of serum protein SAA in rhesus monkeys with secondary amyloidosis. Lab Invest 45: 7–13

121. Doolittle RF (1975) In Putnam FW (ed.), The Plasma Proteins, Vol 2. Academic Press, New York

122. Doolittle RF (1984) Fibrinogen and fibrin. Ann Rev Biochem 53: 195–229

123. Dormandy TL (1978) Free-radical oxidation and anti-oxidants. Lancet i: 647–650

124. Dowton SB, Woods DE, Mantzouranis EC, Colten HR (1985) Syrian hamster female protein: Analysis of female protein primary structure and gene expression. Science 228: 1206–1208

125. Doyle MJ, Halsall HB, Heineman WR (1984) Enzyme-linked immunoadsorbent assay with electrochemical detection for α_1-acid glycoprotein. Anal Chem 56: 2355–2360

126. Dyck RF, Lockwood M, Kershaw M, McHugh N, Duance V, Baltz ML, Pepys MB (1980) Amyloid P-component is a constituent of normal human glomerular basement membrane. J Exp Med 152: 1162–1174

127. Enholm C, Teppo A-M, Ohisalo JJ, Maury CPJ (1985) Human high-density lipoprotein associated amyloid A protein. Structural characteristics, relation to apo A-I and A-II concentrations, and plasma clearance kinetics in the rat. Scand J Rheumatol 14: 201–208

128. Eriksen N, Benditt EP (1980) Isolation and characterization of the amyloid-related apoprotein (SAA) from human high density lipoprotein. Proc Natl Acad Sci USA 77: 6860–6864

129. Eriksen N, Benditt EP (1986) Serum amyloid A (apo SAA) and lipoproteins. Methods Enzymol 128: 311–320

130. Eriksson S (1965) Studies in alpha 1-antitrypsin deficiency. Acta Med Scand 177 (Suppl 432): 1–85

131. Etlinger HM, Coe JE (1986) Complement activation by female protein, the hamster homologue of human C-reactive protein. Int Arch Allergy Appl Immunol 81: 189–191

132. Evans GW, Cornatzer NF, Cornatzer WE (1970) Mechanism for hormone-induced alterations in serum ceruloplasmin. Am J Physiol 218: 613–615

133. Evans GW, Majors PF, Cornatzer WE (1970) Induction of ceruloplasmin synthesis by copper. Biochem Biophys Res Comm 41: 1120–1125

134. Evans GW, Myron DR, Cornatzer NF, Cornatzer WE (1970) Age-dependent alterations in hepatic subcellular copper distribution and plasma ceruloplasmin. Am J Physiol 218: 298–302

135. Evans GW, Wiederanders RE (1968) Effect of hormones on ceruloplasmin and copper concentrations in the plasma of the rat. Am J Physiol 214: 1152–1154

136. Exner T, Burridge J, Power P, Rickard KA (1979) An evaluation of currently available methods for plasma fibrinogen. Am J Clin Pathol 71: 521–527

137. Fagerhol MK (1968) The Pi-system. Genetic variants of serum α_1-antitrypsin. Ser Haematol 1, (Suppl 1): 153–161

138. Feinman RD, ed. (1983) Chemistry and biology of α_2-macroglobulin. Ann NY Acad Sci 421: 1–478

139. Feldman BF, Madewell BR, O'Neill S (1981) Disseminated intravascular coagulation: antithrombin, plasminogen, and coagulation abnormalities in 41 dogs. J Am Vet Med Assoc 179: 151–154

140. Feldman SR, Gonias SL, Pizzo SV (1985) Model of α_2-macroglobulin structure and function. Proc Natl Acad Sci 82: 5700–5704

141. Feldman SR, Rosenberg MR, Ney KA, Michalopoulos G, Pizzo SV (1985) Binding of α_2-macroglobulin to hepatocytes: Mechanism of in vivo clearance. Biochem Biophys Res Commun 128: 795–802

142. Ferard G, Goester C, Klumpp T, Metais P (1980) Evaluation of immunonephelometry of C-reactive protein in serum. Clin Chem 26: 782–783

143. Fiedel BA, Gewurz H (1986) Cleaved forms of C-reactive protein are associated with platelet inhibition. J Immunol 136: 2551–2555

144. Fiedel BA, Ku CSL (1986) Further studies on the modulation of blood coagulation by human serum amyloid P component and its acute phase homologue C-reactive protein. Thromb Haemostasis 55: 406–409

145. Fiedel BA, Ku CSL, Izzi JM, Gewurz H (1983) Selective inhibition of platelet activation by the amyloid P-component of serum. J Immunol 131: 1416–1419

146. Fiedel BA, Simpson RM, Gewurz H (1982) Effects of C-reactive protein on platelet function. Ann NY Acad Sci 389: 263–271

147. Fischer CL, Gill C, Forrester MG, Nakamura R (1976) Quantitation of "acute-phase proteins" postoperatively. Am J Clin Pathol 66: 840–846

148. Franks JJ, Kirsch, RE, Frith LO'C, Purves LR, Franks WT, Franks JA, Mason P, Saunders SJ

(1981) Effect of fibrinogenolytic products D and E on fibrinogen and albumin synthesis in the rat. J Clin Invest 67: 575–580

149. Frazer JM, Nathoo SA, Katz J, Genetta TL, Finlay TH (1985) Plasma protein and liver mRNA levels of two closely related murine α_1-protease inhibitors during the acute phase reaction. Arch Biochem Biophys 239: 112–119

150. Fuchs HE, Pizzo SV (1983) Regulation of factor Xa *in vitro* in human and mouse plasma and *in vivo* in mouse. J Clin Invest 72: 2041–2049

151. Ganrot K (1973) α_2-acute phase globulin in rat serum. Purification, determination and interaction with trypsin. Biochim Biophys Acta 295: 245–251

152. Ganrot K (1973) Plasma protein response in experimental inflammation in the dog. Res Exp Med 161: 251–261

153. Ganrot K (1973) Rat α_2-acute phase globulin, a human α_2-macroglobulin homologue: Interaction with plasmin and trypsin. Biochim Biophys Acta 322: 62–67

154. Ganrot K (1974) Plasma protein pattern in acute infectious diseases. Scand J Clin Lab Invest 34: 75–81

155. Ganrot PO (1966) Determination of α_2-macroglobulin as trypsin-protein esterase. Clin Chim Acta 14: 493–501

156. Ganrot PO (1972) Variation of the concentrations of some plasma proteins in normal adults, in pregnant women and in newborns. Scand J Clin Lab Invest 29 (Suppl 124): 83–88

157. Gauthier F, Mouray H (1976) Rat α_2 acute-phase macroglobulin. Isolation and physicochemical properties. Biochem J 159: 661–665

158. Gavotto AC, Palma JA, Villagra SB (1985) Interactions of prostaglandin E_1, bradykinin and histamine and the increase of plasma fibrinogen in rats. Prostaglandins 30: 879–886

159. Gentry PA, Liptrap RM (1981) Influence of progesterone and pregnancy on canine fibrinogen values. J Small An Pract 22: 185–194

160. Gertz MA, Sipe JD, Skinner M, Cohen AS, Kyle RA (1984) Measurement of murine serum amyloid P component by rate nephelometry. J Immunol Methods 69: 173–180

161. Gewurz H, Mold C, Siegel J, Fiedel B (1982) C-reactive protein and the acute phase response. Adv Int Med 27: 345–372

162. Giclas PC, Manthei U, Strunk RC (1985) The acute phase response of C3, C5, ceruloplasmin, and C-reactive protein induced by turpentine pleurisy in the rabbit. Am J Pathol 120: 146–156

163. Glibetic MD, Baumann H (1986) Influence of chronic inflammation on the level of mRNA for acute-phase reactants in the mouse liver. J Immunol 137: 1616–1622

164. Gliemann J, Davidsen O, Sottrup-Jensen L, Sonne O (1985) Uptake of rat and human α_2-macroglobulin-trypsin complexes into rat and human cells. FEBS Letters 188: 352–356

165. Göhler K, Schade R, Hirschelmann R, Martin A, Weidhase R (1986) Modulation of α_2-acute phase globulin serum concentration in turpentine- and immune complex-challenged rats by dexamethasone

and adrenaline: Evidence for a synergistic mode of action. Biomed Biochim Acta 45: 661–672

166. Goldstein IM, Kaplan HB, Edelson HS, Weissmann G (1979) Ceruloplasmin. A scavenger of superoxide anion radicals. J Biol Chem 254: 4040–4045

167. Gonias SL, Balber AE, Hubbard WJ, Pizzo SV (1983) Ligand binding, conformational change and plasma elimination of human, mouse and rat α-macroglobulin proteinase inhibitors. Biochem J 209: 99–105

168. Gordon AH (1976) The α-macroglobulins of rat serum. Biochem J 159: 643–650

169. Gordon AH, Limaos EA (1979) Effects of bacterial endotoxin and corticosteroids on plasma concentrations of α_2 macroglobulin, haptoglobin and fibrinogen in rats. Br J Exp Pathol 60: 434–440

170. Gordon AH, Limaos EA (1979) Human blood and rabbit peritoneal leucocytes as sources of endogeneous mediators. Br J Exp Pathol 60: 441–446

171. Gorevic PD, Cleveland AB, Franklin EC (1982) The biologic significance of amyloid. Ann NY Acad Sci 389: 380–393

172. Gorevic PD, Levo Y, Frangione B, Franklin EC (1978) Polymorphism of tissue and serum amyloid A (AA and SAA) proteins in the mouse. J Immunol 121: 138–140

173. Got R, Cheftel R-I, Font J, Moretti J (1967) Étude de l'α_1-macroglobuline du serum de lapin. III. Biochimie de la copule glucidique. Biochim Biophys Acta 136: 320–330

174. Got R, Mouray H, Moretti J (1965) Étude biochimique de l'α_1-macroglobuline de serum de lapin. I. Preparation et propriétés physicochimiques. Biochim Biophys Acta 107: 278–285

175. Gozzard DI, Liu Yin JA, Delamore IW (1986) The clinical usefulness of C-reactive protein measurements. Br J Haematol 63: 411–414

176. Grannis GF (1970) Plasma fibrinogen: Determination, normal values, physiopathologic shifts, and fluctuations. Clin Chem 16: 486–494

177. Greene ND, Damian RT, Hubbard WJ (1971) The identification of α_2-macroglobulin in the mouse. Biochim Biophys Acta 236: 659–663

178. Gregoriadis G, Morell AG, Sternlieb I, Scheinbert IH (1970) Catabolism of desialylated ceruloplasmin in the liver. J Biol Chem 245: 5833–5837

179. Gressner AM, Peltzer B (1984) Amidolytic and immuno-nephelometric determination of α_1-proteinase inhibitor and α_2-macroglobulin in serum with calculation of specific inhibitor activities in health and disease. J Clin Chem Clin Biochem 22: 633–640

180. Griswold DE, Hillegass L, Antell L, Shatzman A, Hanna N (1986) Quantitative Western blot assay for measurement of the murine acute phase reactant, serum amyloid P component. J Immunol Methods 91: 163–168

181. Gutteridge JMC (1985) Inhibition of the Fenton reaction by the protein caeruloplasmin and other copper complexes. Assessment of ferroxidase and radical scavenging activities. Chem Biol Interactions 56: 113–120

182. Gutteridge JMC, Winyard PG, Blake DR, Lunec J, Brailsford S, Halliwell B (1985) The behavior of caeruloplasmin in stored human extracellular fluids

in relation to ferroxidase II activity, lipid peroxidation and phenanthroline-detectable copper. Biochem J 230: 517–523

183. Hallen J, Laurell C-B (1972) Plasma protein pattern in cirrhosis of the liver. Scand J Clin Lab Invest 29 (Suppl 124): 97–103

184. Hantgan R, McDonagh J, Hermans J (1983) Fibrin assembly. Ann NY Acad Sci 408: 344–365

185. Hart DA, Stein-Streilein J (1981) Hamster lymphoid cell responses in vitro. Adv Exp Med Biol 134: 7–22

186. Haverback BJ, Dyce B, Bundy HF, Wirtschafter SK, Edmondson HA (1962) Protein binding of pancreatic proteolytic enzymes. J Clin Invest 41: 972–980

187. Hayashida K, Okubo H, Noguchi M, Yoshida H, Kangawa K, Matsuo H,Sakaki Y (1985) Molecular cloning of DNA complementary to rat α_2-macroglobulin mRNA. J Biol Chem 260: 14224–14229

188. Hellerstein MK, Sasak V, Ordovas J, Munro HN (1985) Isolation of alpha-1-acid glycoprotein from human plasma using high-performance liquid chromatography. Anal Biochem 146: 366–371

189. Henry RJ, Chiamori N, Jacobs SL, Segalove M (1960) Determination of ceruloplasmin oxidase in serum. Proc Soc Exp Biol Med 104: 620–624

190. Hickman J, Aswell G, Morell AG, Van den Hamer CJA, Scheinbert IH (1970) Physical and chemical studies of ceruloplasmin. VIII. Preparation of N-acetylneuraminic acid-l-^{14}C labelled ceruloplasmin. J Biol Chem 245: 759–766

191. Hind CRK, Collins PM, Baltz ML, Pepys MB (1985) Human serum amyloid P, a circulating lectin with specificity for the cyclic 4,6-pyruvate acetal of galactose: Interactions with various bacteria. Biochem J 225: 107–111

192. Hind CRK, Collins PM, Renn D, Cook RB, Caspi D, Baltz ML, Pepys MB (1984) Binding specificity of serum amyloid P component for the pyruvate acetal of galactose. J Exp Med 159: 1058–1069

193. Hirschelmann R, Schade R, Bekemeier H (1980) 6-sulphanilamidoindazole arthritis of rats: Relation between acute-phase proteins, degree of arthritis and treatment with soybean trypsin inhibitor. Agents Actions 10: 431–434

194. Hoffman JS, Benditt EP (1983) Plasma clearance kinetics of the amyloid-related high density lipoprotein apoprotein, serum amyloid protein (Apo-SAA), in the mouse. Evidence for rapid ApoSAA clearance. J Clin Invest 71: 926:934

195. Hol PR, van Ederen AM, Snel FWJJ, Langeveld JPM, Veerkamp JH, Gruys E (1985) Activities of lysosomal enzymes and levels of serum amyloid A (SAA) in blood plasma of hamsters during casein induction of AA-amyloidosis. Br J Exp Pathol 66: 279–292

196. Holtzman NA, Gaumnitz BM (1970) Identification of an apoceruloplasmin-like substance in the plasma copper-deficient rats. J Biol Chem 245: 2350–2353

197. Holtzman NA, Gaumnitz BM (1970) Studies on the rate of release and turnover of ceruloplasmin and apoceruloplasmin in rat plasma. J Biol Chem 245: 2354–2358

198. Hsieh HS, Frieden E (1975) Evidence for ceruloplasmin as a copper transport protein. Biochem Biophys Res Comm 67: 1326–1331

199. Hudig D, Sell S (1979) Isolation, characterization and radioimmunoassay of rat alpha-macrofeto-protein (acute phase α_2-macroglobulin). Molec Immunol 16: 547–554

200. Hulman G, Fuller M, Pearson HJ, Bell PRF (1986) An accurate, simple and rapid test for detecting elevated levels of C-reactive protein in serum by agglutination of fat emulsion. Clin Chim Acta 156: 337–340

201. Hunt DM, (1974) Primary defect in copper transport underlies mottled mutants in the mouse. Nature 249: 852–854

202. Husebekk A, Skogen B, Husby G, Marhaug G (1985) Transformation of amyloid precursor SAA to protein AA and incorporation in amyloid fibrils in vivo. Scand J Immunol 21: 283–287

203. Ihrig J, Kleinerman J, Rynbrandt DJ (1971) Serum antitrypsins in animals. Studies of species variations, components, and the influence of certain irritants. Am Rev Resp Dis 103: 377–389

204. Ikehara Y, Miyasato M, Ogata S, Oda K (1981) Multiple forms of rat-serum α_1-protease inhibitor. Involvement of sialic acid in the multiplicity of three original forms. Eur J Biochem 115: 253–260

205. Ikuta T, Okubo H, Ishibashi, Okumura Y, Hayashida K (1986) Human lymphocytes synthesize C-reactive protein. Inflammation 10: 223–232

206. Imlah P (1964) Inherited variants in serum ceruloplasmins of the pig. Nature 203: 658–659

207. Ishibashi H, Shibata K, Okubo H, Tsudua-Kawamura K, Yanase T (1978) Distribution of α_1-antitrypsin in normal, granuloma, and tumor tissues in rats. J Lab Clin Med 91: 576–583

208. James K, Baum LL, Vetter ML, Gewurz H (1982) Interaction of C-reactive protein with lymphoid cells. Ann NY Acad Sci 389: 274–285

209. Jamieson JC, Ashton FE (1973) Studies on acute phase proteins of rat serum. III. Site of synthesis of albumin and α_1-acid glycoprotein and the contents of these proteins in liver microsome fractions from rats suffering from induced inflammation. Can J Biochem 51: 1034–1045

210. Jamieson JC, Ashton FE (1973) Studies on acute phase proteins of rat serum. IV. Pathway of secretion of albumin and α_1-acid glycoprotein from liver. Can J Biochem 51: 1281–1291

211. Jamieson JC, Ashton FE, Friesen AD, Chou (1972) Studies on acute phase proteins of rat serum. II. Determination of the contents of α_1-acid glycoprotein, α_2-macroglobulin, and albumin in serum from rats suffering from induced inflammation. Can J Biochem 50: 871–880

212. Jamieson JC, Friesen AD, Ashton FE, Chou B (1972) Studies on acute phase proteins of rat serum. I. Isolation and partial characterization of an α_1-acid glycoprotein and an α_2-macroglobulin. Can J Biochem 50: 856–870

213. Jeejeebhoy KN, Bruce-Robertson A, Ho J, Sodtke U (1972) The effect of cortisol on the synthesis of rat plasma albumin, fibrinogen and transferrin. Biochem J 130: 533–538

214. Jeppsson J-O, Franzen B (1982) Typing of genetic variants of α_1-antitrypsin by electrofocusing. Clin Chem 28: 219–225

215. Johansson BG, Kindmark C-O, Trell EY, Wollheim FA (1972) Sequential changes of plasma proteins after myocardial infarction. Scand J Clin Lab Invest 29 (Suppl 124): 117–126

216. John DW, Miller LL (1969) Regulations of net biosynthesis of serum albumin and acute phase plasma proteins. J Biol Chem 244: 6134–6142

217. Kammermann B, Gmur J, Stunzi H (1971) Afibrinogenamie beim Hund. Zentralbl Veterinaermed Reihe A 18: 192–205

218. Kampschmidt RF, Mesecher M (1985) Interleukin-1 from P388D₁: Effect upon neutrophils, plasma iron, and fibrinogen in rats. Proc Soc Exp Biol Med 179: 197–200

219. Kampschmidt FR, Upchurch HF, Pulliam LA (1982) Characterization of a leukocyte-derived endogenous mediator responsible for increased plasma fibrinogen. Ann NY Acad Sci 389: 338–353

220. Kaplan MH, Volanakis JE (1974) Interaction of C-reactive protein complexes with the complement system. I. Consumption of human complement associated with the reaction of C-reactive protein with pneumococcal C-polysaccharide and with the choline phosphatides, lecithin and sphingomyelin. J Immunol 112: 2135–2147

221. Karpatkin M, Howard L, Karpatkin S (1984) Studies of the origin of platelet-associated fibrinogen. J Lab Clin Med 104: 223–237

222. Kazal LA, Grannis GF, Tocantins LM (1964) In Tocantins LM, Kazal LA (eds), Blood Coagulation, Hemorrage and Thrombosis. Grune & Stratton, New York

223. Kernoff L, Colman J (1982) Neutropenia fails to prevent the acute phase stimulation of fibrinogen synthesis. Thromb Res 28: 47–57

224. Kessler CM, Bell WR (1979) Regulation of fibrinogen biosynthesis: Effect of fibrin degradation products, low-molecular-weight peptides of fibrinogenolysis, and fibrinopeptides A and B. J Lab Clin Med 93: 758–767

225. Kessler CM, Bell WR (1980) Stimulation of fibrinogen systhesis: A possible functional role of fibrinogen degradation products. Blood 55: 40–47

226. Killingsworth LM, Killingsworth CE (1981) In Spiegel HE (ed), Clinical Biochemistry: Contemporary Theories and Techniques, Vol 1. Academic Press, New York

227. Kobayashi S, Nagasawa S (1974) Protease inhibitors in guinea pig serum. I. Isolation of two functionally different trypsin inhibitors from guinea pig serum. Biochim Biophys Acta 342: 372–381

228. Koepke JA (1980) Standardization of fibrinogen assays. Scand J Haematol Suppl 37: 130–138

229. Kohayakawa M, Inoue K (1986) Augmentation of PAF-induced human platelet activation by C-reactive protein. Thromb Res 41: 649–657

230. Koj A (1968) The measurement of absolute and relative synthesis rates of fibrinogen in vivo. Biochim Biophys Acta 165: 97–107

231. Koj A (1974) In Allison AC (ed), Structure and Function of the Plasma Proteins, Vol 1, Plenum Press, New York

232. Koj A, Dubin A, Kasperczyk H, Bereta J, Gordon AH (1982) Changes in the blood level and affinity to concanavalin A of rat plasma glycoproteins during acute inflammation and hepatoma growth. Biochem J 206: 545–553

233. Koj A, Hatton MWC, Wong KL, Regoeczi E (1978) Isolation and partial characterization of rabbit plasma α₁-antitrypsin. Biochem J 169: 589–596

234. Koj A, McFarlane AS (1968) Effect of endotoxin on plasma albumin and fibrinogen synthesis rates in rabbits as measured by the (¹⁴C) carbonate method. Biochem J 108: 137–146

235. Koj A, Regoeczi E (1978) Effect of experimental inflammation on the synthesis and distribution of antithrombin III and α₁-antitrypsin in rabbits. Br J Exp Pathol 59: 473–481

236. Koj A, Regoeczi E (1981) Differential inhibition of serine proteinases by rabbit alpha-1-proteinase inhibitors. Int J Pept Protein Res 17: 519–526

237. Kojima E, Mitsuno T, Osawa T (1986) Immunological effects of mouse ceruloplasmin. J Pharmacobiol Dyn 9: 101–109

238. Koo PH (1978) Tumor suppression of α-macroblobulins of mice. Fed Proc 37: 1337

239. Koo PH (1982) Characterization of growth-inhibitory activities associated with an α-macroglobulin of mice. Cancer Res 42: 1788–1797

240. Kuehn L, Rutschmann M, Dahlmann B, Reinauer H (1984) Proteinase inhibitors in rat serum. Purification and partial characteriztion of three functionally distinct trypsin inhibitors. Biochem J 218: 953–959

241. Kueppers F, Lee CC, Fox RR, Mills JK (1984) Genetic heterogeneity of rabbit alpha-1-antitrypsin. Genetics 106: 695–703

242. Kulkarni AB, Reinke R, Feigelson P (1985) Acute phase mediators and glucocorticoids elevate α₁-acid glycoprotein gene transcription. J Biol Chem 260: 15386–15389

243. Kuranda MJ, Aronson NN Jr (1983) tissue locations for the turnover of radioactively labelled rat orosomucoid in vivo. Arch Biochem Biophys 224: 526–533

244. Kushner I (1981) In Kelley WN (ed), Textbook of Rheumatology. WB Saunders, Philadelphia

245. Kushner I (1982) The phenomenon of the aucte phase response. Ann NY Acad Sci 389: 39–48

246. Kushner I, Feldman G (1978) Control of the acute phase response. Demonstration of C-reactive protein synthesis and secretion by hepatocytes during acute inflammation in the rabbit. J Exp Med 148: 466–477

247. Kushner I, Gequrz H, Benson MD (1981) C-reactive protein and the acute-phase response. J Lab Clin Med 97: 739–749

248. Kushner I, Volanakis JE, Gewurz H (eds) (1982) C-reactive protein and the plasma protein response to tissue injury. Ann NY Acad Sci 389: 1–479

249. Kuta AE, Baum LL (1986) C-reactive protein is produced by a small number of normal human peripheral blood lymphocytes. J Exp Med 164: 321–326

250. LaMontagne LR, Gauldie J, Befus AD, McAdam KPWJ, Baltz ML, Pepys MB (1984) The acute phase response in parasitic infection. Nippostrongylus brasiliensis in the mouse. Immunology 52: 733–741

251. LaMontagne L, Gauldie J, Koj A (1981) Ontogeny and tissue distribution of alpha-1-antitrypsin of the mouse. Biochim Biophys Acta 662: 15–21

252. Laurell C-B (1972) Electroimmunoassay. Scand J Clin Lab Invest 29 (Suppl 124); 21–37

253. Laurell C-B, Jeppsson J-O (1975) In Putnam FW (ed), The Plasma Proteins, Vol 1. Academic Press, New York

254. Laurell C-B, Kullander S, Thorell J (1969) Plasma protein changes induced by sequential type of contraceptive steroid pills. Clin Chim Acta 25: 294–296

255. Le PT, Mortensen RF (1986) Induction and regulation by monokines of hepatic synthesis of mouse serum amyloid P-component (SAP). J Immunol 136: 2526–2533

256. Le PT, Muller MT, Mortensen RF (1982) Acute phase reactants of mice I. Isolation of serum amyloid P-component (SAP) and its induction by a monokine. J Immunol 129: 665–672

257. Lebreton De VT, Gutman N, Mouray H (1970) Les α-macroglobulines du lapin au cours de la reaction inflammatoire. Clin Chim Acta 30: 603–607

258. Levo Y, Wollner S (1985) Effects of serum amyloid P-component on human lymphocytes. Int Arch Allergy Appl Immunol 77: 322–325

259. Li JJ, McAdam KPWJ (1984) Human amyloid P-component: An elastase inhibitor. Scand J Immonol 20: 219–226

260. Li JJ, McAdam KPWJ, Bausserman LL (1982) The regulatory role of acute phase reactants on human immune responses. Ann NY Acad Sci 389: 456

261. Li JJ, Pereira MEA, DeLellis RA, McAdam KPWJ (1984) Human amyloid P-component: A circulating lectin that modulates immunological responses. Scand J Immunol 19: 227–236

262. Liao Y-C J, Taylor JM, Vannice JL, Clawson GA, Smuckler EA (1985) Structure of the rat α₁-acid glycoprotein gene. Mol Cell Biol 5: 3634–3639

263. Liu T-Y, Robey FA, Wang C-M (1982) Structural studies on C-reactive protein. Ann NY Acad Sci 389: 151–162

264. Lopaciuk S, McDonagh RP, McDonagh J (1978) Comparative studies on blood coagulation Factor XIII (40141). Proc Soc Exp Biol Med 158: 68–72

265. Lowell CA, Stearman RS, Morrow JF (1986) Transcriptional regulation of serum amyloid A gene expression. J Biol Chem 261: 8453–8461

266. MacIntyre SS, Schultz D, Kushner I (1983) Synthesis and secretion of C-reactive protein by rabbit primary hepatocyte cultures. Biochem J 210: 707–715

267. Manolis A, Cox DW (1980) Purification of rat ceruloplasmin: Characterization and comparison with human ceruloplasmin. Prep Biochem 10: 121–132

268. Mannhalter JW, Borth W, Eibl MM (1986) Modulation of antigen-induced T-cell proliferation by α₂M-trypsin complexes. J Immunol 136: 2792–2799

269. Marguerie GA (1983) The fibrinogen-dependent pathway of platelet aggregation. Ann NY Acad Sci 408: 556–566

270. Marhaug G (1983) Three assays for the characterization and quantitation of human serum amyloid A. Scand J Immunol 18: 329–338

271. Maudsley S, Hind CRK, Munn EA, Buttress N, Pepys MB (1986) Isolation and characterization of guinea-pig serum amyloid P-component. Immunology 59: 317–322

272. McAdam KPWJ, Li J, Knowles J, Foss NT, Dinarello CA, Rosenwasser LJ, Selinger MJ, Kaplan MM, Goodman R (1982) The biology of SAA: Identification of the inducer, in vitro synthesis, and heterogeneity demonstrated with monoclonal antibodies. Ann NY Acad Sci 389: 126–136

273. McAdam KPWJ, Sipe JD (1976) Murine model for human secondary amyloidosis: Genetic variability of the acute-phase serum protein SAA response to endotoxins and casein. J Exp Med 144: 1121–1127

274. McCombs ML, Bowman BH (1970) Electrophoretic comparison of ceruloplasmin types in ten primate species. Texas Rep Biol Med 28: 69–74

275. McNamara PJ, Brouwer KR, Gillespie MN (1986) Autocoid binding to serum proteins. Interaction of platelet activating factor (PAF) with human alpha-1-acid glycoprotein (AAG). Biochem Pharmacol 35: 621–624

276. Meek RL, Hoffman JS, Benditt EP (1986) Amyloidgenesis. One serum amyloid A isotype is selectively removed from the circulation. J Exp Med 163: 499–510

277. Mega T, Lujan E, Yoshida A (1980) Studies on the oligosaccharide chains of human α₁-protease inhibitor. II. Structure of oligosaccharides. J Biol Chem 255: 4057–4061

278. Meier H, MacPike AD (1968) Levels and heritability of serum ceruloplasmin activity in inbred strains of mice. Proc Soc Exp Biol Med 128: 1185–1190

279. Melamies L (1983) Rapid quantification of C-reactive protein by centrifugal analysis. Clin Chem 29: 696–697

280. Menache D (1983) Congenital fibrinogen abnormalities. Ann NY Acad Sci 408: 121–129

281. Millar HR, Simpson JG, Stalker AL (1971) An evaluation of the heat precipitation method for plasma fibrinogen estimation. J Clin Pathol 24: 827–830

282. Minnich M, Kueppers F, James H (1984) Alpha-1-antitrypsin from mouse serum: isolation and characterization. Comp Biochem Physiol 78B: 413–419

283. Miyanaga O, Okubo H, Kudo J, Ikuta T, Hirata Y (1982) Effect of α₂-macroglobulin on the lymphocyte response. Immunology 47: 351–356

284. Mold C, DuClos TW, Nakayama S, Edwards KM, Gewurz H (1982) C-reactive protein reactivity with complement and effects on phagocytosis. Ann NY Acad Sci 389: 251–259

285. Mold C, Kingzette M, Gewurz H (1984) C-reactive protein inhibits pneumoncoccal activation of the alternative pathway by increasing the interaction between Factor H and C3b. J Immunol 133: 882–885

286. Mold C, Nakayama S, Holzer TJ, Gewurz H, DuClos TW (1981) C-reactive protein is protective against Streptococcus pneumoniae infection in mice. J Exp Med 154: 1703–1708

287. Monnet D, Feger J, Biou D, Durand G, Cardon P, Leroy Y, Fournet B (1986) Effect of phenobarbital on the oligosaccharide structure of rat α₁-acid glycoprotein. Biochim Biophys Acta 881: 10–14

288. Morley JJ, Kushner I (1982) Serum C-reactive protein levels in disease. Ann NY Acad Sci 389: 406–417

289. Morse JO (1978) Alpha 1-antitrypsin deficiency (part 1). New Engl J Med 299: 1045–1048

290. Morse JO (1978) Alpha 1-antitrypsin deficiency (part 2). New Engl J Med 299: 1099–1105

291. Mortensen RF, Beisel K, Zeleznik NJ, Le PT (1983) Acute-phase reactants of mice. II. Strain dependence of serum amyloid P-component (SAP) levels and response to inflammation. J Immunol 130: 885–889

292. Mortensen RF, Le PT, Taylor BA (1985) Mouse serum amyloid P-component (SAP) levels controlled by a locus on chromosome 1. Immunogenetics 22: 367–375

293. Mortensen RF, Marcelletti JF, Johnson CS, Furmanski P (1982) Human C-reactive protein (CRP): A selective regulator of bone marrow monocyte progenitor cells. Ann NY Acad Sci 389: 457–458

294. Mouray H, Got R, Moretti J (1965) Étude biochimique de l'α1-macroglobuline du serum de lapin. II. Metabolisme. Biochim Biophys Acta 107: 286–293

295. Muller-Berghaus G, Moeller R-M, Mahn I (1978) Fibrinogen turnover in pregnant rabbits during the first and last thirds of gestation. Am J Obstet Gynecol 131: 655–660

296. Mullins RE, Miller RL, Hunter RL, Bennett B (1984) Standardized automated assay for functional α_1-antitrypsin. Clin Chem 30: 1857–1860

297. Myerowitz RL, Chrambach A, Rodbard D, Robbins JB (1972) Isolation and characterization of mouse serum alpha 1-antitrypsins. Anal Biochem 48: 394–409

298. Nagashima M, Urban J, Schreiber G (1980) Intrahepatic precursor form of rat α1-acid glycoprotein. J Biol Chem 255: 4951–4956

299. Nakagawa H, Suzuki K, Yamaki K, Tsurufuji S (1984) Changes in functional ceruloplasmin concentrations of plasma and exudate and the effect of exogenous ceruloplasmin on the carrageenin-induced inflamamtion in rats. J Pharm Dyn 7: 755–759

300. Nakagawa H, Watanabe K, Tsurufuji S (1984) Changes in serum and exudate levels of functional macroglobulins and anti-inflammatory effect of α_2-acute phase macroglobulin on carrageenin-induced inflammation in rats. Biochem Pharmacol 33: 1181–1186

301. Nathoo SA, Finlay TH (1986) Immunological and chemical properties of mouse α_1-protease inhibitors. Arch Biochem Biophys 246: 162–174

302. Nathoo S, Rasums A, Katz J, Ferguson WS, Finlay TH (1982) Purification and properties of two different α_1-protease inhibitors from mouse plasma. Arch Biochem Biophys 219: 306–315

303. Nilehn J-E, Ganrot PO (1967) Plasmin, plasmin inhibitors and degradation productions of fibrinogen in human serum during and after intravenous infusion of streptokinase. Scand J Clin Lab Invest 20: 113–121

304. Nilsson LA (1968) Comparative testing of precipitation methods for quantification of C-reactive protein in blood serum. Acta Pathol Microbiol Scand 73: 129

305. Northemann W, Heisig M, Kunz D, Heinrich PC (1985) Molecular cloning of cDNA sequences for rat α_2-macroglobulin and measurement of its transcription during experimental inflammation. J Biol Chem 260: 6200–6205

306. Noyer M, Dwulet FE, Hao YL, Putnam FW (1980) Purification and characterization of undegraded human ceruloplasmin. Anal Biochem 102: 450–458

307. O'Donnell MR, Slichter SJ, Weiden PL, Storb R (1981) Platelet and fibrinogen kinetics in canine tumors. Cancer Res 41: 1379–1383

308. Ohlsson K (1971) Interactions in vitro and in vivo between dog trypsin and dog plasma protease inhibitors. Scand J Clin Lab Invest 28: 219–223

309. Ohlsson K (1971) Isolation and partial characterization of two related trypsin binding α-macroglobulins of dog plasma. Biochim Biophys Acta 236: 84–91

310. Okubo H, Shibata K, Ishibashi H, Kudo J, Ikuta T, Tsuda-Kawamura K (1982) Acute phase proteins—dynamics in inflammatory or tumor-bearing animals. Fukuoku Acta Med 73: 146–154

311. Okumura Y, Kuda J, Ikuta T, Kurokawa S, Ishibashi H, Okubo H (1985) Influence of acute-phase proteins on the activity of natural killer cells. Inflammation 9: 211–219

312. Orena SJ, Goode CA, Linder MC (1986) Binding and uptake of copper from ceruloplasmin. Biochem Biophys Res Commun 139: 822–829

313. Osaki S, Johnson DA (1969) Mobilization of liver iron by ferroxidase (ceruloplasmin). J Biol Chem 244: 5757–5758

314. Osaki S, Johnson DA, Frieden E (1971) The mobilization of iron from the perfused mammalian liver by a serum copper enzyme, ferroxidase I. J Biol Chem 246: 3018–3023

315. Osmand AP, Friedenson B, Gewurz H, Painter RH, Hofmann T, Shelton E (1977) Characterization of C-reactive protein and the complement subcomponent Clt as homologous proteins displaying cyclic pentameric symmetry (pentraxins). Proc Natl Acad Sci USA 74: 739–743

316. Osmand AP, Mortensen RF, Siegel J, Gewurz H (1975) Interactions of C-reactive protein with the complement system. III. Complement-dependent passive hemolysis initiated by CRP. J Exp Med 142: 1065–1077

317. Owen CA (1971) Metabolism of copper 67 by the copper-deficient rat. Am J Physiol 221: 1722–1727

318. Palma JA, Gavotto AC, Villagra TA (1983) Effects of diethylstilbesterol, 17 beta estradiol, and progesterone on plasma fibrinogen levels in rats submitted to tissue injury (laparotomy). J Trauma 23: 132–135

319. Palma JA, Gavotto AC, Villagra SB (1983) Effects of the administration of progesterone and adrenal medullectomy on the plasma fibrinogen levels in rats with surgical injury (laparotomy). Arch Int Physiol Biochim 91: 81–85.

320. Panrucker DE, Lai POW, Lorscheider FL (1983) Distribution of acute-phase α_2-macroglobulin in rat

fetomaternal compartments. Am J Physiol 245: E138–142

321. Panrucker DE, Lorscheider FL (1982) Isolation and purification of rat acute-phase α_2-macroglobulin. Biochim Biophys Acta 705: 174–183

322. Panrucker DE, Lorscheider FL (1982) Radioimmunoassay of rat acute-phase α_2-macroglobulin. Biochim Biophys Acta 705: 184–191

323. Panrucker DE, Lorscheider FL (1983) Synthesis of acute-phase α_2-macroglobulin during inflammation and pregnancy. Ann NY Acad Sci 417: 117–124

324. Parfentjev IA, Johnson ML, Clifton EE (1953) The determination of plasma fibrinogen by turbidity with ammonium sulfate. Arch Biochem Biophys 46: 470–480

325. Parks JS, Rudel LL (1983) Metabolism of the serum amyloid A proteins (SAA) in high-density lipoproteins and chylomicrons of nonhuman primates (Vervet monkey). Am J Pathol 112: 243–249

326. Pepys MB (1979) Isolation of serum amyloid P-component (protein SAP) in the mouse. Immunology 37: 637–641

327. Pepys MB, Baltz ML (1983) Acute phase proteins with special reference to C-reactive protein and related proteins (pentaxins) and serum amyloid A protein. Adv Immunol 34: 141–212

328. Pepys MB, Baltz ML, deBeer FC, Dyck RF, Holford S, Breathnach SM, Black MM, Tribe CR, Evans DJ, Feinstein A (1982) Biology of serum amyloid P component. Ann NY Acad Sci 389: 286–297

329. Pepys MB, Baltz M, Gomer K, Davies AJS, Doenhoff M (1979) Serum amyloid P-component is an acute-phase reactant in the mouse. Nature 278: 259–261

330. Pepys MB, Baltz ML, Musallam R, Doenhoff MJ (1980) Serum protein concentrations during *Schistosoma mansoni* infection in intact and T-cell deprived mice. I. The acute phase proteins, C3 and serum amyloid P-component (SAP). Immunology 39: 249–254

331. Pepys MB, Dash AC, Fletcher TC, Richardson N, Munn EA, Feinstein A (1978) Analogues in other mammals and in fish of human plasma proteins, C-reactive protein and amyloid P-component. Nature 273: 168–170

332. Pepys MB, Dash AC, Markham RE, Thomas HC, Williams BD, Petrie A (1978) Comparative clinical study of protein SAP (amyloid P-component) and C-reactive protein in serum. Clin Exp Immunol 32: 119–124

333. Pepys MB, deBeer FC, Dyck RF, Hind C, Lanham JG, Fagan EA, Maton PN, Starke I, Fox K, Allan R, Hodgson H, Chadwick VS, Hughes GRU, Goldman J, Catovsky D, Galton D, Kirkler D, Maseri A, Mallya RK, Berry H, Hamilton EDB, Mace BEW (1982) Clinical measurement of serum C-reactive protein in the monitoring and differential diagnosis of inflammatory diseases and tissue necrosis and in the recognition and management of intercurrent infection. Ann NY Acad Sci 389: 459–460

334. Pepys MB, Rogers SL (1980) Complement-independence of the acute-phase production of serum amyloid P-component (SAP) in mice. Br J Exp Pathol 61: 156–159

335. Pepys MB, Rowe IF, Baltz ML (1985) C-reactive protein: Binding to lipids and lipoproteins. Int Rev Exp Pathol 27: 83–111

336. Perier C, Chamson A, Engler R, Frey J (1983) Evolutionary changes in acute-phase proteins in alcoholic hepatocellular diseases. Clin Chem 29: 45–47

337. Pesce MA, Bodourian SH (1982) Nephelometric measurement of ceruloplasmin with a centrifugal analyzer. Clin Chem 28: 516–519

338. Poole S, Gordon AH, Baltz M, Stenning BE (1984) Effect of bacterial endotoxin on body temperature, plasma zinc and plasma concentrations of the acute phase protein serum amyloid P component in mice. Br J Exp Pathol 65: 431–439

339. Poulik MD (1968) Heterogeneity and structure of ceruloplasmin. Ann NY Acad Sci 15: 476–501

340. Poulik MD, Weiss ML (1975) In Putnam FW (ed), The Plasma Proteins, Vol 2. Academic Press, New York

341. Pressac M, Magnier C, Amyard P (1986) Concurrent immunoassay of C-reactive protein and orosomucoid by random access analysis. Clin Chem 32: 1386–1389

342. Princen HMG, Moshage HJ, deHaard HJW, vanGemert PJL, Yap SH (1984) The influence of glucocorticoid on the fibrinogen mRNA content of rat liver *in vivo* and in hepatocyte suspension culture. Biochem J 220: 631–637

343. Princen HMG, Moshage HJ, Emeiss JJ, DeHaard HJW, Nieuwenhuizen W, Yap SH (1985) Fibrinogen fragments X, Y, D and E increase levels of plasma fibrinogen and liver mRNAs coding for fibrinogen polypeptides in rats. Thromb Haemost 53: 212–215

344. Rabinovitch RA, Koethe SM, Kalbfleisch JH, Preheim LC, Rytel MW (1986) Relationships between alternative complement pathway activation, C-reactive protein, and pneumococcal infection. J Clin Microbiol 23: 56–61

345. Ragan HA, Nacht S, Lee GR, Bishop CR, Cartwright GE (1969) Effect of ceruloplasmin on plasma iron in copper-deficient swine. Am J Physiol 217: 1320–1323

346. Ramadori G, Sipe JD, Colten HR (1985) Expression and regulation of the murine serum amyloid A (SAA) gene in extrahepatic sites. J Immunol 135: 3645–3647

347. Ramadori G, Sipe JD, Dinarello CA, Mizel SB, Colten HR (1985) Pretranslational modulation of acute phase hepatic protein synthesis by murine recombinant interleukin 1 (IL-1) and purified human IL-1. J Exp Med 162: 930–942

348. Rastogi SC, Clausen J (1985) Kinetics of inhibition of mitogen-induced proliferation of human lymphocytes by α_2-macroglobulin in serum-free medium. Immunobiology 169: 37–44

349. Ratnoff OD, Menzie C (1951) A new method for determination of fibrinogen in small samples of plasma. J Lab Clin Med 370: 316–320

350. Raynes JG, Cooper EH (1983) Comparison of serum amyloid A protein and C-reactive protein concentrations in cancer and non-malignant disease. J Clin Pathol 36: 798–803

351. Regoeczi E, Hobbs KR (1969) Fibrinogen turnover in pregnancy. Scand J Haematol 6: 175–178

352. Regoeczi E, Koj A, Lam LSL (1980) Synthesis and catabolism of rabbit α_1-antitrypsins F and S. Biochem J 192: 929–934

353. Reinke R, Feigelson P (1985) Rat α_1-acid glycoprotein. Gene sequence and regulation by glucocorticoids in transfected L-cells. J Biol Chem 260: 4397–4403

354. Ricca GA, Hamilton RW, McLean JW, Conn A, Kalinyak JE, Taylor JM (1981) Rat α_1-acid glycoprotein mRNA. J Biol Chem 256: 10362–10368

355. Ricca GA, McLean JW, Taylor JM (1982) Kinetics of induction of α_1-acid glycoprotein. Ann NY Acad Sci 389: 88–103

356. Ricca GA, Taylor JM (1981) Nucleotide sequence of rat α_1-acid glycoprotein messenger RNA. J Biol Chem 256: 11199–11202

357. Riley RF, Coleman MK (1970) Isolation of C-reactive proteins of man, monkey, rabbit and dog by affinity chromatography on phosphorylated cellulose. Clin Chim Acta 30: 483–496

358. Riley RF, Zontine W (1972) Further observations on the properties of dog C-reactive protein and the C-reactive protein response in the dog. J Lab Clin Med 80: 698–703

359. Rinderknecht H, Geokas MC (1973) On the physiological role of α_2-macroglobulin. Biochim Biophys Acta 295: 233–244

360. Ritchie DG, Fuller GM (1983) Hepatocyte-stimulating factor: A monocyte-derived acute-phase regulatory protein. Ann NY Acad Sci 408: 490–500

361. Ritchie RF (1979) In Henry JB (ed), Clinical Diagnosis and Management by Laboratory Methods. W. B. Saunders, Philadelphia

362. Robey FA, Jones KD, Steinberg AD (1985) C-reactive protein mediates the solubilization of nuclear DNA by complement in vitro. J Exp Med 161: 1344–1356

363. Robey FA, Jones KD, Tanaka T, Lieu T-Y (1984) Binding of C-reactive protein to chromatin and nucleosome core particles: A possible physiological role of C-reactive protein. J Biol Chem 259: 7311–7316

364. Robey FA, Liu T-Y (1981) Limulin: A C-reactive protein from *Limulus polyphemus*. J Biol Chem 256: 969–975

365. Rordorf-Adam C, Serban D, Pataki A, Grüninger M (1985) Serum amyloid P component and auto-immune parameters in the assessment of arthritis activity in MRL/lpr/lpr mice. Clin Exp Immunol 61: 509–516

366. Rordorf C, Schnebli HP, Baltz ML, Tennent GA, Pepys MB (1982) The acute-phase response in (NZB x NZW) F_1 and MRL/1 mice. J Exp Med 156: 1268–1273

367. Rose PE, Johnson SA, Meakin M, Mackie PH, Stuart J (1981) Serial study of C-reactive protein during infection in leukaemia. J Clin Pathol 34: 263–266

368. Rosenberg M, Roegner V, Becker FF (1976) Isolation and characterization of two α_1-protease inhibitors in rat serum. Am Rev Resp Dis 113: 779–785

369. Rosenthal CJ, Franklin EC (1975) Variation with age and disease of an amyloid A protein-related serum component. J Clin Invest 55: 746–753

370. Rosenthal CJ, Sullivan LM (1979) Serum amyloid A to monitor cancer dissemination. Ann Int Med 91: 383–390

371. Rowe IF, Baltz ML, Soutar AK, Pepys MB (1984) In vivo turnover studies of C-reactive protein and lipoproteins in the rabbit. Clin Exp Immunol 58: 245–252

372. Ryden L (1972) Comparison of polypeptide-chain structure of four mammalian ceruloplasmins by gel filtration in guanidine hydrochloride solutions. Eur J Biochem 28: 46–50

373. Ryden L, Bjork I (1976) Reinvestigation of some physiochemical and chemical properties of human ceruloplasmin (ferroxidase). Biochemistry 15: 3411–3417

374. Salonen E-M, Vartio T, Hedman K, Vaheri A (1984) Binding of fibronectin by the acute phase reactant C-reactive protein. J Biol Chem 259: 1496–1501

375. Samols D, MacIntyre SS, Kushner I (1985) Studies of translatable mRNA for rabbit C-reactive protein. Biochem J 227: 759–765

376. Sarcione EJ, Bogden AE (1966) Hepatic synthesis of alpha$_2$ (acute phase)-globulin of rat plasma. Science 153: 547–548

377. Sarcione EJ, Bohne M (1969) Synthesis of alpha$_2$ (acute phase) globulin by fetal and neonatal rat liver *in vitro*. Proc Soc Exp Biol Med 131: 1454–1456

378. Sarlo KT, Mortensen RF (1985) Enhanced interleukin-1 (IL-1) production mediated by mouse serum amyloid P-component. Cell Immunol 93: 398–405

379. Schade VR (1980) Quantitative development of IgG and alpha-2-acute phase protein (alpha-2-AP) during the lifespan of female and male laboratory rats (Rattus Norvegicus Berkenhout, 1769). Z Versuchstierk 22: 113–121

380. Schade R, Gotz F, Porstmann B, Friedrich A, Nugel E (1982) The acute phase proteins of the rat, their regulation by hormones and biological significance. Agents Actions Suppl 10: 213–231

381. Schalm OW, Jain NC, Carroll EJ (1975) Veterinary Hematology, 3rd ed. Lea & Febiger, Philadelphia

382. Schmid K (1975) In Putnam FW (ed), The Plasma Proteins, Vol 1. Academic Press, New York

383. Schmid K, Kaufmann H, Isemura S, Bauer F, Emura J, Motoyama T, Ishiguro M, Nanno S (1973) Structure of α_1-acid glycoprotein. The complete amino acid sequence, multiple amino acid substitutions, and homology with immunoglobulins. Biochemistry 12: 2711–2724

384. Schreiber G, Aldred AR, Thomas T, Birch HE, Dickson PW, Guo-fen T, Heinrich PC, Northemann W, Howlett GJ, De Jong FA, Mitchell A (1986) Levels of messenger ribonucleic acids for plasma proteins in rat liver during acute experimental inflammation. Inflammation 10: 59–66

385. Seaman AJ, Malinow MR (1968) Blood clotting in nonhuman primates. Lab Anim Care 18: 80–84

386. Selinger MJ, McAdam KPWJ, Kaplan MM, Sipe JD, Vogel SN, Rosenstreich DL (1980) Monokine-

induced synthesis of serum amyloid A protein by hepatocytes. Nature 285: 498–500

387. Senju O, Takagi Y, Uzawa R, Iwasaki Y, Suzuki T, Gomi K, Ishii T (1986) A new immunoquantitative method by latex agglutination-application for the determination of serum C-reactive protein (CRP) and its clinical significance. J Clin Lab Immunol 19: 99–103

388. Serban D, Rordorf-Adam C (1986) Quantitation of serum amyloid P component by an enzyme-linked immunoassay. J Immunol Methods 90: 159–164

389. Serbource-Goguel Seta N, Durand G, Corbic M, Agneray J, Feger J (1986) Alterations in relative proportions of microheterogenous forms of human α₁-acid glycoprotein in liver disease. J Hepatol 2: 245–252

390. Sheedlo HJ, Beck ML (1982) Electrophoretic analysis of the plasma and urinary proteins and the ceruloplasmin oxidase activity of heterozygous tortoiseshell Mo^to/+) female mice (Mus musculus). Comp Biochem Physiol 71B: 309–311

391. Shephard EG, Van Helden PD, Strauss M, Böhm L, DeBeer FC (1986) Functional effects of CRP binding to nuclei. Immunology 58: 489–494

392. Shibata K, Okubo H, Ishibashi H, Tsuda K (1977) Rat α₁-acid glycoprotein. Purification and immunological estimation of its serum concentration. Biochim Biophys Acta 495: 37–45

393. Shibata K, Okubo H, Ishibashi H, Tsuda-Kawamura K, Yanase T (1978) Rat α₁-acid glycoprotein: Uptake by inflammatory and tumor tissues. Br J Exp Pathol 59: 601–608

394. Siegel J, Osmand AP, Wilson MF, Gewurz H (1975) Interactions of C-reactive protein with the complement system. II. C-reactive protein-mediated consumption of complement by poly-L-lysine polymers and other polycations. J Exp Med 142: 709–721

395. Singh PP, Gervais F, Skamene E, Mortensen RF (1986) Serum amyloid P-component-induced enhancement of macrophage listericidal activity. Infect Immun 52: 688–694

396. Sipe JD, Ignaczak TF, Pollock PS, Glenner GG (1976) Amyloid fibril protein AA: Purification and properties of the antigenically related serum component as determined by solid phase radioimmunoassay. J Immunol 116: 1151–1156

397. Sipe JD, Vogel SN, Ryan JL, McAdam KPWJ, Rosenstreich DL (1979) Detection of a mediator derived from endotoxin-stimulated macrophages that induces the acute phase serum amyloid A response in mice. J Exp Med 150: 597–606

398. Sipe JD, Vogel SN, Sztein MB, Skinner M, Cohen AS (1982) The role of interleukin 1 in acute phase serum amyloid A (SAA) and serum amyloid P (SAP) biosynthesis. Ann NY Acad Sci 389: 137–149

399. Sottrup-Jensen L, Stepanik TM, Kristensen T, Lonblad PB, Jones CM, Wierzbicki DM, Magnusson S, Domdey H, Wetsel RA, Lundwall A, Tack BF, Fey GH (1985) Common evolutionary origin of α₂-macroglobulin and complement components C3 and C4. Proc Natl Acad Sci 82: 9–13

400. Srai SKS, Burroughs AK, Wood B, Epstein O (1986) The ontogeny of liver copper metabolism in the guinea pig: Clues to the etiology of Wilson's disease. Hepatology 6: 427–432

401. Starcher B, Hill CH (1966) Isolation and characterization of induced ceruloplasmin from chick serum. Biochim Biophys Acta 127: 400–406

402. Starkey PM, Barrett AJ (1982) Evolution of α₂-macroglobulin. The demonstration in a variety of vertebrate species of a protein resembling human α₂-macroglobulin. Biochem J 205: 91–95

403. Stein-Streilein J, Hart DA (1981) Isolation and characterization of hamster alpha₂ macroglobulin. Adv Exp Med Biol 134: 111–119

404. Stolc V (1984) Genetic polymorphism of ceruloplasmin in the rat. J Hered 75: 414–415

405. Stolc V, Kunz HW, Gill TJ (1983) Polymorphism of malic dehydrogenase, methemoglobin reductase, ceruloplasmin, and catalase in the rat. Transplant Proc 15: 1679–1680

406. Sur J, Chatterjee T, Datta AG (1979) Studies on the effects on some biogenic amines on plasma fibrinogen level of rats and rabbits. Biochem Pharmacol 28: 1597–1600

407. Suzuki Y, Sinohara H (1986) Isolation and characterization of α-macroglobulin from guinea pig plasma. J Biochem 99: 1655–1665

408. Swick RA, Cheeke PR, Buhler DR (1982) Subcellular distribution of hepatic copper, zinc and iron and serum ceruloplasmin in rats intoxicated by oral pyrrolizidine (senecio) alkaloids. J An Sci 55: 1425–1430

409. Syin C, Gotschlich EC, Liu T-Y (1986) Rabbit C-reactive protein: Biosynthesis and characterization of cDNA clones. J Biol Chem 261: 5473–5479

410. Sztein MB, Vogel SN, Sipe JD, Murphy PA, Mizel SB, Oppenheim JJ, Rosenstreich DL (1981) The role of macrophages in the acute-phase response: SAA inducer is closely related to lymphocyte activating factor and endogenous pyrogen. Cell Immunol 63: 164–176

411. Takahara H, Nakamura Y, Yamamoto K, Sinohara H (1983) Comparative studies on the serum levels of α-1-antitrypsin and α-macroglobulin in several mammals. Tohoku J Exp Med 139: 265–270

412. Takahara H, Nakayama H, Sinohara H (1980) Purification and characterization of rat plasma α-1-antitrypsin. J Biochem 88: 417–424

413. Takahara H, Sinohara H (1982) Mouse plasma trypsin inhibitors. Isolation and characterization of α-1-antitrypsin and contrapsin, a novel trypsin inhibitor. J Biol Chem 257: 2438–2446

414. Takahara H, Sinohara H (1983) Inhibitory spectrum of mouse contrapsin and α₁-antitrypsin against mouse serine proteases. J Biochem 93: 1411–1419

415. Takahashi M, Yokota T, Yamashita Y, Ishihara T, Uchino F (1985) Ultrastructural evidence for the synthesis of serum amyloid A protein by murine hepatocytes. Lab Invest 52: 220–223

416. Takahashi N, Ortel TL, Putnam FW (1984) Single-chain structure of human ceruloplasmin: The complete amino acid sequence of the whole molecule. Proc Natl Acad Sci USA 81: 390–394

417. Tanner AR, Collins AL, Bull FG (1985) The clinical value of rapid C-reactive protein measurement in cerebrospinal fluid. Clin Chim Acta 147: 267–272

418. Tatsuta E, Sipe JD, Shirahama T, Skinner M, Cohen AS (1983) Different regulatory mechanisms for serum amyloid A and serum amyloid P synthesis by cultured mouse hepatocytes. J Biol Chem 258: 5414–5418

419. Tavassoli M, Kishimoto T, Kataoka M (1986) Liver endothelium mediates the hepatocyte's uptake of ceruloplasmin. J Cell Biol 102: 1298–1303

420. Thomas T, Schreiber G (1985) Acute-phase response of plasma protein synthesis during experimental inflammation in neonatal rats. Inflammation 9: 1–7

421. Thompson RA, Sukumaran KD, Rajagopalan K (1985) Inappropriate responses to *Mycobacterium leprae* infections-C-reactive protein in man and serum amyloid P in mice. Clin Exp Immunol 61: 329–335

422. Thompson WL, Abeles FB, Beall FA, Dinterman RE, Wannemacher RW (1976) Influence of the adrenal glucocorticoids on the stimulation of synthesis of hepatic ribonucleic acid and plasma acute-phase globulins by leucocytic endogenous mediator. Biochem J 156: 25–32

423. Tillett WS, Francis T (1930) Serological reactions in pneumonia with a non-protein somatic fraction of pneumococcus. J Exp Med 52: 561–571

424. Tobias PS, McAdam KPWJ, Ulevitch RJ (1982) Interactions of bacterial lipopolysaccharide with acute-phase rabbit serum and isolation of two forms of rabbit serum amyloid A. J Immunol 128: 1420–1427

425. Turner R, Liener IE (1977) α_1-antitrypsin in rat and man: A comparison of structure, biosynthesis, and degradation. Fed Proc 36: 765

426. Ungar-Waron H, Gluckman A, Spira E, Waron M, Trainin Z (1978) Ceruloplasmin as a marker of neoplastic activity in rabbits bearing the VX-2 carcinoma. Cancer Res 38: 1296–1299

427. Ungar-Waron H, Gluckman A, Trainin Z (1982) The source of increased serum coeruloplasmin activity in rabbits bearing the VX-2 carcinoma. J Comp Pathol 92: 331–336

428. Van den Hamer CJA, Morell AG, Scheinberg IH, Hickman J, Aswell G (1970) Physical and chemical studies on ceruloplasmin. IX. The role of galactosyl residues in the clearance of ceruloplasmin from the circulation. J Biol Chem 245: 4397–4402

429. VanGool J, Boers W, deNie I (1978) Inhibitory effects of rat α_2 macrofetoprotein (α_MFB), an acute phase globulin, on galactosamine hepatitis. Exp Molec Pathol 29: 228–240

430. VanGool J, Ladiges NCJJ, Boers W (1982) Inhibition of polymorphonuclear leukocyte chemotaxis by α-macrofetoprotein, an acute-phase reactant of the rat. Inflammation 6: 127–135

431. VanGool J, Schreuder J, Ladiges NCJJ (1974) Inhibitory effect of foetal α_2 globulin, an acute phase protein, on carrageenin oedema in the rat. J Pathol 112: 245–262

432. VanGool J, VanVugt H, deNie I (1986) Acute phase reactants enhance CCl_4 induced liver cirrhosis in the rat. Exp Mol Pathol 44: 157–168

433. Vannice JL, Taylor JM, Ringold GM (1984) Glucocorticoid-mediated induction of α_1-acid glycoprotein: Evidence for hormone-regulated RNA processing. Proc Natl Acad Sci USA 81: 4241–4245

434. VanRuijven IAM, Nieuwenhuizen W (1978) Purification of rat fibrinogen and its constituent chains. Biochem J 169: 653–658

435. VanVugt H, VanGool J, de Ridder L (1986) α_2 macroglobulin of the rat, an acute phase protein, mitigates the early course of endotoxic shock. Br J Exp Pathol 67: 313–319

436. Verbanac KM, Heath EC (1983) Biosynthesis and processing of rat α_1-antitrypsin. Arch Biochem Biophys 223: 149–157

437. Versavel C, Feve A, Esnard F, Lebreton de Vonne T, Mouray H (1983) The evolution of α-1 and α-2-macroglobulin in levels in the serum of rabbit fetus and newborn. Comp Biochem Physiol 75-B: 701–702

438. Vetter ML, Gewurz H, Baum LL (1986) The effects of C-reactive protein on human cell-mediated cytotoxicity. J Leukocyte Biol 39: 13–25

439. Viedma JA, de la Iglesia A, Parera M, Lopez MT (1986) A new automated turbidimetric immunoassay for quantifying α_1-antitrypsin in serum. Clin Chem 32: 1020–1022

440. Voelkel EF, Levine L, Alper CA, Tashjian AH (1978) Acute phase reactants ceruloplasmin and haptoglobin and their relationship to plasma prostaglandins in rabbits bearing the VX_2 carcinoma. J Exp Med 147: 1078–1088

441. Volanakis JE, Kaplan MD (1971) Specificity of C-reactive protein for choline phosphate residues of pneumococcal C-polysaccharide. Proc Soc Exp Med Biol 136: 612–614

442. vonArdenne M, Chaplain RA (1973) The inhibitory effect of α-2-macroglobulin on tumor growth. Experientia 29: 1271–1272

443. Wadsworth C, Fasth A, Wadsworth E (1985) A critical analysis of commercially available latex particle reagents for C-reactive protein (CRP) slide agglutination tests. J Immunol Methods 83: 29–36

444. Waites GT, Bell AM, Bell SC (1983) Acute phase serum proteins in syngeneic and allogeneic mouse pregnancy. Clin Exp Immunol 53: 225–232

445. Wannemacher RW, Pekarek RS, Thompson WL, Curnow RT, Beall FA, Zenser TV, DeRubertis FR, Beisel WR (1975) A protein from polymorphonuclear leukocytes (LEM) which affect the rate of hepatic amino acid transport and synthesis of acute-phase globulins. Endocrinology 96: 651–661

446. Weimer HE, Benjamin DC (1965) Immunochemical detection of an acute-phase protein in rat serum. Am J Physiol 209: 736–744

447. Weimer HE, Roberts DM, Comb JC (1972) Genetic differences in the α 2-AP (acute phase) globulin response to a phlogogenic stimulus in albino rats. Br J Exp Pathol 53: 253–257

448. Weiner AL, Cousins RJ (1983) Hormonally produced changes in caeruloplasmin synthesis and secretion in primary cultured rat hepatocytes. Biochem J 212: 297–304

449. Weisman S, Goldsmith B, Winzler R, Lepper MH (1961) Turnover of plasma orosomucoid in man. J Lab Clin Med 57: 7

450. Werner M (1969) Serum protein changes during the acute phase reaction. Clin Chim Acta 25: 299–305

451. Westrom BR, Karlsson BW, Ohlsson K (1983) Immuno-cross-reactivity between α-macroglobulins from pig, dog, rat and man including human pregnancy-associated α2-glycoprotein. Hoppe-Seyler's Z Physiol Chem 364: 375–381

452. Whicher JT, Chambers RE, Higginson J, NAshef L, Higgins PG (1985) Acute phase response of serum amyloid A protein and C-reactive protein to the common cold and influenza. J Clin Pathol 38: 312–316

453. Whisler RL, Newhouse YG, Mortensen RF (1983) CRP-mediated modulation of human B cell colony development. J Immunol 130: 248 253

454. Whisler RL, Proctor VK, Downs EC, Mortensen RF (1986) Modulation of human monocyte chemotaxis and procoagulant activity by human C-reactive protein (CRP). Lymphokine Res 5: 223–228

455. Williams RC (1982) C-reactive protein binding to lymphocyte subpopulations in human disease states. Ann NY Acad Sci 389: 395–404

456. Williams JE, Cypher JJ, Mosesson MW (1985) Evidence that production of platelet fibrinogen is synchronous with platelet production in the turpentine-induced acute phase response. J Lab Clin Med 106: 343–348

457. Woloski BMR NJ, Gospodarek E, Jamieson JC (1985) Studies on monokines as mediators of the acute phase response. Effects on sialyltransferase, albumin, α1-acid glycoprotein, and β-N-acetylhexosaminidase. Biochem Biophys Res Comm 130: 30–36

458. Wood DD, Gammon M, Staruch MJ (1982) An ELISA assay for murine amyloid A and serum amyloid A utilizing monoclonal antibodies. J Immunol Meth 55: 19–26

459. Wood M (1986) Plasma drug binding: implications for anesthesiologists. Anesth Analg 65: 786–804

460. Wright SD, Craigmyle LS, Silverstein SC (1983) Fibronectin and serum amyloid P-component stimulate C3b- and C3bi-mediated phagocytosis in cultured human monocytes. J Exp Med 158: 1338–1343

461. Wycoff HD (1970) Production of fibrinogen following an endotoxin injection. Proc Soc Exp Biol Med 133: 940–943

462. Yamamoto K-I, Shiroo M, Migita S (1986) Diverse gene expression for isotypes of murine serum amyloid A protein during acute phase reaction. Science 232: 227–229

463. Yamamoto K, Sinohara H (1984) Regulation by sex hormones of serum levels of contrapsin and α1-antiprotease in the mouse. Biochim Biophys Acta 798: 231–234

464. Yamamoto K, Takahara H, Sinohara H (1981) Developmental changes in the levels of alpha-1-antitrypsin and contrapsin in the mouse serum. Biochem Int 3: 617–620

465. Yamamoto K, Tsujino Y, Saito A, Sinohara H (1985) Concentrations of murinoglobulin and α-macroglobulin in the mouse serum: Variations with age, sex, strain, and experimental inflammation. Biochem Int 10: 463–469

466. Yasuhara M, Fujiwara J, Kitade S, Katayama H, Okumura K, Hori R (1985) Effect of altered plasma protein binding on pharmacokinetics and pharmacodynamics of propranolol in rats after surgery: Role of alpha-1-acid glycoprotein. J Pharmacol Exp Ther 235: 513–520

467. Zahedi K, Mortensen RF (1986) Macrophage tumoricidal activity induced by human C-reactive protein. Canc Res 46: 5077–5083

468. Zeineh RA, Barrett B, Niemirowski L, Fiorella BJ (1972) Turnover rate of orosomucoid in the dog with sterile abscess. Am J Physiol 222: 1326–1332

469. Zuckerman SH, Surprenant YM (1986) Simplified micro ELISA for the quantitation of murine serum amyloid A protein. J Immunol Methods 92: 37 43

11

Clinical Enzymology

WALTER E. HOFFMANN, DVM, PhD, JOHN KRAMER, DVM, PhD, A. R. MAIN, PhD,* and
J. L. TORRES, PhD

The activities of serum enzymes in many diseases of humans and animals have been investigated extensively. Observations of these changes have proven to be important in diagnosing diseases and in determining the patient's prognosis.

Several reviews discuss the diagnostic value of changes in serum enzymes in animals (39,176). These studies generally are based on clinical observations of such changes in experimentally induced or naturally occurring diseases. The data and observations thus obtained are most useful in further investigations of the animal species in which the original studies were conducted. We do not mean to minimize species differences, but it is hoped that from the information and concepts presented, extrapolations and predictions can be applied to species in which less definitive work has been carried out.

The concentration of enzymes in serum depends on the rate of enzyme release from tissue into blood and its subsequent removal from the blood. Obviously, a significant factor affecting the amount of enzyme released from tissue is its concentration in tissue. Tissues with greater concentrations of an enzyme are more likely to contribute that enzyme to serum than are tissues with little or no concentration. In the dog, for

example, serum alanine aminotransferase is a specific and sensitive indicator of hepatocellular disease because it is found in high concentrations only in the liver.

However, the magnitude of increase of an enzyme in serum is not always a reflection of the quantity of the enzyme in the tissue from which it is derived. Alkaline phosphatase, for example, is markedly elevated in hepatobiliary disorders and virtually never elevated in renal disease, yet the concentration of the enzyme is many-fold higher in renal tissue than in liver tissue. The accessibility of liver alkaline phosphatase to blood and the increased synthesis of the enzyme during cholestasis allow alkaline phosphatase to increase dramatically in hepatic disease; however, in the kidney, tubular disease results in release of the enzyme into urine and thus is inaccessible to blood (62). The tissue concentration of many of the commonly used diagnostic enzymes of several species is listed in tabular form elsewhere (39,58).

The cellular location and mechanism by which an enzyme is released and reaches blood affect the increase of the enzyme in blood. In some cases cytoplasmic enzymes can be released directly into the blood through damaged cell membranes, as with alanine aminotransferase from hepatocytes. Other cytoplasmic enzymes whose tissues do not have direct accessibility to the bloodstream may first be released into

---

*Deceased.

237

interstitial fluid and carried by the lymphatics to the bloodstream, as are the muscle enzymes. Creatine kinase is a good example. Enzymes such as gamma glutamyl transpeptidase of biliary epithelial cells or the proximal tubular epithelial cells of kidney are inaccessible to the bloodstream and are lost in bile or urine. In addition, gamma glutamyl transferase and alkaline phosphatase are membrane enzymes and not easily released. However, as will be discussed, in cholestasis two factors come into play to allow serum increases of biliary enzymes. Retention of bile allows solubilization of a membrane-bound enzyme by bile acids, and regurgitation of bile between the lateral surfaces of the hepatocyte membranes allows accessibility to the blood.

Drugs and physiologic changes such as age also play an important role in the serum activity of various enzymes in health and disease. The well-recognized increase in alkaline phosphatase in dogs being treated with glucocorticosteroids is an example of enzyme induction as the result of a drug.

Numerous additional factors affect the rate and magnitude of enzyme release from tissue. The extent, rapidity, and susceptibility of tissue injury affect the rate and extent of release of an enzyme. The molecular weight of an enzyme may determine when and how the enzyme is leaked from the cell, but the molecular weight might also determine the rate of clearance of the enzyme from blood, if the enzyme is small enough to pass through the glomerulus. The rate of synthesis of the enzyme in tissue will affect the increase in blood. Also, if injury to tissue results in cellular proliferation, more cells will be available to release their enzymes to blood.

As already indicated, the rate of removal from the blood is also an important factor in determining the magnitude of enzyme increase in the blood in disease, the persistence of the enzyme increase, and thus the diagnostic and prognostic value of that enzyme. Intestinal alkaline phosphatase in the dog is cleared from blood so rapidly (T1/2 < 6 minutes) that it is thought to offer no diagnostic value. Arginase is also cleared fairly rapidly (T1/2 < 80 minutes), yet it remains in the blood sufficiently long to be of diagnostic value in acute disease. This rapid clearance is beneficial in that it allows assessment of the direction of the disease. Rapidly decreasing serum enzyme activity indicates a good prognosis. Other enzymes, such as alanine aminotransferase, with half-lives of days rather than minutes or hours, offer diagnostic value during as well as after the initial tissue insult. In addition, these longer-lived enzymes may in some cases be more sensitive in detecting chronic and/or low grade disease because the longer half-life allows accumulation of the enzyme in blood when enzyme leakage from tissue is only minimal. Minimal elevations of alanine aminotransferase are often seen in dog serum in several conditions during which serum arginase is in the normal range because of its rapid clearance from blood.

Many enzymes exist in multiple forms (isoenzymes); this finding has little importance in regulating the concentration of serum enzymes but may have considerable importance in determining the value of an enzyme as a diagnostic tool. A specific isoenzyme or a defined pattern of isoenzymes is often indicative of the organ from which it is derived. Examples of this are lactic acid dehydrogenase, creatine phosphokinase, and alkaline phosphatase.

In light of the foregoing discussion an attempt will be made to include in this chapter information or reference to the source of information dealing with tissue concentration, cellular location, drug effects, mechanism of release, half-life in the bloodstream, and isoenzymes for each of the enzymes discussed.

HEPATIC ENZYMES OF CLINICAL IMPORTANCE

Clinical enzymology as it relates to diagnosis of liver disease may be conveniently but not completely broken down into two areas of discussion: (1) the study of enzymes, sometimes referred to as parenchymal enzymes, whose presence in serum reflects loss of hepatocyte membrane integrity or necrosis of hepatocytes, and (2) the study of "biliary enzymes" whose presence in serum reflects abnormalities of the biliary system such as obstruction, proliferation, inflammation, or neoplasia. Although there are numerous enzymes that are reported to fall into one of these two categories and probably numerous enzymes that remain to be evaluated, this section will deal with those enzymes that have been investigated most extensively and are accepted for their role as clinical markers of hepatocellular or hepatobiliary disease.

ALANINE AMINOTRANSFERASE

Alanine aminotransferase (EC 2.6.1.2) (ALT), which is commonly known as glumatic pyruvic transaminase, catalyzes the reaction: L-alanine + alpha - ketoglutarate → pyruvate + L - glutamate. The measurement of ALT activity in serum has been used extensively to assess hepatic necrosis/hepatocellular integrity in man, dog, cat, and several laboratory animals but is of no value for this purpose in large domestic animals such as horse, cow, and sheep. The diagnostic value of ALT has been studied more thoroughly than that of any enzyme with the exception of alkaline phosphatase.

Tissue Distribution

The tissue concentration as well as the tissue specificity of ALT is of obvious importance in determining the presence and extent of hepatocellular disease in various laboratory animal species. In the dog, the activity of ALT per gram of liver tissue is approximately five times greater than that in any other tissue, with the next highest activity per gram of tissue being found in the heart (58,63,357). Similar findings were reported for the rat, ferret, and mouse in which 3 to 10 times greater activities of ALT were found in liver tissue than in tissue from any other organ (39,58). On the basis of tissue concentration of ALT, this enzyme would show little or no organ specificity in the guinea pig, rabbit, monkey, and baboon as there is as much or nearly as much ALT activity in heart muscle per gram of tissue as there is in liver (58). In addition, the activity of ALT in liver tissue in the guinea pig and rabbit is less than half that found in the dog, mouse, and rat liver on a per gram basis, suggesting that the sensitivity of the enzyme as an indicator of hepatocellular disease is also reduced.

There is a continuing effort to determine the magnitude of loss of hepatocellular integrity from the ALT activity in serum. This determination may be affected by the variability of tissue concentrations of ALT among individual animals. The activity of ALT per gram of tissue in a group of 10 dogs amounted to a 20 per cent difference between lowest and highest (334). There was no difference between lobes of the liver of the same dog. The difference in liver content of ALT between animals could be the

result of many factors, one of which is protein content in the diet. With an increase of protein in the diet of rats there is as much as a threefold increase in liver ALT activity (37,46). In hepatocellular damage this increase in liver ALT activity probably would have been reflected in serum. There also is as much as a five- to sevenfold increase in ALT activity in liver tissue of fasted rats, probably as a result of gluconeogenesis (268).

Cellular Location

It is well recognized that ALT is found in both the cytoplasm and mitochondria. Considerable difference exists in the distribution of the enzyme between these two compartments when various organs from the same species or the same organs from different species are compared. The cytosol to mitochondrial ratio of ALT in the rat heart is approximately 50:1, whereas the ratio is 5:1 in the rat liver (73). The differences between species are demonstrated in the observation that the ratio of cytosol to mitochondrial ALT in guinea pig liver is approximately 0.5:1, whereas in the rat liver it is 5:1 (73,275).

Isoenzymes

Although the isoenzymes of ALT have not been studied as extensively as those of aspartic aminotransferase (AAT), evidence of a soluble or cytoplasmic isoenzyme and a mitochondrial isoenzyme of ALT is conclusive. The soluble form has been purified to homogeneity and its physiochemical and kinetic properties have been studied (296). However, the mitochondrial form is more labile, resulting in only limited knowledge of its properties. The isoenzymes have been separated by isoelectric focusing with the pI of the soluble enzyme from rat, guinea pig, and human liver and from rat and pig kidney ranging from 4.8 to 5.7, whereas the mitochondrial ALT from the same tissues has a pI ranging from 6.7 to 7.5 (275). Additional reported differences in the physiochemical and kinetic properties of the two isoenzymes along with the pI data indicate that ALT from mitochondria and that from cytoplasma are two different proteins (73).

The similarity of the cyotplasmic enzyme obtained from different organs indicates that the isoenzymes have no organ specificity but rather are specific for the cell compartment from which they are derived. This apparently has not been explored from a diagnostic standpoint. Considering the instability of the mitochondrial isoenzyme, separation of the isoenzymes may not be diagnostically fruitful.

Little is known about the mitochondrial isoenzyme of ALT from man. At least two groups of investigators (162,275) have been unable to isolate mitochondrial ALT, possibly because of the instability of the enzyme in livers obtained at autopsy.

Although most studies of the ALT isoenzymes have concentrated on differences in the mitochondrial and soluble isoenzymes, there is also evidence that different forms of the soluble enzyme may exist. In rat liver, two soluble isoenzymes have been demonstrated by DEAE-cellulose column chromatography and polyacrylamide gel electrophoresis (243). One form is predominant in the immature rat, the other is predominant in the senescent rat, whereas both isoenzymes are present in the adult rat.

Half-Life

Experimental data regarding the clearance rate of ALT from blood are variable. Intravenous injection of a crude extract of normal dog liver into normal dogs has resulted in a half-life in the bloodstream of approximately 3 hours (357), approximately 20 hours in a second study (258), and 45 hours in a third study (95). Partially purified (100-fold) dog liver ALT showed a half-life in the bloodstream of 60 hours in a fourth study (96). Rabbit liver ALT has an intravenous half-life of approximately 5 hours in the rabbit (11), whereas pig heart ALT has a half-life of approximately 10 hours when injected into the mouse (193). Although the difference in clearance rate in different species may be attributed to species differences, the marked variation of half-life (3 vs 60 hours) in the dog is more difficult to understand. If semilogarithmic plotting of ALT acitivity is begun 4 to 5 days after carbon tetrachloride (CCl_4) intoxication of dogs, the half-life calculated is most consistent with the 45 to 60 hours reported (142). Although these data may overestimate the half-life because of continued leakage of ALT from cells, the return of arginase (which has a short half-life of approximately 80 minutes) to pre-dose activity by this time would suggest that leakage of ALT

has abated, and an estimate of a half-life of 45 to 60 hours is the most realistic value (142).

The manner in which ALT is removed from blood is unknown, but removal of the spleen or intravenous administration of India ink to block the reticuloendothelial system has no effect on the half-life (96). There is no apparent excretion of ALT into the urine, indicating the kidney is probably not the means by which ALT is removed from blood.

Organ Disease

The release of ALT from cells into serum during hepatic disease is well documented. Positive correlations of the degree of necrosis to serum ALT activity have been made in dog (330), rabbit (304), and rat (24,67). Although ALT is released from cells during necrosis, ALT also can be "leaked" from cells without morphologic evidence of cell damage. In perfused rat liver in which the degree of hypoxia can be controlled, cytoplasmic enzymes are leaked from the cell at a rate inversely proportional to their molecular weight (287), indicating that leakage of enzymes such as ALT may occur without necrosis of the cell. Following ligation of the bile duct of dogs, there was poor correlation between serum ALT activity and the morphologic changes observed (330). There was essentially no evidence of necrosis, yet 5 to 6 days after ligation, there was as much as a 25-fold increase in serum ALT. The bile salt and cholesterol retention which occurs following bile duct ligation, may change the lipid composition of the hepatocyte membrane, resulting in increased permeability. The increase in serum cholesterol and serum ALT activity paralleled one another following ligation (330).

Carbon tetrachloride (CCl_4) is the toxin most commonly used to create hepatocellular damage. Studies with this toxin have provided most of our information regarding alterations in serum ALT activity during hepatocellular necrosis. The increase in serum ALT activity is proportional to the dose in both rabbit (304) and rat (175). Repeated administration of CCl_4 over a prolonged period results in a decrease in peak serum ALT activity (304), thought to be a result of decreased functional liver mass.

The magnitude of increase of serum ALT following CCl_4-induced hepatotoxicity is a result not only of leakage or release from the cell in rats, but also of new synthesis of the enzyme (240). Administration of the protein synthesis inhibitor cycloheximide along with CCl_4 blocked synthesis of ALT in liver and reduced the increase of ALT in serum after 24 hours by as much as 75 per cent.

Peak activity of ALT following a single dose of CCl_4 has been reported to occur at 24 hours, in the rabbit (304), within 24 to 48 hours in the dog (231), or at 58 hours in the dog (357). Peak activities of ALT associated with or secondary to cholestasis were not observed until 5 or more days after obstruction in the dog (123,330).

As indicated previously, experimental data for the clearance rate of ALT are variable, so that the duration of increased serum ALT activity at this time is best obtained from experiments that provide an acute but single insult to the liver. There seems to be considerable species variation in the duration of increased ALT activity. In rabbits treated with CCl_4, there was a 100-fold elevation of ALT activity by 24 hours with a return to normal by 96 hours (304). This rapid return to normal correlates well with the reported half-life of 5 hours for the rabbit. The elevation of ALT activity following CCl_4 intoxication in the dog persists from 9 to 23 days (64,123,231). This finding correlates with the reported half-life of 45 to 60 hours. Elevations of ALT activity induced by hyperthermia in rats returned to normal in 72 to 96 hours after reaching a peak at 24 hours (146), suggesting that the clearance rate in the rat is more like that of the rabbit than the dog. The diagnostic and prognostic significance of the duration of increased ALT activity in serum is of obvious importance and will be discussed further in regard to other enzymes later in this chapter.

The effect of the manner of handling mice on serum ALT has been described (315). Serum ALT activity in either normal mice or rats given CCl_4 is approximately three times greater if the mouse is handled by the body than if handled by the tail.

Drug Effects on ALT Activity in Serum and Liver

The list of drugs that cause hepatotoxicity, and thus release ALT into serum is extensive. However, those drugs that cause alterations in ALT activity in liver or serum, or both, without causing hepatotoxicity may be of greater importance in choosing ALT as a diagnostic tool, establishing normals, and interpreting alterations in serum ALT. Glucocorticoids are the most often studied drug in the induction of ALT and are documented to increase ALT in rat liver tissue following treatment (244,268–270,316). Only those steroids that are active as glycogenic agents induce an increase in ALT (268). In 7 days these increases ranged to as much as 13 times greater than ALT activity before treatment. The response was directly related to the dose of corticosteroid administered (270). The hormonally induced increases in activity of hepatic ALT were due to changes in the quantity of enzyme protein (297). There is definite agreement that glucocorticoids induce the soluble or cytoplasmic form of ALT. However, there is less agreement on whether mitochondrial ALT is induced. Induction of mitochondrial ALT may depend on the age of the rat (244,316).

The effect of glucocorticoid treatment on serum ALT activity is less thoroughly studied. It could be expected that the increase in liver ALT would result in increases in serum ALT activity especially during hepatocellular injury. In the dog, increases in serum ALT following glucocorticosteroid treatment reached approximately 30 times pretreatment activity (27,77). There was considerable variation in the response, which may be a result of the synthetic corticosteroid used and the route of administration. To what extent these increases are due to increased synthesis of ALT as opposed to leakage of the enzyme is not known. Little or no necrosis of hepatocytes is seen with corticosteroid treatment; however, the swollen appearance of the hepatocytes, cytoplasmic vacuolization, and glycogen accumulation could result in some leakage of the enzyme from hepatocytes into blood.

An increase in ALT activity in liver was also seen after glucagon administration (25). Because this increase also followed the administration of cyclic AMP and of cyclic AMP activators and inhibitors of phosphodiesterase, it is believed that the effect of glucagon is mediated through cyclic AMP.

The increase in serum ALT activity observed in mice treated with morphine can be totally or partially prevented with hypophysectomy or adrenalectomy, suggesting that morphine has an effect on hepatic function by way of the central nervous system (55). This increase in serum ALT activity may or may not be related to increased ALT synthesis.

Although it is more common to consider drugs that elevate serum ALT activity either through enzyme induction or hepatocellular damage, decreases in ALT also can be observed. Cefazolin treatment of rats resulted in decreased serum ALT activity, which was associated with decreased ALT activity in liver, brain, and kidney (75).

ORNITHINE CARBAMYL TRANSFERASE

Ornithine carbamyl transferase (OCT) (EC 2.1.3.3) catalyzes the reaction: carbamyl phosphate + ornithine → citrulline + phosphate. This enzyme is a urea cycle enzyme and found in all ureotelic animals.

Organ Distribution

Ornithine carbamyl transferase along with arginase is considered a truly liver specific enzyme; however, a small amount of activity is found in the ileum and duodenum (178,258). The activity is approximately 60-fold higher in dog liver than in the ileum or duodenum, indicating OCT activity in the latter organs can essentially be ignored. Similar organ distribution of OCT is found in the rat; however, some OCT activity is also found in kidney (291). Kidney OCT amounts to only 1 to 2 per cent of that found in liver.

Cell Location

Ornithine carbamyl transferase is located entirely in mitochondria. Although it is synthesized extramitochondrially on membrane-free polysomes, it is rapidly transported into mitochondria where it is processed to the mature enzyme (218). The enzyme constitutes about 3 to 4 per cent of total mitochondrial protein (159).

Isoenzymes

There are no reports of isoenzymes of OCT as a result of expression of different genetic loci. In fact, it was clearly shown that OCT from gut and liver is a product of the same gene (349). There are reports of mutations in mice with the x-chromosomal sparse-fur mutations which result in OCT preparations with reduced specific

activity (71,249). This mutation results in OCT with an altered pH optimum, reduced Michaelis Constant (Km) for carbamyl phosphate, and reduced V_{max} and as such it appears to be a good model for studying the molecular basis of similar mutation in man (43).

Intravenous Half-Life

Intravenous infusion of OCT prepared from dog liver into normal dog resulted in only 14 per cent of the activity remaining after 24 hours and only 3 per cent after 48 hours (258), suggesting a half-life of less than 10 hours. This clearance of OCT is considerably more rapid than the clearance of ALT in the same study. A similar rapid clearance of OCT from serum was observed in rats following galactosamine-induced hepatic necrosis (323).

Organ Disease

Hepatic necrosis induced by CCl_4 results in increases of OCT activity several thousandfold greater than that of normal serum activity. In dogs with biliary occlusion there was a 500-fold increase in OCT activity but a much slower return to normal when compared to that in hepatic necrosis (258). Because histologic study of the liver was not performed, it is not possible to correlate severity of the lesion with OCT activity in serum. A 600-fold increase in OCT activity was observed in mice following D-galactosamine–induced hepatic necrosis (323). Increases in serum OCT activity have been observed with experimentally induced hypovolemic shock and were correlated with the severity of the shock (261).

Drug Effects on OCT

Little has been written about the effect of various drugs on OCT induction in the liver. De novo synthesis of OCT is induced in rats with increases in protein consumption and with administration of carbamyl phosphate, the substrate for OCT (291). Because OCT is induced with the need for urea synthesis from ammonia, it is possible that liver OCT will increase with drugs that cause protein catabolism. This may or may not be reflected in normal serum activity.

ARGINASE

Arginase (EC 3.5.3.1), like OCT, is found in the liver of all ureotelic animals. It has received some attention for its value as a diagnostic tool in veterinary medicine, and has considerable potential for being of diagnostic value in both domestic and laboratory animals.

Organ Distribution

Unlike OCT, there are detectable quantities of arginase in red blood cells and in mammary gland and submaxillary salivary gland and in organs including small intestine, pancreas, and kidney in addition to liver. In the rat these organs have less than 10 per cent of the arginase activity per gram of tissue than does liver (135), with kidney having about 4 per cent of the arginase activity when compared to liver (331). The ratio of liver to kidney arginase is high in all species studied, with the highest ratio being found in the dog (241).

The arginase activity in rat liver at birth is approximately 20 per cent of that in adult rat liver (115,136). Arginase activity in the adult rat is not reached until approximately 4 weeks after birth.

Cell Location

Reports on the subcellular location of arginase have suggested that arginase is associated with nuclei, mitochondria, microsomes, and lysosomes. The most recent efforts indicate that arginase is a cytoplasmic enzyme and that previous reports of arginase in various organelles were the result of adsorption of arginase to organelles during isolation procedures (305,314).

Isoenzymes

The isoenzymes of arginase have been studied in greatest detail in man and rat using primarily arginase from liver, kidney, submaxillary gland, and mammary gland. A general conclusion might be that liver arginase in man and rat is similar and in both species is different from that found in all other tissues with the exception of the submaxillary gland. This is somewhat of an oversimplification because there are some species differences. Using antiserum prepared against a purified rat liver arginase, all rat liver arginase is precipitated, suggesting one isoenzyme (106,136,257). This finding is supported by electrophoretic studies which also suggest only one isoenzyme (87,135,257). Using DEAE-cellulose chromatography, liver arginase from numerous species was separated into two forms, with the percentage of each form varying between species (241). In man, two forms of liver arginase can be separated electrophoretically (38,136). The major form is precipitated by rat liver arginase antiserum, whereas the minor form is not, indicating a definite difference between rat and man (136).

Additional differences exist between human and rat arginase. Liver arginase in fetal rat is identical to that in adult rat, whereas in man fetal liver arginase is like that found in kidney. The adult form is not seen until after this fetal period (136). In addition, arginase in fetal rat kidney is like that found in liver. This enzyme disappears at birth and is completely replaced by the adult kidney form of arginase (135).

Arginase from the submaxillary gland is the hepatic type as determined by both electrophoretic and immunologic studies (135,257). Arginase from kidney, intestines, mammary gland, and probably most other tissues is thought to have two forms. These two forms have been studied primarily by electrophoretic and chromatographic means. Whether they are antigenically different is unknown.

Half-Life

To my knowledge there are no studies in which the half-life of arginase in blood of laboratory animals is measured. Intravenous infusion of bovine arginase into two calves resulted in an estimated half-life of 80 minutes (64). Likewise the half-life of arginase in two swine was 129 and 86 minutes (190). If the data that demonstrate the changes in serum arginase activity in the dog following CCl₄ administration (231) are used and certain assumptions made (peak arginase activity at 36 hours of 1,500 U and a return to normal of 1 to 2 U by 84 hours), a crude approximation of a T1/2 of less than 5 hours can be made. This also assumes no continued release of arginase into blood, and arginase activity did not reach 1 to 2 U before 84 hours. Because this is probably not true, the actual T1/2 may be considerably less than 5 hours. Studies of arginase after CCl₄ administration in other species indicate similar kinetics. Regardless of the actual half-life, the rate of removal of arginase is considerably more rapid than that of ALT.

Organ Disease

Many studies have been conducted to evaluate the use of serum arginase as an indicator of hepatic necrosis. These studies demonstrated very low activity in the normal animal and extremely marked elevations in animals with experimentally induced necrosis. The increase in arginase activity from normal levels ranged up to 200-fold in the dog between 1 and 2 days after CCl_4 administration (208,231), with lesser increases in the mouse (49) and rat (52). These increases in serum arginase activity in the rat showed a direct correlation with the dose of CCl_4 and the resultant hepatic necrosis. Although a difference in the magnitude of arginase activity existed among species in which similar doses of CCl_4 were used, the time of maximum arginase activity (1 to 2 days) and the return to normal by 4 days after CCl_4 administration were similar for all species.

The effect of biliary disease or occlusion has been less well studied. The effect of complete bile duct occlusion in the dog resulted in only a transient and minimal increase in arginase activity (232). During this study serum ALT activity was increased as much as 20-fold and remained increased approximately 16 days. These studies with CCl_4 administration and bile duct ligation indicate that arginase is truly a measure of acute hepatic necrosis and provide little apparent help in diagnosing biliary disease. It has been suggested that arginase activity be interpreted in conjunction with ALT activity to gain a better insight in diagnosing the severity and prognosing the direction of the lesion (64). This is based on the fact that arginase returns to normal much more rapidly than does ALT, thereby providing a more immediate indication of the presence of necrosis. Because of its longer half-life, ALT is a better indicator of the magnitude of necrosis.

Drug and Physiologic Effects on Arginase Activity

Arginase is constantly undergoing synthesis and degradation in the liver with a half-life within the hepatocyte of 4 days (284). This rapid turnover allows for rapid changes in arginase in liver when physiologic or pharmacologic stimuli demand it. Cortisone and hydrocortisone cause as much as a threefold increase in liver arginase in 3 to 5 days of treatment (181,254). This increase in liver arginase can be reflected in an increase in serum arginase, as indicated by a twofold increase in serum arginase activity after 3 days of treatment with cortisone (52). Liver arginase decreases as much as 80 per cent following adrenalectomy (115,254).

Consistent changes in liver arginase are also seen with fasting and increasing or decreasing dietary protein intake. Fasting results in a twofold increase in arginase in liver as a result of a decrease in arginase degradation and is reflected in a twofold increase in plasma arginase activity (52). When high dietary intake of protein is changed to low intake, liver arginase decreases as a result of increased arginase degradation as determined by immunoprecipitation (284).

These changes induced by physiologic and pharmacologic stimuli might have little effect on a clinical diagnosis of liver necrosis, but they may result in a statistical difference in studies involving large numbers of animals.

GAMMA GLUTAMYL TRANSPEPTIDASE

Gamma glutamyl transpeptidase (γGT) (EC 2.3.2.2) catalyzes the transfer of gamma glutamyl groups from gamma glutamyl peptides to other peptides, amino acids, and water. It may play a role in amino acid transport or in regulation of tissue glutathione concentration. Indepth reviews of the biochemical and clinical characteristics of this enzyme in both man and animals have been made (42,153,266).

Organ Distribution

Gamma glutamyl transpeptidase in all species is found in highest concentration in kidney, pancreas, and liver. Detectable activity is also found in spleen, lung, intestine, and placenta. In the dog, the pancreas has 69 per cent of the activity found in kidney on a per gram of tissue basis, whereas the liver has only 1.6 per cent of the activity found in kidney (299). Although in all species the kidney appears to have the highest γGT activity per gram of tissue, the comparison between the amount found in other organs varies between species (5,58). For instance, in man, kidney has 10 times the activity found in liver, while the activity in rat kidney is 200 to 300 times higher than that in rat liver (5,89). The dog, mouse, hamster, and rat are similar in that they have lower activity of liver γGT than that found in guinea pig, rabbit, and man (36,212, 313).

There are marked differences in the activity of γGT in adult versus fetal livers. In fetal rat liver, γGT activity is 10 to 30 times higher than that found at 20 weeks of age (34,100). Similar observations have been made in man; however, adult liver γGT activity in man is higher than that in the rat (34). In rat pancreas, γGT activity is lower in newborn and increases approximately fourfold at 20 weeks of age (100).

Cell Location

In kidney, γGT is demonstrated histochemically in the brush border of epithelial cells lining the proximal convoluted tubules (5). In pancreas, the luminal border of cells lining the acini and the pancreatic ducts demonstrates γGT activity (5,107). In rat small intestine, the enzyme is located in brush border membranes of villus cells (66).

The location of liver γGT is of diagnostic interest because of both serum γGT increases as a result of hepatobiliary disease and increases in γGT in preneoplastic cells of liver. Histochemically, γGT is located on the canalicular surface of the parenchymal cells and on biliary cells (69,107). In rat liver, the biliary cells in the portal spaces show γGT activity. When parenchymal cells, Kupffer cells, and biliary cells are isolated independent of one another, a major portion of γGT is found in the biliary cells (78,148,255,319).

Considerable disagreement exists as to whether γGT is a microsomal enzyme or a plasma membrane enzyme. Recent evidence indicates it is associated with the plasma membrane (148,255,319).

Isoenzymes

Isolation and characterization of the isoenzymes of γGT and separation of these isoenzymes by electrophoresis for diagnostic purposes have been complicated by the observation that γGT occurs in many isozymic forms. Rat kidney γGT, isolated by detergent extraction and affinity chromatography and separated by isoelectric focusing, yields 12 enzymatically active isoenzymes (317). Rat mammary gland yields 12 γGT isoenzymes (154), and 10 isoenzymes have been identified in human serum of individuals with hepatic cancer (171). The manner in which γGT is isolated and the techniques used to separate dramatically alter the results. The multiple isoenzymes formed are a result of varying carbohydrate, primarily sialic acid, attached to the enzyme (317).

Isolated rat kidney γGT is in an aggregate form that has a molecular weight of over 200,000 daltons (d) and contains other proteins (317). When separated from the rest of these proteins, γGT has a molecular weight of 68,000 d and is made up of two subunits of 46,000 and 22,000 d molecular weight.

Rat liver γGT has been less well studied because normal rat liver contains only small amounts of the enzyme. The γGT from rat hepatomas and hyperplastic nodules is immunologically identical to rat kidney γGT but has a light and heavy subunit which differs from the rat kidney γGT by having a greater sialic acid concentration (91,322). Differences in kidney γGT and that from hepatocellular carcinoma membranes have been detected with monoclonal antibodies. This is likely a result of carbohydrate microheterogeneity (120).

Increased γGT in serum following bile duct ligation has been compared to γGT in bile by polyacrylamide electrophoresis (150). In bile a major large molecular weight isoenzyme and a minor low molecular weight isoenzyme are found. The large molecular weight enzyme can be converted to the small molecular weight enzyme with papain. Serum contains both of these forms as well but in reverse concentration. The hypothesis is that retention of bile causes release from biliary cells by detergent action of the large molecular weight form of γGT which is converted to the small molecular weight isoenzyme during translocation into blood.

In summary, it is suggested that the polypeptide portions of various isoenzymes of γGT are similar or possibly identical. The isoenzymes may result from changes in sialyltransferase activity of the cell from which the γGT is derived, aggregation of γGT with other proteins and lipids, and possibly techniques used to isolate and separate the γGT.

Half-Life

Little definitive information can be found regarding the rate of clearance of γGT from the serum of man or animals. The nearly parallel increase and decrease of γGT activity with alkaline phosphatase after bile duct ligation in the dog and the known half-life of alkaline phosphatase might suggest a half-life of γGT in the order of 2 to 3 days.

Organ Disease

The diagnostic use of γGT has been directed towards its value as an indicator of cholestasis and its association with precancerous changes in the liver. Because the enzyme is found primarily on biliary cells in normal liver, necrosis of hepatocytes results in little or no change in serum γGT activity in the dog (123,232).

Increases in γGT activity following bile duct ligation were seen in all species studied. In dog and rat, this increase was evident until termination of the experiments, some of which were carried out as long as 23 days (72,180, 232,299,348). Bile duct ligation in the dog resulted in an increase in serum γGT activity which nearly paralleled that of alkaline phosphatase but showed less relative change. The livers of dogs with either complete or partial biliary obstruction showed approximately a sixfold increase in γGT above normal (72,299). In the rat, the initial increase in serum γGT activity was not associated with an increase in γGT in the liver, in fact there was a small decrease in the specific activity of liver γGT (348). By 7 days, however, there was an increase in specific activity of γGT in both biliary and parenchymal cells. It was thought that the initial increase in serum γGT activity reflected a release of γGT from nonparenchymal cells as a result of membrane solubilization by bile acids. The proliferation of biliary epithelium after a few days increased the liver γGT and provided an additional source for the continual increase in serum γGT. These conclusions are supported by more recent data which showed that rats treated with alpha-naphthylisothiocyanate, which specially causes necrosis of biliary epithelial cells, resulted in increased serum γGT (184). In addition, chronic feeding of alpha-naphthylisothiocyanate resulted in a time-dependent increase in serum γGT activity which correlated

with quantitative increases in hepatic bile duct volume determined by morphometric means.

Bile duct ligation in the guinea pig results in a somewhat different pattern of increase of serum γGT activity (149). There is an initial 10- to 20-fold increase in serum γGT activity at 3 to 6 hours after ligation which drops to approximately an eightfold elevation by 3 days. The initial increase is not prevented by cycloheximide, indicating that this increase is not due to increased synthesis. It is suggested that as in the rat, the initial increase in serum γGT is a result of solubilization of biliary γGT by the retained bile acids. This idea is supported by the parallel increase in serum bile acids, absence of increased synthesis of γGT, and a decrease in γGT in liver tissue. Also, large molecular weight γGT was found in serum 3 hours after ligation, which suggests that membrane complexes were released by bile salts. The difference in the serum pattern of γGT activity between guinea pig and rat or dog probably lies in the fact that the normal guinea pig has much higher γGT activity in liver than does the rat or dog, and thus there is initially more γGT available for release into serum.

Although kidney has the highest concentration of γGT, renal disease probably does not cause increases in serum γGT activity. Ligation of the ureters in rabbits did not result in an increase in serum γGT activity (4).

In addition to serum changes in γGT activity associated with cholestasis, there are well-documented increases in the activity of tissue γGT during chemically induced hepatocarcinogenesis (36,51,89,91,198,322). Although normal hepatocytes stain negatively or only faintly for γGT activity, during treatment with hepatocarcinogens the bile canalicular surface of the plasma membrane of hepatocytes stains dramatically for γGT. These carcinogens often induce γGT at an early stage of hepatocarcinogenesis, which can be useful as a biochemical and histochemical marker for preneoplastic hepatocytes.

Drug Effects

Increases in the activity of γGT in liver and plasma as a result of induction of enzyme synthesis are often associated with drugs such as barbiturates (255,265,267,319). Responses to inducing drugs vary among species. Rabbits respond to phenobarbital with a greater increase in liver and serum γGT than do guinea pig and rat. Although the rat shows an increase in liver γGT with phenobarbital, it may show no increase in serum γGT activity (265). In rabbits treated with phenobarbital for 20 days, there was an immediate increase in liver γGT, but increases were not seen in serum until day 18 (319).

Glucocorticoids (dexamethasone and prednisone) cause an increase in serum γGT in the dog (22,72,299). There was a progressive increase in enzyme activity until termination of the experiments. It was suggested that this increase in γGT activity is a result of induced synthesis of the enzyme, but this remains to be proven. There is a concomitant increase in serum bile acids, which might suggest increased solubilization of γGT as well (72).

5'NUCLEOTIDASE

The enzyme 5'nucleotidase (5Nase) (EC 3.1.3.5) catalyzes the hydrolysis of nucleoside 5'-monophosphates. The most commonly used substrate for this enzyme is adenosine monophosphate. The biochemistry, methods of assay, and clinical diagnostic value in man have been reviewed adequately (35,111,112).

Organ Distribution

5'Nucleotidase is found in a large number of tissues of the body including kidney, liver, lung, brain, intestine, pancreas, neutrophils, lymphocytes, skeletal and heart muscle, as well as several others (127,259). Although a quantitative evaluation of all tissues containing 5Nase has not been conducted in one study, it would appear that the highest activities are found in kidney and intestinal mucosae (80,127). On a per milligram of protein basis, liver has less activity than does kidney, but it has equal to or more activity than does lung and brain (80,260).

The diagnostic value of serum 5Nase has centered around increases associated with hepatobiliary disease. Little information is available to suggest a contribution of other tissue to increased serum 5Nase activity; however, it has been suggested that normal serum 5Nase may not be derived from liver (152). The methods used to make this assessment, however, leave room for question. Although virtually all organs contain 5Nase, the hepatobiliary specificity of 5Nase very likely lies in the observation that it is a membrane-bound enzyme which requires treatment with detergents or bile acids for release. The environment in the liver and biliary tree during disease provides the appropriate conditions for its release. This suitable environment is not provided in other organs with a high complement of 5Nase activity.

As previously indicated, γGT in rat liver decreases with age. In regard to 5Nase, the opposite is true: 5Nase increases with age to adulthood (34,85). The adult rat liver has three times the 5Nase activity of the neonate liver and six times the activity of the fetal liver.

Cellular Location

5'Nucleotidase is found predominantly as a membrane enzyme. Early studies suggested that a considerable amount of the enzyme may be associated with the nuclei, but recent studies confirm that a major position of the enzyme is the microsomal membranes which were defined as including endoplasmic reticulum and plasma membranes (306). Further purification of plasma membranes resulted in an eightfold increase in specific activity. Although it cannot be concluded that all membrane 5Nase resides in the plasma membrane, it is accepted that at least a major portion does. The 5Nase requires deoxycholate or triton detergents plus deoxycholate to allow solubilization, which offers another indication of its association with membranes. These results support previous histochemical demonstration of 5Nase activity in plasma membranes limiting the bile canaliculi and sinusoids of the liver (235). 5'Nucleotidase is an ectoenzyme (307,321,328) with approximately one third of the enzyme, including the active site, accessible to outer surface of the cell (27).

There also appears to be a soluble 5Nase fraction and a fraction associated with the lysosomal membrane which appear different from the plasma membrane enzyme (112). Quantitatively these fractions would appear to be considerably less significant than the plasma membrane 5Nase.

5'Nucleotidase has been reported in hepatocytes, Kupffer cells, and biliary epithelial cells. In rat liver, based on specific activity, Kupffer cells contain four times the amount of enzyme as biliary epithelial cells and 10 times the amount found in hepatocytes (348). Bile duct ligation did not increase the biliary or Kupffer cell specific activity of 5Nase as it did that of alkaline phosphatase.

Isoenzymes

Evidence indicates that 5Nase exists in multiple forms. In the rat and mouse, there is histochemical evidence for a form with greatest activity at pH 5 and another form with greatest activity at pH 7.0 to 7.5 (126). Five different zones of activity could be identified on agarose electrophoresis after extraction in the presence of butanol (127). More recent evidence indicates that partially purified 5Nase from rat liver, spleen, kidney, heart, lung, brain, and skeletal muscle exhibited the same pH optimum, was inhibited by conanavalin A, and was inhibited in an identical manner by antibody to liver 5Nase (260). Although there may be multiple forms of 5Nase, these forms may well be a result of variation of lipid and carbohydrate associated with the protein molecule and could be artifacts created by the method of isolation. In any event, there is little indication at this point that the separation of isoenzymes would be of diagnostic value.

Organ Disease

Increases in serum 5Nase activity are of value in the diagnosis of biliary disease in man and animals (35). It has been reported that increases in serum 5Nase are often found in patients with breast cancer (151), but these increases have not been identified as being from or as a result of the tumor.

Increases in serum 5Nase activity after bile duct ligation in the rat are similar to increases in γGT and ALP activity; however they are not identical. The initial increase more closely parallels that of ALP, with maximum activity reported to occur at 24 hours (180). This initial increase in serum 5Nase activity was not accompanied by an increase in liver 5Nase as described for ALP and was not affected by inhibitors of protein synthesis. This increase in serum 5Nase activity was suggested to be as a result of solubilization of membrane-bound 5Nase by bile salts and regurgitation of the enzyme into the blood. At 48 hours, liver 5Nase activity began to increase. This increase was considered a result of proliferation of biliary cells (180) and it nearly paralleled the increase in γGT activity in liver. That the increase in liver 5Nase activity is a result of proliferation of the biliary cells and not increased synthesis of the enzyme within the cell is supported by the demonstration that 5Nase was not increased in isolated membranes from cholestatic rats (303).

5'Nucleotidase is a less commonly used diagnostic enzyme than ALP or γGT; however, there is no conclusive evidence in laboratory animals that it is a less effective diagnostic enzyme than ALP or γGT. In man there are conflicting reports, some of which suggest it is less commonly elevated in hepatobiliary disease than are γGT and ALP, whereas other reports indicate it is equally as efficient an indicator of hepatobiliary disease (111).

Drug Induction

Considerably less effort has been directed toward the effect of various drugs on 5Nase than on γGT and ALP. There is evidence that thyroxin increases serum and tissue 5Nase activity in the rat (80). Chronic ethanol administration in rats increased serum 5Nase activity while depressing liver activity (229). The γGT activity was increased in both serum and liver.

ALKALINE PHOSPHATASE

The alkaline phosphatases (ALPs) (EC 3.1.3.1) are enzymes that hydrolyze a wide range of monophosphates at an alkaline pH. The in vivo function of this enzyme is not known. Hundreds of articles are published each year dealing in some way with ALP, making this by far the most studied, clinically important enzyme. In-depth reviews of various aspects of this enzyme exist (92,124).

Organ Distribution

Alkaline phosphatase may be considered ubiquitous in that it is found in most or all tissues of the body. On a per gram of tissue basis, intestinal mucosa contains the highest concentration of ALP activity followed by kidney (58, 166,170,223), whereas other tissues contain considerably less ALP activity. Serum activities of ALP in disease are generally not a reflection of tissue ALP activities. For example, liver has less than 1 per cent of the activity of ALP per gram of tissue as compared to intestine in the dog, yet liver is by far the greater contributor to serum ALP in disease.

Cellular Location

Alkaline phosphatase is generally located on the absorptive or secretory surface of cells. This enzyme is primarily a plasma membrane enzyme; however, some activity is found in the endoplasmic reticulum and Golgi apparatus. It is clearly associated with 5Nase, a standard marker for plasma membrane (93). That it is a membrane enzyme is also indicated by the requirement of butanol or detergent in the extraction buffer to solubilize the enzyme.

In kidney, ALP is found in the brush border of proximal convoluted tubules (335). In intestine, ALP is located on the tips of villi especially in the small intestinal mucosa (338). In bone, ALP is found in the osteoblast. Liver ALP is located primarily in membranes bordering the bile canaliculus; however, some activity is seen on the sinusoidal surface of the hepatocyte as well (93,158,336). In the dog, corticosteroid-induced ALP is also located primarily along the bile canalicular surface of hepatocytes (282).

Isolated cells from rat liver showed a major portion of ALP associated with Kupffer cells, but after bile duct ligation most of the increase in activity was associated with biliary and parenchymal cells (348).

Isoenzymes

Literally hundreds of publications have dealt with detection, separation, and characterization of the isoenzymes of ALP with the primary purpose of enhancing the diagnostic usefulness of increases in serum ALP activity. Identification and characterization of ALP isoenzymes found in various tissues have been carried out to gain understanding of the genetic expression of this enzyme as well as to determine its usefulness as a marker for oncogenesis. Most of these studies have used electrophoresis, sensitivity to heat and various other inhibitors, and reactivity with antiserum to identify or characterize the various isoenzymes. These studies have resulted in identification of numerous isoenzymes in normal, diseased, and neoplastic tissues from several species of animals.

The ALP isoenzymes are as a result of both the expression of different gene loci and the differences in posttranslational modifications of the enzyme. In man, chimpanzee, and orangutan, there are at least three genes coding for alkaline phosphatase; one for the polymorphic placental form, one for the intestinal form, and another for the form found in liver, kidney, bone, and most other tissues (114,128). In other mammalian species studied, there are two major genes coding for ALP; one for the intestinal ALP and the other for hepatic, renal, osseous, and most other tissue ALPs including placental ALP (113,128,214). Although the ALP isoenzymes expressed by these genes just described are currently of major interest to us, there may be additional genes expressing ALP found in the testes and lungs of some species (128). The isoenzymes expressed by the three major genes in man and higher primates and the two major genes of other mammals are different antigenically, enzymatically, and biochemically. The isoenzymes identified from various tissues, but which are a result of the same gene expression (ALP derived from liver and bone), are usually antigenically and enzymatically similar. They cross-react with antiserum produced against one or the other ALP, and their activity is inhibited equally by one or more of the inhibitors of ALP such as L-phenylalanine, levamisole, and homoarginine. These isoenzymes are a result of posttranslational modification of the protein molecule which is organ specific. The posttranslational modifications involve primarily the carbohydrate portion of the molecule. The electrophoretic migration of the isoenzymes in various media is generally altered as a result of these posttranslational changes.

Liver ALP from all species, except rabbit, is a heat-labile (56°C) enzyme, extremely sensitive to inhibition by levamisole but less sensitive to inhibition by L-phenylalanine. The carbohydrate portions of the enzyme are terminated with sialic acid, allowing the enzyme to migrate rapidly on electrophoresis. In the rat liver there may be two forms of ALP which can be separated by electrophoretic mobility, susceptibility to heat treatment, and response to digestion with neuraminidase (3). Increased serum ALP following bile duct ligation in the rat is identical to normal liver ALP (263). Rat hepatoma ALP appears similar to normal rat liver ALP with the possible addition of carbohydrate, especially sialic acid (165). Two or more forms of mouse liver ALP have also been reported (169). There appears to be only one form of dog liver ALP (282).

Rabbit liver ALP is made up of two isoenzymes separable by DEAE-cellulose chromatography (230,281). Peak one represents approximately 30 per cent of the total activity and is nearly completely inhibited by low concentrations of levamisole similar to the liver isoenzyme of other species. Peak two represents approximately 70 per cent of the total activity and is insensitive to low concentrations of levamisole as is the intestinal isoenzyme of other species. This suggests the two isoenzymes are from different genes and indicates the rabbit may be the only species normally producing two distinct phenotypes of ALP in the liver.

The ALP from bone is antigenically and enzymatically similar to liver ALP. It generally has a slower migration on cellulose acetate electrophoresis and is more susceptible to heat inactivation (143,224). The ALP from rat osteosarcoma, calvarium, kidney, and placenta showed no significant difference in amino acid composition and identity in the first 20 N-terminal amino acids (225).

Kidney ALP is often found in multiple forms, possibly as a result of modifications in the carbohydrate portion of the molecule or of different gene expression. Although kidney ALP is generally considered an expression of the liver/bone ALP gene, there is in man an ALP that is antigenically identical to intestinal ALP in addition to liver-like ALP (174). In the rat and dog, however, kidney ALP is more than likely a result of expression of the liver ALP gene (233,280). Heterogeneity in these two species is probably a result of variation in carbohydrate content, especially sialic acid. Rabbit kidney ALP can also be separated into multiple forms with considerable difference indicated between two of the forms (253). Recent evidence indicates that two forms of rabbit kidney ALP are separable by DEAE-cellulose chromatography and are nearly identical to the two forms found in liver and just described herein (230,281). Kidney ALP is almost never seen in serum; however, it is found in urine and may be of diagnostic value in detecting acute tubular necrosis (250).

The ALP expressed by intestine is more heat stable than that expressed by bone, liver, or kidney (224). It is generally considered an asialoglycoprotein and therefore does not migrate on cellulose acetate or agarose electrophoresis to the extent that liver ALP does. In the adult dog, however, ALP extracted from intestine contains some sialic acid (283). Rabbit intestinal ALP has been reported to have sensitivity to levamisole identical to that of liver and kidney peak two (230) or intermediate between that of peak one and two of liver and kidney (281). Separation of rabbit intestinal ALP with DEAE-cellulose chromatography results in one broad peak which is likely the result of bacterial glycosidase action on the carbohydrate portion of ALP. Clarification of the isoenzyme forms of intestinal ALP awaits monoclonal antibody to facilitate purification of the enzyme(s) and characterization (281). Two to three electrophoretic forms of intestinal ALP are found in extractions of rat small intestine (197,227). These forms are considered to be a result of either aggregation or limited proteolysis of the enzyme.

As previously mentioned, placental ALP in laboratory animals including some primates is coded by the gene expressing the liver and bone ALP (113,214). In the dog this enzyme appears to be an asialoglycoprotein because it has little migration on electrophoresis and is unaffected by neuraminidase treatment.

In the dog there exists an additional isoenzyme referred to as corticosteroid-induced ALP which is produced in the liver during glucocorticoid treatment (79). On cellulose acetate electrophoresis this isoenzyme has a greater anodal migration than do any of the normal ALP isoenzymes. This isoenzyme is a highly glycosylated form of the intestinal-type ALP because it is antigenically similar with both polyclonal and monoclonal antibody, responds to heat, levamisole, and L-phenylalanine inhibition in the same manner as does intestinal ALP, and has nearly identical amino acid composition, identical N-terminal amino acid sequence and peptide maps but has considerably less N-acetylglucosamine, mannose, galactose, and sialic acid (283,340). This enzyme has not been reported in other species, but it has similar properties to that ALP found in some human hepatocellular carcinomas (140).

The extensive literature on additional isoenzymes of ALP associated with neoplastic cells in man is adequately reviewed elsewhere (92). In general, these represent expression of one of the existing isoenzymes in cells in which it is not normally found. A large portion of this work has centered around the expression of placental ALP in tumor tissue.

Half-Life

The clearance rate and mechanism of clearance of intestinal ALP have been investigated to the greatest degree. Primary interest in the clearance of intestinal ALP arises from the presence of this isoenzyme in serum of rats and man after ingestion of a fat-laden meal (167,192). Increases do not occur in all humans and may be related to blood type and secretor status. Intestinal ALP has not been observed in significant quantities in the serum of dogs.

Intestinal ALP isoenzyme is an asialoglycoprotein that is cleared from the circulation in minutes. After intravenous infusion into either dogs or rats, intestinal ALP is cleared in a biphasic manner with a T1/2 for the initial phase being less than 5 minutes (29,144,289, 352). The second phase of clearance occurs more slowly and can be abolished with concurrent taurcholate infusion in the rat (277). The rapid initial clearance of dog intestinal ALP is accomplished via the liver by recognition by asialoglycoprotein receptors on hepatocytes of terminal galactose units on the carbohydrate portion of the molecule, followed by endocytosis and destruction by lysosomes (289,290). A small portion of the infused intestinal ALP is secreted into bile (277,289). The second slower phase is thought to be a result of exocytosis of a portion of the previously endocytosed intestinal ALP (277). Taurcholate may enhance this exocytosis and might partially explain why intestinal ALP is found in serum for a few hours postprandially when enterohepatic circulation of bile salts is at a maximum.

Clearance of other isoenzymes of ALP has been studied less thoroughly. Early studies indicated that in the dog, liver ALP isoenzyme had a half-life of approximately 6 days (53,68). These clearance studies involved creation of increased serum ALP activity either by bile duct ligation followed by relief of biliary obstruction or by infusion of serum from dogs with biliary obstruction into normal dogs. More recent studies confirm this general approximation of the half-life of liver ALP (29,144).

The half-life of corticosteroid-induced ALP in the dog is approximately 3 days and is nearly identical to that of normal liver isoenzyme (144). Removal of sialic acid from the liver and corticosteroid-induced ALP reduces the half-life from 3 days to less than 6 minutes. This rapid clearance of these asialophosphatases is more than likely a result of the mechanism shown for the removal of intestinal ALP.

The half-life of placental and renal ALP in dogs is also less than 6 minutes (144). It is speculated that these also have nonsialated terminal galactose units, allowing them to be removed by receptor-mediated endocytosis in the liver.

In man the placental ALP isoenzyme has a half-life of approximately 6 days (59). The bone isoenzyme of ALP appears to have a half-life somewhat less than that of placental ALP, but it was not determined because of an inadequate number of experiments. Complete clearance required 4 days. In the dog, bone ALP half-life is reported to be approximately 3 minutes for phase one and 17 to 49 minutes for phase two (29).

Organ Disease

Normal serum ALP activity in man originates from bone, liver, and intestine, and in pregnant women from placenta. Bone and intestinal ALPs are also observed in the rat; however, liver ALP may be absent in normal rat serum (262). The ALP activity in normal dog serum is predominately hepatic in origin with only a small portion attributed to bone (279); however, based on binding experiments with monoclonal antibody to intestinal ALP and bromotetramisole inhibitor studies, the presence of a small amount of intestinal-like ALP in serum is likely (10).

Increases in serum ALP activity derived from bone are generally associated with osteogenesis. In puppies the increase in serum ALP activity is two to four times that seen in adult dogs and is primarily that derived from bone (143). Increases are minimal or nonexistent in dogs with localized tumors involving bone.

Intestinal ALP isoenzyme is commonly seen in the rat after a fat-laden meal (192,278,352). The increase in the intestinal ALP isoenzyme in serum, reaching a maximum at 7 hours, was dependent on transport of fat across the villous cell in the presence of bile salts and on normal intestinal lymphatic drainage. It is thought that this increased intestinal ALP in serum is derived from a soluble fraction of ALP found in the cytoplasm of villous cells (352).

Increases in liver ALP isoenzyme in serum as a result of hepatocellular necrosis or cellular leakage are minimal, showing only a one- to twofold elevation (123,231). This minimal increase more than likely reflects the low concentration of ALP in hepatocytes when compared to cytoplasmic enzymes such as ALT and arginase and reflects the need for solubilization of ALP from the membrane before its release into serum.

The mechanism by which ALP activity is elevated in serum during cholestasis does not involve retention in serum of ALP from other sources, but it does involve the regurgitation of liver ALP in bile plus solubilization of additional membrane ALP from bile canalicular membranes and increased synthesis of ALP in hepatocytes and biliary epithelial cells. As with 5Nase, the release or solubilization of ALP from the membrane by the bile acids is an important aspect of the increase in serum ALP activity. Increases in ALP activity in liver also occur following CCl_4 intoxication and partial hepatectomy; however, there is no increase in serum ALP activity, supporting the concept that membrane solubilization is necessary for the release of ALP and to increase serum ALP activity (289).

The mechanism by which ALP reaches the serum may involve release of the membrane-bound ALP into bile, diffusion between the lateral membranes through tight junctions, and release directly into the bloodstream without being carried through lymphatics (23,158). Increased ALP in liver during bile stasis is a result of increased synthesis because the increase can be prevented by inhibitors of protein synthesis and because techniques using immunoprecipitation of the ALP protein show an increase in ALP protein following bile duct ligation (163,173,285). Increased ALP synthesis results from an enhanced rate of translation of mRNA because ALP mRNA concentration remains unchanged during cholestasis (295). This increased ALP synthesis during biliary stasis may well be the result of increased bile acid concentration, especially taurocholate (130,131).

In the rat, marked elevations of ALP activity are seen as early as 6 to 7 hours following bile duct ligation, with a maximum increase of 7- to 10-fold greater than normal at 12 to 24 hours (23,163,164,180,286,292). In the dog, however, marked elevations are not seen for nearly 24 hours and maximum elevations are not seen for 4 to 7 days (123,142,232,299). These maximum serum values can reach 30 to 40 times normal serum ALP activity. The difference in time of response between the dog and rat probably reflects the absence of a gallbladder in the rat.

Drug Effects

Drugs causing increases in rat serum and liver ALP activity include cortisol, glycine, phosphorylcholine, phosphotidylcholine, phenobarbital, diphenytoin, ethinyl estradiol, clofibrate, theophylline, caffeine, and papaverine (116, 239,342). The effect of ALP activity of most of these drugs can be blocked by inhibitors of RNA and protein synthesis. Thus, the increase in ALP activity is a result of new ALP protein synthesis and not of activation or enhancement of pre-existing enzyme molecules.

The most notable and most often studied example in the dog is induction caused by cortisol or one of the synthetic corticosteroids. Increased ALP in serum and liver during prolonged corticosteroid therapy is a common finding and is of clinical significance because of the routine use of corticosteroids in veterinary medicine. Increases in serum ALP begin within a few days after initiation of therapy and rise dramatically to as much as 40 to 50 times normal serum activity (22,72,79,143). This increase involves the induction of the corticosteroid-induced ALP isoenzyme which has previously been discussed.

PANCREATIC ENZYMES

Several enzymes of the pancreas have been evaluated for their suitability in diagnosing pancreatic disease. Routinely, however, amylase and lipase are the standards on which other diagnostic procedures have been based. This section will deal with only amylase and lipase.

AMYLASE

Alpha-amylase (EC 3.2.1.1) is a low molecular weight enzyme (45,000 d) that cleaves α-D-(1-4) glycan linkage of starch and glycogen. It is by far the most thoroughly studied pancreatic enzyme of diagnostic importance and has been in use longer than has any other enzyme in clinical chemistry.

Organ Distribution

Amylase is found in extremely high concentration in the pancreas of virtually all laboratory animals. The salivary gland of the adult rat and mouse has nearly as high amylase activity on a per gram of tissue basis as does pancreas; however, the salivary glands of the dog, rabbit, and neonatal rat have less than 0.1 per cent the amylase activity found in the pancreas (125,191,251). Amylase is found in the small intestine of most animals studied; however, only the rat has appreciable quantities. Liver amylase activity is extremely low in most species (191,251); however, there is considerable information that suggests normal serum amylase is of hepatic origin. In the mouse and rat, synthesis of hepatic amylase can be inhibited with puromycin or cycloheximide which results in a reduction in serum amylase (125,201–203). The liver apparently does not accumulate amylase but secretes it into plasma, much as it does albumin. The intracellular half-life of amylase in liver is approximately 4 hours. The rabbit liver produces little or no amylase, which is reflected in low serum amylase activities (201). The dog liver produces amylase and it may be a major source of normal serum amylase (228,234). The amylase extracted and purified from canine liver has properties suggesting it is true amylase (215). Pancreatectomy has resulted in only minimal to 50 per cent decreases in serum amylase (40,226,234). However, hepatectomy resulted in a steady decrease in serum amylase, suggesting the major portion of serum amylase is derived from liver.

Cell Location

Rat liver amylase is primarily associated with the microsomal fraction of the cell (45,217). A major portion of the enzyme was of a latent form which could be activated four- to sixfold by sonication or the addition of detergent. In the pancreas, amylase is associated with zymogen granules (70).

Isoenzymes

Numerous efforts have been made to determine and identify isoenzymes of amylase in serum and various tissues of laboratory and domestic animals. Unfortunately, there is considerable confusion and variability in the results obtained. Results depend on the techniques used to separate the isoenzymes and on the assay procedure used to identify amylase. For example, the saccharogenic procedures for amylase measure the formation of reducing sugars. In the dog, maltase or glucosidases produce an increase in reducing sugars but are not true amylases. The use of starch-containing agarose slabs on which the electrophoretic strip is incubated and the slabs then stained with iodine to identify the areas of hydrolyzed starch also produce confusing results. Albumin apparently binds the starch, giving the impression that an isoenzyme of amylase exists in the albumin region of the electrophoretic strip. The number of isoenzymes in the various tissues of different species and the origin of normal serum amylase is not well defined. Contradictions are found throughout the literature. The discussion in this section will touch on some of the observations made, but they should not be accepted as absolute in all cases.

In the dog, essentially two isoenzymes have been identified by cellulose acetate electrophoresis (309). One is associated with the gamma globulin region, is extracted from the intestinal mucosa, and is the predominant amylase in normal serum. The other isoenzyme is associated with the beta globulins on electrophoresis, is found in pancreas and uterus, and is absent from or present in small quantities in normal serum. Hepatic amylase was not identified on electrophoresis. These data suggest that pancreas is not the source of normal serum amylase, as was previously suggested; however, this does not prove or disprove the liver as the source of normal amylase.

With acrylamide gel, the pancreatic amylase of dogs could be separated into four bands of activity (251). Serum contained only one band, which corresponded to one of the pancreatic bands. Two serum isoamylases could be identified with paper electrophoresis, one major fraction migrating in the gamma globulin region and the other in the alpha globulin region (294). Pancreatectomy resulted in a reduction in gamma globulin-associated amylase. These results appear to directly contradict the results of studies using cellulose acetate electrophoresis as previously discussed. Two amylases were isolated from dog serum using Sephadex G-75 column chromatography; however, one of these fractions proved to be an alpha-glucosidase and not a true amylase (97). Using agar gel, only one isoenzyme of amylase was identified in dog serum (325). In a recent study using agarose electrophoresis four isoamylases were found in normal dog serum with fraction three (from anode) identified as pancreas specific and as the fraction with the greatest increase following experimentally induced pancreatitis (220).

With paper electrophoresis coupled to the saccharogenic assay of amylase, rabbit and guinea pig serum showed only one isoenzyme of amylase, whereas rat showed two isoenzymes (294). Electrophoresis of rat serum amylase on acrylamide gel resulted in two bands of amylase activity whose migration was identical to that of two of the three bands of activity seen in salivary gland extracts (229). The pancreatic amylase of rat produced only one fraction. An electrophoretic comparison of isomylases in numerous species indicates that the isoamylases of serum and urine of the prairie dog are most similar to those of man (356).

The amylase isoenzymes have not reached the diagnostic importance seen with other enzymes such as ALP and creatine phosphokinase. This may be due in part to the confusing and contradictory results, just described. Additional information regarding the amylase isoenzymes is reviewed elsewhere (204).

Half-Life

Removal of amylase from blood in all species is relatively rapid. Values for the half-life of amylase in the normal dog range from 1 to 5 hours (14,147,350). Plasma half-life of rabbit pancreatic and parotid gland amylase was 97 and 95 minutes, respectively (272). In the mouse, the half-life may be even shorter because all of the intravenously injected amylase was removed within 2 hours.

The mechanism of clearance from blood has been studied extensively which has resulted in some confusion and obvious species differences. In man a sizable portion of amylase is found in urine, and increases in blood amylase are found when the glomerular filtration rate is reduced. The dog has been used as a model to study the mechanism of amylase clearance, but its mode of clearance may be considerably different from that in man. Decreases in glomerular filtration rate in the dog result in increases in serum amylase, and nephrectomy does result in an increased half-life from 5 to 14 hours. However, less than 1 per cent of pancreatic amylase infused in normal dogs is found in urine (147). Because the infused amylase in the nephrectomized dogs was eventually cleared, additional means of clearing amylase must exist. Other reports suggest that nephrectomy has no such effect and suggest that a major portion of amylase is cleared by another mechanism (226). One means of clearance may be found in the liver. Amylase infused into dogs was rapidly cleared, resulting in a concurrent increase in amylase in liver which could be prevented by blocking the reticuloendothelial system (139). In the mouse, a major portion of infused pancreatic amylase was found in urine; however, infused salivary gland amylase was not found in urine (191). Bilateral nephrectomy in the rabbit significantly slowed the plasma clearance of amylase (272). In the rabbit, urinary excretion of salivary gland amylase was greater than that of pancreatic amylase.

Organ Disease

Because amylase is found in greatest quantities in the pancreas, it is generally used to diagnose pancreatitis. In experimentally induced pancreatitis, maximal increases of approximately eight times normal were seen at 24 to 48 hours (44,209). Amylase activity returned to normal in 3 to 5 days in five of six dogs in one study and in 8 days in the other study. This rapid return to normal may be expected based on the short half-life of amylase.

In clinical cases, serum amylase activity greater than two times normal with no evidence of renal disease is highly suggestive of pancreatitis (90). The value of serum amylase activity in the clinical diagnosis of canine pancreatitis has been questioned (310). Only 4 of 16 dogs with histologic evidence of pancreatitis had serum amylase activity greater than the mean plus 2 standard deviations for normal dogs. It was suggested from this study that lipase activity was a much more sensitive indicator of pancreatitis than was amylase activity. In addition, 8 of 16 dogs without pancreatitis had elevated serum amylase activity. These dogs with elevated amylase activity had a variety of diseases including renal disease, diabetes mellitus, lymphosarcoma, and hemangiosarcoma. Elevation of serum amylase activity in renal disease is a common occurrence. Dogs with renal vessel ligation showed a 60 per cent increase in serum amylase activity in 48 hours (147). Mean increases in serum amylase activity in both surgically induced and spontaneously occurring renal disease in dogs reached 2.5-fold greater than normal amylase (247).

In rats, in which the liver is thought to play an important role in serum amylase regulation, serum amylase activity decreases when the rats are treated with such hepatotoxins as CCl_4, endotoxin, and lead acetate. This decrease in serum amylase activity is consistent with the hypothesis that the liver synthesizes amylase and secretes it but does not store it. Distal ligation of the main biliary-pancreatic duct in the rat caused serum amylase activity to increase approximately sixfold in 24 to 48 hours. By 72 hours, these values had returned to normal (105, 298).

Drug Effects

Numerous drugs have been studied to determine their importance or effect on both the pancreas and pancreatic enzymes. The drug of considerable interest is cortisone because of the normal endogenous increase in stressful situations and its routine administration in several clinical entities. Neonatal rats responded to cortisol administration with an increase in pancreatic amylase, but a similar increase was not seen in adult rats treated with cortisol (182,298). However, 34 of 36 rabbits treated with cortisone showed mild to marked increases in serum amylase activity (311).

For many years it was accepted that the dog responded to cortisol or ACTH with increased serum amylase activity (54). However, clinical studies suggest that the stress associated with surgery does not affect normal amylase activity (90). More recently, treatment of normal dogs with both small doses and large doses of dexamethasone has resulted in a statistical decrease in serum amylase activity (242). Similar observations have been made in dogs treated with prednisolone (94,189).

LIPASE

The lipase (E.C. 3.1.1.3) of interest in the diagnosis of pancreatic disease is a low molecular weight enzyme (42,000 d) that acts at an oil/water interface to hydrolyze triglycerides. Assay methods generally use an incubation medium consisting of an emulsion of long chain triglycerides in buffer. Such assays minimize the activity of nonspecific esterases, whereas water-soluble artificial substrates tend to measure the esterases rather than true pancreatic lipase. Experimental data pertaining to pancreatic lipase must always be evaluated in light of the assay procedure used.

Isoenzymes

The existence of esterases and lipases of non-pancreatic origin and different substrate requirements complicate the questions of isoenzymes of lipase. If there are multiple forms or isoenzymes of pancreatic lipase, it has not been confirmed to my knowledge.

Half-Life

The intravenous half-life of lipase after infusion of pancreatic juice or pancreatic extract in the dog is approximately 2 to 3 hours (147,350). As with amylase, this rapid clearance rate in the dog does not result in significant quantities in urine. Approximately 1 per cent of the lipase of infused pancreatic juice was found in urine (350). The kidney may play a part in clearance of lipase, because the half-life of infused lipase increased from 2 to 11 hours after nephrectomy (147). Tubular metabolism of the filtered lipase may prevent its appearance in urine.

Organ Disease

Though serum lipase activity as assayed by the oil suspension assay has not been confirmed as being specific for pancreatic disease, its primary purpose in the clinical laboratory is to diagnose pancreatitis. Increases in serum lipase activity in experimentally induced pancreatitis in the dog generally occur at 24 to 48 hours, with increases up to 50 times over baseline activity (44,209).

These increases and subsequent decreases generally paralleled the rise and fall of serum amylase activity.

The effectiveness of serum lipase versus amylase activity determinations in diagnosing pancreatitis is often debated. A recent clinical study of these two enzymes in the dog suggests that lipase activity is more sensitive in diagnosing pancreatitis because 15 of 18 dogs with histologic evidence of pancreatitis had elevated serum lipase activity (310). However, as many as 19 of 74 dogs without pancreatitis also had elevated lipase activity. Increases in lipase activity were seen in such conditions as diabetes mellitus, adenocarcinoma of the small intestine, lymphosarcoma, glomerulitis, Cushing's disease, and bile duct carcinoma. These data indicate that serum lipase activity may be more sensitive than serum amlyase activity in detecting pancreatitis but is more likely to give false-positive results as well.

A three- to fourfold increase in serum lipase was seen in both surgically induced and spontaneously occurring renal disease (247). There was no relationship among increments in serum lipase activity and inulin clearance and serum creatinine or urea nitrogen concentration.

Drug Effects

As with several other clinically important enzymes, the drugs that are of considerable importance in altering serum lipase activity are the corticosteroids. Dexamethasone-treated dogs had mean lipase activity as much as four times over baseline activity (242). Similar results have been obtained with prednisolone-treated dogs without histologic evidence of pancreatitis (94,180). These results suggest that lipase determinations are of little diagnostic value in corticosteroid-treated dogs.

SERUM ENZYMES AS DETECTORS OF MYOPATHIES

Muscle is the major soft tissue mass of the body and contains high concentrations of enzymes. Aldolase (ALS; EC 4.1.2.13), aspartate aminotransferase (AST; EC 2.6.1.1), lactate dehydrogenase (LDH; EC 1.1.1.27), and creatine kinase (CK; EC 2.7.3.2) have all been used as serum markers of myopathies. Of these four enzymes, only total serum CK, CK isoenzymes, and LDH

isoenzymes are now regarded to have sufficient muscle specificity and sensitivity to be used as diagnostic aids. Aldolase, AST, and total LDH have sufficient activity in other tissue to render an increase in their serum activity as nonspecific. In addition, red blood cells have high total AST and LDH activity, with an LDH isoenzyme pattern similar to that of cardiac muscle. Therefore, serum used to measure AST and LDH isoenzymes must be free of hemolysis and promptly separated from erythrocytes, as enzymes can be released from the RBCs into serum (104).

The activities of the various tissue enzymes used in diagnostic enzymology have not been measured in all the species with which we are concerned. However, in those studies in which one or more of the foregoing enzymes have been measured in muscle, the relative quantitative relationship remains the same among species (39,145,156,168,170,288). Relative changes in activity of these enzymes in serum following altered physiologic activity or pathology of muscle tissue are also similar when species comparisons are made. However, the basal value and magnitude of change of serum enzyme activities may vary between species. In some cases these differences may be a result of the assay procedure used, whereas in others it may be a true physiologic difference. An example of quantitative differences in serum enzyme activities as a result of physiologic differences between species is CK activity in hypothyroidism. Man has elevated CK activity in the hypothyroid state, where as hypothyroid rats do not (48,118,119,122,236). However, as just alluded to, CK demonstrates the most specificity for muscle in the majority of species studied.

Soluble enzymes of muscle leak into the plasma in proportion to their concentration, severity of cellular damage, and amount of tissue damaged (288). Numerous soluble enzymes occur in muscle, but because LDH and CK isoenzymes are soluble in high concentrations and have different isoenzyme profiles in cardiac and skeletal muscle, they are the more commonly used markers of muscle damage (104,157,176, 183). Increased serum CK and LDH enzymes are proportional to the size of an infarct (30,65,137,141,264,300). Currently, serum enzyme activity assays do not permit the differentiation of a large mass of reversible tissue damage from a smaller mass of irreversible damage. With the advent of immunoassays for enzyme concentration it may become possible to measure the mitochondria CK (CKm) to specifically characterize irreversible cell damage (74,264).

Although there are tissues other than muscle that contain the LDH isoenzymes, only cardiac muscle, with the exception of RBCs, produces an isoenzyme profile that is readily recognizable and organ specific under clinical conditions. Isoenzyme profiles of CK activity also allow the differentiation of skeletal and cardiac muscle injury with better sensitivity and specificity than do LDH isoenzymes. Before the use of CK isoenzyme profiles, it was impossible to distinguish the hypoxia of aerobic exercise from that of myocardial diseases (9,157,176,183). The increase in CK with exercise is inversely proportional to the amount of training of the subject, with lower changes associated with better trained subjects (9). Steroidal anti-inflammatory drugs reduce these changes by a poorly understood mechanism thought to involve improved muscle membrane stability (157,183,337). Convulsions and shivering cause an increase in muscle activity with resultant enzyme release. Assays currently in use are sensitive enough to detect the muscle damage associated with the intramuscular injection of drugs and the migration of parasites through muscle (34,341).

Primary genetic and acquired muscle diseases of man, ranging from myocardial infarction to inherited muscular dystrophies, are the best documented examples of changes in serum muscle enzyme profiles (183). Although the dog and most laboratory animals are not susceptible to spontaneous myocradial infarction, the dog and rat have been used extensively as experimental models of spontaneous myopathies in man (8,76,121,133,177,211,216,341,343). Changes in serum muscle enzyme profiles in spontaneous myopathies in man occur in primary muscle disorders, but less so or not at all in neuromuscular disorders. Marked elevation of serum CK activity is observed in dogs with a hereditary muscle disorder resembling Duchen muscular dystrophy in humans (326). However, in other hereditary muscle disorders in dogs, hamsters, and mice, increases in muscle-specific enzymes in serum are not observed (133). In dogs with neuromuscular disorders, the basal serum CK is lower than that in nonaffected dogs because of their reduced muscle mass (177). In these dis-

orders the rate of release from the reduced muscle mass when compared to that of normal animals may be lower, whereas the rate of degradation by the reticuloendothelial system may be the same, resulting in lower basal serum CK activity. Malignant hyperthermia in pigs and dogs, and nutritional myopathies attributable to vitamin E and/or selenium deficiency in dogs, mice, rats, and rabbits, result in elevation of serum CK before the disorder is clinically evident (8,176,237,329). It is evident that there are numerous causes for increases in muscle enzymes in plasma. Some of these are more the result of physiologic processes, such as muscular activity, than of pathologic processes, and the investigator must be aware of the general state of the subjects under study before any conclusion concerning the change is drawn.

Inheritance and development play an important role in the isoenzyme profiles. The enzymes' subunits are coded for by different genes which may be expressed at different times during ontogeny. Both LDH and CK isoenzyme profiles in heart muscle change as gestation progresses. The embryonic mouse heart has predominantly LDH-5 and CK-BB in early gestation and by birth has a pedominantly LDH-1 and 2, and CK-MB (88,176,264). In mice, skeletal muscle changes from a predominance of CK-BB in early gestation to CK-MM by birth. These changes must be considered when serum enzyme profiles of fetuses are studied. Genetic variation of CK, LDH, and aldolase occurs in mice. Both structural and processor genes are responsible for this variation, which can result in changes in activity as well as electrophoretic mobility. Therefore, it is important that reference values for comparative studies be established for the strain as well as the species of animal being studied.

Subcellular location of enzymes is generally studied by fractionation procedures, histochemistry, or both. Results of fractionation procedures must be interpreted with caution. In vitro enzymes, as charged particles, may bind to other soluble or insoluble fractions to which they were not exposed in vivo. Therefore, the subcellular location of an enzyme is not as easy to document as is the major tissue of origin (145).

The development of immunoassays for various enzymes is and will continue to enhance the diagnostic value of serum enzymes. Immunoassays allow the measurement of enzyme concentration rather than enzyme activity, which may be advantageous if an enzyme is highly unstable and quickly loses activity after being released from the cell. In addition, immunoassays may be designed to be more non-sensitive than measurement of enzyme activity and, in the case of some enzymes, can be specific for measuring an isoenzyme that could not be identified by conventional means. Measurement of enzyme activity as generally determined is not species specific and has allowed rapid application of diagnostic enzyme measurements to laboratory animals. The need for species-specific immunoassays and/or the validation of immunoassays prepared for one species and used in another may not allow for a rapid application of immunoassays to all laboratory animals.

Aldolase (EC 4.1.2.13; D-fructose-1,6-diphosphate; D-glyceraldehyde-3-phosphate lyase)

For many years, aldolase (ALS) was the muscle-specific serum enzyme of choice in biomedical science. It was replaced by serum CK because liver could also be a major source of serum ALS. Muscle and liver of vertebrates contain high specific ALS activity with appreciably lesser amounts in all other tissues. Aldolase, a soluble cytosolic enzyme, catalyzes a reversible step in the hexose portion of the glycolytic pathway and therefore plays a role in glycolysis, the pentosephosphate recycling pathway, and gluconeogenesis (31,145,157).

The ALS molecule is a tetramer that can exist as five isoenzymes. The ALS-A_4 is primarily found in skeletal muscle, ALS-B hybrids in liver, ALS-A-C hybrids in heart muscle, and ALS-C_4 in brain and embryonic tissue. These various forms have different substrate specificity for fructose 1,6-diphosphate (FDP) and fructose 6-phosphate (F6P). Muscle ALS-A_4 has a marked preference for FDP over F6P. The recognition and ability to assay for ALS isoenzymes may aid in improving the muscle specifity of serum ALS as a diagnostic aid for myopathies. However, with the greater sensitivity and vast accumulated knowledge of serum CK value as a muscle-specific serum enzyme, it is doubtful that ALS will ever return to its former popularity as a serum marker of myopathies (13).

Lactate Dehydrogenase (EC 1.1.1.27; L-lactate-NAD-oxidoreductase)

Lactate dehydrogenase (LDH) is a soluble, cytosolic, tetrameric enzyme with five isoenzymes made up of M and H subunits and a sixth of C subunits. The molecular weight of the enzyme is 134,000 d. The reduction of pyruvate to lactate is the favored direction of the reaction of this enzyme, but the in vitro assay generally measures the formation of NADH from the oxidation of lactate to pyruvate. Substrate specificity is greatest for pyruvate, but also nearly as high for alpha-hydroxybutyrate reduction to alpha-oxobutyrate. The greater the amount of H subunit, the greater the substrate specificity for alpha-hydroxybutyrate over pyruvate. Total serum alpha-hydroxybutyrate dehydrogenase (HBD) activity is thought to be LDH-H_4 and possibly LDH-H_3,M_1 isoenzymes, two of the five LDH isoenzymes with the greatest amount of H subunit. Synonymous with LDH-H_4 is LDH-1 and with LDH-M_4, LDH-5, with the other forms named between these two homolgous tetramers dependent upon the subunit content and electrophoretic mobility (31,145, 157).

Elevated total serum LDH activity is a mark of tissue damage but not of any specific tissue. Lactic dehydrogenase isoenzyme profiles, to some extent, are tissue specific. The electrophoretic separation of the isoenzymes to determine this profile is a clinical laboratory procedure used to characterize myocardial infarction. Most LDH activity in heart muscle is of the LDH-H_4 and LDH-H_3M_1 types. Heat instability and HBD determination as a ratio of total serum LDH activity are less commonly used for quantitating LDH-H_4. Red blood cells have LDH isoenzyme profiles similar to those of heart muscle, whereas in skeletal muscle LDH-M_3,H_1 and LDH-M_4 predominate. The LDH isoenzymes in a hemolyzed serum sample can mimic the profile seen as a result of cardiomyopathy or can mask that seen with a skeletal muscle disorder. Therefore, care must be taken to avoid hemolysis and the resulting superimposition of the RBCs LDH isoenzyme profile on the normal serum profile and that of the organ being evaluated.

Differences in the various LDH isoenzyme profiles could theoretically be used to identify any damaged organ; however, this is not the case. Extensive study of LDH isoenzyme profiles in human medicine has revealed that LDH isoenzyme profiles have efficacy only as a diagnostic aid in cardiac infarctions, and even then it is generally recommended that CK isoenzyme determination be used to complement the information obtained from the LDH change. In veterinary medicine, spontaneous cardiac infarction occurs in primates but not in other commonly encountered species. Other cardiomyopathies occur in all species, and serum LDH isoenzyme profile or serum HBD activity could have a place in their diagnosis.

Disappearance of the activity of LDH isoenzymes in vitro and in vivo varies with the specific isoenzyme, and in turn, limits their value as diagnostic aids. Immunoassay of LDH isoenzymes within tissue has demonstrated that their turnover rates within the cell vary with their type. In addition, clearance time of human LDH isoenzymes in serum also varies appreciably. The LDH-H_4 has a half-life in serum of 113 ± 35 hours, and skeletal-muscle derived LDH-M_4 has a 10 ± 1 hour half-life. The CK half-life of 15 ± 3 hours is appreciably shorter than that of LDH-H_4, which is evident in cases of myocardial infarction in which LDH-H_4 remains at peak values for more than 3 days but CK returns to basal values in 2 to 3 days.

Stability of the LDH isoenzymes in vitro mirrors that observed in vivo clearance times. The LDH-M_4 and M_3H_1 contain four and three M subunits and appear to have appreciable cold lability that can be stabilized with NAD or glutathione. These two isoenzymes in tissue extracts are lost if frozen overnight. At room temperature for 2 to 3 days, little serum LDH activity is lost, but if they must be kept longer, they should be kept at 4°C with NAD or glutathione added. Plasma containing EDTA, heparin, or serum can be used for the LDH assay, but oxalate inhibits LDH activity. The sample must have no hemolysis and must be well centrifuged to eliminate platelets and their accompanying LDH enzyme. Drugs causing tissue damage can result in increased serum LDH values, but no drugs have been identified that cause specific modification of the enzyme's activity (351). Urea is an inhibitor of LDH and subjects with azotemia may have falsely decreased LDH values.

Creatine Kinase (EC 2.7.3.2; adenosine triphosphate: creatine-N-phosphotransferase

Creatine kinase (CK), also known as creatine phosphokinase (CPK), is a dimer of two subunits, B and M, which can form three isoenzymes: CK-BB, CK-MB, and CK-MM, each with a molecular weight of 84,000 d. These three isoenzymes are found in high concentration in the cytosol of striated muscle and in very small amounts elsewhere. The CK-MM dominates in skeletal muscle, CK-MB in heart muscle, and CK-BB in brain. These three isoenzymes transfer high energy phosphate from creatine phosphate to adenosine diphosphate in the formation of adenosine triphosphate. The M-line region of myofibrillar contractile protein appears to be a major site of CK activity. A fourth CK isoenzyme, CKm, is located on the inner mitrochondrial membrane and functions in the transfer of high energy P_i from mitochondrial-generated adenosine triphosphate through the mitochondrial inner membrane to CK (31,145,157,264).

These CK isoenzymes are very unstable in serum in vitro and have short in vivo half-lives (less than 15 hours). This instability limited their value in diagnostic procedures until it was discovered that the addition of sulfhydryl compounds such as cystine and glutathione in the serum or assay preparation would regenerate nearly all of the lost activity. This loss in activity in vitro appears to be the result of reduction in the enzymes' own sulfhydryl groups. Immunoassays for the inactive CK in serum revealed that it is present long after its activity is gone. When regenerating sulfhydryl compounds are added to the CK assay, the enzyme can be measured in serum or heparinized plasma frozen for months. Many early investigators used assays that did not contain the reactivating sulfhydryl groups, and their publications contain CK values that are appreciably lower than those observed with the new assay procedures. Magnesium is required for CK activity, and plasma containing chelating anticoagulants cannot be used for assay (264).

When serum is diluted with water or saline, the amount of CK activity in the diluted sample frequently exceeds the proportional amount observed in the undiluted sample, a result of the dilution of a plasma inhibitor. The magnitude of increase may be threefold. At least one inhibitor of CK is uric acid. In most species of mammals, serum uric acid values are low, but in man and other primates there are conditions in which it may become high and interfere with the assay.

Electrophoretic separation of the CK isoenzymes is the most common method of determining their activity. In this semiquantitative method, total serum CK activity is first measured and then the relative density of the stain produced by the activity of each isoenzyme separated is determined and converted to a relative proportion of the total CK activity. Immunoassay procedures for human and dog CK have been developed to measure the amount of enzyme present rather than the amount of activity. These immunoassays have increased the sensitivity of CK detection 1,000-fold. There is no cross-reactivity between the antibodies in the CK of these two species.

Developmental changes in tissue CK isoenzyme profiles occur from birth on, and similar changes can be anticipated in the serum into which these enzymes leak (88,264). Skeletal muscle CK isoenzymes of fetal mice during gestation change from predominantly CK-BB to CK-MB to CK-MM by birth. Therefore, serum CK isoenzyme profiles of the fetus can also be expected to change during gestation. Adult human skeletal muscle CK isoenzyme profiles revert to the fetal CK-MB patterns in a number of poorly understood diseases. In addition, marathon runners have increased serum CK-MB activity which is thought to arise not from heart, but rather from skeletal muscle that has altered CK isoenzyme profiles. Total serum CK activity can increase in neurologic disorders, but the isoenzyme pattern is generally that of CK-MB or CK-MM, possibly as a result of various magnitudes of involuntary muscle contraction. Future development of the more sensitive immunoassays for CK-BB may permit the early detection of neurologic disorders. Cerebrospinal fluid CK activity does increase in various forms of encephalomalacia, but the increase in proportion to the amount of tissue damage is not constant (347).

Aspartate Aminotransferase (EC 2.6.1.1.; L-aspartate: 2-oxoblutarate aminotransferase

Aspartate aminotransferase (AST) is better known as glutamate oxaloacetate transaminase (GOT). However, current usage has shifted to AST in closer compliance with the EC standards of nomenclature. There are two isoenzymes of AST, cytosolic and mitochondrial, and they demonstrate high amounts of activity in nearly all tissues (22). Both cardiac and skeletal muscles have a great amount of AST activity, but because other soft tissues also do, AST has little tissue specificty. Red blood cells have an appreciable amount of AST activity, and hemolysis results in masking of activity from other tissues. Although serum AST activity does increase markedly in cardiac disorders of dogs and mice and in exercised rats, so does the more specific CK, leaving little or no need for AST as a marker of muscle disease (9,39,65, 211,274,300,329,341). However, because it does increase, AST remains a general marker of soft tissue damage and is followed with more specific tissue enzyme markers. In addition, it is cleared more slowly from plasma than is CK and may assist in the late detection of a myopathy.

Assay procedures for AST may be direct colorimetric or fluorometric end point determinations or kinetic. The assay procedure forms oxaloacetate, which in high concentrations is an inhibitor of the reaction. Therefore, a coupled indirect procedure converts oxaloacetate to malate and stoichiometrically forms NADH. This latter reaction is generally measured as a kinetic procedure. Stability of AST is very good, with little change in serum activity in at least 3 days at room temperature, 7 days refrigerated, and 30 days frozen.

ACETYLCHOLINESTERASES

The only known function of cholinesterase (ChE) (EC 3.1.1.7) is concerned with nerve transmission and, in particular, with hydrolysis by ChE of the neurotransmitter acetylcholine at the postsynaptic membrane of cholinergic neurons. In addition to nerve tissue (47), these enzymes occur in many nonneural tissues (332), including the blood, where their activities are measured to monitor poisoning by a variety of compounds, including organophosphates and carbamate insecticides. Their activities are also measured to monitor the effects of various drugs, including those affecting cholinergic neurons, and also certain diseases. Clinical investigations involving ChE would first require a suitable method for determining ChE activities. It would be tempting to prescribe a current protocol and let it go at that. However, the method described would probably not be directly applicable to the particular species, tissue, or problem in hand. The reason is that ChE varies widely with respect to properties, specific activities, and distribution in various tissues and species. In addition, more than one type of ChE frequently occurs in a single tissue, which complicates the assay. Thus, the clinician will have to adapt available methods to the special needs of his or her own problem. The present section attempts to provide briefly a background that will help in making such adaptations. Finally, note that the literature on these poorly understood enzymes is vast, numbering over 20,000 papers and several hundred books and monographs, and it is controversial.

Nomenclature

The name "acetylocholinesterase" (AChE) was first used by Augustinsson and Nachmansohn (20) to distinguish this class of cholinesterase (ChE) from the second major class, Psi ChE (pseudocholinesterase) described later. AChEs have also been named "specific" ChE (2), "true" ChE (3), "c-type" ChE (4), and ChE I (5). Although these terms are still used occasionally, acetylcholinesterase is now the generally accepted name.

Distribution

Acetylcholinesterases occur in a wide variety of mammalian tissues (302) and often coexist with Psi ChEs (206). Ord and Thompson (238), for example, found AChEs in widely varying amounts in 15 different rat tissues, including brain, diaphragm, and suprarenal gland where the AChE predominated. This section is concerned primarily with the AChEs in the blood erythrocytes of mammals of clinical interest. The relative activities vary widely depending on the species (Table 11.1), being greatest in human and bovine erythrocytes and least in cats, chickens, ducks and pigeons (206). AChE also occurs in the blood plasma of the rabbit (195,207). However, Psi ChE, not AChE, is the cholinesterase usually associated with blood plasma.

Relationship to Psi ChE

Acetylcholinesterase is now distinguished from other ChEs primarily on the basis of substrate and inhibitor specificity and kinetics and secondarily on the basis of location and function. Although both AChE and Psi ChE are now considered to have closely similar structures and functions, this was not always so. The present attitude is typified by Vigney et al (333), who recently wrote, "We would therefore like to suggest that the two enzyme systems (EC 3.1.1.8 and EC 3.1.1.7 enzymes) fulfill very similar physiological functions. The precise requirements for acetylcholine hydrolysis would be met in various systems, by different combinations of the two genetically distinct, yet structurally similar enzymes."

Recently, the complete amino acid sequence of an AChE from the ray, *Torpedo californica* was inferred from the sequence of a complimentary DNA clone (293). The complete amino acid sequence of human serum Psi ChE was also recently elucidated, in this case by Edman degradation of purified peptides (188). Comparison of the amino acid sequence of human serum Psi ChE with the amino acid sequence of AChE from the electric organ of Torpedo California shows considerable homology. The two proteins have 574 and 575 amino acids per subunit. The primary structure shows 309 identical amino acids. Both enzymes show significant homology with the C-terminal portion of bovine thyroglobulin. The active site serine of human serum Psi ChE is located 198 residues from the amino terminus (188). The active site serine of Torpedo AChE is located 200 residues from the amino terminus (293). The location of other residues important to the activity of AChE and of Psi ChE is not yet known.

Purification

Most AChEs, including the erythrocyte enzyme, are membrane bound, which, together with their scarcity, has made purification difficult. The problem of solubilizing the enzyme (273) has, in recent years, been understood and solved (102,199,200). It has been shown that the AChE from Torpedo electric organ is anchored to the membrane through a specific interaction with the head group of one or more phospha-

Table 11.1. Acetylcholinesterase Activities of Various Mammalian Erythrocytes and Platelets Relative to Human Erythrocyte Acetylcholinesterase (AChE)

Species	From Reference 354		From Reference 50 by Psi pH Method 210
	Erythrocyte AChE	Platelet AChE	Erythrocyte AChE
Man	100	0	100
Monkey	...	...	64
Chimpanzee	...	...	70.7
Rabbit	21	179	5.2
Rat	12	192	...
Guinea pig	32	22	13.7
Dog	...	...	7.7
Cow	88	2	...
Horse	30	68	...
Cat	1.4	248	2
Goat	...	...	12.4
Pig	...	...	16.4

tidylinositol molecules (102). Quantitative solubilization of the AChE from Torpedo electric organ can be achieved in the absence of detergent by treatment with a phosphatidylinositol-specific phospholipase C from *Staphylococcus aureus* (102). The human erythrocyte AChE has also shown indications of being linked in this novel fashion (102). Evidence is accumulating that other enzymes, such as alkaline phosphatase, are likewise membrane bound in this way (172).

Final purification of the solubilized enzyme has been aided greatly by the use of affinity gels including phenyltrime-thylammonium (PAT) (80) and methylacridinium (MAC) (81–83). These affinity gels are not available commercially, and there were problems synthesizing the MAC gels (57), but these have largely been overcome (339). The efficacy of MAC gel affinity chromatography in the purification of AChE from chicken, rat, calf, and human brain and from the electric organ of the electric fish *Torpedo marmorata* has been investigated (327). In most instances, MAC columns retained over 90 per cent of the enzyme. The synthesis of an unquaternized MAC ligand (ie, AC ligand) has been described (318). The AC ligand can be prepared without the troublesome quaternization reaction and coupled to the gel by an easier carbodiimide route. The AC ligand provides an affinity column equaling quaternized MAC columns. These affinity gels offer a convenient method of physically separating and partially purifying AChE.

Structure

Solubilized eel AChE occurs predominantly as an llS tetramer of molecular weight 230,000 to 300,000 d (194,301). The quaternary structure is considered to consist of four identical (α) subunits arranged as an $(\alpha_2)_2$ dimer of dimers (271). The α_2 dimers are held by noncovalent bonds to form the tetramer. The α subunits forming the α_2 dimer are joined by disulfide bonds in addition to noncovalent bonds. The tetramer is assumed to have four active sites, one on each subunit (99); however, there is disagreement about both the number of active sites (185) and whether or not the subunits are identical (186). Reports of monomeric cholinesterases are rare (284,345).

Substrate Specificity

Although the AChE activities of the erythrocytes of different species vary widely, the substrate specificity patterns appear to be similar. Acetylcholinesterases hydrolyze a wide variety of aromatic and aliphatic carboxylic and thiocarboxylic esters in addition to choline esters. However, acetylcholine is usually the best substrate in terms of both binding (K_m) and relative V_{max} values. A typical substrate specificity pattern based on velocities at optimal substrate concentrations or on V_{max} is given in Table 11.2.

Turnover Numbers

It may be worth noting that the turnover numbers (TON) of the AChEs of different species

Table 11.2. Relative Specificities of Mammalian Erythrocyte Acetylcholinesterase and Eel Acetylcholinesterase Toward Selected Substrates

Substrate	Relative Activity (Acetylcholine = 100) (Source)	Reference No.
Acetylcholine	100	
n-Propionylcholine	87 (human), 78 (horse), 79 (eel)	1,6,84
n-Butyrylcholine	2 (human), 2.3 (horse), 12 (eel)	1,6,84
iso-Butyrylcholine	46 (horse)	6
n-Valerylcholine	3.3 (horse)	6
iso-Valerylcholine	0.19 (horse)	6
Benzoylcholine	1.5 (human)	1
D,L-Acetyl-β-methylcholine	33 (human)	1
L(+)Acetyl-β-methylcholine	54 ( )	28
D(−)Acetyl-β-methylcholine	0 ( )	28
Acetylthiocholine	83 (bovine), 85 (eel)	84,179
D,L-Acetyl-β-methylthiocholine	82 (eel)	134
Phenyl acetate	113 (eel)	179
3:3-Dimethylbutyl acetate	60 (human)	1
Triacetin	42 (human)	1
Tributyrin	2 (human)	1

appear to vary widely, from 10,000 min^{-1} in rat (32) to 278,000 min^{-1} in ox (61). The TON of human erythrocyte AChE was 171,000 min^{-1} compared with 13,000 min^{-1} for horse and 50,000 min^{-1} for dog AChE (32), suggesting that the molar concentration of AChE in the erythrocytes of species with relatively low activities may, in fact, be greater than that in the erythrocytes of some species characterized by high activities. For example, the erythrocyte activity of the horse is 30 times that of humans (Table 11.1), but the molar concentration of AChE would be four times greater in horse than in human erythrocytes on the basis of their TONs.

Kinetics

The substrate and inhibition kinetics of AChE tend to be complex, but certain features are well understood. The reaction at low concentrations of acetylcholine and many other substrates can be described by the following scheme:

$$EOH + R_1\overset{O}{\overset{\|}{C}}\!\!-\!OR_2 \overset{K_s}{\rightleftharpoons} (EOH\,R_1\overset{O}{\overset{\|}{C}}\!\!-\!OR_2)$$

$$\overset{k_2}{\to} EO\overset{O}{\overset{\|}{C}}R_1 \overset{k_3}{\to} EOH + R_1\overset{O}{\overset{\|}{C}}\!\!-\!O + H$$

where EOH is AChE and the OH is on an activated seryl residue.

$(EOH\,R_1\overset{O}{\overset{\|}{C}}OR_2)$ is the reversible binding or Michealis complex,

$EO\overset{O}{\overset{\|}{C}}\!\!-\!R_1$ is the acylated AChE, and K_s is the substrate binding equilibrium constant and is equal to K_m when $k_3 \gg k_2$. The acylation and deacylation rate constants are k_2 and k_3, respectively. K_m is

$$\frac{(k_{-1}+k_2)}{k_1}\frac{k_3}{(k_2+k_3)}$$

whereas V_{max} is $[E]_{total}k_2 k_3/(k_2+k_3)$.

With eel AChE, k_3 is rate limiting, and it follows that no acetate ester can be characterized by a V_{max} value greater than that of acetylcholine with this particular AChE.

At acetylcholine concentrations greater than about 1 to 3 mM, depending on conditions, the activity tends to decrease with inceasing substrate concentration [S]. The v against [S] plots are then hump-shaped, giving an optimal velocity (v_{opt}) at a corresponding $[S]_{opt}$. Although not all substrates show inhibition at high substrate concentrations, some of clinical interest do, including acetylthiocholine (134) and acetyl β-methylcholine (16). Because inhibition occurs at higher substrate concentrations, methods for determing AChE activities employ substrate concentrations at or below $[S]_{opt}$. The K_m values characterizing AChE hydrolysis of acetylcholine, acetylthiocholine, and acetyl-β-methylcholine are typically close to 1×10^{-4} M, whereas $[S]_{opt}$ values are usually 1×10^{-3} M or greater.

Early reports (222) indicated that divalent metal ions, particularly Mg^{++}, were necessary for AChE activity. However, subsequent studies (98,345) showed clearly that Mg^{++}, although mildly activating, was not essential. Despite this, many methods for determining activity continue to include Mg^{++}, usually 0.02 M in the substrate media.

Determination of AChE Activities

Manometric (11,30), titrimetric (17,155,308), spectrophotometric (86,103,138) and change in pH methods (210) have been used to determine AChE activity. The preceding literature references are mostly to original papers describing these methods. The numerous subsequent papers (18,19) describe modifications or adaptations of these original methods for a particular study. Almost any of the papers previously referenced for example, have used or adapted one of these original methods.

Manometric Methods

Recent modifications of the original manometric method of Ammon (12) generally use a Warburg apparatus to measure the rate of CO_2 gas liberated from a reaction of sodium bicarbonate with the acid liberated from ester hydrolysis. The method tends to be tedious, insensitive, and imprecise.

Titrimetric Methods

There are two types of titrimetric methods. The one most commonly used titrates the acid liberated from ester hydrolysis with standard alkali (155,308). The original method of Stedman and Stedman (308) employed an indicator; more recent methods (155) employ continuous titration of the acid librated by standard alkali at constant pH using pH-stats. pH-Stat titrations are sensitive and can be made reasonably precise ($\pm$ 1 per cent) with proper attention to detail. They have the advantage of being able to use almost any substrate except those that are highly insoluble. A fairly sophisticated apparatus of the type made by Radiometer of Copenhagen or by Metrohm is required. The second titrimetric method (17) titrates the sulfhydryl groups liberated when thiocholine esters are split by AChE. A standard I_2, thiosulfate titration system is employed, but this method is not widely used.

Spectrophotometric Methods

There are two well known spectrophotometric methods. The Hestrin (138) hydroxyamic acid method measures the unreacted acetylcholine rather than the products of its hydrolysis. The AChE and acetylcholine are allowed to react for a predetermined time (5 to 60 minutes), usually at 37°C. After incubation, the solution containing unreacted acetylcholine (or other ester) is mixed with alkaline hydroxylamine solution, and after 1 minute it is acidified. The reaction is:

$$R_1\overset{\displaystyle O}{\overset{\|}{C}}\!\!-\!\!O\!\!-\!\!R_2 + NH_2OH$$
$$\text{ester} \qquad \text{hydroxylamine}$$

$$R_1\overset{\displaystyle O}{\overset{\|}{C}}\!\!-\!\!N\overset{\displaystyle H}{\overset{|}{O}}H + R_2\!\!-\!\!OH$$
$$\text{hydroxyamic acid} \qquad \text{alcohol}$$

The hydroxyamic acid is then reacted with ferric chloride. The brown ferric hydroxymate complex is quantitated at 540 nm. This method was used most notably in the brilliant investigations of Wilson and his group, which revealed the hydrolytic mechanism of the AChE-catalyzed reactions (344) and also produced the AChE dephosphorylating agent 2-PAM (pyridine-2-adloxime methiodide) (56,346). It has also found clinical application (33,246), but it does not appear to be widely used.

The second method is probably the method of choice for most clinical investigations (187). It was introduced by Ellman et al (86), and uses 5'5-dithiobis(2-nitrobenzoic acid) (DTNB) to react with the free SH group on the thiocholine liberated by hydrolysis of the substrate acetylthiocholine. The reaction is:

buffers and careful calibration are essential. One problem with this method is the difficulty of converting the ΔpH units to standard units of enzyme activity (eg, micromole per minute). The method has been adapted for using small blood samples (43).

Complications from the Presence of Other Esterases

Determination of erythrocyte AChE in whole blood is complicated by the presence in the

$$CH_3\overset{\overset{O}{\|}}{C}-S-CH_2\overset{+}{N}(CH_3)_3 + H_2O \xrightarrow{AChE} CH_3\overset{\overset{O}{\|}}{C}-O + 2\overset{+}{H} + S-CH_2CH_2-\overset{+}{N}(CH_3)_3$$

(acetylthiocholine)   (thiocholine)

$$NO_2\text{—}\langle O \rangle\text{—}S-S-\langle O \rangle\text{—}NO_2 \rightarrow NO_2-\langle O \rangle\text{—}S + NO_2-\langle O \rangle\text{—}S-S-CH_2CH_2\overset{+}{N}(CH_3)_3$$

COO^- ... COO^- ... COO^- ... COO^-

(DTNB)   Yellow product measured
                                                (5-thio-2-nitro-benzoic acid)

The hydrolysis of acetylthiocholine by AChE occurs at pH 8.0 in the presence of DTNB, so the yellow thionitrophenate, which is measured at 412 nm, is produced stoichiometrically as the acetylthiocholine is hydrolyzed. The progress of hydrolysis can therefore be followed continuously by plotting the changing optical density against time on a recorder. The extinction of the thionitrophenate ion is 13.6 mM^{-1} cm^{-1} at pH 8.0, indicating that the method is very sensitive. Full-scale deflection of the spectrophotometer (OD = 1.0) is achieved by a change of only 0.0735 mM in the acetylthiocholine substrate concentration. In addition to being sensitive, the method is precise and easy to perform, and it can be adapted to measuring activities in a wide variety of tissues.

Change in pH

The change in pH (ΔpH) method of Michel (210) is probably the most widely used clinical method for determining AChE activity. It was developed originally for human blood ChEs, but it can be adapted to blood ChEs of other animals. Like the titrimetric methods (155,308), the ΔpH method measures the H$^+$ produced from hydrolysis of acetylcholine, but it measures it as a function of the change in pH. The selection of

plasma of Psi ChE and sometimes other ChEs and carboxylesterases. This problem is usually overcome by separating the erythrocytes from the plasma by centrifugation. The erythrocytes are washed three or four times with physiologic saline and then lysed by the addition of saponin (210,246). The AChE activity is determined with the lysed solution using acetylcholine or acetylthiocholine as substrate. The carboxylesterase also present in erythrocytes does not hydrolyze acetylcholine.

Specific Substrate

Alternative procedures using the specific substrate acetyl-β-methylcholine have been used. Acetyl-β-methylcholine is readily hydrolyzed by AChE, but not by mammalian Psi ChE (205). It may therefore be used to determine AChE in the presence of Psi ChE, but caution should be exercised because some ChEs do hydrolyze it at significant rates. It should also be noted that acetyl-β-methylthiocholine is *not* specific for AChE, as it is readily hydrolyzed by Psi ChE (117).

Psi ChE Inhibitors

Both AChE and Psi ChE can be differentiated by a number of specific inhibitors. These include organophosphates such as DFP (diisopropylphosphofluoridate), Mipafox® [bis(isopropylamino)fluorophosphine oxide], and Iso-OMPA (tetraisopropylpyrophosphoramide) (6) which inhibit Psi ChE selectively; however, the degree of selectivity varies widely from species to species (248). Because inhibition by organophosphates is progressive with time, they can also inhibit AChE. Experience with organophosphate inhibition is therefore recommended before using these inhibitors. A number of selective reversible inhibitors of Psi ChE have been used including quinidine (86), Astra 1397® [10 - (1 - diethylaminopropionyl)phenothiazine hydrochloride] (17), and ethopropazine [10(2 - diethylaminopropyl)phenothiazine hydrochloride] (117,276). The addition of these inhibitors in the appropriate concentrations to the substrate solution inhibits Psi ChE but not AChE, which can then be determined specifically.

AChE Inhibitors

Conversely, there are a number of compounds that inhibit AChE but not Psi ChE. Most of these are bis-quaternary compounds patterned after the structural feature of tubocurarine, which Barlow and Ing (26) found to be the symmetrically positioned quaternary nitrogens on the iso-quinolinium rings, separated by 14 Å. A number of such compounds exist, but only a few that seem to have found particular favor will be mentioned. One is 284C51 [1,5-bis(4-allyldimethylammonium phenyl)pentane - 3 - one diiodide] (21), which inhibits AChE over 200,000 times better than it does Psi ChE. Another is WIN 8077 or ambenonium [N,N'-bis(diethyl - 2 - chlorobenzylammoniummethyl)oxanide dichloride] (15), and finally there is 3116 CT [bis(3-dimethylamino-5-hydroxyphenoxy)-1,3-propane dimethiodide (101), which also inhibits AChE over 200,000 times better than it does Psi ChE. The addition of appropriate concentrations of one of these compounds to substrate solutions permits specific estimation of Psi ChE activity in the presence of AChE.

PLASMA CHOLINESTERASES

Many aspects of plasma ChE, including distribution, structure, kinetics, relationship to AChE, and inhibitors, and many literature references have necessarily been covered in whole or in part in section on AChE. Precisely the same methods are used to determine Psi ChE as AChE, the only differences being in the selection of substrates and/or inhibitors and in sample preparation. The mechanism of hydrolytic reaction is identical for the two ChEs, except that high substrate concentrations tend to activate rather than inhibit Psi ChE. An exception is benzoylcholine, which inhibits Psi ChE at high concentrations. The K_m values characterizing Psi ChE hydrolysis of choline esters tend to be in the same order of magnitude (10^{-4} to 10^{-5}M) as for AChE, earlier reports to the contrary. The major differences not previously covered are in the naming of the enzyme and its substrate specificity.

Nomenclature

Unlike the AChEs, the Psi ChEs have no generally accepted name. Mendel and Rudney (206) introduced the name "pseudocholinesterase" because they believed that AChE was specific for choline esters, whereas Psi ChE was nonspecific because it hydrolyzed noncholine as well as choline esters. They were incorrect, of course, concerning the choline-ester specificity of AChE (Table 11.1). In addition, results with the differential Psi ChE inhibitor, Nu 683 [the dimethyl carbamate of (2-hydroxy-5-phenylbenzyl) trimethylammonium bromide], suggested to them that "Psi ChE plays no essential part in the hydrolysis of acetylcholine *in vivo*" (132). However, Glick (110) and others have objected to the name "pseudocholinesterase," and in view of current views on the relationship of Psi ChE to AChE and on the function of Psi ChE (333), the choice of the prefix "pseudo" seems unfortunate. Sturge and Whittaker (312) and others suggested the name butyrocholinesterase based on the preferred substrate of this enzyme, and many current authors (7), including the present one (195), prefer the name butyrylcholinesterase (BuChE) for human and horse plasma ChE. The problem with BuChE as a name is that the plasma ChEs of several species, such as the rat, are propionyl rather than butyryl specific (324). The Psi ChE has also been called "nonspecific" ChE (110,333), s type ChE (355), and ChE II (16). The use of Psi ChE as a name has the advantage that it can be used

Table 11.3 Specificity of Horse or Human Serum Pseudocholinesterase Toward Selected Substrates

Substrate	Relative Activity (Acetylcholine = 100) (Source)	Reference
Acetylcholine	100	
Propionylcholine	170 (human)	129
Butyrylcholine	330 (human)	129
Benzolcholine	35 (human)	2
D,L-Acetyl-β-methylcholine	1 (human)	2
L(+)Acetyl-β-methylcholine	2 (horse)	108
D(−)Acetyl-β-methylcholine	0 (horse)	108
Acetyl-β-methylthiocholine	50 (horse)	109
Acetylthiocholine	140 (human)	32
Phenyl acetate	91 (human)	219
3:3-Dimethylbutyl acetate	35 (human)	2
Triacetin	14 (human)	2
Tributyrin	45 (human)	2

to apply to this type of ChE in all tissues and sera and also that it is well recognized. However, the implications of the prefix "pseudo" gives a highly inaccurate description of this enzyme, and it would seem wise to find another name.

Substrate Specificity

The substrate specificity patterns of horse and human serum Psi ChE are given in Table 11.3. The specificity patterns of the two enzymes are similar with respect to the substrates shown. However, the substrate specificity patterns of Psi ChE from other species vary widely (Table 11.4). Eight of the 12 species of Psi ChEs are butyrate specific, whereas four are propionyl specific, including hamster, rat, chicken, and mouse. One further point of interest is the observation of Meyers (221) that the Psi ChE specificity patterns of a single species did not appear to vary greatly between the Psi ChEs in the tissues of the given species; however, this point needs further study.

Determination of Psi ChE Activities

The methods used to determine AChE can also be used with Psi, ChE, and most of them have been. This is particularly true of the ΔpH method (210), the Ellman et al method (86), the manometric method (12,33), and the pH-stat titrimetric method (155). The chief difference may be the choice of substrate, which typically is butyrylcholine or butyrylthiocholine (86).

Table 11.4. Species Variation of Substrate Specificity Patterns with Respect to Four Acylcholine Esters (Recalculated from Myers [221])

Species	(Choline-Ester Activity Relative to Acetylcholine = 100)			
	Acetyl	Propionyl	Butyryl	Benzoyl
	Butyryl Specific			
Dog	100	150	253	60
Horse	100	161	231	28
Cat	100	111	211	27
Man	100	155	192	36
Duck	100	139	153	25
Squirrel	100	122	144	14
Ferret	100	122	139	28
Pig	100	72	122	17
	Propionyl Specific			
Hamster	100	153	128	24
Rat	100	211	119	17
Chicken[a]	100	147	83	6
Mouse	100	139	75	11

[a] Chicken brain AChE hydrolyzes propionylcholine faster than acetylcholine, but does *not* hydrolyze butyrylcholine.

Besides being a better substrate, butyrylcholine is specific for Psi ChE (Tables 11.3 and 11.4). Acetylcholinesterase does not hydrolyze butyrylcholine, but it appears to bind quite tightly to AChE and in this sense is a fairly respectable inhibitor (256).

Several additional methods might be mentioned, including the β-carbonaphthoxycholine method (256), the ultraviolet, benzoylcholine method (160,161), the *o*-nitrophenylbutyrate method (196), and the ultraviolet, acetylthiocholine method. All have been in clinical use at one time or another and some may still be (41). In the authors' opinion, the DTNB method of Ellman et al (86) is the method of choice for routine clinical screening, whereas the pH-state titrimetric method is an excellent reference method.

Recently, a method was described for the determination of Psi ChE activities using acetylcholine as substrate (320). The method is based on the liberation of acetate from acetylcholine by Psi ChE and the conversion of the acetate to acetylphosphate and ADP in the presence of ATP by acetate kinase. The produced ADP is coupled with pyruvate kinase and lactate dehydrogenase in the presence of phosphoenolpyruvate and NADH. The amount of NADH consumed is determined by the absorbance at 340 nmol. The results show good correlation with those obtained by the usual methods.

REFERENCES

1. Adams DH (1949) The specificity of human erythrocyte cholinesterase. Biochim Biophys Acta 3: 1–14
2. Adams DH, Whittaker VP (1949) The cholinesterases of human blood. I. The specificity of the plasma enzyme and its relationship to the erythrocyte cholinesterase. Biochim Biophys Acta 3: 358–366
3. Adeniyi FA, Heaton FW (1982) Heterogeneous nature of alkaline phosphatase from rat liver. Comp Biochem Physiol 72B: 221–226
4. Adjarou D, Popov S, Ivanov E (1976) Studies on the mechanism of the changes in serum liver γ-glutamyl transpeptidase activity. Enzyme 21: 1–7
5. Albert Z, Orlowski J, Orlowski M, Szewczuk A (1964) Histochemical and biochemical investigations of gamma-glutamyl transpeptidase in the tissues of man and laboratory rodents. Acta Histochem 18: 78–89
6. Aldridge WN (1953) The differentiation of true and pseudocholinesterase by organo-phosphorus compounds. Biochem J 53: 62–67
7. Allemand P, Bon S, Massoulie J, Vigny M (1981) The quaternary structure of chicken acetylcholinesterase and butyrylcholinesterase; effect of collagenase and tryspin. J Neurochem 36: 860–867
8. Allen W, Berrett S, Harding J, Patterson D (1970) Plasma levels of muscle enzymes in the pietrain pig in relation to the acute stress syndrome. Vet Rec 87: 410–411
9. Altland P, Highman B (1961) Effects of exercise on serum enzyme values and tissues or rats. Am J Physiol 201: 393–395
10. Amacher DE, Smith DJ, Martz LK, Hoffmann WE (1987) Characterization of alkaline phosphatase in canine serum. Enzyme 37: 141–149
11. Amelung D (1960) Untersuchungen zur Grösse der Eliminationsgeschwindigkeit von Fermenteu aus deru Kaninchen-serum. Zeitschrift Physiol Chem 318: 219–228
12. Ammon R (1933) Die fermentative Spaltung des Acetylcholins. Pflügers Arch Physiol 233: 486–491
13. Andrews M, McIlwain P, Eveleth D (1961) Serum transaminase and aldolase during migration of larval ascaris serum in swine. Am J Vet Res 22: 1026–1029
14. Appert HE, Dimbiloglu M, Paireut FW, Howard JM (1968) The disappearance of intravenously injected pancreatic enzymes. Surg Gynecol Obstet 127: 1281–1287
15. Arnold A, Soria AE, Kerchner FK (1954) A new anticholinesterase oxamide. Proc Soc Esp Biol (NY) 87: 393–394
16. Augustinsson K-B (1948) Cholinesterases. A study in comparative enzymology. Acta Physiol Scand 15: 1–182
17. Augustinsson K-B (1955) A titrimetric method for the determination of plasma and red blood cell cholinesterase activity using thiocholine esters as substrates. Scand J Clin Lab Invest 7: 284–290
18. Augustinsson K-B (1957) In Glick D (ed), Methods of Biochemical Analysis, Vol 5. Interscience Publishers, New York, pp 1–63
19. Augustinsson K-B (1971) In Glick D (ed), Methods of Biochemical Analysis, Supplemental Vol. Interscience Publishers, New York, pp 217–275
20. Augustinsson K-B, Nachmansohn D (1949) Distinction between acetylcholine-esterase and other choline ester-splitting enzymes. Science 110: 98–99
21. Austin L, Berry WK (1953) Two selective inhibitors of acetylcholinesterase. Biochem J 54: 695–700
22. Badylak SF, VanVleet JF (1981) Sequential morphologic and clinicopathologic alteration in dogs with experimentally induced glucocorticoid hepatopathy. Am J Vet Res 42: 1310–1318
23. Baker AL, Hauser SC (1978) Alkaline phosphatase activity in lymph and serum of bile duct ligated rats. Digestion 18: 103–109
24. Balozs T, Murray TK, McLaughlin JM, Grice HC (1961) Hepatic tests in toxicity studies on rats. Toxical Appl Pharmacol 3: 71–79
25. Banerjec BB, Bhadra R, Datta AG (1983) Effect of glucagon on alanine 2-oxoglutarate aminotransferase. Biochem Biophys Res Comm 115: 506–511
26. Barlow RB, Ing HR (1948) Curare-like action of polymethylene bioquaternary ammonium salts. Nature (London) 161: 718
27. Baron MD, Pope B, Luzio JP (1986) The membrane topography of ecto-5′-nucleotidase in rat hepatocytes. Biochem J 236: 495–502
28. Beckett AH (1967) Stereospecificity in the reactions of cholinesterase and the cholinoreceptor. Ann NY Acad Sci 144: 675–688
29. Bengmark S, Olsson R (1974) Elimination of alka-

line phosphatases from serum in dog after intravenous injection of canine phosphatases from bone and intestine. Act Chir Scand 140: 1–6

30. Berezov T, Budyakova G, Levin F (1979) Enzymes and isoenzymes of heart muscle during aneurysm formation after myocardial infarction. Ind Clin Enzymology 61: 173–182

31. Bergmeyer H, Bernt E, Gawehn K, Michal G (1971) In Bergmeyer H (ed), Methods of Enzymatic Analysis, 2nd ed. Academic Press, New York

32. Berry WK (1951) The turnover number of cholinesterase. Biochem J 49: 615–620

33. Bockendahl H, Ammon R (1965) In Bergmeyer H-U (ed), Cholinesterases 3(b) Section CII. Methods of Enzymatic Analysis. Academic Press, New York, pp 771–775

34. Bodansky H, Greengard O, Den T (1980) Pulmonary and hepatic activities of membrane-bound enzymes in man and rat. Enzyme 25: 97–101

35. Bodansky O, Schwartz MK (1968) 5'-Nucleotidase. Adv Clin Chem 11: 227–328

36. Boelsterli U (1979) Gamma-glutamyl transpeptidase (GGT): An early marker for hepatocarcinogens in rats. Trends Pharm Sci 1: 47–49

37. Bolter CP, Critz JB (1974) Plasma enzyme activities in rats with diet-induced alterations in liver enzyme activities. Experientia 30: 1241–1243

38. Bovcic O, Straus B (1976) Separatoin of arginase isoenzymes from human tissue by agar gel electrophoresis. J Clin Chem Clin Biochem 14: 533–535

39. Boyd JW (1962) The comparative activities of some enzymes in sheep, cattle, and rats: Normal serum and tissue levels and changes during experimental liver necrosis. Res Vet Sci 3: 256–268

40. Boyd TF, Traad EB, Byrne JJ (1961) Serum amylase levels in experimental intestinal obstruction. J Surg Res 1: 128–131

41. Brard PE, Nix MS (1968) Modification of a test paper procedure for the determination of human serum cholinesterase activity. Arch Environ Health 17: 986–989

42. Braun JP, Rico AG, Benard P, Burgot-Sacaze V (1977) La gammaglutamyltransferase. Ann Biol Clin 35: 433–457

43. Briand P, Francois B, Rabier D, Cathelmian L (1982) Ornithine transcarbamylase deficiencies in human males: Kinetic and immunochemical classification. Biochim Biophys Acta 704: 110–106

44. Brobst D, Ferguson AB, Carter JM (1970) Evaluation of serum amylase and lipase activity in experimentally induced pancreatitis in the dog. J Am Vet Med Assoc 157: 1697–1702

45. Brosemer RW, Rutter WJ (1961) Liver amylase. I. Cellular distribution and properties. J Biol Chem 236: 1253

46. Burnette MA, Babcock MS (1978) Hepatic transaminase in protein restricted rats: Development of a controlled model. J Nutr 108: 458–464

47. Burton BK (1986) Positive amniotic fluid acetycholinesterase: Distinguishing between open spina bifida and ventral wall defects. Am J Obstet Gynecol 155: 984–986

48. Butenandt O (1968) Serum enzyme activity in hypothyroidism. Israel J Med Sci 4: 285–289

49. Cacciatore L, Antoniello S (1971) Arginase activity of mouse serum and liver tissue in some conditions of experimental liver damage. Enzymologia 41: 112–120

50. Callahan JF, Kruckenberg SM (1967) Erythrocyte cholinesterase activity of domestic and laboratory animals: Normal levels in nine species. Am J Vet Res 28: 1509–1512

51. Cameron R, Kellen J, Kolin A, Malkin A, Farber E (1978) γ-glutamyl transferase in putative premalignant liver cell populations during hepatocarcinogenesis. Cancer Res 38: 823–829

52. Cargil CF, Shields RP (1971) Plasma arginase as a liver function test. J Comp Pathol 81: 447–454

53. Carr JL, Foote FS (1944) Alkaline and acid phosphatase levels in serum of dogs after ligation of common bile duct. Arch Surg 49: 44–50

54. Challis TW, Reid LC, Hinton JW (1957) Study of some factors which influence the level of serum amylase in dogs and humans. Gastroenterology 33: 818–822

55. Chang YH, Ho IK (1979) Effects of acute and continuous morphine administration on serum glutamate oxaloacetate transaminase and glutamate pyruvic transaminase activities in the mouse. Biochem Pharm 28: 1373–1377

56. Childs AF, Davies DR, Green AL, Rutland JP (1955) The reactivation of oximes and hydroxamic acids of cholinesterase inhibited by organophosphorus compounds. Biol J Pharm 10: 462–465

57. Christopher JP, Kurlanksi L, Millar DB, Chignell C (1978) On the homogeneity of ll-S acetyl cholinesterase. Biochim Biophys Acta 525: 112–121

58. Clampitt RB, Hart RJ (1978) The tissue activities of some diagnostic enzymes in ten mammalian species. J Comp Pathol 88: 607–621

59. Clubb JS, Neale FC, Posen S (1965) The behavior of infused human placental alkaline phosphatase in human subjects. J Lab Clin Med 66: 443–507

60. Cohen JA, Kalsbeek F, Warringa MGPJ (1949) The significance of butyrylcholine in the testing of cholinesterase-containing preparations. Acta Brev Neerl Physiol 17: 32–39

61. Cohen JA, Oosterbann RA, Warringa MGPJ (1955) The turnover number of aliesterase, pseudo and true cholinesterase and ten combinations of these enzymes with diisopropylflourophosphonate. Biochim Biophys Acta 18: 228–235

62. Conzelman G, Gribble D (1973) Urinary excretion of β-glucuronidase after administration of neomycin to rats: A preliminary report. Toxicol Appl Pharm 26: 158–160

63. Cornelius CE, Bishop J, Switzer J, Rhode EA (1958) Serum and tissue transaminase activities in domestic animals. Cornell Vet 49: 116–126

64. Cornelius CE, Douglas GM, Gronwall RR, Freedland RA (1963) Comparative studies on plasma arginase and transaminases in hepatic necrosis. Cornell Vet 53: 181–191

65. Crawley G, Sevenson M (1963) Blood serum enzymes as diagnostic aids in canine heart disease. Am J Vet Res 24: 1270–1271

66. Curthorp NP, Shapiro R (1975) γ-glutamyl transferase in intestinal brush border membranes. FEBS Letters 58: 230–233

67. Cutler MC (1974) The sensitivity of function tests in detecting liver damage in the rat. Toxicol Appl Pharm 28: 349–357

68. Dalgaard JB (1952) Serum phosphatase after transfusion of phosphatase-rich blood into normal dogs. Acta Physiol Scand 22: 192–199

69. Daoust R (1982) The histochemical demonstration of γ-glutamyl transpeptidase activity in different populations of rat liver cells during azo dye carcinogenesis. J Histochem Cytochem 30: 312–316

70. DeDuve C, Wattiamx R, Baudhiun P (1962) Distributions of enzymes between subcellular fractions in animal tissues. Adv Enz 24: 291–358

71. DeMars R, LeVan S, Trend BL, Russell LB (1976) Abnormal ornithine carbamyl transferase in mice having the sparse-fur mutation. Proc Natl Acad Sci 73: 1693–1697

72. DeNova RC, Prasse KW (1983) Comparison of serum biochemical and hepatic functional alterations in dogs treated with corticosteroids and hepatic duct ligation. Am J Vet Res 44: 1703–1709

73. DeRosa G, Swick RW (1975) Metabolic implications of the distribution of the alanine aminotransferase isoenzymes. J Biol Chem 250: 7961–7967

74. Desjardins P (1982) Creatine kinase isoenzymes. Clin Chem News, March 1982: 12–14

75. Dhami MSI, Drangova R, Farkas R, Balozs T, Feurer G (1979) Decreased aminotransferase activity of serum and various tissue in the rat after cefazolin treatment. Clin Chem 25: 1263–1266

76. DiBartola S, Tasker J (1977) Elevated serum creatine phosphokinase: A study of 53 cases and a review of its diagnostic usefulness in clinical veterinary medicine. J Am An Hosp Assoc 13: 744–753

77. Dillon AR, Spano JS, Powers RD (1980) Prednisolone induced hematologic, biochemical and histologic changes in the dog. J Am An Hosp Assoc 16: 831–837

78. Ding JL, Smith GD, Peters TJ (1981) Purification and properties of γ-glutamyl transferase from normal rat liver. Biochim Biophys Acta 657: 334–343

79. Dorner JL, Hoffmann WE, Long GB (1974) Corticosteroid induction of an isoenzyme of alkaline phosphatase in the dog. Am J Vet Res 35: 1457–1458

80. Drozdz M, Kucharz E, Koslowski A (1975) Studies on 5-nucleotidase activity in blood serum, tissue and liver mitochondrial fraction of normal, hypo- and hyperthyroid rats. Endokrinologie 65: 328–332

81. Dudai Y, Silman I (1975) Acetylcholinesterases. Methods Enzymol 34: 571–580

82. Dudai Y, Silman I, Kalderon N, Blumberg S (1972) Purification by affinity chromatography of acetylcholinesterase from electric organ tissue of the electric eel subsequent to tryptic treatment. Biochim Biophys Acta 268: 138–157

83. Dudai Y, Silman I, Shinitzky M, Blumberg S (1972) Purification by affinity chromatography of the molecular forms of acetylcholinesterase present in fresh electric organ tissue of electric eel. Proc Natl Acad Sci USA 69: 2400–2403

84. Ecobischan DJ, Israel Y (1967) Characterization of the esterases from electric tissue of *electrophorus* by starch-gel electrophoresis. Can J Biochem 45: 1099–1105

85. El-Aaser AA, Reid E (1969) Phosphatase activities in rat liver before and after birth. Histochem J 1: 439–458

86. Ellman GL, Courtney KD, Andres V Jr, Featherstone RM (1961) A new rapid colorimetric determination of acetylcholinesterase activity. Biochem Pharm 7: 88–95

87. Farron F (1973) Arginase isoenzymes and their detection by catalytic staining in starch gel. Anal Biochem 53: 264–268

88. Felder M (1980) Biochemical and development genetics of isoenzymes in the mouse, *Mus musculus*. Isozymes: Current topics in biological and medical research 4: 2–69

89. Fiala S, Fiala ES (1973) Activation by chemical carcinogens of γ-glutamyl transpeptidase in rat and mouse liver. J Natl Cancer Inst 51: 151–158

90. Finco DR, Stevens JB (1969) Clinical significance of serum amylase activity in the dog. J Am Vet Med Assoc 155: 1686–1691

91. Fischer G, Lilienblum W, Ullrich D, Bock KW (1986) Immunohistochemical differentiation of γ-glutamyl transpeptidase in focal lesions and in zone 1 of rat liver after treatment with chemical carcinogens. Carcinogenesis 7: 1405–1410

92. Fishman MH (1974) Perspectives on alkaline phosphatase isoenzymes. Am J Med 56: 617–650

93. Fishman WH, Lin CW (1973) Membrane phosphohydrolases, metabolic conjugation and metabolic hydrolysis. Academic Press, New York, p 387

94. Fittscen C, Bellamy JEC (1984) Prednisone treatment alters the serum amylase and lipase activities in normal dogs without causing pancreatitis. Can J Comp Med 48: 136–140

95. Fleisher GA, Wakim KG (1956) Transaminase in canine serum and cerebrospinal fluid after carbon tetrachloride poisoning and injection of transaminase concentrates. Proc Staff Meet, Mayo Clinic 31: 640

96. Fleisher GA, Wakim KG (1963) The fate of enzymes in body fluids: An experimental study. Disappearance rates of glutamic-pyruvic transaminase under various conditions. J Lab Clin Med 61: 76–85

97. Franzini C, Bonini PA (1967) Amylolytic enzymes in dog serum. Experientia 23: 373–374

98. Friess SL, Wilson IB, Cabib E (1954) On the Mg (II) activation of acetylcholinesterase. J Am Chem Soc 76: 5156–5157

99. Froede HC, Wilson IB (1971) In Boyer PD (ed), The Enzymes, 3rd ed, Vol 5. Acetylcholinesterase. Academic Press, New York, pp 87–114

100. Fujiwara K, Katgal SL, Lombardi B (1982) Influence of age, sex and cancer on the activities of γ-glutamyl transpeptidase and of dipeptidyl aminopeptides IV in rat tissues. Enzyme 27: 114–118

101. Funke A, Bagot J, Depierre F (1954) Anticholinesteraiques. I. Synthèse de diphenoxyalkanes porteurs d'une ou deux fonctions phenoliques libres. CR Acad Sci (Paris) 239: 329–331

102. Futerman AN, Fiorimi RM, Roth E, Low MG, Silman I (1985) Physiological behavior and

structural characteristics of membrane bound acetylcholinesterase from Torpedo electric organ. Biochem J 226: 369–377

103. Gal EM, Roth E (1957) Spectrophotometric methods for determination of cholinesterase activity. Clin Chem Acta 2: 316–326

104. Gerlach U (1971) In Bergmeyer H (ed), Methods of Enzymatic Analysis, 2nd ed, Vol I. Academic Press, New York

105. Gingold JL, DiPasquale G (1976) Serum amylase in rats following the administration of endotoxin. Toxical Appl Pharm 36: 603–606

106. Glass DG, Knox WB (1973) Arginase isoenzymes of rat mammary gland, liver and other tissues. J Biol Chem 248: 5785–5789

107. Glenner GG, Folk JE, McMillan PJ (1962) Histochemical demonstration of γ-glutamyl transpeptidase-like activity. J Histochem Cytochem 10: 481–489

108. Glick D (1939) Cholinesterase and the theory of chemical mediation of the nerve impulse. J Gen Physiol 21: 431–438

109. Glick D (1939) Further studies on the specificity of choline esterase. J Biol Chem 130: 527–534

110. Glick D (1945) The controversy on cholinesterases. Science 102: 100–102

111. Goldberg DM (1972) 5'-Nucleotidase: Recent advances in cell biology, methodology and clinical significance. Digestion 8: 87–99

112. Goldberg DM (1976) Biochemical and clinical aspects of 5'-nucleotidase in gastroenterology. Front Gastrointest Res 2: 71–108

113. Goldstein DJ, Rogers CF, Harris H (1980) Expression of alkaline phosphatase loci in mammalian tissues. Proc Natl Acad Sci USA 77: 2857–2860

114. Goldstein DJ, Rogers C, Harris H (1982) Evolution of alkaline phosphatases in primates. Proc Natl Acad Sci USA 79: 879–883

115. Gopalakrishna R, Nagarajan B (1979) Effect of growth and differentiation on distribution of arginase and arginine in rat tissue. Ind J Biochem Biophys 16: 66–68

116. Gopinath C, Rombout PJA, VanVersendaal RG (1978) Serum alkaline phosphatase elevation in female rats treated with ethinyl estradiol. Toxicology 10: 91–102

117. Gordon JJ (1948) N-diethylaminoethylphenothiazine: A specific inhibitor of pseudo-cholinesterase. Nature 162: 146

118. Graig F, Ross G (1963) Serum creatine phosphokinase in thyroid disease. Metab Clin Exp 12: 57–59

119. Graig F, Smith J (19650 Serum creatine phosphokinase activity in altered thyroid states. J Clin Endocrinol Metab 25: 723–731

120. Green JA, Cook ND, Manson MM (1986) Monoclonal antibodies against rat kidney γ-glutamyl transpeptidase show species and tissue specificity. Biochem J 238: 913–917

121. Griffiths I, Duncan I (1973) Myotonia in the dog: A report of four cases. Vet Rec 93: 184–188

122. Griffiths P (1963) Creatine phosphokinase levels in hypothyroidism. Lancet i: 894

123. Guelfi JF, Braun JP, Benard P, Rico AG, Thouvenot JP (1982) Value of so-called cholestasis markers in the dog: An experimental study. Res Vet Sci 33: 309–312

124. Gutman AB (1959) Serum alkaline phosphatase activity in diseases of the skeletal and hepatobiliary systems. Am J Med 27: 875

125. Hammerton K, Messer M (1971) The origin of serum amylase. Electrophoretic studies of isoamylases of the serum, liver, and other tissues of adult and infant rats. Biochim Biophys Acta 244: 441–451

126. Hardonk MJ (1968) Distribution of 5-nucleotidase in tissues of rat and mouse. Histochemie 12: 1–17

127. Hardonk MJ, DeBoer HGA (1968) III. Determinations of 5-nucleotidase isoenzymes in tissue of rat and mouse. Histochemie 12: 29–41

128. Harris H (1982) Multilocus enzyme systems and the evaluation of gene expression: The alkaline phosphatases as a model example. The Harvey Lectures, Series 76, Academic Press, New York, pp 95–125

129. Hastings FL (1966) The study of horse and human serum cholinesterase substrate reactions. PhD thesis, North Carolina State University, Raleigh, NC

130. Hatoff DE, Hardison WGM (1979) Induced synthesis of alkaline phosphatase of bile acids in rat liver cell culture. Gastroenterology 77: 1062–1067

131. Hatoff DE, Hardison WGM (1981) Bile acids modify alkaline phosphatase induction and bile acid secretion pressure after bile duct obstruction in the rat. Gastroenterology 80: 666–672

132. Hawkins RD, Gunter JM (1946) Studies on cholinesterase. 5. The selective inhibition of pseudo-cholinesterase in vivo. Biochem J 40: 192–197

133. Hegreberg G (1979) In Andrews E, Ward B, Altman N (eds), Spontaneous Animal Models of Human Disease, Vol II. Academic Press, New York

134. Heilbronn E (1959) Hydrolysis of carboxylic esters of thiocholine and its analogues. 3. Hydrolysis catalyzed by acetylcholine esterase and butyrylcholine esterase. Acta Chemica Scand 13: 1547–1560

135. Herzfeld A, Raper SM (1976) The heterogeneity of arginases in rat tissue. Biochem J 153: 469–478

136. Herzfeld A, Rosenoer V, Raper SM (1976) Glutamate dehydrogenase, alanine aminotransferase, thymidine kinase, and arginase in fetal and adult human and rat liver. Pediat Res 10: 960–964

137. Hess J, MacDonald R, Frederick R (1964) Serum creatine phosphokinase (CPK) activity in disorders of heart and skeletal muscle. Ann Int Med 61: 1015–1028

138. Hestrin S (1949) The reaction of acetylcholine and carboxylic acid derivatives with hydroxylamine and its analytical application. J Biol Chem 180: 249–261

139. Hiatt N, Bonorris G (1966) Removal of serum amylase in dogs and the influence of reticuloendothelial blockade. Am J Physiol 210: 133–138

140. Higashino K, Otani R, Kudo S, Yamamura Y (1977) A fetal intestinal type alkaline phosphatase in hepatocellular carcinoma tissue. Clin Chem 23: 1615–1623

141. Hillis L, Braunwald E (1977) Myocardial ischemia. N Engl J Med 296: 1034–1041

142. Hoffmann WE Unpublished data

143. Hoffmann WE, Dorner JL (1975) Separation of isoenzymes of canine alkaline phosphatase by cellulose acetate electrophoresis. J Am An Hosp Assoc 11: 283–285

144. Hoffmann WE, Dorner JL (1977) Disappearance rate of intravenously injected canine alkaline phosphatase isoenzymes. Am J Vet Res 38: 1553–1555

145. Holmes R, Master C (1979) Subcellular localization of isoenzymes. Isoenzymes: Current topics in biological and medical research 3: 53–114

146. Hubbard RW, Criss REL, Elliot LP, Kelly EC, Matthew WT, Bowers WD, Leav I, Mager M (1979) Diagnostic significance of selected serum enzymes in a rat heatstroke model. J Appl Physiol Resp Environ Exercise Physiol 46: 334–339

147. Hudson EB, Strombeck DR (1978) Effects of functional nephrectomy on the disappearance rates of canine serum amylase and lipase. Am J Vet Res 39: 1316–1321

148. Huseby N (1979) Subcellular localization of γ-glutamyl transferase activity in guinea pig liver. Effects of phenobarbital on the enzyme activity levels. Clin Chem Acta 94: 163–171

149. Huseby NE, Vik T (1978) The activity of γ-glutamyl transferase after bile duct ligation in guinea pig. Clin Chem Acta 88: 385–392

150. Inoue M, Hayashida S, Hosomi F, Huriuchi S, Morino Y (1980) The molecular forms of γ-glutamyl transferase in bile and serum of icteric rats. Biochim Biophys Acta 615: 70–78

151. Ip C, Dao T (1978) Alterations in serum glycosyltransferases and 5'-nucleotidase in breast cancer patients. Cancer Res 38: 723–728

152. Isea FS, Mullock BM, Hinton R (1976) 5'-Nucleotidase in liver plasma membrane and in the serum of normal and jaundiced rats. Biochem Soc Trans 4: 55–58

153. Ivanov E, Krastev L, Adjarov D, Chernev K, Apostolov I, Dimitrov P, Drenska E, Stefanova M, Pramatarovv (1976) Studies on the mechanism of the changes in serum and liver γ-glutamyl transpeptidase activity. Enzyme 21: 8–20

154. Jaken S, Mason M (1978) Difference in the isoelectric focusing patterns of γ-glutamyl transpeptidase from normal and cancerous rat mammary tissue. Proc Natl Acad Sci 75: 1750–1753

155. Jenson-Holm J, Lansen HH, Miethers K, Moller KO (1959) Determination of the cholinesterase activity in blood and organs by automatic titration, with some observations on serious errors of the method and remarks of the photometric method. Acta Pharm Toxicol 15: 384–394

156. Jordan J (1977) Normal laboratory values in beagle dogs of twelve to eighteen months of age. Am J Vet Res 38: 509–513

157. Kachmar J, Moss D (1976) In Tietz N (ed), Fundamentals of Clinical Chemistry. WB Saunders, Philadelphia

158. Kako M, Toda G, Torii M, Kimura H, Miyake K, Suzuki H, Oda T (1980) Electron microscopic studies on hepatic alkaline phosphatase in experimentally induced biliary obstruction of the rat. Gastroent Jap 15: 600–605

159. Kalousek F, Francois B, Rosenberg LE (1978) Isolation and characterization of ornithine transcarbamylase from normal human liver. J Biol Chem 253: 3939–3944

160. Kalow W, Genest K (1957) A method for the determination of atypical forms of human serum cholinesterase. Determinations of dibucaine numbers. Can J Biochem 35: 339–349

161. Kalow W, Lindsey HA (1955) A comparison of optical and manometric methods for the assay of human serum cholinesterase. Can J Biochem 33: 568–574

162. Kamoda N, Minatogawa Y, Nakamura M, Nakanishi V, Okundo E, Kido R (1980) The organ distribution of human alanine-2-oxoglutarate aminotransferase and alanine-glyoxalate aminotransferase. Biochem Med 23: 25–34

163. Kaplan MM, Ohkubo A, Quaroni EG, Sze-Tu D (1983) Increased synthesis of rat liver alkaline phosphatase by bile duct ligation. Hepatology 3: 368–376

164. Kaplan MM, Righetti A (1970) Induction of rat liver alkaline phosphatase: The mechanism of the serum elevation in bile duct obstruction. J Clin Invest 49: 508–516

165. Kawahara S, Ogata S, Ikehara Y (1982) Chemical and immunological characterization of rat ascites hepatoma alkaline phosphatase: A comparison with the liver enzyme. J Biochem 91: 201–210

166. Kay HD (1928) The phosphatases of mammalian tissues. Biochem J 22: 855–866

167. Keiding NR (1966) Intestinal alkaline phosphatase in human lymph and serum. Scand J Clin Lab Invest 18: 134–140

168. Keller P (1981) Enzyme activities in the dog: Tissue analysis, plasma values, and intracellular distribution. Am J Vet Res 42: 575–582

169. Kinnett DG, Wilcox FH (1982) Partial characterization of two liver alkaline phosphatases that require manganese for activity. Int J Biochem 14: 977–981

170. Knox W (1976) Enzyme Patterns in Fetal, Adult, and Neoplastic Rat Tissue, 2nd ed. S Karger, Switzerland

171. Kojima J, Kanatani M, Nakamura N, Koshiwagi T, Tohjoh F, Akiyama M (1980) Electrophoretic fractionation of serum γ-glutamyl transpeptidase in human hepatic cancer. Clin Chem Acta 106: 165–172

172. Kolata G (1985) Novel protein/membrane attachment. Science 229: 850

173. Komoda T, Kumegawa K, Yasima T, Tamura G Alpers DH (1984) Induction of rat hepatic and intestinal alkaline phosphatase activity produced by bile from bile duct-ligated animals. Am J Physiol 246: G393–G400

174. Korngold L (1977) Further characterization of alkaline phosphatases of human kidney and urine. Int Arch Allergy Appl Immunol 54: 300–307

175. Korsrud GO, Grice HC, McLaughlin JM (1972) Sensitivity of several serum enzymes in detecting carbon tetrachloride induced liver damage in rats. Toxicol Appl Pharmacol 22: 474–483

176. Kramer J (1980) In Kaneko J (ed), Clinical Bio-

chemistry of Domestic Animals. Academic Press, New York

177. Kramer J, Hegreberg G, Bryan G, Meyers K, Ott R (1976) A muscle deficiency of Labrador retrievers characterized by deficiency of type II muscle fibers. J Am Vet Med Assoc 169: 817–820

178. Krebs H, Eggleston LV, Knivett VA (1955) Arsenolysis and phosphorolysis of citrulline in mammalian liver. Biochem J 59: 185–193

179. Krupka RM (1966) Hydrolysis of neutral substrates of acetylcholinesterase. Biochemistry 5: 1983–1988

180. Kryszewski AJ, Neale G, Whitefield JB, Moss DW (1973) Enzyme changes in experimental biliary obstruction. Clin Chem Acta 47; 175–182

181. Kumar AN, Kalyankar GD (1984) Effect of steroid hormones on age dependent changes in rat arginase isoenzymes. Exp Gerontol 19: 191–198

182. Kumegawa M, Maeda N, Yajima T, Takuma T, Ikeda E, Hanai H (1980) Permissive role of L-thyroxime in induction of pancreatic amylase by cortisol in neonatal rats. J Endocrinol 86: 497–500

183. Laudahn G (1971) In Bergmeyer H (ed), Methods of Enzymatic Analysis, 2nd ed, Vol I. Academic Press, New York

184. Leonard TB, Neptun DA, Popp JA (1984) Serum gammaglutamyltransferase as a specific indicator of bile duct lesions in the rat liver. Am J Pathol 16: 262–269

185. Leuzinger W (1971) The number of catalytic sites in acetylcholinesterase. Biochem J 123: 139–141

186. Leuzinger W, Goldberg M, Calvin E (1969) Molecular properties of acetylcholinesterase. J Mol Biol 40: 217–225

187. Lewis PJ, Lowing RK, Gompert D (1981) Auto mated discrete kinetic method for erythrocyte acetylcholinesterase and plasma cholinesterase. Clin Chem 27: 926–929

188. Lockridge O, Bartela CF, Vaughan TA, Wong C, Norton S, Johnson L (1987) Complete amino acid sequence of human cholinesterase. J Biol Chem 262: 549–557

189. Long GB (1974) The effects of prednisolone administration on circulating blood cells, serum proteins and serum enzymes in the normal dog. PhD Thesis, University of Illinois, Urbana, IL

190. Lovell RA, Hoffmann WE, Valentine WM, Lund LA, Dahlem AM, Carmichael WW, Beasley VR (1987) Arginase activity in twelve tissues and serum, serum arginase half-life, and changes in serum arginase activity following administration of microcystin-A (cyanoginosin-LR) in swine. Submitted to Am J Vet Res

191. MacKenzie PI, Mosser M (1976) Studies on the origin and excretion of serum α-amylase in the mouse. Comp Biochem Physiol 54B: 103–106

192. Madsen WB, Tuba J (1952) On the source of alkaline phosphatase in rat serum. J Biol Chem 195: 741–750

193. Mahy BWJ, Rowson KEK, Parr CW (1967) Studies on the mechanism of action of Riley Virus IV. The reticuloendothelial system and impaired plasma enzyme clearance in infected mice. J Exp Med 125: 277–288

194. Main AR (1976) In Goldberg AM, Hanin I (eds),

Structure and Inhibitors of Cholinesterase. Biology of Cholinergic Function. Raven Press, New York, p 269–353

195. Main AR, McKnelly SC, Burgess-Miller SK (1977) A subunit-sized butyrylcholinesterase present in high concentrations in pooled rabbit serum. Biochem J 167: 367–376

196. Main AR, Miles KE, Braid PE (1961) The determination of human serum cholinesterase activity with o-nitrophenylbutyrate. Biochem J 78: 769–776

197. Malik N, Butterworth PJ (1976) Molecular properties of rat intestinal alkaline phosphatase. Biochim Biophys Acta 446: 105–114

198. Manson MM, Smith AG (1984) Effect of hexachlorobenzene on male and female rat hepatic gammaglutamyltranspeptidase levels. Cancer Lett 22: 227–234

199. Massoulié J, Rieger F (1969) L'acetylcholinesterase des organes electriques des poissons (torpille et gymnote); complexes membranaires Eur J Biochem 11: 441–455

200. Massoulié J, Rieger F, Tsuji S (1970) Solubilization de l'acètylcholinesterase des organes electrique de gymnote. Eur J Biochem 14: 430–439

201. McGeachin RL, Abshier WM, O'Leary K (1978) The effects of puromycin and actinomycin D on the serum and liver amylase levels in the mouse, rabbit, and rat. Carbohydrate Res 61: 425–429

202. McGeachin RL, Johnson WD (1964) The in vivo effect of puromycin on amylase levels in the serum liver, salivary glands and pancreas of the rat. Arch Biochem Biophys 107: 534–536

203. McGeachin RL, Potter BA, Potts ER (1978) The inhibition of amylase synthesis in the isolated perfused rat liver by cycloheximide and dinitrophenol. Biochem Med 20: 353–356

204. Meites S, Rogols S (1971) Amylase isoenzymes. CRC Crit Rev Clin Lab Sci 2: 103–138

205. Mendal B, Mundell DB, Rudney H (1943) Studies on cholinesterase. 3. Specific tests for true cholinesterase and pseudo-cholinesterase. Biochem J 37: 473–476

206. Mendel B, Rudney H (1943) Studies on cholinesterases. 1. Cholinesterase and pseudo-cholinesterase. Biochem J 37: 59–63

207. Mendel B, Rudney H (1945) Some effects of salts on true cholinesterase. Science 102: 616–617

208. Mia AS, Koger HD (1978) Direct colorimetric determinations of serum arginase in various domestic animals. Am J Vet Res 39: 1381–1383

209. Mia AS, Koger HD, Tierney MM (1978) Serum values of amylase and pancreatic lipase in healthy mature dogs and dogs with experimental pancreatitis. Am J Vet Res 39: 965–969

210. Michel HO (1949) An electrometric method for the determination of red blood cell and plasma cholinesterase activity. J Lab Clin Med 34: 1564–1568

211. Michelson A, Russell E, Hartman P (1955) Dystrophia muscularis: A hereditary primary myopathy of the house mouse. Proc Natl Acad Sci 41: 1079–1084

212. Milne EM, Doyey DL (1985) Gammaglutamyltransferase and its multiple forms in the tissues and sera of normal dogs. Res Vet Sci 39: 385–387

213. Minic-Oka J, Cupic Z, Japundzic I (1971) Effect of adrenal function on level of hepatic and extra-hepatic arginase. Experientia 27: 1477–1478

214. Moak G, Harris H (1979) Lack of homology between dog and human placental alkaline phosphatases. Proc Natl Acad Sci USA 76: 1948–1951

215. Moore WE, Cunningham BA (1976) Comparative properties of canine hepatic and pancreatic amylase. Bull Am Soc Vet Lin Pathol 5: 11–12

216. Moore W, Fieldman B (1974) The use of isoenzymes in small animal medicine. J Am An Hosp Assoc 10: 420–429

217. Mordoh J, Krisman CR, Parodi AJ, Leloir LF (1968) Some properties of rat liver amylase. Arch Biochem Biophys 127: 193–199

218. Morita T, Mori M, Ikeda F, Tatibana M (1982) Transport of carbamyl phosphate synthetase I and ornithine transcarbamylase into mitochondria. J Biol Chem 257: 10547–10550

219. Mounter LA, Whittaker VP (1953) The hydrolysis of esters of phenol by cholinesterases and other esterases. Biochem J 54: 551–559

220. Muntangh RJ, Jacobs RM (1985) Serum amylase and isoamylases and their origins in healthy dogs and dogs with experimentally induced acute pancreatitis. Am J Vet Res 46: 742–747

221. Myers DK (1953) Studies on cholinesterase. 9. Species variation in the specificity patterns of the pseudo-cholinesterase. Biochem J 55: 67–69

222. Nachmansohn D (1940) Action of ions on choline esterase. Nature 145: 513–514

223. Nagode LA, Frajola WJ, Loeb WF (1966) Enzyme activities in canine tissues. Am J Vet Res 27: 1385–1393

224. Nagode LA, Koestner A, Steinmeyer CL (1969) Organ identifying properties of alkaline phosphatase from canine tissues. Clin Chem Acta 26: 45–54

225. Nair BC, Johnson DE, Majeska RJ, Rodkey JA, Bennett CD, Roden GA (1987) Rat alkaline phosphatase. II. Structural similarities between the osteosarcoma, bone, kidney, and placenta isoenzymes. Arch Biochem Biophys 254: 28–34

226. Nakashima Y, Hachinen A, Apport HE, Howard JM (1980) The contribution of pancreas and kidney in regulating serum amylase levels in dogs. Gastroenterol Jap 15: 475–479

227. Nakasaki H, Matsushima T, Sato S, Kawachi T (1979) Purification and properties of alkaline phosphatase from the mucosa of rat small intestine. J Biochem 86: 1225–1231.

228. Neuman GJ, Skupp S, Farrar JT (1964) Studies on canine liver amylase. Biochim Biophys Acta 85: 296–303

229. Nishimura M, Teschke R (1982) Effects of chronic alcohol consumption on the activities of liver plasma membrane enzymes: Gamma-glutamyl transferase, alkaline phosphatase and 5'-nucleotidase. Biochem Pharm 31: 377–381

230. Noguchi T, Yamashita Y (1987) The rabbit differs from other mammalian in the tissue distribution of alkaline phosphatase isoenzymes. Biochem Biophys Res Comm 143: 15–19

231. Noonan NE (1980) Variations of plasma enzymes in the pony and the dog after carbon tetrachloride administration. Am J Vet Res 42: 674–678

232. Noonan NE, Meyer DJ (1979) Use of plasma arginase and the γ-glutamyl transpeptidase as specific indicators of hepatocellular or hepatobiliary disease in the dog. Am J Vet Res 40: 942–947

233. Nose K (1976) Purification and characterization of alkaline phosphatase from rat kidney. J Biochem 79: 283–288

234. Nothman MM, Callow AD (1971) Investigations on the origin of amylase in serum and urine. Gastroenterology 60: 82–89

235. Novikoff AB, Essner E (1960) The liver cell (some new approaches to its study). Am J Med 29: 102–131

236. Nuttall F (1968) Tissue and serum creatine kinase activity in hypothyroid rats. J Endocrinol 42: 495–499

237. Olson R (1967) Are we looking at the right enzyme systems? Am J Clin Nutr 20: 604–611

238. Ord MG, Thompson RHS (1950) The distribution of cholinesterase types in mammalian tissues. Biochem J 46: 346–352

239. Panchenko SV, Popova SV, Antonenkov VD (1982) Inducing effect of clofibrate on alkaline phosphatase and histidine-glyoxylate aminotransferase in rat liver. Experientia 33: 433–434

240. Pappas NJ (1986) Source of increased serum aspartate and alanine aminotransferase: Cycloheximide effect on carbon tetracholride hepatotoxicity. Clin Chem Acta 154: 181–190

241. Parembska Z, Baranczyk A, Jachimowicz J (1971) Arginase isoenzymes in liver and kidney of some mammals. Acta Biochem 18: 79–85

242. Parent J (1982) Effects of dexamethasone on pancreatic tissue and on serum amylase and lipase activities in dogs. J Am Vet Med Assoc 180: 743–746

243. Patnaik SK (1979) Changes in the sub-types of soluble alanine aminotrasferase in the liver of rats during development and aging. Cell Biol Int Reports 3: 607–614

244. Patnaik SK, Kanungo MS (1977) Age-related expression of alanine aminotransferase isoenzymes in normal and hydrocortisone-treated rats. Ind J Biochem Biophys 14: 245–246

245. Pekarthy JM, Short J, Lansing AI, Lieberman I (1972) Function and control of liver alkaline phosphatase. J Biol Chem 247: 1767–1774

246. Pilz W (1965) In Bergmeyer HH (ed), Acetylcholinesterase 3(b) Section CII. Methods of Enzymatic Analysis. Academic Press, New York, pp 765–770

247. Polzin DJ, Osborne CA, Stevens JB, Hayden DW (1983) Serum amylase and lipase activities in dogs with chronic primary renal failure. Am J Vet Res 44: 404–410

248. Pree DJ, Townsend JL, Archibald DE (1987) Sensitivity of acetylcholinesterase from aphelenchusanema to organo-phosphorus and carbonate pesticides. J Neonatal 19: 188–193

249. Quieshi J, Letcute J, Ouellet R (1979) Ornithine transcarbamylase deficiency in mutant mice. I. Studies on characterization of enzyme defect and

suitability as an animal model of human disease. Pediat Res B: 807–811

250. Raab WP (1972) Diagnostic value of urinary enzyme determination. Clin Chem 18: 5–25

251. Rajasingham R, Bell JL, Baron DN (1971) A comparative study of the isoenzymes of mammalion α-amylase. Enzyme 12: 180–186

252. Ralston JS, Rush RS, Doctor BP, Wolfe AD (1985) Acetylcholinesterase from fetal bovine serum. J Biol Chem 260: 4312–4318

253. Ramados CS, Selvom R, Shanmugasundaram KR, Shanmugasundaram ERB (1977) Alkaline phosphatase from rabbit kidney: Studies on the catalytic properties of its multiforms. J Biochem 81: 1813–1823

254. Rao SS, Kanungo MS (1974) Age-dependent induction of arginase in the liver of rats. Ind J Biochem Biophys 11: 208–212

255. Ratansavanh D, Tazi A, Galteau MM, Siest G (1979) Localization of γ-glutamyl transferase in subcellular fractions of rat and rabbit liver: Effect of phenobarbital. Biochem Pharm 28: 1363–1365

256. Ravin HA, Tsou KC, Seligman AM (1951) Colorimetric estimation and histochemical demonstration of serum cholinesterase. J Biol Chem 191: 843–857

257. Reddi PK, Knox WE, Herzfeld A (1975) Types of arginase in rat tissue. Enzyme 20: 305–314

258. Reichard H (1959) Ornithine carbamyl transferase in dog serum on intravenous injection of enzyme, choledochus ligation and carbon tetrachloride poisoning. J Lab Clin Med 53: 417–425

259. Reis J (1940) The specificity of phosphomonoesterases in human tissue. Biochem J 48. 548–551

260. Riemer BL, Widnell CC (1975) The demonstration of a specific 5'-nucleotidase activity in rat tissue. Arch Biochem Biophys 171: 343–347

261. Riemert C, Häcker R, Scheuch DW (1978) Aktivität der Ornithinkarbamyl-Transferase im experimentellen hämorrhagischeu Schock des Hundes. Z Med Labor Diagn 19 218–222

262. Righetti AB-B, Kaplan MM (1971) The origin of the serum alkaline phosphatase in normal rats. Biochim Biophys Acta 230: 504–509

263. Righetti AB-B, Kaplan MM (1974) Properties of rat liver alkaline phosphatase before and after bile duct ligation. Proc Soc Exp Biol Med 145: 726–728

264. Roberts R (1979) Creatine kinase isozymes as diagnostic and prognostic indices of myocardial infarction. Isozymes: Current topics in biological and medical research 3: 115–154

265. Roomi MW, Goldberg DM (1981) Comparison of γ-glutamyl transferase induction by phenobarbital in the rat, guinea pig and rabbit. Biochem Pharm 30: 1563–1571

266. Rosalki SB (1975) Gamma-glutamyl transpeptitase. Adv in Clin Chem 17: 53–107

267. Rosalki SB, Tarlow D, Ran D (1971) Plasma γ-glutamyl traspeptidase elevation in patients receiving enzyme inducing drugs. Lancet 2: 376–377

268. Rosen F (1959) The specificity of the glutamic pyruvic transaminase response. Endocrin 65: 256–264

269. Rosen F (1963) Enzymes in tissues responsive to corticosteroids. Canc Res 23: 1447–1458

270. Rosen F, Roberts NR, Nichol CA (1959) Glucocorticosteroids and transaminase in four conditions associated with gluconeogenesis. J Biol Chem 234: 476–480

271. Rosenberry TL, Chen YT, Bock E (1974) Structure of 11 S acetylcholinesterase subunit composition. Biochem 13: 3068-3079

272. Rosenblum JL, Niesen TE, Roab BK, Alpers DH (1983) Fate of circulating isoamylase in the rabbit. Am J Physiol 244: G254–G250

273. Rothenberg MA, Nachmansohn D (1947) Studies on cholinesterase. III. Purification of the enzyme from electric tissue by fractional ammonium sulphate precipitation. J Biol Chem 168: 223–231

274. Ruesegger P, Nyrick I, Freiman A, LaDue J (1959) Serum activity patterns of glutamic oxaloacetic transaminase, glutamic pyruvic tranaminase and lactic dehydrogenese following graded myocardial infarctions in dogs. Circ Res 7: 4–10

275. Ruscak M, Orlicky J, Zubor V (1982) Isoelectric focusing of the alanine aminotransferase isoenzymes from the brain, liver and kidney. Comp Biochem Physiol 71: 141–144

276. Rush RS, Main AR, Kilpatrick BF, Faulkner G (1981) Inhibition of two monomeric butyrylcholinesterases from rabbit liver by chlorpromazine and other drugs. J Pharm Exp Ther 216: 586–591

277. Russel FGM, Weitering JG, Oosting R, Groothuis GMM, Hardonk MJ, Meijer DKF (1983) Influence of taurcholate on hepatic clearance and biliary excretion of asialointestinal alkaline phosphatase in the rat in vivo and in isolated perfused rat liver. Gastroenterology 85: 225–234

278. Saini PK, Posen S (1969) The origin of serum alkaline phosphatase in the rat. Biochim Biophys Acta 177: 42–49

279. Saini PK, Saini SK (1978) Immunochemical study of canine intestinal, hepatic and osseous alkaline phosphatase. Am J Vet Res 39: 1506–1509

280. Saini PK, Saini SK (1978) Origin of serum alkaline phosphatase in the dog. Am J Vet Res 39: 1510–1513

281. Sanecki RK, Cechner S, Martin L, Hoffmann WE (1987) Characterization of rabbit ALP isoenzymes. In preparation

282. Sanecki RK, Hoffmann WE, Gelberg H, Dorner JL (1987) Subcellular location of corticosteroid-induced alkaline phosphatase in canine hepatocytes. Vet Pathol 24: 296–301

283. Sanecki RK, Hoffmann WE, Kuhlenschmidt MS, Dorner JL (1987) The canine corticosteroid-induced alkaline phosphatase: Subcellular location, purification by monoclonal antibody affinity chromatography and biochemical comparisons to the intestinal and hepatic isoenzymes (abstr). Vet Clin Pathol 16: 8

284. Schimke RT (1964) The importance of both synthesis and degradation in the control of arginase in rat liver. J Biol Chem 239: 3808–3817

285. Schlaeger R (1975) The mechanism of the increase in the activity of liver alkaline phosphatase in experimental cholestasis: Measurement of an increased enzyme concentration by immunochemical titration. Z Klin Chem Klin Biochem 13: 277–281

286. Schlaeger R, Harx P, Kattermann R (1982) Studies on the mechanism of the increase in serum alkaline phosphatase activity in cholestasis: Significance of the hepatic bile and concentration for the leakage of alkaline phosphatase from rat liver. Enzyme 38: 3–13

287. Schmidt E, Schmidt FW (1967) Release of enzyme from the liver. Nature 213: 1125–1126

288. Schmidt E, Schmidt F (1971) In Bergmeyer H (ed), Methods of Enzymetric Analysis, 2nd ed, Vol I. Academic Press, New York

289. Scholtens HB, Hardonk MS, Meijer DKF (1982) A kinetic study of hepatic uptake of canine intestinal alkaline phosphatase in the rat. Liver 2: 1–13

290. Scholtins HB, Meijer DKF, Hardonk MJ (1982) A histochemical study on the distribution of injected canine intestinal alkaline phosphatase in rat liver. Liver 2: 14–21

291. Schiut KE, Dickie MW (1973) Induction of enzyme activity during fetal development. Biol Neonate 23: 171–179

292. Schulz BO, Schlaeger R (1979) Evidence for an enhanced de novo synthesis of alkaline phosphatase in cholestatic rat liver using immunotitration and precursor incorporation techniques. Enzyme 24: 173–180

293. Schumacker M, Camp S, Manlet Y, Newton M, MacPhee-Quigley K, Taylor P (1986) Primary structure of *Torpedo Californica* acetylcholinesterase deduced from its cDNA sequence. Nature 319: 407–409

294. Searcy RL, Hayaski S, Berk JE, Stern H (1966) Electrophoretic behavior of serum amylase in various mammalian species. Proc Soc Exp Biol Med 122: 1291–1295

295. Seetharam S, Sussman NL, Komoda T, Alpers DH (1986) The mechanism of elevated alkaline phosphatase activity after bile duct ligation in rat. Hepatology 6: 374–380

296. Segal HL, Matsuzawa T (1970) L-alanine aminotransferase (rat liver). In Tabar H, Tabar CW (eds), Methods in Enzymology, Vol XVII. Academic Press, New York, pp 153–159

297. Segal HL, Rosso RG, Hopper S, Weber MM (1962) Direct evidence for an increase in enzyme level as the basis for the glucocorticoid-induced increase in glutamic-alanine transaminase activity in rat liver. J Biol Chem 237: PC3303–3305

298. Short DW (1961) The effects of drugs upon experimental pancreatitis in the rat. Br J Surg 48: 446–454

299. Shull RM, Hornbuckle W (1979) Diagnostic use of serum γ-glutamyl transferase in canine liver disease. Am J Vet Res 40: 1321–1324

300. Siegal S, Bing R (1956) Plasma enzyme activity in myocardial infarction in dog and man. Proc Soc Exp Biol Bed 91: 604–607

301. Sikoran JL, Grassi J, Bon S (1985) Synthesis *in vitro* of precursors of the catalytic subunits of acetylcholinesterase (EC 3.1.1.7) from *Torpedo mormorata* and *Electrophorus electricus*. Eur J Biochem 145: 519–524

302. Silver A (1974) The biology of cholinesterases. Frontiers of Biology, Vol. 36. North Holland, Amsterdam

303. Simon FR, Arias IM (1973) Alterations of bile canalicular enzymes in cholestasis. A possible cause of bile secretory failure. J Clin Invest 52: 765–774

304. Sinha KP, Saran A (1972) Serum transaminase levels during the course of repeated administration of carbon tetrachloride to rabbits. Ind J Med Res 60: 1378–1385

305. Skrzypek-Osiecka I, Rahden-Staron I, Porembska Z (1980) Subcellular localization of arginase in rat liver. Acta Biochim Pol 27: 203–208

306. Song CS, Bodansky O (1967) Subcellular localization and properties of 5'-nucleotidase in the rat liver. J Biol Chem 242: 694–699

307. Stanley KK, Edwards MR, Luzio JP (1980) Subcellular distribution and movement of 5'-nucleotidase in rat cells. Biochem J 186:59–69

308. Stedman E, Stedman E, Easson LH (1932) CCXLY choline-esterase. An enzyme present in the blood serum of the horse. Biochem J 26: 2056–2066

309. Stickle JE, Carlton WW, Boon GD (1979) Isoamylase in clinically normal dogs. Am J Vet Res 41: 506–509

310. Strombeck DR, Farver T, Kaneko JJ (1981) Serum amylase and lipase activities in the diagnosis of pancreatitis in dogs. Am J Vet Res 42: 1966–1970

311. Stunpf HH, Wilens SL, Sornoza C (1956) Pancreatic lesions and peripancreatic fat necrosis in cortisone treated rabbits. Lab Invest 5: 224–235

312. Sturge LM, Whittaker VP (1950) The esterase of horse blood. I. The specificity of horse plasma cholinesterase and ali-esterase. Biochem J 47: 518–525

313. Sulakhe SJ, Lautt WW (1985) The activity of hepatic γ-glutamyltranspeptidase in various animal species. Comp Biochem Physiol 82B: 263–264

314. Sumitani A (1977) Immunological studies of liver arginase in man and various kinds of vertebrates. Hiroshima J Med Sci 26: 59–80

315. Swain LK, Taylor HW, Jersey GC (1985) The effect of handling techniques on serum ALT activity in mice. J Appl Toxicol 5: 160–162

316. Swich RW, Barnstein PL, Stange JL (1965) The metabolism of mitochondrial proteins. II. The response of isozymes of alanine aminotransferase to diet and hormones. J Biol Chem 240: 3341–3345

317. Tate SS, Meister A (1976) Subunit structure and isozymic forms of γ-glutamyl transpeptidase. Proc Natl Acad Sci 73: 2599–2603

318. Taylor J, Almond W, Himel C (1983) Affinity chromatography of acetylcholinesterase from *Electrophorus electricus*: A new 9-alkylominoacridine affinity ligand. J Chrom 257: 225–284

319. Tazi A, Galteau M-M, Siest G (1980) γ-glutamyltransferase of rabbit liver: Kinetic study of phenobarbital induction and *in vitro* solubilization by bile salts. Toxcol Appl Pharm 55: 1–7

320. Tomita K, Kamei S, Shiraishi T, Hoshinomoto Y, Yanamaka M (1986) UV spectrophotemetric method for determination of cholinesterase activity with acetylcholine as a substrate. Appl Biochem 7: 303–310

321. Trams EG, Lauter CJ (1974) On the sidedness of plasma membrane enzymes. Biochim Biophys Acta 345: 180–197

322. Tsuchida S, Hoshino K, Sato T, Ito N, Sato K

(1979) Purification of γ-glutamyl transferase from rat hepatomas and hyperplastic nodules and comparison with the enzyme from rat kidney. Canc Res 39: 4200–4205

323. Tsuda M, Taketani T, Sawamura T, Shiozaki Y, Tokunaga R, Sameshima Y (1985) Release of hepatic mitochondrial ornithine transcarbomylase into the circulation in D-galactosamine-treated rats. Identification of serum ornithine transcarbomylase as the intact form of the mitochondrial enzyme. J Biochem 97: 1391–1399

324. Unaleami S, Suzuki S, Nakanishi E, Iclinoke K, Hirata M, Tanimoto Y (1987) Comparative studies of multiple forms of serum cholinesterase in various species. Ex An 36: 199–204

325. Vacikova A (1971) Comparitive study on some amylase in mammalian blood serum. Comp Biochem Physiol 40A: 975–978.

326 Valentine BA, Cooper BJ, de Lahunta A (1986) Muscular dystrophy in the Golden Retriever dog (abstr). Proceed Amer Col Vet Pathol 37th annual meeting, New Orleans, LA, p 174

327. Vallette FM, Muller D, Massoulic J (1983) Comparative affinity chromatography of acetylcholinesterases from fine vertebrate species. J Chromat 257: 289–296

328. Van den Bosch R, Geuze HJ, du Maine ATP, Stous GJ (1986) Transport and metabolism of 5'-nucleotidase in a rat hepatoma cell line. Eur J Biochem 160: 49 54

329. Van Vleet J (1975) Experimentally induced vitamin E-selenium deficiency in the growing dog. J Am Vet Med Assoc 166: 769–774

330. Van Vleet JF, Alberts JO (1968) Evaluation of liver function tests and liver biopsy in experimental carbon tetrachloride intoxication and extrahepatic bile duct obstruction in the dog. Am J Vet Res 29: 2119–2131

331. Venkatakrishnan G, Roghupathi S, Reddy R (1983) A comparative polyacrylamide gel electrophoresis study of arginase in vertebrate tissues. Enzyme 39: 145–152

332. Vidal C, Munoz-Delgado E, Yague-Guirao A (1987) Acetylcholinesterase in membrane fractions derived from sarcotubular system of skeletal muscle: Presence of monomoric acetylcholinesteral in sarcoplasmic reticulum and transverse tubule membrane. Neurochem Int 10: 329–338

333. Vigny M, Gisiger V, Massoulie J (1978) "Non-specific" cholinesterases and acetylcholinesterase in rat tissues: Molecular forms, structural and catalytic properties and significance of the two enzymes. Proc Natl Acad Sci USA 75: 2588–2592

334. Visser MP, Krill MTA, Muijtjens AMM, Willems GM, Hermens WTH (1981) Distributions of enzymes in dog heart and liver: Significance for assessment of tissue damage from data on plasma enzyme activities. Clin Chem 27: 1845–1850

335. Wachstein M, Bradshaw M (1965) Histochemical localization of enzyme activity in the kidneys of three mammalian species during their post natal development. J Histochem Cytochem 13: 44–56

336. Wachstein M, Meisel E (1957) Histochemistry of hepatic phosphatases at a physiological pH with special reference to the demonstration of bile canaliculli. Am J Clin Pathol 27: 13–23

337. Wagner J, Critz B (1968) The effect of prednisolone on the serum creatine phosphokinase response to exercise. Proc Soc Exp Biol Med 128: 716

338. Watanabe K, Fishman WH (1964) Application of the stereo inhibitor L-phenylalanine to enzyme morphology of intestinal alkaline phosphatase. J Histochem Cytochem 12: 252–260

339. Webb G, Clark DG (1978) Acetylcholinesterase: Differential affinity chromatographic purification of 11S and 18S plus 14S forms; The importance of multiple-site interactions and salt concentrations. Arch Biochem Biophys 191: 278–288

340. Wellman ML, Hoffman WE, Dorner JL, Mock RE (1982) Comparison of the steroid-induced, intestinal and hepatic isoenzymes of alkaline phosphatase in the dog. Am J Vet Res 43: 1204–1207

341. Wentink G, van der Lindi-Sepman J, Meijer A, Kamphaisen H, van Vorstenbosch C, Hartman W, Hendricks H (1972) Myopathy with a possible recessive X-linked inheritance in a litter of Irish terriers. Vet Pathol 9: 328–349

342. Wilfred G, Rao JP (1976) Induction of hepatic alkaline phosphatase: Phosphodiesterase inhibition and adrenaline. Ind J Biochem Biophys 13: 331–334

343. Wilkens R, Hurvitz A (1975) Chemical profiles of feline diseases. J Am An Hosp Assoc 11: 29–41

344. Wilson IB, Bergmann F, Nachmansohn D (1950) Acetylcholinesterase. X. Mechanism of catalysis of acylation reactions. J Biol Chem 186: 781–790

345. Wilson IB, Cabib E (1954) Is acetylcholinesterase a metalloenzyme? J Am Chem Soc 76: 5154–5156

346. Wilson IB, Gensburg S (1955) A powerful reactivator of alkylphosphate inhibited acetylcholinesterase. Biochim Biophys Acta 18: 168–170

347. Wilson J (1977) Clinical application of cerebrospinal fluid creatine phosphokinase determination. J Am Vet Med Assoc 171: 200–202

348. Wootton AM, Neale G, Moss DW (1977) Enzyme activities of cells of different types isolated from livers of normal and cholestatic rats. Clin Sci Mol Med 52: 585–590

349. Wright C, Lingelbach K, Hoogenroad N (1985) Comparison of ornithine transcarbamylase from rat liver and intestine: Evidence for differential regulation of enzyme levels. Eur J Biochem 153: 239–242

350. Yacoub RS, Apport HE, Howard JM (1969) Metabolism of pancreatic amylase and lipase infused intravenously into dogs. Arch Surg 99: 54–59

351. Young D, Pestaner L, Gibberman V (1975) Effects of drugs on clinical laboratory test. Clin Chem 21: 1D–432D

352. Young GB, Friedman S, Yedlin ST, Alpers DH (1981) Effects of fat feeding on intestinal alkaline phosphatase activity in tissue and serum. Am J Physiol 241: G461–468

353. Young GP, Rose IS, Cropper S, Seetharam S, Alpers DH (1984) Hepatic clearance of rat plasma intestinal alkaline phosphatase. Am J Physiol 247: G419–G426

354. Zajicek J (1957) Studies on the histogenesis of blood

platelets and megakaryocytes. Acta Physiol Scand
40 (Supl 138): 1–32

355. Zeller EA, Bessigger A (1943) Uber die Cholinesterase des Geherns und der Erythrocyten. 3. Mitter-
lung über die Beermflussring von Fermentreak-
tionen durch Chemotherapeutica und Pharmaka.
Helv Chim Acta 26: 1619–1630

356. Zimmerman HM, Bank S, Smolow C, Burns G,

Lenduai S (1983) Comparison of electrophoretic
isoamylase patterns among various species. Am J
Gastroenterol 78: 575–578

357. Zinkl JG, Bush RM, Cornelius CE, Freedland RA
(1971) Comparative studies on plasma and tissue
sorbital, glutamic, lactic and hydroxybutyric
dehydrogenase and transaminase activities in the
dog. Res Vet Sci 12: 211–214

12

Endocrine Hormones in Laboratory Animals

LOUIS V. DEPAOLO, PhD and EDWARD J. MASORO, PhD

In its broadest sense, the study of hormones and their actions on target tissues had its origin several hundred years before the birth of Christ. However, the real science of endocrinology began at the turn of the 20th century with the demonstration by Bayliss and Starling (16) that "chemical messages" or hormones elaborated from the duodenal mucosa affected pancreatic exocrine function in the absence of nervous intervention. Thus, the first hormone, secretin, was identified. Since that time, a whole array of hormones has been isolated and characterized both structurally and functionally. However, many more as yet unidentified "chemical messages" await future identification.

In keeping with the overall theme of this book, a major objective of this chapter will be to provide the reader with a comprehensive survey of circulating levels of the major hormones in common laboratory species such as the mouse, rat, hamster, guinea pig, rabbit, dog and non-human primate. Unless stated otherwise, levels will be reported for adult animals with organs intact. For some hormones, levels in sheep, cows, goats, and horses will be presented. Current information on the various methods of hor-

mone analysis will also be presented. Emphasis will be placed on species specificity and the effects of the reproductive cycle on hormone levels. The hormones covered in this chapter will include those elaborated by the gonads as well as the anterior and posterior lobes of the pituitary, thyroid, parathyroid, and adrenal glands.

Because of the limits of space inherent in any book, the gastrointestinal family of hormones, which ironically includes secretin, will not be covered. Insulin and glucagon will be covered in Chapter 8.

METHODS OF HORMONE ANALYSIS

Before beginning this extensive survey, it is pertinent to describe briefly some of the current methods of measuring hormone levels available to the scientist or clinician. Many of these methods are variants of the competitive radioassay procedure. Without question, the most widely used competitive binding assay to quantify hormone levels in blood is the radioimmunoassay (RIA). First described for the hormone insulin by Berson and Yalow (24) in 1959, this procedure can be applied to quantify

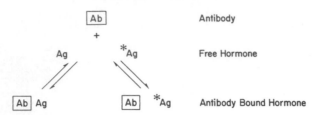

Figure 12.1. Diagrammatic representation of the competition between unlabeled (Ag) and labeled (*Ag) antigen for binding sites on an antibody (Ab) during a radioimmunoassay.

levels of any known hormone whether it be a protein, steroid, or amine. The major advantage of the RIA over the preexisting biologic assay is its increased sensitivity, its ability to detect a smaller quantity of hormone, thus negating the need for large sample volume. Other favorable aspects of the RIA are its greater precision, high specificity, and time and cost efficiency. In recognition of this revolutionary technological advance, Yalow shared the Nobel Prize for Medicine in 1977.

The theory of the RIA is predicated on the competition of radiolabeled (usually iodine or tritium) and nonlabeled antigen (hormone) for recepter binding sites on an antibody (Figure 12.1). Much of the success of an RIA lies in the ability to separate bound from free antigen. This separation may be accomplished by numerous techniques including precipitation of the antigen-antibody complex with a second antibody or absorption of free hormone with dextran-coated charcoal. Regardless of the method employed, the greater the quantity of nonlabeled antigen present in the assay tube, the lower the radioactive counts in the bound fraction. This inverse relationship can be visualized more readily in Figure 12.2 in which a typical standard curve is generated by the addition of increasing quantities of unlabeled hormone to assay tubes containing a fixed amount of labeled hormone. Hormone contents in unknown samples then can be read directly off the curve.

A necessary prerequisite to induce the production of antibody to a hormone is that the hormone be antigenic. However, in the case of steroid and amine hormones which in themselves are nonantigenic (haptens), proteins such as thyroglobulin and albumin may be coupled to the haptens, making the entire conjugate antigenic. To circumvent the need to produce an antibody to the hormone to be assayed, carrier proteins (ie, thyroxine-binding globulin and sex

hormone-binding globulin) or high affinity reactor proteins on target tissues have been used to quantify steroid and thyroid hormones by competitive binding.

Until the last several years, most antibodies were generated in live animals, which resulted in a heterogeneous population of antibodies differing in their affinity and specificity towards the antigen. Recently, the technique of producing monoclonal antibodies has replaced the earlier procedure because of the generation of a more "pure" antibody as well as the capacity to produce enormous quantities of antibody.

Although the advantages of using the RIA were alluded to earlier, one important caveat requires mentioning. The RIA has the ability to measure only immunoreactive hormone, which may or may not accurately reflect the more important level of biologically active hormone. This likely is due to the antibody recognizing only a portion of the hormone molecule. To circumvent this caveat, bioassays may be employed in conjunction with RIAs to provide a qualitative (immunologic vs biologic) analysis of changing hormone levels. In most instances, changes in immunoreactive and biologic hormone levels coincide; however, the magnitude of change in immunoreactive versus biologic activity may differ (Figure 12.3).

Numerous in vivo and in vitro bioassays are available to measure biologic endpoints of most protein hormones, with the in vitro bioassays providing greater sensitivity. The major disadvantages of the bioassays over the RIA are their higher cost and longer length. Furthermore, most bioassays sacrifice the sensitivity and specificity of the RIA.

More recently, the development of a radio-receptor assay (RRA) which combines the sensitivity of an RIA with the biologic significance of a bioassay has provided the investigator with a means to measure changes in functionally

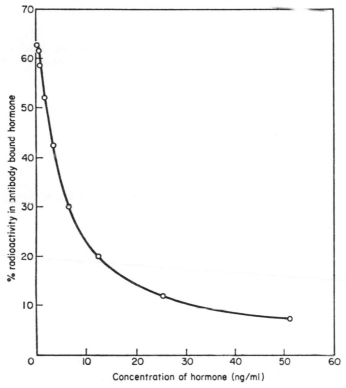

Figure 12.2. Representative standard curve for a radioimmunoassay generated by the addition of increasing amounts of unlabeled hormone to the culture tubes containing a fixed amount of labeled hormone and antibody.

active hormone. Although the RRA adheres to the general principles of competitive radio-assays, receptor sites on target cells are used instead of antibodies or serum proteins. Receptor sites on Leydig cells, granulosa cells, and monocytes have been used in RRAs to quantify levels of luteinizing hormone, follicle-stimulating hormone, and growth hormone, respectively. The only drawback of the RRA is that in some instances the specificity of the receptor may not approach the high specificity of a good antibody.

Finally, other methods besides competitive protein binding assays and bioassays are available to the scientist or clinician for determination of hormone levels including gas chromatography-mass spectrophotometry (GC-MS) and, more recently, high performance liquid chromatography (HPLC) coupled with various detector systems. In comparison to competitive radioassays and bioassays, both techniques provide greater specificity and equal sensitivity, but

they are less cost efficient and sample turnover time is slower. In addition, GC-MS analysis requires that the hormone be volatile and have a molecular weight at or below 1,000 to 2,000 daltons. The application of GC-MS to the measurement of thyroid and peptide hormones in body fluids and tissues has been limited by the instability, involatility, and, in the case of peptide hormones, the large molecular weight of these hormones. Consequently, steroid hormones and biogenic amines are best suited for analysis by GC-MS.

Conversely, HPLC permits separation, detection, and estimation of substances insufficiently stable for GC-MS without the need for transformation into volatile derivatives. Quantification of substances following separation by HPLC has been accomplished by ultraviolet, fluorimetric, electrochemical, and other detectors. Separated fractions may also be analyzed by various competitive protein-binding assay techniques. Although HPLC can be used to

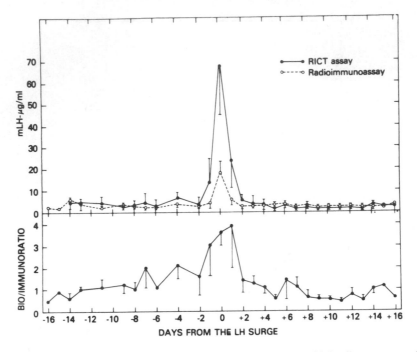

Figure 12.3. Comparison of serum LH levels measured by bioassay (rat interstitial cell testosterone [RICT]) and radioimmunoassay in four ovulatory menstrual cycles of female rhesus monkeys. Individual values were combined by defining the day of the LH surge as day zero. Vertical bars indicate the standard deviation of the mean. No bar is drawn when the number of observations is less than 4. The mean ± standard deviation of the bioimmuno ratio is shown in the lower panel. (With permission from Dufau ML, Hodgen GD, Goodman AL, Catt KJ [1977] Bioassay of circulating luteinizing hormone in the rhesus monkey: Comparison with radioimmunoassay during physiological changes. Endocrinology 100: 1557–1565.)

determine levels of a variety of hormones, steroids and monoamines have been the most extensively studied. High performance liquid chromatography has a distinct advantage over earlier techniques used to measure monoamines (ie, fluorimetric and radioenzymatic assays) in that various amine metabolites, in addition to the native amine, can be separated and quantified. More detailed accounts of these and other techniques of hormone analysis have been published elsewhere (37,125).

DEFINITION OF RHYTHMIC HORMONE PATTERNS

The ability to quantitate hormone levels by RIA in small volumes of plasma or serum has enabled investigators to measure hormone concentrations in small animals more frequently. As a consequence, it is becoming increasingly apparent that most, if not all, major hormones

are secreted into the peripheral circulation in a rhythmic fashion. These rhythmic secretions are examples of biologic rhythms, which in turn are related to the more generalized schema of homeostatic control systems.

Without exception, hormone rhythms originate within the organism and are thus termed endogenous rhythms. However, these rhythms can be entrained to certain environmental cues such as the light-dark cycle. This is especially true in rodents. In addition, endogenous hormone rhythms can be influenced by other endogenous rhythms such as the sleep-wake cycle.

If circulating levels of a particular hormone reach their peak during a specific time of day and reach their trough during another time of that same day, the hormone is said to have a circadian rhythm. In general, these rhythms are highly synchronized among animals within a given species, but they may vary to some degree between species. In some instances hormones may be secreted in an episodic or pulsatile manner with a periodicity of less than 24 hours. This rhythmic secretory profile is termed ultradian and can be superimposed on a more stable circadian rhythm. The pulse frequency of ultradian rhythms may vary from one episode per 20 to 30 minutes to one episode per 3 to 4 hours. Ultradian rhythms are usually less synchronized among animals within a given species than are circadian rhythms. Finally, pulse frequencies of approximately 1 hour are termed circhoral. For more information on hormone rhythms, the reader is referred to the book entitled, "Endocrine Rhythms", edited by Kreiger (178).

PITUITARY HORMONES

Anterior Lobe

Luteinizing Hormone

In the animal species considered in this chapter, luteinizing hormone (LH) acts on the ovary to: (1) promote follicular development; (2) increase estrogen secretion in the preovulatory follicle; (3) cause follicular rupture (ovulation); (4) convert the preovulatory follicle into a corpus luteum following ovulation, and (5) increase progesterone production from the corpus luteum (340). In the male mammal, LH is referred to as interstitial cell-stimulating hormone for its ability to increase the production of testosterone from Leydig cells (340).

Luteinizing hormone is a glycoprotein composed of two peptide chains, an α and a β chain. The amino acid sequences of the α-chain are identical or very similar for all glycoprotein hormones such as follicle-stimulating hormone and thyroid-stimulating hormone (125). In contrast, differences exist between hormones in the amino acid sequences of the β-chain (125). Data obtained from recombination experiments indicate that the β-chain of a glycoprotein hormone is responsible for the specificity of binding to cell receptors, whereas the α-chain may be more directly involved in activation of adenylate cyclase (79). Thus, any cross-reactivity between hormones from different species most likely will reflect structural similarities in the β-chain.

In 1968 Niswender et al (213) developed a highly specific RIA for LH employing antiserum of rabbit origin against ovine LH and purified ovine LH. Because of the high cross-reactivity of antiserum with LH from several species, this RIA has been used to measure circulating LH levels in rat (213), hamster (27), monkey (214), dog (199), and guinea pig (298). A homologous RIA for rat LH using antisera to rat LH and purified radiolabeled rat LH has been employed to measure LH levels in mice (40).

Before beginning a discussion on circulating concentrations of LH, it is imperative to mention that reference standards for determination of anterior pituitary hormone levels may vary among laboratories, making it difficult to compare levels. Although this difficulty has been circumvented somewhat by the availability of reference preparations from the National Hormone and Pituitary Program (NIDDK), some laboratories in the past have chosen to use other reference standards. Moreover, the potency of reference preparations supplied by the NIDDK varies from batch to batch. Therefore, in reporting anterior pituitary hormone levels in this chapter, the appropriate reference preparation will be given.

Circulating LH levels in male rats are reported to be in the range of 10 to 40 ng reference preparation-1(RP-1)/ml (144,159,297). Lowest levels of LH are observed between 0500 and 1100 hours and highest values are attained between 2300 and 0200 hours, indicating a circadian influence on LH release (144,159,297). More recently, frequent sampling of blood from male rats at 5-minute intervals revealed that LH is secreted in an episodic fashion and not in a steady, uninterrupted manner (97). The frequency of pulses averages 1 pulse every 1 to 2 hours. This mode of secretion is attributed to pulsatile release of luteinizing hormone-releasing hormone (LHRH) from the hypothalamus because LHRH antisera or antagonists abolish episodic LH release in castrated rats (98).

Using RP-1 as a standard, LH levels in male mice (69,77), hamsters (320), and dogs (85) are approximately 10 to 40, 10 to 30, and 0.2 to 10 ng/ml, respectively. Mating results in a two- to sixfold increase in LH levels in the rat (163). Basal secretion values for guinea pigs, rabbits, and rhesus monkeys employing other reference standards are 500 ng NIH-S21/ml for guinea pigs (43), 10 to 100 ng WP-360-A/ml for rabbits (207) and 1 to 5 ng WDP-X-47-BC/ml for monkeys (235). Moreover, pulsatility of LH secretion has been demonstrated in dogs (85), rabbits (207), rhesus monkeys (235), and mice (69).

In all other species considered in this chapter, ovulation is preceded by a precipitious increase in circulating LH concentrations. In rats (3, 48), hamsters (54), and mice (40), increases in LH levels from basal levels of 20 to 40 ng RP-1/ml or 0.5 to 1 ng RP-2/ml to 1,500 to 2,000 ng RP-1/ml or 10 to 25 ng RP-2/ml occur during the afternoon of proestrus. In the guinea pig, increases in serum LH levels from 5 to 55 ng RP-1/ml are observed on estrus, shortly before ovulation (74). Contrastingly, increases in serum LH levels from 2 ng/ml to 20 to 30 ng RP-1/ml lasting for 3 days occur several days before to 7 days after estrus in the dog (199). In rhesus monkeys plasma LH levels during the height of the midcycle surge average 50 to 60 ng WDP-X-47-BC/ml (329). Whereas rats, hamsters, mice, guinea pigs, and monkeys are spontaneous ovulators, rabbits release LH only in response to coital stimulation and hence are called reflex ovulators. Peak LH levels averaging 30 to 40 ng AFP-559-B/ml usually are reached 1 to 2 hours after coitus (204).

Follicle-Stimulating Hormone

The principal role of follicle-stimulating hormone (FSH) in the female mammal is to stimulate the growth and development of ovarian follicles (340). In the male, FSH is involved primarily with the latter stages of the spermatogenic process (227).

As with LH, there appears to be considerable cross-reactivity between FSH from various species. Attesting to this statement is the frequent use of the rat FSH RIA kit from the NIDDK for the measurement of FSH levels in hamsters (320), guinea pigs (43), and mice (77).

In the male rat, pituitary FSH secretion exhibits a circadian rhythmicity with low values ranging from 250 to 500 ng RP-1/ml (144,297) and high values between 500 and 900 ng RP-1/ml (144,159). Highest levels are attained during the dark period (144,159,176). In contrast to LH, mating does not alter circulating FSH levels (163). In adult male hamsters, FSH levels are reported to be in the range of 200 to 300 RP-1/ml (277,320), whereas values for circulating FSH in mice are generally 1,000 to 1,200 ng RP-1/ml (39,77). Male guinea pigs exhibit FSH

levels of approximately 100 to 200 ng RP-1/ml (43). Using LER-1909–2 as a reference standard, Resko et al (252) reported levels of FSH in adult male rhesus macaques to be 1 to 3 μg/ml. Finally, Berger et al (22) reported plasma FSH levels in adult male rabbits to be between 2 and 4.5 ng AFP-538-C/ml.

During the rat estrous cycle, basal FSH concentrations approximate 100 to 200 ng RP-1/ml (48) or 2 to 3 ng RP-2/ml (256). Concomitant with the preovulatory LH surge, plasma FSH levels increase to 400 to 600 ng/ml (48) or 5 to 6 ng RP-2/ml (256). These levels are again attained during a secondary increase in FSH levels early on estrous morning. Similar values and profiles were reported for the hamster (54). In contrast, plasma levels of FSH in female mice increase from an average of 80 to 120 ng RP-1/ml to 250 to 300 ng RP-1/ml on proestrus and estrus (262). Croix and Franchimont (74) observed a biphasic increase in serum FSH concentrations during the estrous cycle of guinea pigs; basal levels approximated 40 to 50 ng RP-1/ml, increasing to 300 and 150 ng RP-1/ml during the first and second FSH rise, respectively. However, it should be noted that Blatchley et al (28) failed to observe any significant surge-like increases in FSH in the guinea pig. Rather, increased levels of FSH occurred over a 10-day period during the follicular phase of the cycle (28), which may have been due to the different antisera used for RIA in these studies.

Using a reference standard with a biologic potency of $14 \times$ NIH-FSH-S1 preparation, Weick et al (329) reported that plasma FSH concentrations increased from 10 to 15 ng/ml during the follicular phase of the rhesus monkey menstrual cycle to 160 ng/ml during the midcycle surge of FSH. A perimenstrual increment in FSH levels was also observed with peak levels approximating 40 ng/ml (174). In the rabbit, postcoital increases in serum FSH levels were not observed in one study (88), but Mills et al (204) observed an initial increase in FSH levels 2 hours after coitus followed by a second elevation at 18 to 30 hours postcoitum preceded by a nadir at 12 hours. Peak levels of FSH averaged 5 ng AFP-538-C/ml (baseline levels 2 to 3 ng/ml). As with the guinea pig, this discrepancy may be explained by the use of different antisera in the RIA; the former study (88) used anti-ovine sera, whereas antirabbit sera were employed in the latter study (204).

Prolactin

With regard to the biologic effects of prolactin (PRL), this hormone is undoubtedly the most versatile of all adenohypophyseal hormones. Prolactin in many vertebrates possesses a wide spectrum of effects including those related to osmoregulation, growth, and metabolism (23). However, the most important effects of PRL in mammals are on the reproductive system to: (1) promote the growth and development of the mammary gland; (2) cause milk production during lactation, and (3) maintain corpus luteum function in several species. It is difficult to compare the species specificity of PRL because only the structure of ovine prolactin is known. However, considering chemical similarities, overlapping biologic activities, and immunologic relatedness, it would appear that the various vertebrate prolactins have evolved from a common ancestral molecule or molecules.

Like that of the gonadotropins, PRL secretion in the male rat exhibits a distinct circadian rhythm with peak levels of 80 ng RP-1/ml occurring during the night (144). Values at other times of the day are reported to be between 5 and 30 ng RP-1/ml (144,276,297). In adult male rats, mating results in an immediate increase in serum PRL levels from 40 to 200 ng RP-1/ml. Prolactin levels in undisturbed male mice are reported to be below 1 ng RP-1/ml (39); however, other investigators reported PRL levels to be between 10 and 20 ng RP-1/ml (78,202). In contrast, serum levels of PRL in male hamsters average between 5 and 10 ng RP-1/ml (320). Using a homologous RIA for canine PRL, Knight and colleagues (173) reported average serum PRL levels in male dogs to be about 9.0 ng/ml. Plasma PRL concentrations in male rabbits before mating are 6 ng/ml with no increases observed after coitus (107). Finally, a diurnal rhythm in circulating PRL levels has been discerned in both female (243) and male (234) rhesus monkeys. Prolactin levels were higher during the night ($\bar{x}$ = 10 to 20 ng WDP-1-49-29/ml) than during the day ($\bar{x}$ = 4 to 10 ng/ml).

As with LH and FSH, PRL levels in blood increase precipitously during the afternoon of proestrus in rats (48) and hamsters (15). Using a homologous rat RIA, plasma PRL levels increase from 15 to 30 ng RP-1/ml to 200 to 300 ng RP-1/ml in the rat (48) and from 10 to 15 ng RP-1/ml to 30 ng RP-1/ml in the hamster (15) on proestrus. In contrast, a midcycle surge of PRL was not detected during the monkey menstrual cycle (243). In anestrous bitches, serum PRL levels average 12.6 ng/ml (173). Using the rabbit PRL standard from the NIDDK, plasma PRL levels average 10 ng/ml in female rabbits (107).

Growth Hormone:

Although overall body growth is dependent on growth hormone (GH), some forms of growth such as increases in muscle mass and hair growth are independent of GH. The growth-promoting effects of GH are manifest on bone and soft tissues. The effects of GH on the growth of bone occur principally on chondrogenesis and calcification (122). Growth hormone also promotes symmetric enlargement of soft tissue mass in proportion to skeletal growth (122). Of a metabolic nature, GH (1) decreases protein degradation and accelerates protein synthesis, (2) minimizes glucose consumption by muscle and adipose tissue, and (3) increases mobilization of free fatty acids from adipose tissue depots (122).

Sequential blood collection over a 24-hour period has disclosed an ultradian rhythm in GH secretion in rats with GH secretory episodes occurring at approximately 3-hour intervals (91,295; Figure 12.4). Peak values of GH ranged between 100 and 200 ng RP-1/ml, whereas trough values approximated 1 ng RP-1/ml (295). This ultradian rhythm appears to be entrained by the light-dark cycle because this rhythm becomes "free-running" in rats exposed to constant light (295). Secretory profiles of GH did not differ among various days of the rat estrous cycle; however, frequency of GH pulses as well as trough values were higher in female than in male rats (91).

Using purified rat GH for iodination, anti-rat GH, and a standard hamster pituitary homogenate, Borer and Kelch (34) reported serum GH concentrations in hamsters to be about 30 mg/ml. In contrast, GH levels in male and female mice were reported to range from 1 to 2 ng/ml (202) to 60 to 90 ng/ml (78). The biologic potency of the GH standard preparation in the aforementioned studies was 3.1 USP units per milligram. It is not known whether an ultradian

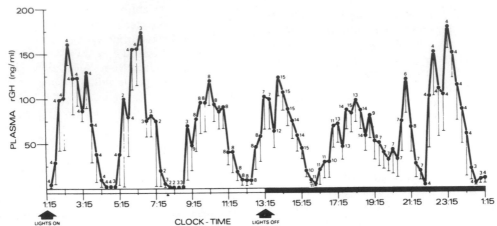

Figure 12.4. Ultradian rhythm in mean plasma growth hormone levels of rats during a 24-hour period with 12 hours of light and dark. Numbers indicate number of animals sampled at each time point. Vertical lines represent standard error of the mean (with permission from Tannenbaum and Martin [295]).

rhythm for GH secretion exists in mice or hamsters.

Levels of GH in dogs measured by a homologous RIA averaged 2 ng/ml (94). Using the rat GH kit, single determinations of GH levels in rabbits of different strains ranged between 6 and 20 ng RP-1/ml (268). In most strains, GH levels in female rabbits were slightly higher than those in male rabbits (268). Similar to rats, GH secretion in male rhesus monkeys is pulsatile with episodes occurring every 3 to 6 hours (240). Using the reference preparation WDP-V111–61–46, peak GH concentrations often exceeded 20 ng/ml with trough values approaching 1 ng/ml (240). However, in striking contrast to the rat, the ultradian GH rhythm in primates is linked to the sleep-awake cycle rather than to the light-dark cycle (242).

Thyroid-Stimulating Hormone

As its name implies, thyroid-stimulating hormone (TSH) increases the secretion of thyroid hormones from the thyroid gland. Specifically, TSH promotes iodine trapping, iodination of thyroglobulin, and the elaboration of thyroglobulin itself (122). These actions of TSH appear to be independent because inhibition of one synthetic phase does not affect the other processes (122).

Expressed in terms of the rat RP-1 standard, levels of TSH in male rats are between 400 and 600 ng/ml (203,306). In female rats, Othenweller

and Hedge (221) reported a diurnal variation in TSH secretion with peak values of about 200 ng RP-1/ml (basal levels 100 ng/ml) occurring at the onset of lights on. As with GH, basal TSH levels did not vary during the rat estrous cycle (81).

Using the rat TSH kits provided by the NIDDK, circulating TSH levels in hamsters (314) and mice (218) are reported to be approximately 300 ng RP-1/ml. In contrast, serum TSH levels in euthyroid dogs are reported to be 7.0 ng/ml with a range of 2.7 to 7.9 ng/ml using a homologous RIA for canine TSH (246). Gianella-Neto et al (115) determined that TSH levels in adult male rhesus monkeys averaged 2.5 microinternational unit equivalents per milliliter during a 24-hour period using a double antibody RIA for human TSH and a rhesus monkey pituitary preparation WDP-X-103–30. Furthermore, levels of the hormone in rhesus macaques lacked a circadian rhythm and were not influenced by the sleep-awake cycle (115). Finally, circulating TSH levels in rabbits (185) and guinea pigs (309) measured by bioassay (per cent increase in blood levels of radiolabeled iodine) were reported to be 40 to 100 and less than 320 μU/ml, respectively.

Adrenocorticotropic Hormone

Adrenocorticotropic hormone (ACTH) is a peptide consisting of the first 39 amino acids of a postulated larger pro-ACTH molecule (95). The remainder of the pro-ACTH molecule forms β-lipotropin. The major physiologic function of ACTH is the stimulation of glucocorticoid secretion from the zona fasciculata of the adrenal cortex (122).

In contrast to nanogram and microgram quantities of hormone per milliliter of blood for the previous five adenohypophyseal hormones, each milliliter of blood contains picogram quantities of ACTH. Synthetic (1–39) ACTH is used as a reference standard in place of the crude preparations of LH, FSH, PRL, GH, and TSH used in the RIA. Under resting conditions, ACTH levels in extracted plasma of male rats measured by RIA range from 30 to 100 pg/ml (68,332). Although afternoon plasma ACTH levels were higher than morning levels, the differences were not significant (332). Using a bioassay that measures radioimmunoassayable cortisol production by guinea pig adrenal gland slices, it has been possible to detect femtogram amounts of ACTH in the plasma of various animal species (42). Values for the rat average 40 pg/ml, not different from levels obtained by RIA (68,332). Concentrations of ACTH in the plasma of guinea pigs, rabbits, and hamsters using this bioassay average 23, 25, and 41 pg/ml (42). Basal ACTH levels in conscious dogs measured by RIA approximated those reported in other species (93). Finally, morning levels of plasma ACTH in mice were reported to be 2.66 ng/ml, whereas afternoon levels were 5.44 ng/ml indicative of a circadian variation in ACTH secretion in this species (93).

Posterior Lobe

Vasopressin (Antidiuretic Hormone)

Vasopressin is a nonapeptide that is secreted by the neurophypophysis. The major action of vasopressin is to return water of the glomerular filtrate to the body which it accomplishes by increasing the permeability of the distal tubules and collecting ducts of the kidney to water. This action plays an important role in the regulation of body fluid osmolality and extracellular fluid volume. At pharmacologic concentrations vasopressin increases arterial blood pressure, thus its name. The recent development of RIA procedures has made it possible to reliably measure the concentrations of vasopressin in the plasma and serum of laboratory animal models.

The basal serum vasopressin concentration in a variety of common laboratory rat strains has been reported to range from 1 to 8 pg/ml (86,112,132,171,172,180,278,288). There appears to be no appreciable sex difference and little difference between common laboratory strains. However, the male of the WKY strain does appear to have higher basal levels than do most other strains with the concentration in the WKY strain ranging from 7.5 to 15 pg/ml (73). It should be noted that the state of hydration markedly influences the concentration of plasma vasopressin. Also, anesthesia increases the concentration of plasma vasopressin, and anesthesia combined with surgery increases it even further (10). Vasopressin is not detectable in the plasma of homozygous Brattleboro rats (142).

The basal concentration of plasma vasopressin in unanesthetized male rhesus monkeys ranges from 0.5 to 16 pg/ml (9). An average value for the ketamine-restrained male rhesus monkey was reported to be 3.2 pg/ml (26). The average basal plasma vasopressin value for awake female rhesus monkeys was 4.3 pg/ml (135); however, if the animals were water loaded, the concentration fell to 1.5 pg/ml and if water was restricted for 3 days, it rose to 25.5 pg/ml. The plasma vasopressin concentration in anesthetized *Macaca fuscicularis* monkeys ranged from 1.3 to 13 pg/ml (117) and in anesthetized baboons (*Papio cynocephalus*) it ranged from 30 to 40 pg/ml (334).

There are many studies on the plasma or serum vasopressin concentrations in both awake and anesthetized dogs; most studies reported values between 0.5 and 10 pg/ml (12,25,70,129, 165,182,183,244,247,321,322,326,331,337). However, in some studies, values well in excess of 10 pg/ml were found (13,169,258,272,325). It is interesting that in all studies on awake dogs the concentration was less than 10 pg/ml. Thus, anesthesia may be part of the reason for the wide range of reported values. However, many studies with anesthetized dogs also reported values well below 10 pg/ml, suggesting that the state of hydration also may be a major reason for the variation in findings. Guo et al (129) reported that in conscious dogs given water at will, the plasma vasopressin concentration ranged from 2.5 to 10 pg/ml, but when the water was withheld for 64 hours, the range was 12.5 to 25 pg/ml.

Leighton et al (184) reported the plasma vasopressin concentration in male rabbits to average 0.89 pg/ml, whereas other investigators reported values well in excess of 10 pg/ml (29,271). This difference may relate to the effects of hydration and/or anesthesia (184). Serum vasopressin concentration in mature female sheep was reported to range from 1 to 4 pg/ml (330,343). In cattle, plasma vasopressin concentration ranged from 3 to 25 pg/ml depending on the state of hydration (17) and in the horse from 0 to 5 pg/ml (249).

Oxytocin

Oxytocin is a nonapeptide that is secreted by the neurohypophysis. Oxytocin causes contraction of the myoepithelial cells of the mammary gland, resulting in the ejection of milk. Oxytocin also is involved in labor by means of stimulating uterine contractions. Recent developments in the radioimmunoassay of oxytocin have begun to yield reliable data on its concentration in the plasma or serum of laboratory animal models.

The basal plasma oxytocin concentration reported for rats (male Wistar and both sexes of Long-Evans) ranged from 4 to 10.5 pg/ml (92,180). One group reported that water deprivation for 24 hours doubled the plasma oxytocin concentration (86), whereas another group found no effect (92). Water deprivation for 72 hours has been reported to result in plasma oxytocin concentrations in excess of 70 pg/ml.

The basal concentration of oxytocin in the plasma of conscious female rhesus monkeys has been reported to range between 30 and 60 pg/ml (100). It was higher in the middle of the menstrual cycle than at other periods of the cycle. A recent report (157) involving both sexes of rhesus monkeys gave a range of plasma concentrations of 5 to 10 pg/ml.

In nursing guinea pigs, low levels of plasma oxytocin (≤ 5 pg/ml) were found when the animals were not nursing their young. However, the concentration increased to more than 50 pg/ml during milk ejection (257). In male rabbits the plasma concentration of oxytocin was reported to range from 10 to 20 pg/ml (287) and a similar range was found for pregnant female rabbits (217).

In female sheep, the plasma concentration of oxytocin ranged between 1 and 50 pg/ml (266, 274,327). Moreover, a complex relationship

Table 12.1. Concentration of Total and Free T_4 and T_3 in Adult Sprague-Dawley Rats[a]

Substance	Serum Concentration
Total T_4	5.53 ± 0.40 $\mu g/dl$[b]
Free T_4	2.212 ± 0.055 ng/dl
Total T_3	89.48 ± 4.63 ng/dl
Free T_3	208.49 ± 8.55 pg/dl

[a] Compiled from data of Walker et al (323).
[b] Mean $\pm$ standard error.

was found between the stage of the estrous cycle and the plasma concentration of oxytocin.

The basal plasma oxytocin concentration in heifers was reported to range between 0.5 and 6.4 pg/ml with a complex relationship to the estrous cycle (264). Basal concentration in dairy cows before milking was reported to range from 0.5 to 2.5 pg/ml (264). The basal concentration of oxytocin in the bull was found to be less than 3 pg/ml (265) and in pigs it ranged from 4 to 54 pg/ml (307).

In male dogs the plasma concentration of oxytocin ranged from 0 to 30 pg/ml and in female dogs from 4 to 73 pg/ml (307). In plasma of anesthetized female cats it ranged from 11 to 33 pg/ml (224).

THYROID HORMONES

The thyroid gland secretes the iodinated amino acids thyroxine (T_4) and triiodothyronine (T_3); however, from one third to one half of the T_3 in blood is generated outside the thyroid gland by the deiodination of T_4. The mechanism of action of thyroid hormone is not known but it is known that in its absence, metabolic rate declines, central nervous system function declines—indeed, the function of almost all organ systems is disturbed. The total plasma or serum concentrations of T_4 and T_3 may be determined by radioimmunoassays and the concentrations of free T_4 and free T_3 are measured by equilibrium dialysis or sephadex binding methods.

There is a wealth of literature on the plasma or serum concentrations of T_4 and T_3 in the common laboratory rat strains. In most studies (109,181,210,238,260,336) with adult male Sprague-Dawley rats, the T_4 concentration ranged between 3 and 7 $\mu g/dl$; a similar range was found with adult female Sprague-Dawley rats (67,109,273,305). Studies (45,118, 154,181,279,290) with adult male Wistar rats showed a T_4 concentration range from 2.5 to 7 $\mu g/dl$ plasma or serum. The serum T_4 concentration of adult male Long-Evans rats was reported to be 5.1 ± 0.4 $\mu g/dl$ ($\bar{x}\pm1$ SE) (145) and that of adult female Long-Evans rats to be 4.9 ± 0.1 SE $\mu g/dl$ (58). The concentration of T_4 in the serum of the male Black-hooded/Ztn rat was reported as 3.2 ± 0.1 SE $\mu g/dl$ (336).

The serum or plasma concentration of T_3 in the male Sprague-Dawley rat was found to range between 25 and 100 ng/dl (109,181,210, 238,260) and that of adult female Sprague-Dawley rats between 80 and 100 ng/dl (67,109). In male Wistar rats, the serum or plasma T_3 concentration ranged from 30 to 100 ng/dl (45, 118,154,279,290). For the male Long-Evans rat, the serum T_3 concentration averaged 66 ± 3.5 (SE) ng/dl (145) and for the female Long-Evans rat 83 ± 3 ng/dl (58). For the male Fischer 344 rat, the serum T_3 concentration ranged from 50 to 90 ng/dl (111) and for the male Black-hooded/Ztn it averaged 54.9 ± 2.9 (SE) ng/dl (336).

Studies have also been carried out in which both total T_3 and T_4 and free T_3 and T_4 were measured (58,154,323). Data from Walker et al (323) from adult Sprague-Dawley rats shown in Table 12.1 are typical of the findings.

It has also been shown that there is a diurnal rhythm in the plasma or serum T_3 and T_4 concentrations in rats (153,221). The peak concentration occurs during the light phase of the light-dark cycle and the minimum concentration during the dark phase.

Stewart et al (286) reported the plasma T_4 concentration for the following strains of male mice: BALB/c, 7.4 ± 0.5 SE $\mu g/dl$; CBA/Fa Carr, 6.1 ± 0.4 SE $\mu g/dl$; C57B1/Fa, 5.2 ± 0.4 SE $\mu g/dl$; C3H, 4.6 ± 0.3 SE $\mu g/dl$; and Peru, 4.0 ± 0.3 SE $\mu g/dl$. The serum T_4 concentration for male DDY mice was reported as 6.5 ± 0.4 (SE) $\mu g/dl$ and the T_3 concentration as 138 ± 7 (SE) ng/dl (59) and the values in the lean C57B1/6J ob/ob mice were similar, the serum T_4 being 6.6 ± 0.6 (SE) $\mu g/dl$ and the T_3 127.8 (SE)±5.3 ng/dl (205). The concentration range for T_4 in Swiss-Webster (324) mice was reported as 5.5 to 6.5 $\mu g/dl$ and 3.5 to 6.5 $\mu g/dl$ for C3H/HeC mice (338); the T_3 concentration range in these mice strains was reported as 65 to 80 ng/dl and 75 to 115 ng/dl, respectively. The mean plasma values plus or minus the standard deviation for male ICR mice were reported as 4.7 ± 0.3 $\mu g/dl$ total T_4 and 71.6 ± 5.2 ng/dl total T_3 (46).

In hamsters, serum or plasma T_4 concentrations ranged between 3 and 7 $\mu g/dl$ and plasma T_3 concentrations between 30 and 80 ng/dl (313–316). In guinea pigs, the range for total serum T_4 was 2.1 to 2.5 $\mu g/dl$ and that of free T_4 2.1 to 3.8 ng/dl (250). A recent study (52) reported somewhat different values. For the male guinea pig total plasma T_4 was 2.9 ± 0.6 $\mu g/dl$, free T_4 1.26 ± 0.41 ng/dl, total T_3 39 ± 17 ng/dl, and free T_3 0.257 ± 0.035 ng/dl, and for the female guinea pig total plasma T_4 was 3.2 ± 0.7 $\mu g/dl$, free T_4 1.33 ± 0.25 ng/dl, total T_3 44 ± 10 ng/dl, and free T_3 0.260 ± 0.059 ng/dl (all values are means $\pm$ standard deviations).

There are many studies on the serum or plasma concentrations of T_3 and T_4 in the rhesus monkey. The T_4 concentration has ranged from 0.8 to 6.6 $\mu g/dl$ for males and 1.3 to 7.6 $\mu g/dl$ for females and the T_3 concentration from 54 to 115 ng/dl for males and 65 to 295 ng/dl for females (115,155,237,250). Free T_4 has been reported to range from 0.4 to 1.0 ng/dl in male rhesus monkeys (237,250).

Measurements have also been made on other nonhuman primates. For squirrel monkeys, the serum T_4 concentration ranged from 1.7 to 5.1 $\mu g/dl$ for males and from 1.0 to 7.3 $\mu g/dl$ for females and for T_3, the range was 21 to 92 ng/dl for males and 20 to 168 ng/dl for females (156). The range of serum T_4 concentrations for the African green monkey was 3.9 to 5.7 $\mu g/dl$ for males and 3.0 to 8.4 $\mu g/dl$ for females, for the Talapoin monkey it was 1.8 to 3.4 $\mu g/dl$ for males and 3.0 to 4.2 $\mu g/dl$ for females, and for the male chimpanzee it was 3.7 to 5.9 $\mu g/dl$ (155). The serum T_3 concentrations for the same primate species were 91 to 178 ng/dl for the male and 94 to 350 ng/dl for the female African green monkey, 107 to 170 ng/dl for the male and 127 to 180 ng/dl for the female Talapoin monkey, and 87 to 155 ng/dl for the male chimpanzee (155). The concentrations for the female baboon (*Papio cynocephalus*) were 9.9 ± 2.2 $\mu g/dl$ (SD) for T_4 and 121 ± 18 ng/dl (SD) for T_3 (192).

Reported values for serum T_4 in the rabbit ranged from 1.7 to 2.4 $\mu g/dl$ and for serum T_3 130 to 143 ng/dl (291). Anderson and Brown (6) reported the following mean serum T_4 concentrations for cats: males, 2.5 $\mu g/dl$; castrated males, 3.2 $\mu g/dl$; females, 4.0 $\mu g/dl$; castrated females, 2.6 $\mu g/dl$, but in each case the range was great. The results of other studies on cats are in general agreement (138,140,158,187,251).

The serum T_3 concentration for cats has been reported to range between 60 and 200 ng/dl (140). The serum or plasma total T_4 concentration for normal dogs ranges from 1.5 to 3.6 μg/dl (19) and the free T_4 concentration from 0.6 to 3.9 ng/dl (90). Serum T_3 concentrations for normal dogs range from 48 to 154 ng/dl (19). Total T_4 was found to range from 0.2 to 0.6 μg/dl and total T_3 from 25 to 75 ng/dl of plasma in a recent report of a study on greyhound dogs (226).

The concentration of T_4 in goats ranged from 2 to 17 μg/dl (7,158). The following have been reported for the serum concentrations of T_4 and T_3 in castrated male sheep (31): total T_4, 6.3 ± 8.1 (SE) μg/dl; free T_4, 1.3 ± 0.01 (SE) ng/dl; total T_3, 70 ± 8 (SE) ng/dl and free T_3, 0.12 ± 0.01 (SE) ng/dl. These data are in agreement with other reports in the literature (310). Serum T_4 values for female sheep have ranged from 3.2 to 4.6 μg/dl for total T_4 and 1.3 to 22 ng/dl for free T_4 (250).

Blum and Kunz (32) reported the following data on plasma T_3 and T_4 concentrations of 279- to 423-kg steers: total T_4 from 4.0 to 5.1 μg/dl; free T_4 from 1.2 to 1.6 ng/dl; total T_3 from 117 to 136 ng/dl; and free T_3 from 0.260 to 0.330 ng/dl. Similar data have been reported for young bulls (304). It was reported that heifers have a serum T_4 concentration of 6 to 8 μg/dl (275) and a plasma T_3 concentration of 150 to 200 ng/dl (11). The plasma T_4 concentration of nonlactating cows ranged from 5.7 to 7.7 μg/dl (269).

Published reports show horses to have a serum total T_4 concentration of 0.3 to 4 μg/dl (57,158,208,250,299), serum T_3 of 60 to 100 ng/dl (208,269), and serum free T_4 concentration of 1.2 to 2.2 ng/dl (250). The serum total T_4 concentration for pigs was reported to average 2.1 μg/dl (158). In a recent report of a study of female pigs the following ranges of plasma concentrations were reported (339): total T_4, 4.8 to 6.1 μg/dl; free T_4, 1.5 to 1.9 ng/dl; total T_3, 26 to 48 ng/dl.

CALCIUM-REGULATING HORMONES

The major hormones involved in the regulation of calcium and phosphorus metabolism are parathyroid hormone, calcitonin, and 1,25-dihydroxyvitamin D. These hormones play an important role in the control of bone mass.

Parathyroid Hormone

Parathyroid hormone (PTH) is secreted by the chief cells of the parathyroid gland. Parathyroid hormone is a polypeptide comprised of 84 amino acids. The main action of PTH is to promote bone resorption, but it also increases renal Ca^{+2} reabsorption, decreases renal phosphate reabsorption, and increases the generation of 1,25-dihydroxyvitamin D from 25-hydroxyvitamin D by the kidney.

The radioimmunoassay is the primary method for the measurement of plasma or serum PTH levels. There have been problems with this method of assay because some procedures may measure inactive fragments of PTH in addition to the intact hormone. Assays detecting the C-terminal region are hazardous because biologically inactive C-terminal fragments accumulate in plasma. Assays detecting the N-terminal region are likely to provide physiologically reliable results.

Sound data on the plasma or serum PTH concentrations of laboratory rats have been collected. In male Sprague-Dawley rats, the PTH concentration was reported to range from 140 to 180 pg/ml (336), whereas in female Sprague-Dawley rats, it ranged from less than detectable (ie, <50 pg/ml) to 400 pg/ml (300). The range reported for the serum PTH concentration in male Wistar rats was 200 to 600 pg/ml (248) and for female Wistar rats 50 to 150 pg/ml with no relationship to stage of estrous cycle (71). The range reported for male Fischer 344 rats was 300 to 700 pg/ml (284), for male Sherman rats 70 to 180 pg/ml (47), and for Black-hooded/Ztn rats 148 ± 5 (SE) pg/ml (336). A marked increase in plasma PTH concentration occurred with increasing age in male Fischer 344 rats (162), which may explain the higher levels in 12- to 18-month-old Fischer rats compared to those in Wistar and Sprague-Dawley rats of the same age (161).

Little reliable information is available on the plasma or serum PTH concentrations of other commonly used laboratory animal models. However, there are good data on goats and cattle. In female goats, serum PTH concentrations have been reported to range from 500 to 900 pg/ml (190). In steers, the reported plasma PTH concentrations ranged from 200 to 400 pg/ml (30) and in cows from 10 to 500 pg/ml (33). Based on C-terminal radioimmunoassay of serum PTH concentration, ponies had a range of 200 to 1,500 pg/ml (96). The plasma concentration of PTH was 322 ± 33 (SE) pg/ml in dogs (200,201), but insufficient information was provided to evaluate the physiologic validity of the immunoassay used. A more recent study (127) showed that radioimmunoassay of plasma PTH levels in dogs yields much higher values than do bioactivity assays.

Calcitonin

Calcitonin is secreted by the C cells of the thyroid gland. The hormone is a peptide consisting of 32 amino acids. The main action of calcitonin is to inhibit the resorption of bone. Its concentration in serum or plasma is determined by radioimmunoassay.

There is a considerable body of data on rats, with wide variation in the findings. The recent report of Kalu et al (160) indicates that this wide range may be due to failure of the investigators to recognize the effect of age on the concentration of calcitonin. Kalu et al reported that in male Fischer 344 rats there is a progressive increase in the concentration of serum calcitonin from below detectable levels (<90 pg/ml) at 6 weeks of age to more than 14,000 pg/ml at 27 months of age. Peng and Garner (230) reported that 9-month-old Fischer 344 rats have serum calcitonin levels ranging from 200 to 1,000 pg/ml and that the range in 6.5-month-old females was 300 to 3,800 pg/ml and in 15-month-old females 200 to 16,500 pg/ml. With Wistar rats, Roos et al (259) report a range of 200 to 500 pg/ml for 6- to 8-month-old males, 400 to 900 pg/ml for 12- to 14-month-old males, 450 to 1,100 pg/ml for 6- to 8-month-old females, and 700 to 1,800 pg/ml for 12- to 14-month-old females. Gürkan et al (130) reported 6-month-old female Wistar rats to have a plasma calcitonin concentration of 210 ± 50 (SD) pg/ml and 9-month-old males to have a value of 210 ± 60 (SD) pg/ml. Work with 3-month-old female Wistar rats also indicates that the stage of the estrous cycle influences the concentration of plasma calcitonin with minimum levels occurring during proestrus (71). One-month-old male Sprague-Dawley rats had serum calcitonin levels of about 100 pg/ml (4).

Talmage et al (293) also showed that serum calcitonin levels were much higher in rats that were feeding than in those not feeding, and Hirsch and Hagaman (137) found that the stage of light cycle also influenced the plasma calcitonin concentration.

The serum calcitonin concentration range reported for adult male Holtzman rats was 500 to 1,500 pg/ml (229). The concentration for adult male Long-Evans rats was reported to be 440 ± 160 (SD) pg/ml (311).

There is little reliable information on plasma calcitonin concentration in other species of laboratory animals. There are some data on primates, with that of the adult female rhesus monkey being reported to range from 135 to 374 pg/ml (134). Adult female normally cycling baboons (*Papio cynocephalus anubis*) have levels of 45 to 80 pg/ml. Adult female New Zealand white rabbits 8 months of age or older have values that range between 1,125 and 1,200 pg/ml (245).

1,25-Dihydroxyvitamin D

Vitamin D is converted in the liver to 25-hydroxyvitamin D which is transported to the kidney where it is converted to 1,25-dihydroxyvitamin D. It is the 1,25-dihydroxyvitamin D that is the biologically active form and its generation and secretion by the kidney must be considered an endocrine function of the kidney. The most important action of 1,25-dihydroxyvitamin D is the promotion of intestinal calcium absorption, but it also appears to be involved in calcium mobilization from bone and in calcium reabsorption by the kidney. The major methods used to measure serum 1,25-dihydroxyvitamin D are competitive radioassays and high pressure liquid chromatography (82,83,149,212).

The following data have been reported on the plasma or serum concentrations of 1,25-dihydroxyvitamin D in commonly used rat strains: male Wistar rats, 79 ± 7 (SE) pg/ml (303); male Wistar rats, 120 ± 24 pg/ml; and female Wistar rats, 96 ± 17 (SD) pg/ml (216); male Sherman rats, 46 ± 14 (SE) pg/ml by one group of investigators (47) and 101 ± 15 (SE) pg/ml by another (101); male Sprague-Dawley rats, 75 ± 4 (SE) pg/ml (191). The reason for the broad range may relate primarily to the fact that low dietary calcium levels increase the plasma concentration of 1,25-dihydroxyvitamin D (303).

The concentration of 1,25-dihydroxyvitamin D in the plasma of brown lemurs was reported to average 65.2 ± 25.1 (SE) pg/ml for males and

65.9 ± 21.3 (SE) pg/ml for females (126). The concentrations of this hormone averaged 38.0 ± 10.4 (SD) pg/ml for cows, 35.9 ± 30.0 (SD) pg/ml for sheep, and 60.3 ± 7.2 (SD) pg/ml for pigs (143). Dogs were reported to have a serum 1,25-dihydroxyvitamin D concentration of 26 ± 5 (SE) pg/ml (200,201) by one group and 23 ± 3 (SE) pg/ml (148) by another group. The serum concentration of 1,25-dihydroxyvitamin D ranged from 100 to 400 pg/ml in young pigs (99). The concentration of 1,25-dihydroxyvitamin D in the serum of 1-year-old New Zealand rabbits was 37 ± 5 (SD) pg/ml (60).

ADRENAL HORMONES

Cortex

The adrenal cortex secretes steroid hormones. Physiologically, the most important classes of hormones secreted are the glucocorticoids and the mineralocorticoids.

Glucocorticoids

The glucocorticoids secreted by the adrenal cortex of mammalian species are cortisol, corticosterone, or a mixture of the two. The primary functions of the glucocortiocids relate to their regulatory roles in carbohydrate, protein, and fat metabolism. They also play an important role in enabling the organism to withstand stress. The major methods currently in use to measure glucocorticoids in serum or plasma use radioimmunoassays or fluorometric assays.

The major glucocorticoid secreted by the adrenal cortex of the laboratory rat is corticosterone. Because there is marked diurnal variation in the serum or plasma concentration of corticosterone, the time at which a blood sample is withdrawn in relation to the light cycle is critical (76). In addition, when rats are fed meals at a specific time of day, plasma corticosterone levels peak just before food presentation and decrease during ingestion of the meal (76).

With male Sprague-Dawley rats fed at will, the maximum concentration of circulating corticosterone is reached late in the light phase to the beginning of the dark phase and the minimum concentration at the end of the dark phase to the middle of the light phase (75,120,136,301). The mean maximum corticosterone concentrations in several studies ranged from 15 to 23 μg/dl and the mean minimum concentration from 1 to 6 μg/dl (75,120,136,301). In one study, free corticosterone (ie, that not bound to plasma proteins) was measured and its concentration showed the same diurnal pattern as that of total corticosterone with maximum values averaging 4.3 μg/dl and the minimum value being 0.1 μg/dl (75). Similar data were reported for male Wistar rats (141,270).

A similar diurnal concentration pattern is also observed in female rats (maximum values averaging 70 μg/dl and minimum values 17 μg//dl). It should be noted that the corticosterone concentrations were determined fluorometrically (72). The highest plasma corticosterone concentrations were seen during proestrus and the lowest during diestrus (72).

The major glucocorticoid in the plasma of mice is corticosterone. With male mice (Louisiana State University Colony) the maximum plasma corticosterone concentration of 9 μg/dl was seen at the start of the dark period and minimum concentration of 5 μg/dl was observed shortly before the end of the dark period (222). Contrastingly, in female mice (BD₂F₁ strain) the minimum concentration of 13.5 μg/dl was seen at the start of the dark period and the maximum concentration of 40 μg/dl occurred well into the dark period (267). Whether this relates to a sex difference or to the fact that male mice were provided 14 hours of light and 10 hours of dark while the female mice were provided 8 hours of light and 16 hours of dark is not known.

Hamsters have significant plasma levels of both corticosterone and cortisol (223). In one study (223), total glucocorticoids in the plasma of male hamsters 5.5 hours after the onset of light was 1.77 ± 0.10 (SE) μg/dl with a ratio of corticosterone to cortisol of 3.53 ± 0.47 (SE) μg/dl. In another study (38) plasma cortisol at the start of the light cycle was 2.75 ± 0.44 (SD) μg/dl for male hamsters and 0.33 ± 0.04 μg/dl for female hamsters.

The major plasma glucocorticoid for guinea pigs and rabbits is cortisol. With male guinea pigs, peak cortisol concentration occurred late in the light phase and again late in the dark phase, whereas minimum concentrations occurred early in the light phase and again in the middle of the dark phase; total plasma cortisol concentration ranged from 5 to 30 μg/dl (108, 114) and free plasma cortisol concentration from 0.6 to 5.8 μg/dl (108). Rabbits sampled early in the morning were found to have a plasma cortisol concentration of 3.2 ± 0.6 (SE) $\mu g/dl$ (282).

The adrenal cortex of dogs secretes cortisol as the major glucocorticoid. There is no marked diurnal variation in serum or plasma cortisol concentration in dogs (167). The concentration was found to range from 0.34 to 13.5 $\mu g/dl$ in the plasma or serum of dogs (18,56,80,84, 102,119,123,166,168,188,232,233,255,282,292, 308). The adrenal cortex of cats also primarily secretes cortisol. There is little information about the diurnal pattern of serum or plasma cortisol concentration in cats. The range of concentrations reported is 1.7 to 19.8 $\mu g/dl$ (50,55,113). Anesthetized cats have lower concentrations than do cats manually restrained (50).

The adrenal cortex of nonhuman primates secretes cortisol as the major glucocorticoid. In the male rhesus monkey, there is a well-defined diurnal pattern of plasma cortisol concentration. Highest levels occur near the beginning of the light period and minimum values near the start of the dark cycle. The highest diurnal concentrations ranged from 15 to 35 $\mu g/dl$ and lowest from 6 to 20 $\mu g/dl$ (53,87,189,234,241). A similar diurnal pattern was reported for female rhesus monkeys with the maximum values being 36.5 ± 4.6 (SE) $\mu g/dl$ and the lowest 12.1 ± 3.2 (SE) $\mu g/dl$ (285). For female baboons, plasma cortisol concentration was 31 ± 4 (SE) $\mu g/dl$ (231).

The range of plasma cortisol concentrations reported for male *Macaca fascicularis* monkey is 10 to 40 $\mu g/dl$ with no mention of the diurnal pattern (51). A similar range was reported for male talapoin monkeys from which blood was drawn late in the light cycle (89). No difference was found in plasma cortisol concentration between male and female talapoin monkeys (341). The plasma cortisol concentration range for adult female squirrel monkeys sampled in the morning was 25 to 150 $\mu g/dl$ (121) and for male squirrel monkeys 100 to 200 $\mu g/dl$ (289). The range of serum cortisol concentration reported for female chimpanzees in the early follicular phase of the menstrual cycle sampled early in the morning was 25 to 35 $\mu g/dl$ (124). In the female African green vervet, plasma cortisol levels ranged from 20 to 70 $\mu g/dl$, with peak levels occurring about 1 hour after feeding (197). The male Titi monkey had a plasma cortisol

concentration of 34 ± 4 (SE) $\mu g/dl$ and the female 46 ± 9 (SE) $\mu g/dl$, with the percentage free being 42 and 31, respectively (170).

In pigs, about 80 per cent of the plasma glucocorticoids were cortisol and 20 per cent corticosterone (35). The peak concentration for cortisol occurred in the morning (1 to 4 $\mu g/dl$) and minimum concentration in the afternoon (0.5 to 3.5 $\mu g/dl$) (35,302). Cortisol comprised about 90 per cent of the plasma glucocorticoids in horses and corticosterone about 10 per cent (35). The maximum concentration for cortisol occurred at about 8 AM (2.8 ± 0.5 (SE) $\mu g/dl$ for mares) and minimum concentration at about 10 PM (0.5 ± 0.1 (SE) $\mu g/dl$ for mares) (35), but there is a seasonal effect (116). A more recent report (151) shows the peak concentration in mares to be 6.1 ± 0.1 (SE) $\mu g/dl$ and the nadir 2.6 ± 0.4 (SE) $\mu g/dl$.

The major plasma glucocorticoid in sheep is cortisol. In ewes, the peak concentration occurred in the early morning and the lowest concentration during the dark; the concentration ranged from undetectable to 2.6 $\mu g/dl$ (196,239). In rams kept in 14 hours of light (0600 to 2000 hours), peak concentration of plasma cortisol was found at 1600 hours (range 0.47 to 0.72 $\mu g/dl$) and minimum concentration at 2000 hours (range 0.16 to 0.59 $\mu g/dl$) (139). The basal plasma cortisol concentrations reported for cows ranged from 0.2 to 1 $\mu g/dl$ (209) and for male pygmy goats from 0.3 to 1.5 $\mu g/dl$ (146).

Mineralocorticoids

The mineralocorticoid secreted by the adrenal cortex is aldosterone. The major action of aldosterone is its role in the maintenance of Na^+ and K^+ homeostasis. The primary procedure for measuring the plasma or serum concentration of aldosterone is the radioimmunoassay.

There is much information on the serum or plasma aldosterone concentration in laboratory rats. Data from male Sprague-Dawley rats show a distinct diurnal pattern, with the peak concentrations occurring near the end of the light period or start of the dark period and the minimum concentration occurring in the middle of the light period (106,120,136); the minimum concentration ranged from 4 to 11 ng/dl of plasma or serum and the maximum concentration from 12 to 35 ng/dl. At 9 to 10 AM, most male Sprague-Dawley rats have plasma aldosterone concentrations of 10 to 15 ng/dl and most females 25 to 35 ng/dl (294). It should be noted that the sodium content of the diet influences the plasma aldosterone concentration, with rats on low sodium diets having five times the concentration of rats on high sodium diets (176). The plasma concentration for male Fischer 344 rats was reported to be 8.4 ± 1.3 (SE) ng/dl but the time of sampling relative to the light-dark cycle was not reported (283). The concentration of plasma aldosterone for female Long-Evans rats sampled early in the morning was reported to be 29.8 ± 5.0 (SE) ng/dl (228). The plasma concentration of aldosterone for male Wistar rats sampled at 10 AM was 25.4 ± 3.6 (SD) ng/dl (193) and for those sampled in the late morning 26.2 ± 3.7 (SE) ng/dl (1).

Male New Zealand rabbits sampled early in the morning had an average plasma aldosterone concentration of 10.8 ± 1.9 (SE) ng/dl (282). Male rabbits (*Oryctolagus cuniculus*) have plasma aldosterone concentrations that ranged from 20 ng/dl (in the early morning) to 50 ng/dl (in the late afternoon) (318). The range of plasma aldosterone concentrations reported for male dogs was 6 to 31 ng/dl (177,211,282); the lower values were reported for dogs sampled in the morning and the higher values were taken from a study in which the time of sampling was not defined. Female dogs were reported to have plasma aldosterone concentrations that ranged from 4 to 11 ng/dl (5,36).

The plasma concentration of aldosterone in male rhesus monkeys has been reported to range from 2 to 30 ng/dl (26,41,281). Again, the lower values were reported for animals sampled early in the morning and the higher values from studies in which the time of sampling was not reported.

With sheep (rams), a diurnal pattern of plasma aldosterone concentration was reported, with lowest values 3.7 ± 0.5 (SE) ng/dl at midnight and highest values 5.8 ± 0.6 (SE) ng/dl at 9 AM (198). In horses sampled early in the morning, the plasma aldosterone concentration ranged from 1.2 to 4.0 ng/dl (131). Plasma aldosterone concentrations were 5.5 ± 4.3 (SD) ng/dl in normally hydrated goats (Bedoin females) and 13.9 ± 2.3 (SD) ng/dl in dehydrated goats (335).

Adrenal Medulla

The major hormone secreted by the adrenal medulla is epinephrine. However, it also secretes some norepinephrine, but most of the norepinephrine in plasma comes from sympathetic postganglionic fibers. Epinephrine and norepinephrine have a broad spectrum of actions influencing metabolic processes, glandular secretion, and smooth muscle function. Several methods have been used to measure the plasma concentrations of epinephrine and norepinephrine. A currently popular method is the radioenzymatic assay. However, recently, high pressure liquid chromatography has been gaining favor. An older method involved the use of fluorometry.

The literature contains much information on the plasma epinephrine and norepinephrine concentrations of rats. However, much of it must be discarded if basal levels are desired because of the way blood samples were taken. Indeed, the data of Popper et al (236) with male Sprague-Dawley rats make the problem clear. Indwelling arterial catheters permitted blood sampling to take place without disturbing the rat. The following data on plasma epinephrine concentration in picograms per milliliter were obtained: asleep, 180 ± 24 (SE); awake but undisturbed, 253 ± 30 (SE); handled, 460 ± 60 (SE); immobilized, $2,400 \pm 510$ (SE); blood obtained following decapitation, $15,000 \pm 670$ (SE). The data for plasma norepinephrine expressed as picogram per milliliter for the same rats were: asleep, 460 ± 80 (SE); awake but not disturbed, 710 ± 110 (SE); handled, 830 ± 130 (SE); immobilized, $2,800 \pm 710$ (SE); blood following decapitation, $7,600 \pm 779$ (SE). It is clear then that only data in awake undisturbed rats (ie, sampled by indwelling catheter) provide valid basal levels of these catecholamines. Indeed, most studies (164,179,328) with undisturbed male Sprague-Dawley rats have yielded similar data to those of Popper et al. Tapp et al (296) found rapid oscillations in the plasma catecholamine concentrations in male Sprague-Dawley rats that were frequently sampled between 0845 and 1630 hours. In that study, the plasma norepinephrine concentration ranged between 150 and 2,200 pg/ml and the epinephrine concentration between 100 and 8,000 pg/ml.

McCarty and Kapin (195) studied the basal

concentrations of the catecholamines in male rats of many strains. For epinephrine, the concentrations in picograms per milliliter were: SHR (spontaneously hypertensive), 545 ± 37; SP-SHR (stroke prone spontaneously hypertensive), 427 ± 79 (SE); WKY (Wistar-Kyoto), 354 ± 46 (SE); Sprague-Dawley, 337 ± 41 (SE); Osborne-Mendel, 419 ± 63 (SE); Brown-Norway, 337 ± 78 (SE); and Charles River Wistar, 258 ± 15 (SE). For norepinephrine, the concentrations in picograms per milliliter for the same strains were: SHR, 540 ± 52 (SE); SP-SHR, 517 ± 62 (SE); WKY, 438 ± 79 (SE); Sprague-Dawley, 376 ± 40 (SE), Osborne-Mendel, 449 ± 46 (SE); Brown-Norway, 376 ± 40 (SE); and Charles River Wistar, 318 ± 23 (SE). Many of these strains were studied by others with similar results (103,110,219). A similar range of basal concentrations was also reported for male Fischer 344 rats (128,194) and for female Wistar-Kyoto rats (225). In recent studies (152, 319) somewhat lower values have been reported with plasma epinephrine and norepinephrine of 78 ± 18 (SE) pg/ml and 196 ± 23 (SE) pg/ml, respectively, for male Holtzman rats and 110 ± 10 (SE) pg/ml and 180 ± 20 (SE) pg/ml, respectively, for male Wistar rats.

Bronson and Dejardins (39) reported that for awake, apparently undisturbed male CB_6F_1 mice, the plasma epinephrine concentration ranged from undetectable to 200 pg/ml and the norepinephrine concentration from 30 to 300 pg/ml. The concentration of plasma epinephrine for male rabbits was reported to range from 120 to 283 pg/ml and for norepinephrine from 300 to 504 pg/ml (44). In female rabbits, the plasma epinephrine concentration was 329 ± 146 (SD) pg/ml and the norepinephrine concentration 559 ± 104 (SD) pg/ml (215).

In dogs, the basal epinephrine concentration was reported to range from 100 to 400 pg/ml (44,49,165,342) and the basal norepinephrine from 68 to 526 pg/ml (8,44,49,175,341). The basal plasma concentrations for epinephrine in cats ranged from 30 to 113 pg/ml and norepinephrine from 282 to 912 pg/ml (20,21,49). A recent study (147) in which conscious, unanesthetized cats were examined, the plasma norepinephrine was 195 ± 18 (SE) pg/ml and plasma epinephrine 83 ± 10 (SE) pg/ml.

In the male rhesus monkey, the plasma epinephrine and norepinephrine concentrations were found to oscillate rapidly (133,186) with the mean values for epinephrine being 122 ± 14 (SE) pg/ml and for norepinephrine 820 ± 214 (SE) pg/ml. In the pig, the basal epinephrine concentration was reported to be 400 ± 100 (SE) pg/ml and for norepinephrine $400 + 150$ (SE) pg/ml (150) and to range from 210 to 590 pg/ml for epinephrine and from 350 to 650 pg/ml for norepinephrine in another study (333). The range of plasma concentrations reported for cows was 26 to 70 pg/ml for epinephrine and 132 to 180 pg/ml for norepinephrine (44).

SEX STEROID HORMONES

Progesterone

Isolated from swine ovaries in 1928 by Corner and Allen, progesterone is the major steroid hormone responsible for the maintenance of pregnancy. Progesterone secreted by corpora lutea of the ovary is indispensible for normal implantation, and progesterone secreted by corpora lutea and/or placenta is required for retention of the conceptus. During the reproductive cycle, progesterone prepares the estrogen-primed uterus for the nurture and implantation of the newly fertilized ovum. As well, progesterone acts in concert with estradiol-17 β to regulate gonadotropin secretion. Levels of progesterone in serum or plasma are routinely measured by radioimmunoassay. Production and secretion of progesterone occurs in the adrenal gland in addition to the ovaries.

During the 4-day estrous cycle of the female rat, progesterone levels increase on proestrous afternoon concomitant with the preovulatory LH surge from basal levels of 1 to 5 ng/ml to 40 to 50 ng/ml of serum or plasma (48). After declining to basal levels on estrus, a second increase in progesterone levels is evident on the first diestrous day with peak progesterone levels attaining 20 to 30 ng/ml (48). In the hamster, basal progesterone levels during the cycle approach 1 ng/ml with preovulatory increments to 10 to 12 ng/ml on proestrus (54,254). Levels of progesterone between 6 and 8 ng/ml are maintained throughout estrus and most of diestrus, with levels reaching baseline by proestrous morning (254). In cycling mice progesterone levels increase on proestrus from approximately 5 to 35 ng/ml and return to baseline on estrus (262). Rabbits are reflex ovulators and progesterone levels remain under 1 ng/ml in the absence of coitus and ovulation. By 6 hours following coitus or administration of 75 IU of human chorionic gonadotropin and coitus, progesterone levels in the rabbit increase from 1 to 8 ng/ml (104). This increase is short-lived, however, with progesterone levels declining to baseline by 24 hours (104). Levels increase again 1 day later, reach peaks of 15 to 20 ng/ml by day 10, and remain above 1 ng/ml throughout the 16 days of pseudopregnancy or 31 days of pregnancy.

In contrast to the brief (<2 days) life span of the rat, hamster, and mouse corpora lutea, the corpora lutea of the guinea pig estrous cycle and of the monkey menstrual cycle remains functional for approximately 10 days. Progesterone levels during the guinea pig estrous cycle increase abruptly on estrus with peak levels of 9 ng/ml being attained shortly before ovulation (74). A second, more gradual increase in progesterone levels occurs during diestrus with levels reaching 7 to 8 ng/ml between days 8 and 12 of the 16-day estrous cycle (74). Levels of progesterone approximate 1 ng/ml during the remainder of the cycle (74). During the menstrual cycle of both the rhesus and cynomolgus monkey, levels increase slightly to 1 to 2 ng/ml during the preovulatory LH surge. This is followed by a more prolonged and greater increase during the luteal phase (174). Serum progesterone concentrations during the follicular phase are below 1 ng/ml, whereas levels averaging 5 ng/ml are attained by day 9 of the luteal phase (174).

In the dog, the corpora lutea of the 4- to 10-month estrous cycle remain functional following spontaneous ovulation for about 2 to 3 months in the absence of pregnancy and for about 65 days in pregnant bitches (61,64,66). Progesterone levels are below 1 ng/ml during the 1- to 2-week follicular phase, increase to 2 to 4 ng/ml during the preovulatory LH surge, and rise to peak levels of 15 to 80 ng/ml by 15 to 30 days after ovulation (63). Serum progesterone levels then slowly decline during the remainder of the luteal phase and abruptly at parturition (62).

Estradiol-17

In 1923, Allen and Doisy (2) isolated estradiol-17 from the follicular fluid of sow ovaries. The main action of E_2 is to promote the growth

and development of the fallopian tubes, uterus, vagina, and external genitalia (122). Further, E_2 acts on the mammary gland to cause the growth of the duct system (85). In a paracrine role, E_2 secreted from the follicle acts locally to enhance the response of the follicle to FSH (253). Finally, E_2 acts on the hypothalamo-hypophyseal unit to regulate the secretion of gonadotropins and prolactin. Serum or plasma E_2 levels are usually measured by radioimmunoassay.

In every species examined in this chapter, increases in circulating E_2 levels precede preovulatory increments in LH. For example, serum E_2 levels in the rat begin to increase from basal levels below 10 pg/ml on estrus to 20 to 30 pg/ml on the second diestrous day and reach peak levels of 40 to 50 pg/ml on proestrus (280). In the hamster, preovulatory E_2 levels on proestrus are reported to be 300 to 400 pg/ml, declining to basal levels of 5 to 10 pg/ml on estrus (54). Basal E_2 levels in mice were in the range of 1 to 5 pg/ml (262). Basal E_2 levels in preovulatory rabbits approximated 3 pg/ml (105).

In the dog, basal E_2 levels during late anestrus are 2 to 10 pg/ml; E_2 increases during proestrus to reach peak levels of 50 to 150 pg/ml in late proestrus or early estrus, 1 to 3 days before the preovulatory LH peak, and 3 to 5 days before ovulation (61,64). Levels decline during estrus and are 5 to 15 pg/ml during the long luteal phase of nonpregnant bitches, but they have been reported to increase to 20 to 30 pg/ml during pregnancy and fall at parturition (62,66). Levels of E_2 during anestrus have been reported to reach levels up to 50 pg/ml during anestrus (220).

In cats, E_2 levels increase to peaks of 30 to 80 pg/ml before estrus, decline during estrus, and are at basal levels of 2 to 5 pg/ml during interestrus periods and during anestrus (65,317). During the guinea pig estrous cycle, E_2 levels attained values of 70 pg/ml before the LH surge, decreasing to 30 pg/ml during most of diestrus (74). In the rhesus monkey, E_2 levels in the follicular phase increased from 50 to 300 pg/ml before attainment of peak LH concentrations during the periovulatory period (174).

Testosterone

The major effects of testosterone in the male mammal are to: (1) promote the growth, differentiation, and function of the accessory sex organs and external genitalia, the latter through conversion intracellularly to dihydrotestosterone; (2) promote spermatogenesis, specifically the early stages; and (3) regulate gonadotropin secretion through actions mediated centrally and on the anterior pituitary gland (122).

In the male rat, serum testosterone concentrations measured throughout a 24-hour period exhibit a circadian rhythm with peak testosterone levels of approximaty 3 ng/ml being attained between 1330 and 1630 hours (159). Levels below 1 ng/ml were reached at 2130 hours (159). A more detailed examination of plasma testosterone levels in the rat disclosed a trimodal rhythm with average peak levels between 2 and 2.5 ng/ml occurring at 0200, 1200, and 1800 hours (206). Similar to LH and prolactin, serum testosterone levels increased from 1.5 to 3.0 ng/ml 60 minutes after mating (163).

In male mice (77) and hamsters (14), plasma testosterone levels averaged between 1.5 and 2.0 ng/ml. In rabbits, hourly blood collections for 24 or 36 hours revealed episodic fluctuations in serum testosterone levels with peak testosterone values of 3 to 4 ng/ml being attained every 4 to 5 hours (207). Similarly, De Palatis et al (85) observed episodes of increased testosterone secretion in male dogs with a periodicity of 1 to 2 hours. Circulating testosterone values in the dog ranged from 0.4 to 6.0 ng/ml over a 24-hour period. In the male rhesus monkey, Plant (234) reported episodic testosterone secretion during a 24-hour period with levels ranging from 2 to 8 ng/ml. Moreover, the frequency of testosterone pulses in male macaques was higher during the dark than during the light period in accord with a general circadian fluctuation in testosterone levels with higher levels attained during the dark phase (234).

Of interest is a report by Rush and Blake (261) in which serum testosterone concentrations were measured during the rat estrous cycle. These investigators found an increase in testosterone levels on proestrus from 250 pg/ml to 500 to 600 pg/ml followed by a steady decline to reach approximately 100 pg/ml on estrus (261).

REFERENCES

1. Airaksinen MM, Saino EL, Leppoluoto J, Kari L (1984) 6-methoxy-tetrahydro-β-carboline (pino-line): Effects on plasma renin activity and aldosterone, TSH, LH and β-endorphin levels in rats. Acta Endocrinol 107: 525–530

2. Allen E, Doisy EA (1923) An ovarian hormone: A preliminary report on its localization, extraction and partial purification and action in test animals. JAMA 81: 819–827

3. Allen LG, Kalra SP (1986) Evidence that a decrease in opioid tone may evoke preovulatory luteinizing hormone release in the rat. Endocrinology 118: 2375–2381

4. Anast CS, Gardner DW (1985) Elevated circulating immunoreactive calcitonin in the magnesium-deficient normocalcemic rat. Endocrinology 116: 2232–2235

5. Anderson DE, Gomez-Sanchez C, Dietz J (1986) Suppression of plasma renin and aldosterone in stress-salt hypertension in dogs. Am J Physiol 251: R181–R186

6. Anderson JH, Brown BE (1979) Serum thyroxine (T_4) and triiodothyronine (T_3) uptake values in normal adult cats as determined by radioimmunoassay. Am J Vet Res 40: 1493–1494

7. Anderson RR, Haines JR (1975) Thyroid hormone secretion rates in growing and mature goats. J An Sci 40: 1130–1135

8. Arita M, Ueno Y, Suruda H, Mohara O, Nishio I, Masuyama Y (1983) Changes in plasma norepinephrine after intravertebral artery infusion of saralasin in sodium depleted dogs. Jap Circ J 47: 336 341

9. Arnauld E, Czernichow P, Fumoux F, Vincent J (1977) The effects of hypertension and hypovolaemia on the liberation of vasopressin during haemorrhage in the unanaesthetized monkey (*Macaca Mulatta*). Pfluegers Arch 371: 193–200

10. Aziz LA, Forsling ML, Woolf CJ (1981) The effect of intracerebroventricular injections of morphine on vasopressin release in rat. J Physiol 311: 401 409

11. Baccari F Jr, Johnson HD, Hahn GL (1983) Environmental heat effects on growth, plasma T_3 and postheat compensatory effects on Holstein calves. Proc Soc Exp Biol Med 173: 312–318

12. Ball SG, Tree M, Morton JJ, Inglis GC, Fraser R (1981) Circulating dopamine—its effect on the plasma concentrations of catecholamines, renin, angiotensin, aldosterone and vasopressin in the conscious dog. Clin Sci 61: 417–422

13. Bark H, LeRoith D, Nyska M, Glick SM (1980) Elevation in plasma ADH levels during PEEP ventilation in the dog: Mechanisms involved. Am J Physiol 239: E474–E481

14. Bartke A, Goldman BD, Bex FJ, Kelch RP, Smith MS, Dalterio S, Doherty PC (1980) Effects of prolactin on testicular regression and recrudescence in the golden hamster. Endocrinology 106: 167–172

15. Bast JD, Greenwald GS (1974) Serum profiles of follicle-stimulating hormone, luteinizing hormone and prolactin during the estrous cycle of the hamster. Endocrinology 94: 1295–1299

16. Bayliss WM, Starling EH (1902) The mechanism of pancreatic secretion. J Physiol 28: 325–336

17. Becher BA, Bober MB, El-Noutey FD, Johnson HD (1985) Plasma antidiuretic hormone (ADH)

concentrations in cattle, during various water and feed regimens. Comp Biochem Physiol 81A: 755–759

18. Becker MJ, Holland D, Becker DN (1976) Serum cortisol (hydrocortisone) in normal dogs. An J Vet Res 37: 1101–1102

19. Belshaw BE, Rijjuberk A (1979) Radioimmunoassay of plasma T_4 and T_3 in the diagnosis of primary hypothyroidism in dogs. J Am An Hosp Assoc 15: 17–23

20. Bereiter DA, Gaun DS (1986) Potentiation of hemorrhage-evoked catecholamine release by prior blood loss in cats. Am J Physiol 250: E18–E23

21. Bereiter DA, Zaid AM, Gaun DS (1986) Effect of rate of hemorrhage on sympathoadrenal catecholamine release in cats. Am J Physiol 250: E69–E75

22. Berger M, Jean-Faucher C, De Turckheim M, Yeyssiere G, Jean C (1982) Age-related changes in the feedback regulation of gonadotrophin secretion in the immature and adult male rabbit. Acta Endocrinol 100: 18–24

23. Bern HA, Nicoll CS (1968) The comparative endocrinology of prolactin. Rec Prog Horm Res 24: 681–705

24. Berson SA, Yalow RS (1959) Quantitative aspects of the reaction between insulin-binding antibody. J Clin Invest 38: 1996–2016

25. Bie P, Peterson TV, Share L, Gilmore JP (1982) Osmotic control of plasma vasopressin in anesthetized dogs. Acta Physiol Scand 114: 37–43

26. Billman GE, Key MJ, Dickey DT, Kern DC, Keil LC, Stone HL (1983) Hormonal and renal response to plasma volume expansion in the primate Macaca mulatta. Am J Physiol 244: H201–H205

27. Blake CA, Norman RL, Sawyer CH (1973) Validation of an ovine-ovine LH radioimmunoassay for use in the hamster. Biol Reprod 8: 299–305

28. Blatchley FR, Donovan BT, Ter Haar MB (1976) Plasma progesterone and gonadotrophin levels during the estrous cycle of the guinea pig. Biol Reprod 15: 29–38

29. Blessing WW, Sved AF, Reis DJ (1980) Hypertension with elevated plasma vasopressin after lesions of noradrenergic neurons in the rabbit medulla oblongata. Trans Assoc Am Physicians 93: 192–202

30. Blum JW, Fischer JA (1982) Effects of somatostatin on parathyroid hormone levels and on response of parathyroid hormones to β-adrenergic antagonists and hypocalcemia. Acta Endrocrinol 100: 534–538

31. Blum JW, Gingins M, Vitins P, Bickel H (1980) Thyroid hormone levels related to energy and nitrogen balance during weight loss and regain in adult sheep. Acta Endocrinol 93: 440–447

32. Blum JW, Kunz P (1981) Effects of fasting on thyroid hormone levels and kinetics of reverse triiodothyronine in cattle. Acta Endocrinol 98: 234–239

33. Blum JW, Thien R, Fischer JA (1983) Lack of rapid effects of cortisol and parathyroid hormone levels in cattle. Horm Res 17: 49–51

34. Borer KT, Kelch RP (1978) A heterologous radioimmunoassay method for measurement of hamster growth hormone. Neuroendocrinology 25: 65–76

35. Bottoms GD, Roesel OI, Rausch FD, Akins EL (1972) Circadian variation in plasma cortisol and corticosterone in pigs and mares. Am J Vet Res 33: 785–790

36. Bourgoignie JJ, Gavellas G, Van Putten V, Berl T (1985) Potassium-aldosterone response in dogs with chronic renal insufficiency. Miner Electo Metab 11: 150–154

37. Breuer H, Hamel D, Kruskemper HL (eds), (1976) Methods of Hormone Analysis. Wiley & Sons, New York

38. Brinck-Johnson T, Brinck-Johnson K, Kilham L (1981) Gestational changes in hamster adrenocortical function. J Steroid Biochem 14: 835–839

39. Bronson FH, Dejardins C (1982) Endocrine responses to sexual arousal in male mice. Endocrinology 111: 1286–1291

40. Bronson FH, Vom Saal FS (1979) Control of the preovulatory release of luteinizing hormone by steroids in the mouse. Endocrinology 104: 1247–1255

41. Brown RD, Billman GE, Kem DC, Stone HL, Jiang N, Kao P, Hegstad RL (1982) The effects of metoclopromide and dopamine on plasma aldosterone concentration in normal man and rhesus monkey (Macaca mulatta): A new model to study dopamine control of aldosterone secretion. J Clin Endocrinol Metab 55: 828–832

42. Bruni G, Dal Pra P, Segre G (1979) Femtogram determination of ACTH by bioradioimmunoassay. Pharm Res Comm 11: 853–860

43. Buhl AE, Cornette JC (1982) Influence of testosterone, estradiol-17 β and dihydrotestosterone on circulating LH and FSH in castrate male guinea pigs. Biol Reprod 26: 404–412

44. Buhler HU, DaPrada M, Haefely W, Picotti GB (1978) Plasma adrenaline, noradrenaline and dopamine in man and different animal species. J Physiol 276: 311–320

45. Burger AG, Berger M, Wimpfheimer K, Danforth E (1980) Interrelationship between energy metabolism and thyroid hormone during starvation in the rat. Acta Endocrinol 93: 322–331

46. Burgi U, Feller C, Gerber AU (1986) Effects of an acute bacterial infection on serum thyroid hormones and nuclear triiodothyronine receptors in mice. Endocrinology 119: 515–521

47. Bushinsky DA, Favus MJ, Schneider AB, Sen PK, Sherwood LM, Coe FL (1982) Effects of metabolic acidosis on PTH and $1,25(OH)_2D_3$ response to low calcium diet. Am J Physiol 243: F570–F575

48. Butcher RL, Collins WE, Fugo NW (1974) Plasma concentrations of LH, FSH, prolactin, progesterone and estradiol-17 β throughout the 4-day estrous cycle of the rat. Endocrinology 94: 1704–1708

49. Carriere S, Demassieux S, Cardinal J, LeGrimellec C (1983) Release of epinephrine during carotid artery occlusion following vagotomy in dogs. Can J Physiol Pharmacol 61: 495–501

50. Carter KK, Chakraborty PK, Bush M, Wildt DE (1984) Effects of electroejaculation and ketamine-HCl on serum cortisol, progesterone and testosterone in the male cat. J Androl 5: 431–437

51. Castro MI, Rose J, Green W, Lehner N, Peterson D, Taub D (1981) Ketamine-HCl as a suitable anesthetic for endocrine, metabolic and cardio-vascular studies in *Macaca fascularis* monkeys. Proc Soc Exp Biol Med 168: 389–394

52. Castro MI, Sharon A, Young RA, Braverman LE, Emerson CH (1986) Total and free serum thyroid hormone concentrations in fetal and adult pregnant and nonpregnant guinea pigs. Endocrinology 118: 533–537

53. Chambers KC, Resko JA, Phoenix CH (1982) Correlation of diurnal changes in hormones with sexual behavior and age in male Rhesus Macaques. Neurobiol Aging 3: 37–42

54. Chappel SC, Norman RL, Spies IIC (1978) Effects of estradiol on serum and pituitary gonadotropin concentrations during selective elevations of follicle stimulating hormone. Endocrinology 19: 159–166

55. Chastain CB, Graham CL, Nichols CE (1981) Adrenocortical suppression in cats given megestral acetate. Am J Vet Res 42: 2029–2035

56. Chen CL, Kumar MSA, Williard MD, Liao TF (1978) Serum hydrocortisone (Cortisol) values in normal and adrenopathic dogs as determined by radioimmunoassay. Am J Vet Res 37: 1101–1102

57. Chen CL, Riley AM (1981) Serum thyroxine and triiodothyronine concentrations in neonatal foals and mature horses. Am J Vet Res 42: 1415–1417

58. Chen HJ, Walfish PG (1978) Effects of age and ovarian function on the pituitary thyroid system in female rats. J Endocrinol 78: 225–232

59. Chiu SC, Kubota K, Kuzuya N, Ikeda H, Uchimura H, Nagataki S (1983) Effects of prolonged administration of thyrotrophin on serum concentration, release and synthesis of thyroid hormones in mice. Acta Endocrinol 103: 68–75

60. Collette C, Monnier L, Baldet P, Blotman F, Bonnel F, Mirouze J (1986) Effect of methyl prednisolone on 1,25 dihydroxyvitamin D in rabbits. Horm Metab Res 18: 146

61. Concannon PW (1983) In Kirk RW (ed), Current Veterinary Therapy, Small Animal Practice, Vol VIII. WB Saunders, Philadelphia, pp 886–901

62. Concannon PW, Butler WR, Hansel W, Knight PJ, Hamilton JM (1978) Parturition and lactation in the bitch: Serum progesterone, cortisol and prolactin. Biol Reprod 19: 1113–1118

63. Concannon PW, Hansel W, McEntee K (1977) Changes in LH, progesterone and sexual behavior associated with preovulatory luteinization in the bitch. Biol Reprod 17: 604–619

64. Concannon PW, Hansel W, Visek W (1975) The ovarian cycle of the bitch: Plasma estrogen, LH and progesterone. Biol Reprod 12: 112–121

65. Concannon PW, Lein DH (1983) In Kirk RW (ed), Current Veterinary Therapy, Small Animal Practice, Vol VIII. WB Saunders, Philadelphia, pp 932–936

66. Concannon PW, Powers ME, Holder W, Hansel W (1977) Pregnancy and parturition in the bitch. Biol Reprod 16: 517–526

67. Connors JM, Martin LG (1982) Altitude-induced changes in plasma thyroxine 3,5,3'-triiodothyronine and thyrotropin in rats. J Appl Phsyiol 53: 313–315

68. Conte-Devolx B, Oliver C, Giraud P, Castanas E, Boudouresque F, Gillioz P, Millet Y (1982) Adrenocorticotropin, β-endorphin, and corticosterone secretion in Brattleboro rats. Endrocrinology 110: 2097–2100

69. Coquelin A, Bronson FH (1981) Episodic release of luteinizing hormone in male mice: Antagonism by a neural refractory period. Endocrinology 109: 1605–1610

70. Cowley AW Jr, Switzer SJ, Skelton MM (1981) Vasopressin, fluid and electrolyte response to chronic angiotensin II infusion. Am J Physiol 240: R130–R138

71. Cressent M, Elie C, Taboulet J, Moukhtar NS, Milhaud G (1983) Calcium regulating hormones during estrous cycle of the rat. Proc Soc Exp Biol Med 172: 158–162

72. Critchlow V, Liebelt RA, Bar-Sela M, Mountcastle W, Lipscomb HS (1963) Sex difference in resting pituitary adrenal function in the rat. Am J Physiol 205: 807–815

73. Crofton JT, Share L, Shade RE, Allen C, Tarnowski D (1978) Vasopressin in the rat with spontaneous hypertension. Am J Physiol 235: H361–II366

74. Croix D, Franchimont P (1975) Changes in the serum levels of the gonadotrophins, progesterone and estradiol during the estrous cycle of the guinea pig. Neuroendocrinology 19: 1–11

75. D'Agostino JB, Vaeth GF, Henning SJ (1982) Diurnal rhythm of total and free concentrations of serum corticosterone in the rat. Acta Endocrinol 100: 85–90

76. Dallman MF (1984) Viewing the ventromedial hypothalamus from the adrenal gland. Am J Physiol 246: R1–R12

77. Dalterio S, Bartke A, Harper MJK, Huffman R, Sweeney C (1981) Effects of cannabinoids and female exposure on the pituitary testicular axis of mice: Possible involvement of prostaglandins. Biol Reprod 24: 315–322

78. Dalterio SL, Michael SD, Macmillan BT, Bartke A (1981) Differential effects of cannabinoid exposure and stress on plasma prolactin, growth hormone and corticosterone levels in male mice. Life Sci 28: 761–766

79. Daughaday WH (1981) In Williams RH (ed), Textbook of Endocrinolgoy. WB Saunders, Philadelphia

80. DeCoster R, Beerens D, Dom J, Willemsen G (1984) Endocrinological effects of single daily ketoconazole administration in male beagle dogs. Acta Endocrinol 107: 275–281

81. De Lean A, Garon M, Kelly PA, Labrie F (1977) Changes of pituitary thyrotropin releasing hormone (TRH) receptor level and prolactin response to TRH during the rat estrous cycle. Endocrinology 100: 1505–1510

82. DeLeenheer AP, Bauwens RM (1985) Radioimmunoassay for 1,25-dihydroxyvitamin D in serum or plasma. Clin Chem 31: 142–146

83. DeLeenheer AP, Bauwens RM (1985) Comparison of a cystosol radioreceptor assay with a radioimmunoassay for 1,25-dihydroxyvitamin D in serum or plasma. Clin Chem Acta 152: 143–154

84. Dempsher DP, Gann DS (1983) Increased cortisol secretion after small hemorrhage is not attributable to changes in adrenocorticotropin. Endocrinology 113: 86–93

85. De Palatis L, Moore J, Falvo RE (1978) Plasma concentrations of testosterone and LH in the male dog. J Reprod Fert 52: 201–207

86. Dogterom J, Wimersa TB, Swaab DF (1977) Evidence for the release of vasopressin and oxytocin into cerebrospinal fluid: Measurements in plasma and CSF of intact and hypophysectomized rats. Neuroendocrinology 24: 108–118

87. Dubey AK, Puri CP, Puri V, Kumar TCA (1983) Day and night levels of hormones in male rhesus monkeys kept under controlled or constant environmental light. Experiencia 39: 207–209

88. Dufy-Barbe L, Franchimont P, Faure JMA (1973) Time-courses of LH and FSH release after mating in the female rabbit. Endocrinology 92: 1318–1321

89. Eberhart JA, Keverna EB, Meller RE (1983) Social influences on circulating levels of cortisol and prolactin in male talapoin monkeys. Physiol Behav 30: 361–369

90. Eckersall PD, Williams ME (1983) Thyroid function tests in dogs using radioimmunoassay kits. J Small An Pract 24: 525–532

91. Eden S (1979) Age- and sex-related differences in episodic growth hormone secretion in the rat. Endocrinology 105: 555–560

92. Edwards BR, LaRochelle FT Jr, Gellai M (1982) Concentraion of urine by dehydrated Brattleboro homozygotes: Is there a role for oxytocin? Ann NY Acad Sci 394: 497–502

93. Edwardson JA, Hough CAM (1975) The pituitary-adrenal system of the genetically obese (ob/ob) mouse. J Endocrinol 65: 99–107

94. Eigenmann JE, Eigenmann RY (1981) Radioimmunoassay of canine growth hormone. Acta Endocrinol 98: 514–520

95. Eipper BA, Mains RE (1980) Structure and biosynthesis of pro-adrenocorticotropin/endorphin and related peptides. Endo Rev 1: 1–27

96. Elfers RS, Bayly WM, Brobst DF, Reed SM, Liggett HD, Hawker CD, Baylink DJ (1986) Alterations in calcium, phosphorus and C-terminal parathyroid hormone levels in equine acute renal disease. Cornell Vet 76: 317–329

97. Ellis GB, Desjardins C (1982) Male rats secrete luteinizing hormone and testosterone episodically. Endocrinology 110: 1618–1627

98. Ellis GB, Desjardins C, Fraser HM (1983) Control of pulsatile LH release in male rats. Neuroendocrinology 37: 117–183

99. Engstrom GW, Horst RL, Reinhardt TA, Littledike ET (1985) Effect of dietary phosphorus levels on porcine renal 25-hydroxyvitamin D-1 α- and 24R-hydroxylase activities and plasma 1,25-dihydroxyvitamin D concentration. J An Sci 60: 1005–1011

100. Falconer J, Mitchell MD, Mountford LA, Robinson JS (1980) Plasma oxytocin during the menstrual cycle in the rhesus monkey, *Macaca mulatta*. J Reprod Fert 59: 69–72

101. Favus MJ, Coe FL, Kathpalia SC, Poret A, Seu PK, Sherwood LM (1982) Effects of chlorothiazide on 1,25 dihydroxyvitamin D_3, parathyroid hormone, and intestinal calcium absorption in the rat. Am J Physiol 242: G575–G581

102. Feldman EC, Tyrrell JB (1977) Adrenocorticotropic effect of a synthetic polypeptide—alpha 1-24 corticotropin—in normal dogs. J Am An Hosp Assoc 13: 494–499

103. Ferrari P, Picotti GB, Minotti E, Bondiolotti GP, Caravaggi AM, Bianchi G (1981) Plasma concentration of catecholamines of spontaneously hypertensive rats at different ages. Clin Sci 61: 199S–202S

104. Fredericks CM, Anderson WR, Smith CE, Mathur RS (1982) Patterns of periovulatory oviductal motility and progesterone in the unanesthetized rabbit. Biol Reprod 27: 340–350

105. Fredericks CM, Lundquist LE, Mathur RS, Ashton SH, Landgrebe SC (1983) Effects of vasoactive intestinal polypeptide upon ovarian steroids, ovum transport and fertility in the rabbit. Biol Reprod 28: 1052–1060

106. Freeman RH, David JO, Williams GH, Seymour AA (1982) Circadian changes in plasma renin activity and plasma aldosterone concentration in one kidney hypertensive rats. Proc Soc Exp Biol Med 169: 86–89

107. Fuchs A-R, Cubile L, Dawood MY (1981) Effects of mating on levels of oxytocin and prolactin in the plasma of male and female rabbits. J Endocrinol 90: 245–253

108. Fujieda K, Goff AK, Pugeat M, Strott CA (1982) Regulation of the pituitary-adrenal axis and corticosteroid-binding globulin-cortisol interaction in the guinea pig. Endocrinology 111: 1944–1950

109. Fukuda H, Greer, NA, Roberts L, Allen CF, Critchlow V, Wilson M (1975) Nyctohemeral and sex-related variations in plasma thyrotropin, thyroxine, and triiodothyronine. Endocrinology 97: 1424-1431

110. Fushimi H, Inoue T, Namikawa H, Kishino B, Nunotani H, Nishikawa M, Tochino Y, Funakawa S, Yamatodani A, Wado H (1982) Decreased response of plasma catecholamine to stress in diabetic rat. Endocrinol Jap 29: 593–596

111. Gambert SR, Barboriak JJ (1982) Effect of cold exposure on thyroid hormone in Fischer 344 rats of increasing age. J Gerontol 37: 684–687

112. Ganong WF, Shinsako J, Reid IA, Keil LC, Hoffman DL, Zimmerman EA (1982) Role of vasopressin in the renin and ACTH responses to intraventricular angiotensin II. An NY Acad Sci 394: 619–624

113. Garcy AM, Marotta SF (1978) Plasma cortisol of conscious cats during cerebroventricular perfusion with adrenergic, cholinergic and gabanergic antagonists. Neuroendocrinology 25: 343–353

114. Garris M (1986) The ovarian-adrenal axis in the guinea pig: Effects of photoperiod cyclic state and ovarian steroids on serum cortisol levels. Horm Metab Res 18: 34–37

115. Gianella-Neto D, Quabbe H-J, Witt I (1981) Pattern of thyrotropin and thyroxine plasma concentrations during the 24-hour sleep-wake cycle in the male rhesus monkey. Endocrinology 109: 2144-2151

116. Gill J, Kompanowska-Jezierska E, Jakubow K, Kott A, Szumska D (1985) Seasonal changes in the white blood cell system, lysozyme activity and cortisol level in Arabian brood mares and their foals. Comp Biochem Physiol 81A: 511–523

117. Gilmore JP, Zucker IH, Ellington MJ, Richards MA, Share L (1980) Failure of acute intravascular volume expansion to alter plasma vasopressin in the nonhuman primate, *Macaca fasicularis*. Endocrinology 106: 979–982

118. Glass AR, Mellitt R, Burman KD, Wartofsky L, Swerdloff PS (1978) Serum triiodothyronine in undernourished rats: Dependence on dietary composition rather than total calorie or protein intake. Endocrinology 102: 1925–1928

119. Goinz M, Uvnas-Moberg K, Cekan S (1986) Bromocriptine and apomorphine stimulation of cortisol secretion in conscious dogs; Evidence for a stimulatory site located outside the blood brain barrier. Psychopharm 89: 108–112

120. Gomez-Sanchez C, Holland OB, Higgins JR, Kern DC, Kaplan NM (1976) Circadian rhythms of serum renin activity and serum corticosterone, prolactin and aldosterone concentrations in the male rat on normal and low-sodium diets. Endocrinology 99: 567–572

121. Gonzalez CA, Coe CL, Levine S (1982) Cortisol responses under different housing conditions in female squirrel monkeys. Psychoneuroendocrinology 7: 209–216

122. Goodman HM (1974) In Mountcastle VB (ed), Medical Physiology, Vol 2. Mosby, St. Louis

123. Gorski DW, Rao TLK, Glisson SN, Chinthagada M, El-Etr AA (1982) Epidural triamcinolone and adrenal response to hypoglycemic stress in dogs. Anesthesiology 57: 364–366

124. Gosselin RE, Blankstein J, Dent DW, Hobson WC, Fuller GB, Reyes FI, Winter JSD, Faiman C (1983) Effects of naloxone and an enkephalin analog on serum prolactin, cortisol, and gondotrophins in the chimpanzee. Endocrinology 112: 2168–2173

125. Gray CH, Bacharach AL (eds) (1967) Hormones in Blood, Vols 1, 2 and 3. Academic Press, London

126. Gray TK, Lester GE, Moore G, Crews D, Simons EL, Stuart M (1982) Serum concentrations of calcium and vitamin D metabolites in prosimians. J Med Primatol 11: 85–90

127. Grumbaum D, Wexler M, Antos M, Gascon-Barre M, Glotzman D (1984) Bioactive parathyroid hormone in canine progressive renal failure. Am J Physiol 247: E442–E448

128. Güllner HG, Lake CR, Gill JR Jr, Lakatua DJ (1982) Hypokalemia stimulates plasma epinephrine and norepinephrine in the rat. Arch Int Pharmacodyn 260: 78–82

129. Guo GB, Schmid PG, Abboud FM (1982) Effect of digoxin and amino sugar cardiac glycoside (ASI-222) on plasma antidiuretic hormone activity. J Cardiovasc Pharm 4: 730–737

130. Gürkan L, Ekeland A, Gautuik KM, Langeland N, Ronningen H, Solheim LF (1986) Bone changes after castration in rats. Acta Orthop Scand 57: 67–70

131. Guthrie GP Jr, Cecil SG, Darden ED, Kotchen TA (1982) Dynamics of renin and aldosterone in the thoroughbred horse. Gen Comp Endocrinol 48: 296–299

132. Haldar J (1982) Release of antidiuretic hormone by morphine in rats: An *in vivo* and *in vitro* study. Proc Soc Exp Biol Med 169: 113–120

133. Hansen BC, Shielke GP, Jen KLC, Wolfe RA, Movahed H, Pek SB (1982) Rapid fluctuations in plasma catecholamines in monkeys under undisturbed conditions. Am J Physiol 242: E40–46

134. Hargis GK, Reynolds WA, Williams GA, Kamahara W, Jackson B, Bowser EN, Pitkin RM (1978) Radioimmunoassay of calcitonin in the plasma of rhesus monkey and man. Clin Chem 24: 595–601

135. Hayward JN, Pavasuthipaisit K, Perez-Lopez F, Sofroniew MV (1976) Radioimmunoassay of arginine vasopressin in rhesus monkey plasma. Endocrinology 98: 975–981

136. Hilfenhaus M (1976) Circadian rhythm of the renin-angiotensin system in the rat. Arch Toxicol 36: 305–316

137. Hirsch PE, Hagaman JR (1982) Feeding regimen, dietary calcium, and the diurnal rhythms of serum calcium and calcitonin in the rat. Endocrinology 110: 961–968

138. Hoenig M, Ferguson DC (1983) Assessment of thyroid functional reserve in the cat by the thyrotropin-stimulation test. Am J Vet Res 44: 1229–1232

139. Holley DC, Beckman DA, Evans JW (1975) Effect of confinement on the circadian rhythm of ovine cortisol. J Endocrinol 65: 147–148

140. Holzworth J, Theran P, Carpenter JL, Harpster NK, Todoroff RJ (1980) Hyperthyroidism in the cat: Ten cases. J Am Vet Med Assoc 176: 345–353

141. Honma K, Honma S, Hiroshige T (1983) Critical role of food amount for prefeeding corticosterone peak in rats. Am J Physiol 245: R339–R344

142. Horn AM, Robinson ICAF, Fink G (1985) Oxytocin and vasopressin in rat hypophyseal portal blood: Experimental studies in normal and Brattleboro rats. J Endocrinol 104: 221–224

143. Horst RL, Littledike ET, Riley JL, Napoli JL (1981) Quantitation of vitamin D and its metabolites and their plasma concentrations in five species of animals. Anal Biochem 116: 189–203

144. Hostetter MW, Piacsek BE (1977) Patterns of pituitary and gonadal hormone secretion during a 24 hour period in the male rat. Biol Reprod 16: 495–498

145. Huang HH, Steger RW, Meites J (1980) Capacity of old versus young male rats to release thyrotropin (TSH), thyroxine (T_4) and triiodothyronine (T_3) in response to different stimuli. Exper Aging Res 6: 3–12

146. Howland BE, Sanford LM, Palmer WM (1985) Changes in serum levels of LH, FSH, prolactin, testosterone, and cortisol associated with season and mating in male Pygmy goats. J Androl 6: 89–96

147. Hubbard JW, Buchholtz A, Keeton TK, Nathan MA (1986) Plasma norepinephrine concentration reflects pharmacological alteration of sympathetic

activity in the conscious cat. J Auton New Syst 15: 93–100

148. Hulter HN, Halloran BP, Toto RD, Peterson JC (1985) Long-term control of plasma calcitriol concentration in dogs and humans. J Clin Invest 76: 695–702

149. Hummer L, Christiansen C, Tjellesen L (1985) Discrepancy between serum 1,25 dihydroxycholecalciferol measured by radioimmunoassay and cytosol receptor assay. Scand J Clin Lab Invest 45: 725–733

150. Johannson G, Olsson K, Haggendal J, Jonsson L, Thoren-Tolling K (1981) Effect of amygdalectomy on stress-induced myocardial necrosis and blood levels of catecholamines in pigs. Acta Physiol Scand 113: 553–555

151. Johnson AL, Malinowski K (1986) Daily rhythm of cortisol and evidence for a photo-inducible phase for prolactin secretion in non-pregnant mares housed under non-interrupted and skeleton photoperiods. J An Sci 63: 169–175

152. Jones SB, Romana FD (1984) Plasma catecholamines in the conscious rat during endotoxicosis. Circ Shock 14: 189–201

153. Jordan D, Rousset B, Perrin F, Fournier M, Orgiazzi J (1980) Evidence for circadian variations in serum thyrotropin, 3,5,3′-triiodothyronine and thyroxine in the rat. Endocrinology 107: 1245–1248

154. Jurney TH, Smallridge RC, Routledge PA, Shand D, Wartofsky L (1983) Propranolol decreases serum thyroxine as well as triiodothyronine in rats: A protein-binding effect. Endocrinology 112: 727–732

155. Kaack B, Walker L, Brizzee KR, Wolf RH (1979) Comparative normal levels of serum triiodothyronine and thyroxine in nonhuman primates. Lab An Sci 29: 191–194

156. Kaack B, Walker M, Walker L (1980) Seasonal changes in the thyroid hormones of the male squirrel monkey. Arch Androl 4: 113–136

157. Kalin NH, Gibbs DM, Barksdale CM, Shelton SE, Carnes M (1985) Behavioral stress decreases plasma oxytocin concentrations in primates. Life Sci 36: 1275–1280

158. Kallfelz FA, Erali RP (1973) Thyroid function tests in domesticated animals: Free thyroxine index. Am J Vet Res 34: 1449–1451

159. Kalra PS, Kalra SP (1977) Circadian periodicities of serum androgens, progesterone, gonadotrophins and luteinizing hormone-releasing hormone in male rats: The effects of hypothalamic deafferentation, castration and adrenalectomy. Endocrinology 101: 1821–1827

160. Kalu D, Cockerman R, Yu BP, Roos BA (1983) Lifelong dietary modulation of calcitonin levels in rats. Endocrinology 113: 2010–2015

161. Kalu DN, Hardin RH (1984) Age, strain and species differences in circulating parathyroid hormone. Horm Metabol Res 16: 654–657

162. Kalu DN, Hardin RH, Cockerham R, Yu BP (1984) Aging and dietary modulation of rat skeleton and parathyroid hormone. Endocrinology 115: 1239–1247

163. Kamel F, Wright WW, Mock EJ, Frankel AI (1977) The influence of mating and related stimuli on plasma levels of luteinizing hormone, follicle stimulating hormone, prolactin, and testosterone in the male rat. Endocrinology 101: 421–429

164. Katholi RE, Winternitz SR, Oparil S (1982) Decreases in sympathetic nervous system activity and attenuation in response to stress following renal denervation in the one-kidney one-clip Goldblatt hypertensive rat. Clin Exper Hypertens A4: 707–716

165. Keller-Wood ME, Wade CE, Shinsako J, Keil LC, Van Loon GR, Dallmann MF (1982) Insulin-induced hypoglycemia in conscious dogs: Effect of maintaining carotid arterial glucose levels on the adrenocorticotropin, epinephrine and vasopressin responses. Endocrinology 112: 624–632

166. Kemppainen RJ, Filer DV, Sartin JC, Reed RB (1986) Ovine corticotrophin-releasing factor in dogs: Dose-response relationship and effects of dexamethasone. Acta Endocrinol 112: 12–19

167. Kemppainen RJ, Sartin JC (1984) Evidence for episodic but not circadian activity in plasma concentrations of adrenocorticotrophin, cortisol and thyroxine in dogs. J Endocrinol 103: 219–226

168. Kemppainen RJ, Thompson FN, Lorenz MD (1982) Effects of dexamethasone infusion on the plasma cortisol response to cosyntropin (synthetic ACTH) injection in normal dogs. Res Vet Sci 32: 181–183

169. Kimura T, Share L, Wong BC, Crofton JT (1981) Central effects of dopamine and bromocriptine on vasopressin release and blood pressure. Neuroendocrinology 33: 347–351

170. Klosterman LL, Murai JT, Siiteri PK (1986) Cortisol levels, binding and properties of corticosteroid binding globulin in serum of primates. Endocrinology 118: 424–434

171. Knepel W, Nutto D, Henning A, Hertting G (1982) Vasopressin and β-endorphin release after osmotic and non-osmotic stimuli: Effect of naloxone and dexamethasone. Eur J Pharm 77: 299–306

172. Knepel W, Nutto D, Hertting G (1982) Evidence for inhibition by β-endorphin of vasopressin release during fast shock-induced stress in rat. Neuroendocrinology 34: 353–356

173. Knight PJ, Hamilton JM, Scanes CG (1977) Homologous radioimmunoassay for canine prolactin. Acta Endocrinol 85: 736–743

174. Knobil E, Plant TM (1978) In Ganong WF, Martini L (eds), Frontiers in Neuroendocrinology, Vol 5. Raven Press, New York

175. Kopp U, Bradley T, Hjemdahl P (1983) Renal venous outflow and urinary excretion of norepinephrine, epinephrine and dopamine during graded renal nerve stimulation. Am J Physiol 244: E52–E60

176. Kotchen TA, Guthrie GP Jr, Galla JH, Luke R, Welch WJ (1983) Effects of NaCl on renin and aldosterone responses to potassium depletion. Am J Physiol 244: E164–E169

177. Kraut JA, Wish JB, Zoller KM, Weinstein SS, Melby J, Cohen JJ (1982) Aldosterone and the renal response to sulfuric acid feedings in the dog. Am J Physiol 243: F494–F502

178. Kreiger DT (ed) (1979) Endocrine Rhythms. Raven Press, New York

179. Kvetnansky R, Sun CL, Lake CR, Thoa M, Torda T, Kopin IJ (1978) Effects of handling and forced immobilization on rat plasma levels of epinephrine, norepinephrine, and dopamine-β-hydroxylase. Endocrinology 103: 1868–1874

180. Lang RE, Rascher W, Heil J, Unger T, Ganten D (1982) Angiotensin stimulates oxytocin release: Impaired response in rats with genetic hypothalamic diabetes insipidus. Ann NY Acad Sci 394: 147–152

181. Las MS, Surks MI (1981) Dissociation of serum triiodothyronine concentration and hepatic nuclear triiodothyronine-binding capacity in streptozotocin-induced diabetic rats. Endocrinology 109: 1259–1263

182. Ledsome JR, Ngsee J, Wilson N (1983) Plasma vasopressin concentration in the anesthetized dog before, during and after atrial distention. J Physiol 338: 413–421

183. Ledsome JR, Wilson N, Ngsee J (1982) Time course of changes in plasma vasopressin during atrial distension. Can J Physiol Pharm 60: 1210–1218

184. Leighton KM, Kim SL, Wilson N (1982) Arginine vasopressin response to anesthesia produced by halothane, euflurane and isoflurane. Can Anaesth Soc J 29: 563–566

185. Lappaluoto J (1972) Blood bioassayable thyrotropin and corticosterone levels during various physiological and stress conditions in the rabbit. Acta Endocrinol 70 (suppl 165): 1–38

186. Levin BE, Goldstein A, Natelson BH (1978) Ultradian rhythm of plasma noradrenaline in rhesus monkeys. Nature 272: 164–166

187. Ling GV, Lowenstine LJ, Kaneko JJ (1974) Serum thyroxine (T-4) and triiodothyronine (T-3) uptake values in normal adult cats. Am J Vet Res 35: 1247–1249

188. Lathrop CD, Oliver JW (1984) Diagnosis of canine Cushing's syndrome based on multiple steroid analysis and dexamethasone turnover kinetics. Am J Vet Res 45: 2304–2309

189. Lotz WG, Podgorski RP (1982) Temperature and adrenocortical responses in rhesus monkeys exposed to microwaves. J Appl Physiol 53: 1565–1571

190. Marques PR, Williams DD, Shen L, Johnson DC, Baylink DJ, Gale CC (1979) Parathyroid hormone release is not associated with acute sympathetic arousal in goats. Endocrin Res Comms 6: 57–70

191. Matsumato T, Kawanobe Y, Ezawa I, Shibuya N, Hata K, Ogata E (1986) Role of insulin in the increase in serum 1,25 dihydroxyvitamin D concentrations in response to phosphorus deprivation in streptozotocin-induced diabetic rats. Endocrinology 118: 1440–1444

192. Maul DH, Rosenberg DP, Henrickson RV, Kaneko JJ (1982) Response of thyroxine and triiodothyronine to thyroid-stimulating hormone in adult female baboons (Papio cynocephalus). Lab An Sci 32: 267–268

193. Mazzochi G, Robba C, Rebuffat P, Gottardo G, Nussdorfer GG (1985) Effect of somatostatin on the zona glomerulosa of rats treated with angiotensin II or captopril: Stereology and plasma hormone concentrations. J Steroid Biochem 23: 353–356

194. McCarty R (1981) Aged rats: Diminished sympathetic-adrenal medullary responses to acute stress. Behav Neur Biol 33: 204–212

195. McCarty R, Kapin IJ (1978) Sympatho-adrenal medullary activity and behavior during exposure to footshock stress: A comparison of seven rat strains. Physiol Behav 21: 567–572

196. McNatty KP, Cashmore M, Young A (1972) Diurnal variation in plasma cortisol levels in sheep. J Endocrinol 54: 361–362

197. Meis PJ, Rose JC (1983) Plasma cortisol response to feeding in African green vervets. J Med Primatol 12: 49–52

198. Mesbah S, Brudieux R (1982) Diurnal variation of plasma concentrations of cortisol, aldosterone and electrolytes in the ram. Horm Metab Res 14: 320–323

199. Mellin TN, Orczyk GP, Hichens M, Behrman HR (1976) Serum profiles of luteinizing hormone, progesterone and total estrogens during the canine estrous cycle. Theriogenology 5: 175–187

200. Meuten DJ, Segre GV, Capen CC, Kociba GC, Voelkel EF, Levine L, Tashjian AH Jr, Chew DJ, Nagode LA (1983) Hypercalcemia in dogs with adenocarcinoma derived from apocrine glands of the anal sacs. Lab Invest 48: 428–435

201. Meuten DJ, Kociba GC, Capen CC, Chew DJ, Segre GV, Levine C, Tashjian AH Jr, Voelkel EF, Nagode LA (1983) Hypercalcemia in dogs with lymphosarcoma. Lab Invest 49: 553–562

202. Michael SD, Kaplan SB, Macmillan BT (1980) Peripheral plasma concentrations of LH, FSH, prolactin and GH from birth to puberty in male and female mice. J Reprod Fert 59: 217–222

203. Millard WJ, Sagar SM, Badger TM, Carr DB, Arnold MA, Spindel E, Kasting NW, Martin JB (1983) The effects of cysteamine on thyrotropin and immunoreactive β-endorphin secretion in the rat. Endocrinology 112: 518–525

204. Mills TM, Copland JA, Coy DH, Schally AV (1983) Is the postovulatory release of follicle-stimulating hormone in the rabbit mediated by luteinizing hormone-releasing hormone? Endocrinology 113: 1020–1024

205. Mobley PW, Dubuc PU (1979) Thyroid levels in the developing obese-hyperglycemic syndrome. Horm Metab Res 11: 37–39

206. Mock EJ, Norton HW, Frankel AI (1978) Daily rhythmicity of serum testosterone concentration in the male laboratory rat. Endocrinology 103: 1111–1121

207. Moor BC, Younglai EV (1975) Variations in peripheral levels of LH and testosterone in adult male rabbits. J Reprod Fert 42: 259–266

208. Morris DD, Garcia M (1983) Thyroid-stimulating hormone: Response test in healthy horses and effect of phenylbutazone on equine thyroid hormones. Am J Vet Res 44: 503–507

209. Nakao T, Tamamura F, Tsunoda N, Kawata K (1981) Double antibody enzyme immunoassay of cortisol in bovine plasma. Steroids 38: 111–120

210. Nakashima T, Taurog A, Krulich L (1981) Serum

thyroxine, triiodothyronine and TSH levels in iodine-deficient and iodine-sufficient rats before and after exposure to cold. Proc Soc Exp Biol Med 167: 45–50

211. Nicholls MG, Tree M, Livesey JH, Fraser R, Morton JJ, Robertson JIS (1982) Effect of changes in sodium balance on potassium/aldosterone dose-response curves in the dog. Clin Sci 62: 373–380

212. Nicholson GC, Kent JC, Guthridge DH, Retallack RW (1985) Estimation of 1,25 dihydroxyvitamin D by cytoreceptor and competitive protein binding assay without high pressure liquid chromatography. Clin Endocrinol 22: 597–609

213. Niswender GD, Midgley AR, Monroe SE, Reichert LE (1968) Radioimmunoassay for rat luteinizing hormone with anti-ovine LH serum and ovine LH[131]I. Proc Soc Exp Biol Med 128: 807–815

214. Niswender GD, Monroe SE, Peckham WD, Midgley AR Jr, Knobil E, Reichert LE Jr (1971) Radioimmunoassay for rhesus monkey luteinizing hormone (LH) with anti-ovine LH serum and ovine LH[131]I. Endocrinology 88: 1327–1331

215. Nogier R, Nogier P, Menezo Y, Santini R, Khatchadourian C (1982) Influence of skin illumination on plasma biogenic amines in the rabbit. Acupunct Electro-Therap Res Int J 7: 247–253

216. Nyomba BL, Bouillon R, Lissens W, Van Baelin H, De Moor P (1985) 1,25-dihydroxyvitamin D and vitamin D-binding protein are both decreased in streptozotocin-diabetic rats. Endocrinology 114: 2483–2488

217. O'Byrne KT, Ring JPG, Summerlee AJS (1986) Plasma oxytocin and oxytocin neurone activity during delivery in rabbits. J Physiol 370: 501–513

218. Ohtake M, Bray GA, Azukizawa M (1977) Studies on hypothermia and thyroid function in the obese (ob/ob) mouse. Am J Physiol 233: R110–R115

219. Oishi M, Ishiko J, Inagaki C, Takaori S (1983) Release of histamine and adrenaline *in vivo* following intravenous administration of neurotensin. Life Sci 32: 2231–2239

220. Olson PN, Bowey RA, Behrendt MD, Olson JD, Nett TM (1982) Concentration of reproductive hormones in canine serum throughout late anestrus, proestrus and estrus. Biol Reprod 27: 1196–1206

221. Ottenweller JE, Hedge GA (1982) Diurnal variations of plasma thyrotropin, thyroxine, and triiodothyronine in female rats are phase shifted after inversion of the photoperiod. Endocrinology 111: 509–514

222. Ottenweller JE, Meier AH, Russo AC, Frenzke ME (1979) Circadian rhythms of plasma corticosterone binding activity in the rat and the mouse. Acta Endocrinol 91: 150–157

223. Ottenweller, Tapp WN, Burke JM, Natelson BH (1985) Plasma cortisol and corticosterone concentration in the Golden Hamster (*Mesocricetus auratus*). Life Sciences 37: 1551–1558

224. Otteson B, Hansen B, Fahrenkrug J, Fuchs A (1984) Vasoactive intestinal peptide (VIP) stimulates oxytocin and vasopressin release from the neurohypophysis. Endocrinology 115: 1648–1650

225. Pak CH (1981) Plasma adrenaline and nora-

drenaline concentration of spontaneously hypertensive rat. Jap Heart J 22: 987–995

226. Pamenter RW, Boyden TW (1985) One year of ethanol feeding increases circulating thyroid hormones in the dog. J Lab Clin Med 106: 141–146

227. Parvinen M (1982) Regulation of the seminiferous epithelium. Endo Rev 3: 404–417

228. Payet N, Lehoux J (1982) Effect of ACTH or zinc treatment on plasma aldosterone and corticosterone levels and on the *in vitro* steroid output from adrenocortical cells. Can J Biochem 60: 1058–1064

229. Peng T, Garner SC (1979) Hypercalcitoninemia associated with return of serum calcium concentration toward normal in chronically parathyroidectomized rats. Endocrinology 104: 1624–1630

230. Peng T, Garner SC (1980) Sex difference in serum calcitonin in rats as related to feeding, fasting and age. Endocrinology 107: 289–293

231. Pepe GJ, Albrecht ED (1985) The effects of cortisone on the interconversion of cortisol and cortisone in the baboon. J Steroid Biochem 23: 275–278

232. Peterson ME, Gilbertson SR, Drucker WD (1982) Plasma cortisol response to exogenous ACTH in 22 dogs with hyperadenocorticism caused by adrenocortical neoplasia. J Am Vet Med Assoc 180: 542–544

233. Peterson ME, Orth DN, Halmi NS, Zielinsky AC, Davis DR, Chavez FT, Drucker WD (1986) Plasma immunoreactive proopiomelanocortin peptides and cortisol in normal dogs and dogs with Addison's disease and Cushing's syndrome: Basal concentrations. Endocrinology 119: 720–730

234. Plant TM (1981) Time courses of concentrations of circulating gonadotropin, prolactin, testosterone and cortisol in adult male rhesus monkeys (*Macaca mulatta*) throughout the 24 h light-dark cycle. Biol Reprod 25: 244–252

235. Plant TM (1982) Effects of orchidectomy and testosterone replacement on pulsatile luteinizing hormone secretion in the adult rhesus monkey (*Macaca mulatta*). Endocrinology 110: 1905–1913

236. Popper CW, Chiueh CC, Kopin JJ (1978) Plasma catecholamine concentrations in unanesthetized rats during sleep, wakefulness, immobilization and after decapitation. J Pharmacol Exper Therap 202: 144–148

237. Portman OW, Alexander M, Neuringer M (1985) Dietary protein effects on lipoproteins and on sex and thyroid hormones in blood of rhesus monkeys. J Nutr 115: 425–435

238. Potter CL, Sipes G, Russel DH (1983) Hypothyroxemia and hypothermia in rats in response to 2,3,7,8 tetrachlorodibenzo-p-dioxin administration. Toxicol Appl Pharm 69: 89–95

239. Pradier P, Davico MJ, Safwate A, Tournaire C, Dalle M, Barlet JP, Delost P (1986) Plasma adrenocorticotropin, cortisol, and aldosterone responses to ovine corticotrophin-releasing factor and vasopressin in sheep. Acta Endocrinol 111: 93–100

240. Quabbe H-J, Gregor M, Bumke-Yogt C, Eckhof A, Witt I (1981) Twenty-four hour pattern of growth

hormone secretion in the rhesus monkey: Studies including alterations of the sleep/wake and sleep stage cycles. Endocrinology 109: 513–522

241. Quabbe H, Gregor M, Bumke-Vogt C, Harbel C (1982) Pattern of plasma cortisol during the 24-hour sleep/wake cycle in the rhesus monkey. Endocrinology 110: 1641–1645

242. Quabbe H-J, Kroll M, Thomsen P (1983) Dissociation of light onset and wake onset: Effect on rhesus monkey growth hormone secretion. Endocrinology 112: 1828–1831

243. Quadri SK, Spies HG (1976) Cyclic and diurnal patterns of serum prolactin in the rhesus monkey. Biol Reprod 14: 495–501

244. Quillen EWJ, Cowley AW Jr (1983) Influence of volume changes on osmolality-vasopressin relationship in conscious dogs. Am J Physiol 244: H73–H79

245. Quimby FW Personal communication

246. Quinlan WJ, Michaelson S (1981) Homologous radioimmunoassay for canine thyrotropin: Response of normal and X-irradiated dogs to propylthiouracil. Endocrinology 108: 937–942

247. Raff H, Shinsako J, Keil LC, Dallman MF (1983) Vasopressin, ACTH, corticosteriods during hypercapnia and graded hypoxia in dogs. Am J Physiol 244: E453–E458

248. Rayssignier Y, Thomasset M, Garel J, Barlet J (1982) Plasma parathyroid hormone levels and intestinal calcium binding protein in magnesium deficient rats. Horm Metab Res 14: 379–382

249. Redekopp C, Irvine CHG, Donald RA, Livesey JH, Sadler W, Nicholls MG, Alexander SL, Evans MJ (1986) Spontaneous and stimulated adrenocorticotropin and vasopressin pulsatile secretion in the pituitary venous effluent of the horse. Endocrinology 118: 1410–1416

250. Refetoff S, Robin NI, Fang VS (1970) Parameters of thyroid function in serum of 16 selected vertebrate species: A study of PBI, serum T_4, free T_4 and the pattern of T_4 and T_3 binding to serum proteins. Endocrinology 86: 793–805

251. Reimers TJ, Cowan BA, Davidson HP, Colby ED (1981) Validation of radioimmunoassay for triiodothyronine, thyroxine and hydrocortisone (cortisol) in canine, feline and equine sera. Am J Vet Res 42: 2016–2020

252. Resko JA, Jackson GL, Huchkins C, Stadelman H, Spies HG (1980) Cryptorchid rhesus macaques: long term studies on changes in gonadotropins and gonadal steroids. Endocrinology 107: 1127–1136

253. Richards JS, Ireland JJ, Rao MC, Bernath GA, Midgley AR Jr, Reichert LE Jr (1976) Ovarian follicular development in the rat: Hormone receptor regulation by estradiol, follicle stimulating hormone and luteinizing hormone. Endocrinology 99: 1562–1570

254. Ridley K, Greewald GS (1975) Progesterone levels measured every two hours in the cyclic hamster. Proc Soc Exp Biol Med 149: 10–12

255. Rijnbek A, der Kinderen PJ, Thijssen JHH (1968) Investigations on the adrenocortical function of normal dogs. J Endocrinol 41: 387–395

256. Rivier C, Rivier J, Vale W (1986) Inhibin-mediated feedback control of follicle-stimulating hormone secretion in the female rat. Science 234: 205–207

257. Robinson ICAF, Jones PM (1982) Oxytocin and neurophysin in plasma and CSF during suckling in the guinea pig. Neuroendocrinology 34: 59–63

258. Rockhold R, Crofton JT, Wang BC, Share L (1983) Effect of intracarotid administration of morphine and naloxone on plasma vasopressin levels and blood pressure in the dog. J Pharm Exper Ther 224: 386–390

259. Roos BA, Cooper CW, Frelinger AL, Deftos LJ (1978) Acute and chronic fluctuations of immunoreactive and biologically active plasma calcitonin in the rat. Endocrinology 103: 2180–2186

260. Rothwell NJ, Saville ME, Stock JF (1982) Sympathetic and thyroid influences on metabolic rate in fed, fasted and refed rats. Am J Physiol 243: R339–R346

261. Rush ME, Blake CA (1982) Serum testosterone concentrations during the 4-day estrous cycle in normal and adrenalectomized rats. Proc Soc Exp Biol Med 169: 216–221

262. Ryan KD, Schwartz ND (1980) Changes in serum hormone levels associated with male-induced ovulation in group-housed adult female mice. Endocrinology 106: 959–966

263. Saunders A, Terry LC, Audet J, Brazeau P, Martin JB (1976) Dynamic studies of growth hormone and prolactin secretion in the female rat. Neuroendocrinology 21: 193–203

264. Schams D (1983) Oxytocin determination by radioimmunoassay. III. Improvement to subpicogram sensitivity and application to blood levels in cyclic cattle. Acta Endocrinol 103: 180–183

265. Schams D, Baumann G, Leidl W (1982) Oxytocin determination by radioimmunoassay in cattle. III. Effect of mating and stimulation of the genital tract in bulls, cows and heifers. Acta Endocrinol 99: 218–213

266. Schams D, Lahlou-Kassi A, Glatzel P (1982) Oxytocin concentrations in peripheral blood during the oestrous cycle and after ovariectomy in two breeds of sheep with low and high fecundity. J Endocrinol 92: 9–13

267. Scheving LE, Tsai TH, Powell EW, Pasley JN, Halberg F, Dunn J (1983) Bilateral lesions of suprachiasmatic nuclei affect circadian rhythms in ^{3}H-thymidine incorporation into deoxyribonucleic acid in mouse intestinal tract, mitotic index of corneal epithelium and serum corticosterone. Anat Rec 205: 239–249

268. Schindler WJ, Hutchins MO, Laird CW, Fox RR (1974) Effect of strain and sex variation on growth hormone in rabbit serum. Proc Soc Exp Biol Med 147: 820–822

269. Scott IM, Johnson HD, Hahn GL (1983) Effect of programmed diurnal temperature cycles on plasma thyroxine level, body temperature, and feed intake of Holstein dairy cows. Int J Biometeo 27: 47–62

270. Seggie J, Shaw B, Uhlir I, Brown GM (1974) Baseline 24-hour plasma corticosterone rhythm in normal, sham-operated and septally lesioned rats. Neuroendocrinology 15: 51–61

271. Sequeira RP, Raghaven KS, Chaudhury RR (1980) Development and validation of radioimmunoassay of antidiuretic hormone in plasma. Indian J Med Res 72: 365–373

272. Shade RE, Share L (1975) Volume control of plasma antidiuretic hormone concentration following acute blood volume expansion in the anesthetized dog. Endocrinology 97: 1048–1057

273. Sharp SE, Phares CK, Heidrick ML (1982) Immunological aspects associated with suppression of hormone levels in rats infected with pleroceroids of Spirometra mansonoide (cestoda). J Parisitol 68: 993–998

274. Sheldrick EL, Flint APF (1981) Circulating concentrations of oxytocin during the estrous cycle and early pregnancy in sheep. Prostaglandins 22: 631–636

275. Shillo KK, Hansen PJ, Kamwanja LA, Dierschke DJ, Hauser ER (1983) Influence of season sexual development in heifers: Age at puberty as related to growth and serum concentrations of gonadotropins, prolactin, thyroxine and progesterone. Biol Reprod 28: 329–341

276. Shin SH, Chi HJ (1979) Unsuppressed prolactin secretion in the male rat is pulsatile. Neuroendocrinology 28: 73–81

277. Sisk CL, Turek FW (1983) Developmental time course of pubertal and photoperiodic changes in testosterone negative feedback on gonadotropin secretion in the golden hamster. Endocrinology 112: 1208–1216

278. Sladek CD, McNeill TH, Gregg CM, Blair ML, Boggs RB (1981) Vasopressin and renin response to dehydration in aged rats. Neurobiol Aging 2: 293–302

279. Smallridge RC, Glass AR, Wartofsky L, Latham KR, Burman KD (1982) Investigations into the etiology of elevated serum T_3 levels in protein-malnourished rats. Metabolism 31: 538–542

280. Smith MS, Freeman ME, Neill J (1975) The control of progesterone secretion during the estrous cycle and early pseudopregnancy in the rat: Prolactin, gonadotropin and steroid levels associated with rescue of the corpus luteum of pseudopregnancy. Endocrinology 96: 219–226

281. Sowers JR, Eggena P, Phillips D (1982) Effect of metoclopramide and domperidone on aldosterone, 18-hydroxycorticosterone and prolactin secretion in the rhesus monkey. Metabolism 31: 1219–1223

282. Sowers JR, Sharp B, Levin ER, Golub MS, Eggena P (1981) Metoclopramide, a dopamine antagonist, stimulates aldosterone secretion in rhesus monkey but not in dogs or rabbits. Life Sci 29: 2171–2175

283. Sowers JR, Sollars E, Nyby MD, Josberg K, Tuck ML (1981) Hypereninemic hypoaldosteronism in association with neoplasia induced hypercalcemia in the Fischer rat. Metabolism 30: 987–991

284. Spiegel AM, Saxe AW, Deftos LJ, Brennan MF (1983) Humoral hypercalcemia caused by a rat Leydig-cell tumor is associated with suppressed parathyroid hormone secretion and increased urinary cAMP excretion. Horm Metab Res 15: 299–304

285. Spies HG, Norman R, Buhl AE (1979) Twenty-four hour patterns in serum prolactin and cortisol after partial and complete isolation of the hypothalamic-pituitary unit in rhesus monkeys. Endocrinology 105: 1361–1368

286. Stewart AD, Batty J, Harkiss GD (1978) Genetic variation in plasma thyroxine levels and minimal metabolic rates of mouse, Mus musculus. Gen Res 31: 303–306

287. Stoneham MD, Everitt BJ, Hansen S, Lightman SL, Todd K (1985) Oxytocin and sexual behavior in the male rat and rabbit. J Endocrinol 107: 97–106

288. Summy-Long JY, Rosella LM, Keil LC (1981) Effects of centrally administered endogenous opioid peptides on drinking behavior, increased plasma vasopressin concentration and pressor response to hypertonic sodium chloride. Brain Res 221: 343–357

289. Stanton ME, Patterson JM, Levine S (1985) Social influences on conditioned cortisol secretion in the squirrel monkey. Psychoneuroendocrinology 10: 125–134

290. Suzuki Y, Kito K, Uchigata Y, Takata I, Sato T (1982) Maturation of renal and hepatic mono-deiodination of thyroxine to triiodothyronine and postnatal changes of serum thyroid hormones in young rats. Acta Endocrinol 99: 540–546

291. Takagi A, Isozaki Y, Kurata K, Nagataki S (1978) Serum concentrations, metabolic clearance rates, and production rate of reverse triiodothyronine, triiodothyronine and thyroxine in starved rabbits. Endocrinology 103: 1434–1439

292. Takahashi Y, Ebihara S, Nakamura Y, Takahashi K (1981) A model of human sleep-related growth hormone secretion in dogs: Effects of 3, 6, and 12 hours of forced wakefulness on plasma growth hormone, cortisol and sleep stages. Endocrinology 109: 262–272

293. Talmage RV, Doppelt SH, Cooper CW (1975) Relationship of blood concentrations of calcium, phosphate, gastrin and calcitonin to the onset of feeding in the rat. Proc Soc Exp Biol Med 149: 855–859

294. Tang F (1985) Effect of sex and age on serum aldosterone and thyroid hormones in the laboratory rat. Horm Metab Res 17: 507–509

295. Tannenbaum GS, Martin JB (1976) Evidence for an endogenous ultradian rhythm governing growth hormone secretion in the rat. Endocrinology 98: 562–570

296. Tapp WN, Levin BE, Natelson BH (1981) Ultradian rhythm of plasma norepinephrine in rats. Endocrinology 109: 1781–1783

297. Taya K, Igarashi M (1974) Circadian rhythms in serum LH, FSH and prolactin levels in adult male rats. Endocrinol Japon 21: 211–215

298. Terasawa E, Rodriguez JS, Bridson WE, Wiegand SJ (1979) Factors influencing the positive feedback action of estrogen upon the luteinizing hormone surge in the ovariectomized guinea pig. Endocrinology 104: 680–686

299. Thomas CL, Adams JC (1978) Radioimmunoassay of equine serum for thyroxine: Reference values. Am J Vet Res 39: 1239

300. Thomas ML, Forte LR (1982) Serum calcium and parathyroid hormone during the reproductive cycle in normal and vitamin D-deficient rats. Endocrinology 110: 703–707

301. Tobler I, Murison R, Ursin H, Brobely H (1983)

The effect of sleep deprivation and recovery sleep on plasma corticosterone in the rat. Neurosci Letts 35: 297–300

302. Topel DG, Weiss GM, Siers DG, Magilton JH (1973) Comparison of blood source and diurnal variation on blood hydrocortisone, growth hormone, lactate, glucose and electrolytes in swine. J An Sci 36: 531–534

303. Trechsel U, Eisman JA, Fischer JA, Bonjour J, Fleisch H (1980) Calcium-dependent, parathyroid hormone-independent regulation of 1,25 dihydroxyvitamin D. Am J Physiol 239: E119–E124

304. Tveit B, Almlid T (1980) T_4 degradation rate and plasma levels of TSH and thyroid hormones in ten young bulls during feeding conditions and 48 hr of starvation. Acta Endocrinol 93: 435–439

305. Udeschini G (1982) Effect of cold and glucoprivation on TSH and T_4 release in normothermic and hyperthermic rats. Pharm Res Comms 14: 711–718

306. Urman S, Critchlow V (1983) Long term elevations in plasma thyrotropin, but not growth hormone, concentrations associated with lesion-induced depletion of median eminence somatostatin. Endocrinology 112: 659–664

307. Uvnas-Mobert K, Stock S, Erikson M, Linden A, Einarrson S, Kunavongkrit A (1985) Plasma levels of oxytocin increase in response to suckling and feeding in dogs and sows. Acta Physiol Scand 124: 391–398

308. Uvnas Wallensten K, Goiny M, Oriowo MA, Cekan S (1981) Effects of apomorphine and haloperidol on plasma cortisol levels in conscious dogs. Acta Physiol Scand 112: 253–256

309. Valk TW, Taylor RE Jr, Barker SB (1975) Production and measurement of exopthalamus-producing factor in guinea pigs. Endocrinology 96: 151–169

310. Valtorta S, Hahn L, Johnson HD (1982) Effect of high ambient temperature (35 C) and feed intake on plasma T_4 levels in sheep. Proc Soc Exp Biol Med 169: 260–265

311. Van Houten M, Rizzo AJ, Goltzman D, Posner BI (1982) Brain receptors for blood-borne calcitonin in rats: Circumventricular localization and vasopressin-resistant deficiency in hereditary diabetes insipidus. Endocrinology 111: 1704–1710

312. Van Loon GR, Appel NM (1981) Plasma norepinephrine, epinephrine and dopamine responses to intracerebral administration of a metenkephalin analog D-ala²-met-enkephalinamide in rats. Neuroendocrinology 33: 153–157

313. Vaughan GM, Shirani KZ, Vaughan MK, Pruitt BA Jr, Masson AD Jr (1985) Hormonal changes in burned hamsters. Endocrinology 117: 1090–1095

314. Vaughan MK, Powanda MC, Richardson BA, King TS, Johnson LY, Reiter RJ (1982) Chronic exposure to short photoperiod inhibits free thyroxine index and plasma levels of TSH, T_4, triiodothyronine (T_3) and cholesterol in female Syrian hamsters. Comp Biochem Physiol 71A: 615–618

315. Vaughan MK, Richardson BA, Craft CM, Powanda MC, Reiter RJ (1982) Interaction of aging, photoperiod, and melatonin on plasma thyroid hormones and cholesterol levels in female Syrian hamsters (Mesocricetus armatus). Gerontology 28: 345–353

316. Vaughan MK, Richardson BA, Johnson LY, Petterborg LJ, Powanda MC, Reiter RJ, Smith I (1983) Natural and synthetic analogues of melatonin and related compounds. II. Effects on plasma thyroid hormones and cholesterol levels in male Syrian hamsters. J Neurol Trans 56: 279–291

317. Verhage HG, Beamer NB, Brenner RM (1976) Plasma levels of estradiol and progesterone in the rat during polyestrus, pregnancy and pseudopregnancy. Biol Reprod 14: 579–585

318. Vernay M, Marty J, Moalti J (1984) Absorption of electrolytes and volatile fatty acid in the hind-gut of the rabbit. Circadian rhythm of hind-gut electrolytes and plasma aldosterone. Brit J Nutr 52: 419–428

319. Vogel WH, Miller J, DeTurck KH, Routzalin BK Jr (1984) Effects of psychoactive drugs on plasma catecholamines during stress in rats. Neuropharma 23: 1105–1108

320. Vomachka AJ, Greenwald GS (1979) The development of gonadotropin and steroid hormone patterns in male and female hamsters from birth to puberty. Endocrinology 105: 960–966

321. Wade CE, Bie P, Keil C, Ramsay DJ (1982) Osmotic control of plasma vasopressin in the dog. Am J Physiol 243: E287–E292

322. Wade CE, Bie P, Keil C, Ramsay J (1982) Effect of hypertonic intracarotid infusions on plasma vasopressin concentration. Am J Physiol 243: E522–E526

323. Walker P, Dubois JD, Dussault JH (1980) Free thyroid hormone concentrations during postnatal development in the rat. Pediat Res 14: 247–249

324. Walker P, Weichsel ME Jr, Eveleth D, Disher DA (1982) Ontogenesis of nerve growth factor and epidermal growth factor in submaxillary glands and nerve growth factor in brains of immature male mice: Correlation with ontogenesis of serum levels of thyroid hormones. Pediat Res 16: 520–524

325. Wang BC, Share L, Crofton JT (1982) Central infusion of vasopressin decreased plasma vasopressin concentration in dogs. Am J Physiol 243: E365–E369

326. Wang BC, Share L, Crofton JT, Kimura T (1981) Changes in vasopressin concentration in plasma and cerebrospinal fluid in response to hemorrhage in anesthetized dogs. Neuroendocrinology 33: 61–66

327. Webb R, Mitchell MD, Falconer J, Robinson IS (1981) Temporal relationships between peripheral plasma concentrations of oxytocin, progesterone and 13,14 dihydro-15-keto-prostaglandin F_2 during the oestrus cycle and early pregnancy in the ewe. Prostaglandins 22: 443–453

328. Weick BG, Ritter S, McCarty R (1983) Plasma catecholamines in fasted and sucrose supplemented rats. Physiol Behav 30: 247–252

329. Weick RF, Dierschke DJ, Karsch FJ, Butler WR, Hotchkiss J, Knobil E (1973) Periovulatory time courses of circulating gonadotropic and ovarian hormones in the rhesus monkey. Endocrinology 93: 1140–1147

330. Weitzman RE, Fisher DA (1977) Log linear relationship between plasma arginine vasopressin and plasma osmolality. Am J Physiol 233: E37–E40

331. Weitzman RE, Reviczky A, Oddie TH, Fischer DA (1980) Effect of osmolality on arginine vasopressin and renin release after hemorrhage. Am J Physiol 238: E62–E68

332. Wilkinson CW, Shinsako T, Dallman MF (1981) Return of pituitary-adrenal function after adrenal enucleation or transplantation: Diurnal rhythms and responses to ether. Endocrinology 109: 162–169

333. Williams CH, Dozier SE, Buzello W (1985) Plasma levels of norepinephrine and epinephrine during malignant hyperthermia in susceptible pigs. J Chrom 344: 71–80

334. Wilson MF, Brackett DJ, Hinshaw LB, Tompkins P, Archer LT, Benjamin BA (1981) Vasopressin release during sepsis and septic shock in baboons and dogs. Surg Gynecol Obstet 153: 869–872

335. Wittenberg C, Chosniak I, Shkolnik A, Thurau K, Rosenfeld J (1986) Effect of dehydration and rapid rehydration on renal function and on plasma renin and aldosterone levels in the black Bedouin goat. Pflugers Arch 406: 405–408

336. Wong C, Dohler KD. Atkinson MJ, Geerlings H, Hesch R, von zur Muhlen A (1983) Influence of age, strain and season on diurnal periodicity of thyroid stimulating hormone, thyroxine, triiodothyronine and parathyroid hormone in the serum of male laboratory rats. Acta Endocrinol 102: 377–385

337. Wood CE, Shinsako J, Keil LC, Ramsey DJ, Dallman MF (1981) Hormonal and hemodynamic responses to 15 ml/kg hemorrhage in conscious dogs: Responses correlate to body temperature. Proc Soc Exp Biol Med 167: 15–19

338. Wostmann BS, Bruckner-Kardoss E, Pleasants JR (1982) Oxygen consumption and thyroid hormones in germ free mice fed glucose-amino acid liquid diet. J Nutr 112: 552–559

339. Yen JT, Pond WG (1985) Plasma thyroid hormones, growth and carcass measurements of genetically obese and lean pigs as influenced by thyroprotein supplementation. J An Sci 61: 566–572

340. Yen SSC, Jaffe RB (eds), Reproductive Endocrinology: Physiology, Pathophysiology and Clinical Management. WB Saunders, Philadelphia

341. Yodyingyuad U, DeLaRiva C, Abbot DH, Herbert J, Keverne EB (1985) Relationship between dominance hierarchy, cerebrospinal fluid levels of amino transmitter metabolite (5-hydroxyindole acetic acid and homovanillic acid) and plasma cortisol in monkeys. Neuroscience 16: 851–858

342. Young MA, Hintze TH, Vatner SF (1985) Correlation between cardiac performance and plasma catecholamine levels in conscious dogs. Am J Physiol 248: H82–H88

343. Zubrow AB, Daniel SS, Stark RI, Husain MK, James LS (1983) Plasma renin, catecholamines, and vasopressin during nitroprusside-induced hypotension in ewes. Anesthesiology 58: 245–249

13

Liver Function Tests
Bilirubin, Exogenous Dyes, and Urobilinogen

SAMUEL KRUCKENBERG, DVM, PhD and RANDY KIDD, DVM, PhD

Medical scientists are in a continuing search for laboratory tests that provide meaningful information about the status of the liver. Over 100 tests have been developed to estimate liver function in man and animals (14). The numerous functions of the liver and their measurement demonstrate its complex nature. To date no single test has been identified that reflects the functional and morphologic status of the liver. A battery of tests is necessary to assess liver function and often these tests are supplemented by histopathologic studies. Included in these tests are the cholephilic dyes and bilirubin. The use of a battery of liver function tests will aid in the detection of both primary and secondary hepatic disorders; the differentiation of the type of icterus or anemia; the prognostication of the disorder; and investigation of the metabolic observations occurring in specific studies. No single test can be relied upon to differentiate totally the various forms of icterus in animals: prehepatic or hemolytic, hepatocellular and obstructive. Various attempts to relate func-

tional failure to structural changes have been disappointing because more than one anatomic unit of the liver can be involved: parenchymal mass; canalicular, cholangiolar, and extrahepatic biliary system; vascular system; and the reticuloendothelial system.

The intent of this chapter is to present a brief introduction to the measurement of hepatic function in animals as reflected by bilirubin levels in health and disease, to describe the use of the cholephilic dyes sulfobromophthalein (BSP) and indocyanine green (ICG) as liver function tests in animals, and to provide selected references on liver function test in various species.

SULFOBROMOPHTHALEIN

Sulfobromophthalein is one of several phthalein dyes that are eliminated almost exclusively by the liver (7). The rate of BSP removal after its intravenous administration has been widely used in clinical studies of liver disease. An extensive review of the excretion of cholephilic dyes

309

was published (24) which covered the historical aspects, metabolism, physiologic factors, drugs, and diseases that influence the uptake and secretion of the cholephilic dyes as well as analytic methods. Sulfobromophthalein and ICG are the most commonly used cholephilic dyes. Sulfobromophthalein clearance and retention values for various nonhuman primates and for laboratory and domestic animals may be found in the appendix. Cornelius (16) reported that the sensitivity of the BSP test may be affected by fever and competition for excretion by cholates and bilirubin. Many drugs give falsely elevated readings. Fever, shock, and dehydration may also cause false evaluations. Icteric states prevent interpretation of the test. Sulfobromophthalein cannot be used in the differential diagnosis of jaundice because the mechanical effects of biliary obstruction automatically produce retention, and alkaline serum samples containing bile pigments exhibit a red color that prevents the quantitative estimation of BSP (23). Approximately 55 per cent of the functional mass of liver is lost before BSP retention or reduced clearance occurs. The principal lesions that cause this are atrophy and fibrosis (19).

Jablonski and Owen (29) published the preferred names, synonyms, preferred symbols, formulas, or equations used for uptake of dyes from plasma. Fractional disappearance rate (FDR) is the preferred name for fractional clearance or clearance coefficient, logarithmic disappearance rate is the preferred name for clearance coefficient or elimination constant, and half-life is the preferred name for T1/2.

A dose of BSP is given intravenously and the percentage of the dose remaining in the plasma at a given time after the injection is determined (BSP retention test). Tests with multiple samples have been termed "fractional BSP tests." In calculating BSP retention it is necessary to assume the plasma volume to be a constant number of milliliters per kilogram of body weight for that species. In man it is usually assumed that the plasma volume is equal to 50 ml per kilogram of body weight (24). In man an initial dose of 5 mg/kg is taken to give zero-time concentration of 10 mg/dl, so that the percentage of BSP remaining in the plasma is obtained by multiplying the plasma concentration at the given time by 10.

Two methods of conducting the BSP test in animals have been used; *retention*, which is the percentage of BSP remaining in the circulation after a stated number of minutes as compared to the concentration of BSP at time zero, and the T1/2 which is the time required for the serum concentration of BSP to be reduced by one half. A simplified, single sampling retention method in which the BSP concentration is measured at a prescribed time following the administration of a standard dose has been proposed (20).

The clearance method or half-life (T1/2) method of conducting the BSP test requires two or more blood samples. Both samples must be collected during the exponential phase of dye excretion following the uniform mixing of the dye in the plasma. The half-time (T1/2) is calculated by plotting the BSP concentration (log concentration mg/dl) against the time in minutes when the sample was taken. The T1/2 is the time taken to reduce an original concentration to 50 per cent of its value (16).

Cornelius (16) recommends taking several blood samples during the first 15 to 45 minutes, plotting the concentration against time on semi-log graph paper, selecting the exponential phase, and using the resultant slope to calculate the percentage of BSP removed per minute (fractional clearance). In the horse, 1 g of BSP is injected intravenously. Two blood samples are taken at 4-minute intervals between 5 and 9 or 6 and 10 minutes following administration of BSP. The average T1/2 for the horse is 2.8 minutes.

Dog

The BSP test is superior to many other liver function tests in the dog (14). In the dog, the retention test is the most commonly used (23). Five mg/kg are given intravenously and a blood sample is obtained 30 minutes later. Less than 5 per cent retention is normal.

Center et al (11) compared BSP and ICG clearances in the dog. The dosage was 5 mg/kg intravenously for BSP and 1.0 and 1.5 mg/kg for ICG. The half-life of BSP was 4.2 minutes; for ICG it was 9.0 and 8.4 minutes using doses of 1.0 and 1.5 mg/kg, respectively. The disappearance rate (percentage per minute) of BSP was 17.0; for ICG at the 1.0 mg/kg dose level, it was 8.1, and at the 1.5 mg/kg dose level, 8.7. The clearance (ml/min/kg) of BSP was 15.4; for ICG at 1.0 mg/kg, it was 3.7, and for the 1.5

mg/kg dose level, 3.9. The 30-minute retention for BSP was 1.9; for ICG at the 1.0 mg/kg dose level, it was 14.7 and for the 1.5 mg/kg dose level, 11.4. (See the Appendix for additional values and references on the BSP and ICG tests in dogs.)

Cats

Duncan and Prasse (19) recommended that cats as well as dogs be given 5 mg of BSP per kilogram body weight. A blood sample is obtained 30 minutes later and the retention determined. Center et al (12) also compared BSP and ICG clearances in the cat using a BSP dosage of 5 mg/kg of body weight intravenously and in ICG dosage of 1.5 mg per kilogram of body weight. The half-life of BSP was 2.2 minutes and of ICG 3.8 minutes. The disappearance rate (percentage per minute) of BSP was 34.7 and of ICG 19.2. The clearance of BSP was 26.3 ml/m/kg and of ICg 8.6 ml/m/kg. The 30-minute percentage retention for BSP was 0.6 and for ICG 7.3

Nonhuman Primates

The Appendix gives the BSP retention and clearance values for various nonhuman primates. Half-life values of BSP in newborn and 5-day-old *Macaca mulatta* and Alouatta monkeys are given. In chimpanzees a dose of 5 mg/kg is administered intravenously, and approximately 20 per cent retention is noted at 10 minutes; 5 per cent at 20 minutes, and none at 30 minutes in healthy animals. In rhesus monkeys the same dose usually results in less than 1 per cent retention at 30 minutes (range 0 to 9 per cent) (36). Table 13.1 illustrates the effects of disease on BSP tests in nonhuman primates.

Rat

Brauer and Pessotti (7) measured BSP removal both in vivo and in vitro Sprague-Dawley rats. Plasma BSP concentrations in male and female rats were determined 10 minutes after the intravenous administration of BSP (50 mg/kg of body weight). The mean values were 18.4 (SD = 1.1) in the male and 36.5 (SD = 2.9) in the female against a standard of 750 mg BSP per liter of plasma assigned a value of 100. Pretreatment of the rats with India ink or carbon tetrachloride significantly increased the con-

centration of BSP remaining at 10 minutes. The BSP clearance coefficient was 0.091 in 9-week-old rats and 0.133 in 24-week-old rats, the difference being statistically significant. See the Appendix for additional values and references on rats.

Mouse

Kutob and Plaa (31) administered 100 mg of BSP per kilogram intravenously in mice and took blood samples at 15 minutes. The T1/2 for BSP was slightly over 15 minutes. Casals and Olitsky (10) administered 50 mg/kg intraperitoneally in mice and determined plasma concentrations of 0.46 mg/dl at 30 minutes, Williams et al (46) reported a retention of 6.5 per cent at 30 minutes after administering 50 mg/kg intravenously.

Rabbit

Klaassen and Plaa (28) administered BSP in rabbits at 30, 60, and 120 mg/kg of body weight. At 32 minutes the plasma concentrations were 1, 2, and 20 mg/dl, respectively. The overall rate of disappearance of BSP from the blood was 1.8 mg/min per kilogram in the rabbit. The rabbit, like the rat, has a remarkable ability to clear the plasma of BSP when compared to the dog. Comparable degrees of BSP retention in plasma are seen when 60 mg/kg are given intravenously to rats, 60 mg/kg to rabbits, and 15 mg/kg to dogs (28).

INDOCYANINE GREEN

Indocyanine green (Cardio-Green®) is a sensitive test for qualitative and quantitative evaluation of liver function. Half-life increases with increasing dosage. Although unstable in aqueous solution before injection, the dye is stable in plasma and whole blood, permitting later analysis. Indocyanine green is excreted in the bile in the unconjugated form. The Appendix summarizes the literature on ICG, giving the dose of idocyanine green, half-life in minutes, disappearance rate in percentage per minute, clearances in milliliters per minute per kilogram, and 30-minute percentage retention of various laboratory animals.

Table 13.1. Effects of Disease on the BSP Test in Nonhuman Primates

Species	Dose Level (mg/kg)	Percentage of Retention	Condition	Reference No.
Chimpanzee	5	2–8% in 20 min	Normal	18
Chimpanzee	5	0–3% in 40 min	Normal	18
Chimpanzee	5	Up to 43% in 20 min	Hepatitis	18
Chimpanzee	5	Up to 15% in 40 min	Hepatitis	18
Chimpanzee	5	4.7% in 20 min	Normal	46
M mulatta	5	0.9–3.1% in 45 min	Normal	21
M mulatta	5	3.7–8.9% in 45 min	Cirrhosis	21
M mulatta	5	21–46% in 45 min	Cirrhosis	21
M mulatta	5	0.7% in 30 min	Normal	25
M mulatta	5	2.95% in 45 min	Normal	8
M mulatta	5	17.6% in 30 min	Normal	2
M mulatta	5	5% in 30 min	Normal	1
M mulatta	5	35–65% in 30 min	Veno-occlusive	1
M mulatta	5	4.7% in 45 min	Normal	47
M mulatta	5	7.2% in 30 min	Anesthetized	47
M mulatta	5	0–10% in 30 min	Normal	41
M mulatta	5	Up to 80% in 30 min	Yellow fever	41
M mulatta	5	0.25% in 30 min	Normal	9
M mulatta	5	4.77% in 30 min	Schistosomiasis	9
M mulatta (M)	5	1.61% in 30 min	Normal	33
M mulatta (F)	5	1.71% in 30 min	Normal	33
M mulatta		0.70% in 30 min	Normal	34

Dog and Cat

Bonasch and Cornelius (6) published equations for calculating fractional clearance (average rate of plasma removal per minute expressed as a percentage removed per minute or K), T1/2 (half-time value), volume of distribution (plasma volume in milliliters), extraction ratio, and estimated hepatic plasma flow (ml/min). They also plotted dye concentrations (mg/dl) on graph paper with semilogarithmic coordinates and calculated the half-time (T1/2) values. All of their work was performed in dogs given ICG intravenously at a dose schedule of 0.5 mg/kg of body weight.

Center et al (11,12) did extensive studies on ICG in dogs and cats. These results are given in the Appendix and were already discussed with their results of BSP on a comparative basis.

In dogs with bile duct obstruction, Van Vleet and Albert (39) observed impaired ICG clearance with T1/2 values of up to 54.7 minutes. The administration of carbon tetrachloride resulted in ICG half-time of up to 19.95 minutes.

Nonhuman Primates

The plasma clearance of ICG in rhesus monkeys was determined by Vogin et al (41). Half-life values for ICG plasma disappearance in females averaged 1.9 minutes (fractional clearance, 36.5 per cent per minute). In male monkeys, half-life values were 1.3 minutes (fractional clearance 52.9 per cent per minute). The slopes of the clearance curves were observed to be exponentially linear throughout a sampling period of 12 minutes. Pentobarbital anesthesia delayed clearance, possibly by lowering the body temperature. The biliary recovery of ICG was complete by 5 hours after injection with maximal excretion within 2 hours. The arteriohepatic-venous extraction ratio of dye ranged from 21 to 41.

An exponentially linear plasma clearance curve was found in monkeys (164) and dogs (6,30,40,45). More than 96 per cent of the ICG injected into monkeys was recovered in the bile.

In rhesus monkeys that had been anesthetized with pentobarbital sodium, the half-life was 4.8 minutes and for unanesthetized monkeys it was 1.9 minutes. The dosage for monkeys in both groups was 0.5 mg/kg.

Rat and Rabbit

Rats and rabbits have a curvilinear plasma clearance curve (25). Klaassen and Plaa (29) compared the plasma disappearance and biliary excretion of ICG in rats, rabbits, and dogs. Over a 32-minute period, the rate of disappearance was exponential in all three species, and the half-life increased with increasing doses of ICG. Rats were given either 4, 8, 16, 32, or 64 mg/kg; rabbits 8, 16, or 32 mg/kg; and dogs 1, 2, or 4 mg/kg intravenously. The results are given in the Appendix.

Mouse

The dosage of ICG for mice is 10 mg/kg with a half-life of less than 6.0 minutes (36).

BILIRUBIN

Bilirubin is formed when hemoglobin is metabolized by the reticuloendothelial system. Bilirubin is protein bound in the plasma and conjugated in the liver. The complete mechanism by which bilirubin is metabolized by the liver involves at least three processes: the uptake of bilirubin from plasma by the liver cell; the conjugation of bilirubin, primarily with glucoronic acid; and the excretion of conjugated bilirubin into the bile. The physiologic limitations of each of these processes in effecting the normal metabolism of bilirubin by the liver are not known. Hepatic clearance of bilirubin is affected by various factors in the bloodstream, including albumin concentration (7,13), bilirubin binding to erythrocytes (5), and the presence of salicylate, which increases the proportion of nonalbumin-bound bilirubin (4). Bilirubin enters the liver after it is unbound from albumin. It is likely that the affinity for bilirubin resides in the plasma membrane of hepatocytes; however, specific receptor proteins in cytoplasm have been implicated. Increased glucuronyl transferase activity and accelerated clearance of various organic anions have been found after phenobarbital treatment of rats (27). Normally, the rate of hepatic bilirubin uptake is determined by the rate of biliary excretion. Bilirubin is conjugated in the liver mainly with glucuronic acid and to a lesser extent with sulfate and other substances (3). Van den Bergh (32) exposed sera to diazo dyes and found that a color change occurs without the addition of alcohol. This is called the direct reaction and represents conjugated bilirubin. The color change following the addition of alcohol to the sera and the diazo dyes is called the indirect reaction and represents free or unbound bilirubin. The amount of bilirubin in the serum is generally estimated in milligrams per deciliter. Serum bilirubin levels have been used for many years as an indicator of liver function. Values for bilirubin levels of various animals are presented in the Appendix.

Nonhuman Primates

Total serum bilirubin and conjugated bilirubin levels found in various nonhuman primates are given in the appendix. Limited studies and clinical observations on nonhuman primates suggest some similarities to humans in the interpretation of serum bilirubin levels during episodes of hemolytic, hepatic, and obstructive jaundice. However, because serum bilirubin levels reportedly approximate 25 per cent those of man, significant elevations may still not surpass normal human values (38,47).

Dog

Healthy dogs and cats have low serum bilirubin levels (19). High levels of unconjugated bilirubin indicate hemolytic disease in the dog, whereas if more than 50 per cent of the total bilirubin is conjugated, hepatocellular disease is probably present (14). Obstruction of the bile duct system outside the liver results in a greater increase in conjugated bilirubin in the serum (60 to 90 per cent), and this in turn is associated with the presence of a small quantity of free bilirubin.

Cornelius (15) reviewed the biochemical evaluation of hepatic function in the dog. Most of the bilirubin excreted by the liver into the bile is derived from the turnover of erythrocytic hemoglobin. However, 15 per cent of the bilirubin is derived from the catabolism of various hepatic hemoproteins such as cytochrome P-450, peroxidase, and catalase. Hemoglobin released by the red cells is normally transported in the plasma by haptoglobin, an alpha-2 mucoprotein, to the reticuloendothelial cells, where heme is enzymatically degraded first to the biliverdin by heme oxygenase and subsequently to bilirubin by biliverdin reductase. The bilirubin is then transported in the plasma firmly bound to albumin. It next enters the hepatic cell and is bound to ligandin, an intracellular protein, before its conjugation with various sugars. Bilirubin must be conjugated to become water soluble, a process necessary for its excretion into the bile. Any obstruction preventing the excretion of bile pigment results in elevations of conjugated bilirubin in the blood and urine. Bilirubinuria can occur early in hemolytic disease in the dog and need not be due to secondary obstructive processes in the hepatobiliary system (15).

Rat

Gunn (22) reported hereditary acholuric jaundice in a strain of mutant rats, and Malloy and Loewenstein (33) reported on hereditary jaundice in rats. Schmid et al (37) studied congenital jaundice caused by a defect in glucuronide formation in rats (Gunn rat). This jaundice trait was detected in Wistar rats. Schmid et al (37) found that the icterus was nonhemolytic and nonobstructive. No bilirubin glucuronide was demonstrable in the serum, bile, or urine of the affected rats and fecal urobilinogen excretion was greatly reduced. The livers were histologically normal, and the BSP and conjugated bilirubin excretion test results were within normal limits. It was concluded that Gunn rats have a defect in the glucuronyl transferase system. Normal Wistar rats had total bilirubin levels of less than 0.1 mg/dl and Gunn rats had a mean total bilirubin level of 8.09 mg/dl. The Gunn rat has contributed much to the understanding of bilirubin metabolism.

Cutler (17) reported total bilirubin levels of 0.4 mg/dl in normal 9-week-old rats and 0.40 mg/dl in 24-week-old rats. Rats exposed to carbon tetrachloride vapors for 6 weeks or 5 months had bilirubin levels of 0.54 and 0.53 mg/dl.

UROBILINOGEN

Urobilinogen is formed as a result of bacterial action on excreted bile, producing stercobilinogen. Bile and stercobilinogen are involved in the enterohepatic circulation. Stercobilinogen is absorbed in the intestine and is excreted by the kidney as urobilinogen. The presence of urobilinogen indicates that the bile duct is patent and that enterohepatic circulation is occurring. Urobilinogen is present in the urine of normal animals and is increased in conditions in which excessive breakdown of hemoglobin, a feature of hemolytic anemia, is occurring. Urobilinogen can be estimated by the method of

Wallace and Diamond (43), a test not commonly used in veterinary medicine. Antibiotic therapy, which destroys the bacterial flora of the intestinal tract, may reduce the level of urinary urobilinogen. Urobilinogen will break down rapidly if exposed to light. Oxidized urobilinogen (urobilin) does not react with Ehrlich's reagent and therefore may cause a false-negative result.

Urinary urobilinogen (units per 24-hour sample) levels were determined by Cutler (17) using the method of Watson et al (44). Nine-week-old rats had levels of 0.07 and 24-week-old rats had levels of 0.09 units/24 hours.

LIVER FUNCTION TESTS IN RATS

Cutler (17) studied the sensitivity of liver function tests in detecting liver damage in rats. Rats were treated with either carbon tetrachloride or sodium selenate for 5 months. Plasma glucose-6-phosphatase, glutamic-pyruvic transaminase (alanine aminotransferase), cholinesterase, bilirubin concentration, protein fractions, colloidal red flocculation, zinc sulfate turbidity, urine coproporphyrin and urobilinogen determination, BSP, and hippuric acid tests were conducted; relative liver weight and the results of gross and histopathologic examination of the liver were also recorded. The hippuric acid test, the electrophoretic pattern of plasma proteins, and the BSP test were most effective in revealing long-term impairment of liver function. Histopathologic evaluation and the determination of plasma glutamic-pyruvic transaminase were sensitive parameters in detecting structural abnormality. However, liver function tests alone did not give reliable information about structural changes in the liver. Both types of tests are necessary for a satisfactory assessment of hepatic integrity.

REFERENCES

1. Allen JR, Carstens LA (1968) Veno-occlusive disease in rhesus monkeys. Am J Vet Res 29: 1681–1694
2. Anderson DR (1966) Normal values for clinical blood chemistry tests of the *Macaca mulatta* monkey. Am J Vet Res 27: 1484–1489
3. Arias IM, Johnson L, Wolfson S (1961) Biliary excretion of injected conjugated and unconjugated bilirubin by normal and Gunn rats. Am J Physiol 200: 1091–1094
4. Barnhart JL, Clarenburg R (1973) Factors deter-

mining clearance of bilirubin in perfused rat liver. Am J Physiol 225: 497–507

5. Barnhart JL, Clarenburg R (1973) Binding of bilirubin to erythrocytes. Proc Soc Exp Biol Med 142: 1101–1103

6. Bonasch H, Cornelius CE (1964) Indocyanine green clearance: A liver function test for the dog. Am J Vet Res 25: 254–259

7. Brauer RW, Pessotti RL (1949) The removal of bromosulphthalein from blood plasma by the liver of the rat. J Pharmacol Exp Ther 97: 358–370

8. Brooks FP, Deneau GA, Potter HP Jr, Reinhold JG, Norris RG (1963) Liver function tests in morphine-addicted and nonaddicted rhesus monkeys. Gastroenterology 44: 287–290

9. Bruce JI, Warren KS, Sadun EH (1963) Observations on the pathophysiology of schistosomiasis in monkeys. Exp Parasitol 13: 194–198

10. Casals J, Olitsky PK (1946) Tests for hepatic dysfunction of mice. Proc Soc Exp Biol Med 63: 383–390

11. Center SA, Bunch SE, Baldwin BH, Hornbuckle WE, Tennant BC (1983) Comparison of sulfobromophthalein and indocyanine green clearances in the dog. Am J Vet Res 44: 722–726

12. Center SA, Bunch SE, Baldwin BH, Hornbuckle WE, Tennant BC (1983) Comparison of sulfobromophthalein and indocyanine green clearances in the cat. Am J Vet Res 44: 727–730

13. Clarenburg R, Barnhart JL (1973) Interaction of serum albumin and bilirubin at low concentrations. Am J Physiol 225: 493–496

14. Coles EH (1980) Veterinary Clinical Pathology, 3rd ed, WB Saunders, Philadelphia

15. Cornelius CE (1979) Biochemical evaluation of hepatic function in dogs. J Am An Hosp Assoc 15: 259–269

16. Cornelius CE (1980) In Kaneko JJ (ed), Clinical Biochemistry of Domestic Animals. Academic Press, New York

17. Cutler MG (1974) The sensitivity of function tests in detecting liver damage in the rat. Toxicol Appl Pharmacol 28: 349–357

18. Deinhart F, Courtois G, Dherte P, Osterrieth P, Ninane G, Henle G, Henle W (1962) Studies of liver function tests in chimpanzees after inoculation with human infecious hepatitis virus. Am J Hyg 75: 311–321

19. Duncan JR, Prasse KW (1977) Veterinary Laboratory Medicine. Clinical Pathology. Iowa State University Press, Ames, Iowa

20. Everett RM, Harrison SD Jr (1983) Clinical biochemistry. In Foster HL, Small JD, Fox JG (eds), The Mouse in Biomedical Research, Vol III. Academic Press, New York, pp 322–325

21. Gaisford WD, Zuidema GD (1965) Nutritional Laennec's cirrhosis in the *Macaca mulatta* monkey. J Surg Res 5: 220–235

22. Gunn CK (1938) Hereditary acholuric jaundice in a new mutant strain of rats. J Hered 29: 137–139

23. Hoe C (1969) Liver function tests. In Medway W, Prier JE, Wilkinson JS (eds), Textbook of Veterinary Clinical Pathology, Chap 3. Williams & Wilkins Co., Baltimore

24. Jablonski P, Owens JA (1969) The clinical chemistry of bromsulfophthalein and other cholephilic dyes. Adv Clin Chem 12: 309–386

25. Ketterer SG, Weigand BD, Rapoport E (1960) Hepatic uptake and biliary excretion of indocyanine green and its use in estimation of hepatic blood flow in dogs. Am J Physiol 199: 481–484

26. King TO, Gargus JL (1967) Normal blood values of the female monkey (*Macaca mulatta*). Lab An Care 17: 391–396

27. Klaassen CD (1970) Effects of phenobarbital on the plasma disappearance and biliary excretion of drugs in rats. J Pharmacol Exp Ther 175: 289–300

28. Klaassen CD, Plaa GL (1967) Species variation in metabolism, storage and excretion of sulfobromophthalein. Am J Physiol 213: 1322–1326

29. Klaassen CD, Plaa GL (1969) Plasma disappearance and biliary excretion of indocyanine green in rats, rabbits and dogs. Toxicol Appl Pharmacol 15: 374–384

30. Krasavage WJ, Michaelson SM (1965) Indocyanine green-plasma half time clearance (T1/2) in normal beagles. Soc Exp Biol Med Proc 119: 215–218

31. Kutob SD, Plaa GL (1962) Assessment of liver function in mice with bromosulphthalein. J Appl Physiol 17: 123–125

32. Malloy HT, Evelyn KA (1937) The determination of bilirubin with the photoelectric colorimeter. J Biol Chem 119: 481–484

33. Malloy HT, Lowenstein L (1940) Hereditary jaundice in rat. Canad Med Assoc J 42: 122

34. Oser FO, Lang RE, Vogin EE (1970) Blood values in stumptailed macaques (*M. arctoides*) under laboratory conditions. Lab An Care 20: 462–466

35. Petery JJ (1967) Ultramicroanalysis of selected blood components of normal *Macaca mulatta*. Lab An Care 17: 342–344

36. Rossoff IS (1974) Handbook of Veterinary Drugs. Springer, New York

37. Schmid R, Axelrod J, Hammaker L, Swarm RL (1958) Congenital jaundice in rats due to a defect in glucuronide formation. J Clin Invest 37: 1123–1130

38. Steyn DG (1975) Standard serum chemical and haematological values in Chacma baboon (*Papio ursinus*). J South Afr Vet Assoc 46: 235

39. Van Vleet JF, Albert JO (1968) Evaluation of liver function test and liver biopsy in experimental carbon tetrachloride intoxication and extrahepatic bile duct obstruction in the dog. Am J Vet Res 29: 2119–2131

40. Vogin EE, Scott W, Mattis PA (1965) Hepatic clearance of indocyanine green in the beagle. Proc Soc Exp Biol Med 119: 570–573

41. Vogin EE, Moreno OM, Brodie DA, Mattis PA (1966) Indocyanine green clearance in the rhesus monkey (*Macaca mulatta*). J Appl Physiol 21: 1880–1882

42. Wakeman AM, Morrell CA (1932) Chemistry and metabolism in experimental yellow fever in *Macacus rhesus* monkeys. Arch Intern Med 50: 826–833

43. Wallace GB, Diamond JS (1925) The significance of urobilinogen in urine as a test for liver function with description of simple quantitative method for its estimation. Arch Intern Med 35: 698

44. Watson CJ, Schwartz S, Sborov V, Bertie E (1944) Studies of urobilinogen: Simple method for quantitative recording of Ehrlich reaction as carried out with urine and faeces. Am J Clin Pathol 14: 605–615

45. Wheeler HO, Cranston WI, Meltzer JI (1958) Hepatic uptake and biliary excretion of indocyanine green in the dog. Proc Soc Exp Biol Med 99: 11–14

46. Williams JS, Meroney FC, Hutt G, Sadun EH (1966) Serum chemical components in mice determined by the use of ultra micro techniques. J Appl Physiol 21: 1026–1030

47. Wisecup WG, Hodson HH, Hanley WC, Felts PE (1969) Baseline blood levels of the chimpanzee (*Pan troglodytes*). Liver function tests. Am J Vet Res 30: 955–962

48. Zuidema GD, Gaisford WD, Kowalczyz RS, Wolfmen EF Jr, Arbir A (1963) Whole-body hypothermia in ammonia intoxication. Effect on monkeys with portacaval shunts. Arch Surg 87: 578–582

ADDITIONAL REFERENCES
NOT CITED IN TEXT

1. Ahmad NU, Aterman K (1953) Liver function and hepatic necrosis due to deficient diet. Arch Exp Pathol Pharmacol 222: 273–283

2. Altshuler HL, Stowell RE, Lowe RT (1971) Normal serum biochemical values of *Macaca arctoides*, *Macaca fascicularis* and *Macaca radiata*. Lab An Sci 21: 916–926

3. Altshuler HL, Stowell RE (1972) Normal serum biochemical values of *Cercopithecus aethiops*, *Cercocebus atys* and *Presbytis entellus*. Lab An Sci 22: 692–704

4. Anderson JR, Bernirscke K (1966) The armadillo, *Dasypus novemcinctus*, in experimental biology. Lab An Care 16: 202

5. Baetz AL, McLoughlin ME (1983) Serum concentration of bile acids in guinea pigs as an indicator of liver damage caused by aflatoxins. Am J Vet Res 44: 1971–1972

6. Baker HJ, Lindsey JR, Weisbroth SH (1979) The Laboratory Rat, Vol I. Biology and Diseases. Academic Press, New York

7. Baker HJ, Lindsey JR, Weisbroth SH (1980) The Laboratory Rat, Vol II. Research Applications. Academic Press, New York

8. Balabaud C, Saric J, Gonzalez P, Delphy C (1981) Bile collection in free moving rats. Lab An Sci 31: 273–275

9. Barnes CD, Eltherington LG (1973) Drug Dosage in Laboratory Animals. Rev Ed. Univ of California Press, Berkeley

10. Berk PD, Kiang C, Stremmel W, Tavoloni N (1982) A simple procedure for the isolation of bilirubin monoglucuronide and diglucuronide from bile. J Lab Clin Med 99: 539–547

11. Blanckaert N, Gollan J, Schmid R (1980) Mechanism of bilirubin diglucuronide formation in intact rats. J Clin Invest 65: 1332–1342

12. Blumenthal SG, Taggart DB, Rasmussen RD, Ikeda RM, Ruebner BH (1979) Conjugated and unconjugated bilirubins in humans and rhesus monkeys. Biochem J 179: 537–547

13. Brauer RW, Pessotti RL (1950) Hepatic uptake and biliary excretion of bromsulphthalein in the dog. Am J Physiol 162: 565–574

14. Callahan EW Jr, Schmid R (1969) Excretion of unconjugated bilirubin in the bile of Gunn rats. Gastroenterology 57: 134–137

15. Cameron JL, Pulaski EJ, Abei T, Iber FL (1966) Metabolism and excretion of bilirubin-C14 in experimental obstructive jaundice. Ann Surg 163: 330–338

16. Catz C, Yaffe SJ (1968) Barbiturate enhancement of bilirubin conjugation and excretion in young and adult animals. Pediat Res 2: 361–370

17. Clarenburg R, Kao Chi-Chou (1973) Shared and separate pathways for biliary excretion of bilirubin and BSP in rats. Am J Physiol 225: 192–200

18. Cohn C, Levine R, Streicher D (1947) The rate of removal of intravenously injected bromsulphalein by the liver and extra hepatic tissues of the dog. Am J Physiol 150: 299–303

19. Combes B, Stakelum GS (1962) Maturation of sulfobromophthalein sodium-glutathione conjugating system in rat liver. J Clin Invest 41: 750–757

20. Cornelius CE, Himes JA (1973) New concepts in canine hapatic function. J Am An Hosp Assoc 9: 147

21. Cornelius CE, Holm LW, Jasper DE (1958) Bromsulphalein clearance in normal sheep and in pregnancy toxemia. Cornell Vet 48: 305–312

22. Cutler MG (1972) An improved method for measuring the concentration of bromsulphthalein in blood. Clin Chim Acta 40: 503–504

23. Davy CW, Jackson MR, Walker J (1984) Reference intervals for some clinical chemical parameters in the marmoset (*Callithrix jacchus*): Effect of age and sex. Lab An 18: 135–142

24. de la Pena A, Goldzieher JW (1967) Clinical parameters of the normal baboon. Baboon Med Res 2: 379–389

25. de la Pena A, Matthijssen C, Goldzieher JW (1970) Normal values for blood constituents of the baboon (*Papio spp.*). Lab An Care 20: 251–261

26. Deinhardt F, Holmes AW, Capps RB, Popper H (1967) Studies on the transmission of human viral hepatitis to marmoset monkeys. I. Transmission of disease serial passages, and description of liver lesions. J Exp Med 125: 673–688

27. Dooley JF (1979) The role of clinical chemistry in chemical and drug safety evaluation by use of laboratory animals. Clin Chem 25: 345–347

28. Drill VA, Ivy AC (1944) Comparative value of bromsulphalein, serum phosphatase, prothrombin time, and intravenous galactose tolerance tests in detecting hepatic damage produced by carbon tetrachloride. J Clin Invest 23: 209–216

29. Emminger A, Reznik G, Reznik-Schuller J, Mohr U (1975) Differences in blood values depending on age in laboratory bred European hamsters (*Cricetus cricetus*). Lab An 9: 33

30. Evans AS, Evans BK, Sturtz V (1953) Standards for hepatic and hematologic tests in monkeys. Observations during experiments with hepatitis and mononucleosis. Proc Soc Exp Biol NY 82: 437–440

31. Finch CE, Foster JR (1973) Hematologic and serum electrolyte values of the C57BL/6J male mouse in maturity and senescence. Lab An Sci 23: 339–349

32. Foster HL, Small JD, Fox JG (1981) The Mouse in Biomedical Research, Vol I: History, Genetics, and Wild Mice; (1982) Vol II: Diseases; (1983) Vol III: Normative Biology, Immunology, and Husbandry; (1982) Vol IV: Experimental Biology and Oncology. Academic Press, New York

33. Fouts JR, Adamson RH (1959) Drug metabolism in the newborn rabbit. Science 129: 897–898

34. Fox RR, Laird CW, Blau EM, Mitchell HS (1970) Biochemical parameters of clinical significance in rabbits. I. Strain variation. II. Diurnal variation. J Hered 61: 265–268

35. Garcia FG, Hunt RD (1966) The hematogram of the squirrel monkey. Lab An Care 16: 50–51

36. Gartner LM, Arias IM (1969) The transfer of bilirubin from blood to bile in the neonatal guinea pig. Pediat Res 3: 171–180

37. Gartner LM, Lane DL, Cornelius CE (1971) Bilirubin transport by liver in adult *Macaca mulatta*. Am J Physiol 220: 1528–1535

38. Gibson JE, Becker B (1967) Demonstration of enhanced lethality of drugs in hypoexcretory animals. J Pharm Sci 56: 1503–1505

39. Goldbert DM, Ellis G (1978) Mathematical and computer-assisted procedures in the diagnosis of liver and biliary tract disorders. Adv Clin Chem 20: 49–128

40. Goldstein J, Schenker S, Combes B. (1965) Sulfobromophthalein sodium (BSP) conjugation and excretion in neonatal guinea pigs. Am J Physiol 208: 573–577

41. Gollan J, Hammaker L, Licko V, Schmid R (1981) Bilirubin kinetics in intact rats and isolated perfused liver. J Clin Invest 67: 1003–1015

42. Gordon ER, Goresky CA (1980) The formation of bilirubin diglucuronide by rat liver microsomal preparations. Can J Biochem 58: 1302–1310

43. Grodsky GM, Kolb HJ, Fanska RE, Nemechek C (1970) Effect of age of rat on development of hepatic carriers for bilirubin: A possible explanation for physiologic jaundice and hyperbilirubinemia in the newborn. Metabolism 19: 246–252

44. Gronall AG, Bardawill CJ (1952) Study of liver function in dogs. Canad J Med Sci 30: 256–271

45. Gronwall R (1975) Effects of fasting on hepatic function in ponies. Am J Vet Res 36: 145

46. Guelfi JF, Braun JP, Benard P, Rico AG, Thouvenot JP (1982) Value of so called cholestasis markers in the dog: An experimental study. Res Vet Sci 33: 309–312

47. Hallesy D, Benitz KF (1963) Sulfobromophthalein sodium retention and morphological liver damage in dogs. Toxicol Appl Pharmacol 5: 650–660

48. Hargreaves T (1966) Bilirubin, bromsulphthalein and indocyanine green excretion in bile. Quart J Exp Physiol 51: 184–185

49. Hart LG, Guarina AM, Adamson RH (1969) Effect of phenobarbital on biliary excretion of organic acids in male and female rats. Am J Physiol 217: 46–52

50. Heirwegh KPM, Meuwissen JATP, Fevery J (1973) Critique of the assay and significance of bilirubin conjugation. Adv Clin Chem 16: 239–289

51. Himes JA, Cornelius CE (1973) Hepatic excretion and storage of sulfobromophthalein sodium in experimental necrosis in the dog. Cornell Vet 63: 424

52. Holmes AW, Passovoy M, Capps RB (1967) Marmosets as laboratory animals. Lab An Care 17: 41–47

53. Hoerlein BF, Green JE (1950) The bromsulfalein liver function tests as an aid in the diagnosis of canine hepatosis. N Am Vet 31: 662–665

54. Horak W, Grabner G, Paumgartner G (1973) Inhibition of bile formation by indocyanine green. Gastroenterology 64: 1005–1012

55. Hunton DB, Bollman JL, Hoffman HN II (1960) Studies of hepatic function with indocyanine green. Gastroenterology 39: 713–724

56. Hunton DB, Bollman JL, Hoffman HN II (1960) Hepatic removal of indocyanine green. Proc Staff Meet Mayo Clin 35: 752–755

57. Hunton DB, Bollman JL, Hoffman HN II (1961) The plasma removal of indocyanine green and sulfobromophthalein: Effect of dosage and blocking agents. J Clin Invest 40: 1648–1655

58. Hwang SW, Dixon RL (1973) Perinatal development of indocyanine green biliary excretion in guinea pigs. Am J Physiol 225: 1454–1459

59. International Conference on Hepatotoxicity due to Drugs and Chemicals, Fogarty International Center, Washington, DC, November 1977

60. Joe M, Teasdale JM, Miller JR (1962) A new mutation (sph) causing neonatal jaundice in the house mouse. Can J Genet Cytol 4: 219–225

61. Jones RT (1975) Normal values for some biochemical constituents in rabbits. Lab An 9: 143–147

62. Jordorf WR, Maickel RP, Brodie BB (1958) Inability of newborn mice and guinea pigs to metabolize drugs. Biochem Pharmacol 1: 352–355

63. Juhn SK, Haugen J, Steven L (1974) Some chemical parameters of serum cerebospinal fluid, perilymph and aqueous humor of the chinchilla. Lab An Sci 24: 691–695

64. Kaneko JJ (1980) Clinical Biochemistry of Domestic Animals, 3rd ed. Academic Press, New York

65. Katz S, Gilardoni A, Genovese N, Wikinski RW, Cornelius CE, Malinow MR (1968) Liver function studies in free ranging howler monkeys with hepatic pigmentation. Lab An Care 18: 626–630

66. Kitagawa H, Ishihara K, Yokoyama S (1980) Serum total bile acid level in normal dogs. Jpn J Vet Sci 43: 257–260

67. Klaassen CD (1970) Plasma disappearance and biliary excretion of sulfobromophthalein and phenol-3,6-dibromphthalein disulfonate after microsomal enzyme induction. Biochem Pharmacol 19: 1241–1249

68. Klaassen CD (1973) Hepatic excretory function in the newborn rat. J Pharmacol Exp Ther 184: 721–728

69. Klaassen CD (1973) Comparison of the toxicity of chemicals in newborn rats to bile duct-ligated and sham-operated rats and mice. Toxicol Appl Pharmacol 24: 37–44

70. Klaassen CD, Plaa GL (1968) Hepatic disposition of phenol dibromphthalein disulfonate and sulfobromophthalein. Am J Physiol 215: 971–976

71. Klinger W, Sittner J (1976) The sensitivity of the indocyanine green clearance as a liver test after acute injury by carbon tetrachloride and allyl alcohol in 30- and 120-day old rats. Z Versuchstierk Bd 18: 16–24

72. Kozma C, Macklin W, Cummins LM, Mauer R (1974) Anatomy, physiology, and biochemistry of the rabbit. In Weisbroth SH, Flatt RE, Kraus AL (eds), Biology of the Rabbit. Academic Press, New York, pp 50–72

73. Kruckenberg SM (1979) Drugs and dosages. In Baker HJ, Lindsey JR, Weisbroth SH (eds), The Laboratory Rat, Vol I: Biology and Diseases. Academic Press, New York

74. Kruckenberg SM, Cornelius CE, Cook JE (1972) Liver function and disease in primates. In Fiennes RNTW (ed) Pathology of Simian Primates, Part I. Karger, Basel, pp 711–755

75. Ladenson JH, Tsai LB, Michael JM, Kessler G, Joist JH (1974) Serum versus heparinized plasma for 18 common chemistry tests. Am J Clin Pathol 62: 545–552

76. Laird CW (1974) Clinical pathology: blood chemistry. In Melby EC, Altman NH (eds), Handbook of Laboratory Animal Science, Vol II. CRC Press, Cleveland, p 347

77. Larson EJ, Morrill CC (1960) Evaluation of the bromsulfophthalein liver function test in the dog. Am J Vet Res 21: 949

78. Levi AJ, Gatmaitanz, Arias IM (1970) Deficiency of hepatic organic anion-binding protein impaired organic anion uptake by the liver and "physiologic" jaundice in newborn monkeys. N Engl J Med 283 1136–1139

79. Linder GC, Parker RGF, Selzer G (1953) Bromosulphthalein retention in young rats on diets producing liver necrosis. Brit J Exp Pathol 34: 656–660

80. Lloyd JR (1957) Use of a liver function test in the prognosis of ragwort poisoning in cattle. Vet Rec 69: 623

81. Madrid JA, Salido GM, Manas M, Martinez De Victoria E, Mataix FJ (1983) Use of a bidirectional cannula to study biliary secretion in conscious dogs. Lab An 17: 307–310

82. Maillie AJ, Calvo EL, Vaccaro MI, de Caboteau LI, Pivetta OH (1981) An experimental model to study bile and exocrine pancreatic secretion from mice. Lab An Sci 31: 707–709

83. Mann GV, Watson PL, Adams L (1952) Primate nutrition. J Nutr 47: 213–224

84. Maschgan ER (1980) Clinical data for gorillas, organutans and chimpanzees at the Lincoln Park Zoological Gardens. Lincoln Park Zoological Gardens, Chicago, Illinois

85. Mays A Jr (1969) Baseline hematological and blood biochemical parameters of the Mongolian gerbil (Meriones unquiculatus). Lab An Care 19: 838–842

86. McKain KJ (1963) The correlation of liver function tests with the hepatic lesion in dogs fed toxic peanut meal. Cornell University, Ph.D. Thesis

87. McClure HM, Guilland NB, Keeling ME (1973) Clinical pathology data for the chimpanzee and other anthropoid apes. In The Chimpanzee, Vol 6. Basel, Karger

88. McDonagh AF, Palma LA (1980) Hepatic excretion of circulating bilirubin photoproducts in the Gunn rat. J Clin Invest 66: 1182–1185

89. McKibbin JM, Thayer S, Stare FJ (1944) Choline deficiency studies in dogs. J Lab Clin Med 29: 1109–1122

90. Meyer DJ, Noonan NE (1981) Liver tests in dogs receiving anticonvulsant drugs (diphenylhydantoin and primidone). J Am An Hosp Assoc 17: 261–264

91. Meyer DJ (1982) The Liver. Part I. Biochemical tests for evaluation of the hepatobiliary system. Compend Cont Ed 4: 663–674

92. Mills MA, Dragstedt CA (1938) Removal of intravenously injected BSP from the blood stream of the dog. A comparison of removal of intravenously injected bilirubin and that of BSP. Arch Intern Med 62: 216

93. Minette HP, Shaffer MF (1968) Experimental leptospirosis in monkeys. Am Soc Trop Med Hyg 17: 202–212

94. Mitruka BM, Rawnsley HM (1977) Clinical Biochemical and Hematological Reference Values in Normal and Experimental Animals. Masson Publishing Inc., New York

95. Moreland AF (1974) Biological values for various laboratory animals. Lab An Digest 9: 41

96. Morgan HC (1959) A qualitative sulfobromophthalein sodium retention test. J Am Vet Med Assoc 135: 412

97. New AE (1968) In The Squirrel Monkey. Academic Press, New York, pp 418–419

98. Odell GB, Natzschka JC, Storey B (1966) Bilirubin in the liver and kidney in jaundiced rats. Am J Dis Children 112: 351–358

99. Potrepka RR, Spratt JL (1971) Effect of phenobarbital and 3-methylcholanthrene pretreatment on guinea pig hepatic microsomal bilirubin glucuronyltransferase activity. Biochem Pharmacol 20: 861–867

100. Pridgen WA (1967) Values for blood constituents of the African green monkey (Cercopithecus aethiops). Lab An Care 17: 463–468

101. Quick AJ (1939) Intravenous modification of the hippuric acid test for liver function. Am J Digest Dis 6: 716–717

102. Rao GN, Shipley EG (1970) Data on selected clinical blood chemistry tests of adult female rhesus monkeys (M. mulatta). Lab An Care 20: 226–231

103. Rich LJ, Spano JS (1974) Biochemical profiles in small animals: Diseases of pancreas, kidney, and liver. JAAHA 10: 349

104. Richards TG, Tindall VR, Young A (1959) A modification of BSP liver function test to predict the dye content of liver and bile. Clin Sci 18: 499

105. Ricketts WE (1951) Pathological liver with minimal or no change in liver tests. Am J Med Sci 221: 287–292

106. Robertson WG, Mixner JP, Bailey WW Jr, Lennon HD (1957) Determination of liver function, plasma and blood volumes in ketotic cows using bromsulphalein. J Dairy Sci 40: 977

107. Robinson PF, Zeigler RF (1968) Clinical laboratory values for beagle dogs. Lab An Care 18: 39–49

108. Robinson SH, Yannoni C, Nagasawa S (1971) Bilirubin excretion in rats with normal and impaired bilirubin conjugation: Effect of phenobarbital. J Clin Invest 50: 2602–2613

109. Rothstein R, Hunsaker D II (1972) Baseline hematology and blood chemistry of the South American woolly opossum (*Caluromys derbianus*). Lab An Sci 22: 227–232

110. Schall WD (1976) Laboratory diagnosis of hepatic disease. Vet Clin North Am 6: 679

111. Schmid R, Hammaker L (1963) Metabolism and disposition of C14-bilirubin in congenital nonhemolytic jaundice. J Clin Invest 42: 1720–1734

112. Secord DC, Russell JC (1973) A clinical laboratory study of conditioned mongrel dogs and Laborador retrievers. Lab An Sci 23: 567–571

113. Seig A, Heirwegh KPM (1981) Evidence against enzymatic conversion in vitro of bilirubin mono- to bilirubin diglucoronide in preparations from Gunn rat liver. Gastroenterology 80: 1349

114. Sharratt M, Frazer AC (1963) The sensitivity of function tests in detecting renal damage in the rat. Toxicol Appl Pharmacol 5: 36–48

115. Spell JP, Hardy JD (1961) A reappraisal of liver function tests in dogs. Arch Surg 82: 665–667

116. Spiller GA, Spaur CL, Amen RJ (1975) Selected blood values for *Macaca nemestrina* fed semi-purified fiber-free liquid diets. Lab An Sci 25: 341–571

117. Steenbergen W Van, Fevery J (1982) Maximal biliary secretion of bilirubin in the anesthetized rat: Dependence on UDP-glucuronosyl-transferase activity. Clin Sci 62: 521–528

118. Stoll MS, Zenone EA, Ostrow JD (1981) Excretion of administered and endogenous photobilirubins in the bile of the jaundiced Gunn rat. J Clin Invest 68: 134–141

119. Street RP Jr, Highman B (1971) Blood chemistry values in normal *Mystromys albicaudatus* and Osborne-Mendal rats. Lab An Sci 21: 394–398

120. Strombeck DR, Qualls C (1978) Hepatic sulfobromophthalein uptake and storage defect in a dog. J Am Vet Med Assoc 172: 1423–1426

121. Strozier LM, Blair CB, Evans BH (1971) Armadillos. I. Serum chemistry values. Lab An Sci 21: 399–400

122. Svirbely JL, Monaco AR, Alford WC (1946) The comparative efficiency of various liver function tests in detecting hepatic damage produced in dogs by xylidine. J Lab Clin Med 31: 1133

123. Timmons EH, Marques PA (1969) Blood chemical and hematological studies in laboratory confined unanesthetized opossum (*Didelphis virginiana*). Lab An Care 19: 342–344

124. Vogin EE, Moreno OM, Brodie DA, Mattis PA (1966b) Effect of probenecid on indocyanine green clearance. J Pharmacol Exp Ther 152: 509–515

125. Vogin EE, Oser F (1971) Comparative blood values in several species of non-human primates. Lab An Sci 21: 937–941.

126. Vondruska JF (1970) Certain hematologic and blood chemical values in adult stumptailed macaques (*Macaca arctoides*). Lab An Care 20: 97–100

127. Wheeler HO, Epstein RM, Robinson RR, Snell ES (1960) Hepatic storage and excretion of sulfobromophthalein sodium in the dog. J Clin Invest 39: 236–247

128. Wheeler HO, Meltzer JI, Bradley SE (1960) Biliary transport and hepatic storage of sulfobromphthalein sodium in the unanesthetized dog, in normal man and in patients with hepatic disease. J Clin Invest 39: 1131–1144

129. Whelan G, Hoch J, Schenker S, Combes, B (1970) Impaired hepatic disposition of sulfobromphthalein sodium in neonatal guinea pigs: Nature of the defect. J Lab Clin Med 76: 775–780

130. White D, Haidar GA, Reinhold JG (1958) Spectrophotometric measurement of bilirubin concentration in the serum of the newborn by the use of a microcapillary method. Clin Chem 4: 211–251

131. Wilkinson JS (1969) Kidney disease and urine analysis. In Medway W, Prier JE, Wilkinson JS (eds), Textbook of Veterinary Clinical Pathology. Williams & Wilkins, Baltimore.

132. Wirts CW, Cantarow A, Snape WJ, Delserone B (1951) Bile volume and excretion of pigment and bromsulfalein in dogs receiving carbon tetrachloride. Am J Physiol 165: 680–687

133. Yarborough LW, Tollett, JL, Montrey RD, Beattie RJ (1984) Serum biochemical, hematological and body measurement data for common marmosets (*Callithrix jacchus jacchus*). Lab An Sci 34: 276–280

134. Zieve L, Hanson M (1953) Studies of liver function tests. IV. Effect of repeated injections of sodium benzoate on the formation of hippuric acid in patients with liver disease. J Lab Clin Med 42: 872–876

14

Markers of Renal Function and Injury

HARVEY A. RAGAN, DVM

An extensive review of renal physiology is outside the scope of this section. However, a knowledge of normal renal function is essential to the interpretation of serum and urine tests indicative of nephrotoxicity, disease or both. Altered renal function may also have significant effects on other organ systems or, conversely, it may be altered by extrarenal disease processes. Texts on general physiology cover renal function in good detail, and those by Brenner and Rector (12), DeWardener (20), Kinne (52), Vander (112) and Koushanpour (59) review renal physiology very specifically. There are several good texts on the pathophysiologic aspects of renal disease including those of Leaf and Cotran (63), Kurtzman and Martinez-Maldonado (61), Hook (50), Knox (55), Berndt (6), and Schrier (98).

Numerous animal models of acute and chronic renal failure are available for study. Some of the more recent include those of Gabizon et al (35), Walker et al (113), Nakamura et al (75), Newton et al (76), Yokazawa et al (120), Robertson et al (93), and Mackenzie and Asscher (65).

The nephron is the functional unit of the kidney. It consists of two functionally distinct units: the glomerulus, which is basically a vascular bed serving as a diffusion membrane, and the renal tubule, which selectively processes the glomerular ultrafiltrate and maintains homeostasis of the organism. The tubule system accomplishes this function by two general processes: (1) reabsorption of water and solutes from the glomerular filtrate, and (2) secretion of water and specific solutes into the tubular fluid ultimately to be excreted as urine. Thus, the kidneys have a major role in regulation of water, electrolyte, and acid-base balance and in the removal of metabolic waste products and some toxic substances. Analyses of serum and/or urine constituents and the clearance of endogenous or exogenous substances are used to evaluate alterations in renal function or to detect renal lesions.

EXAMINATION OF THE URINE

Urinalysis, in a crude form, was probably the first examination of body fluid to be made in the context of clinical pathology. The monograph on urinalysis by Free and Free (34) has an interesting chapter on the history of urine examination, which indicates that as early as 400 BC Hippocrates' writings made frequent reference to the importance of urinalysis. Many ancient records suggest that certain disease states were associated with changes in urine volume, color, consistency, odor, and even taste. Invention of the microscope added examination of urinary sediment to urology. Quantitative chemical assays of urine composition were not conducted until the 20th century. Initially these were primarily tests for glucose and protein and then more recently for other chemical constituents including numerous enzymes indicating damage at various locations in the nephron. Introduction of "dipstick" chemistry has greatly simplified some aspects of routine urinalysis, and multiparameter automated urinalysis instruments have recently become available.

Basically, routine urinalysis consists of two components: physicochemical tests and microscopic examination of the urinary sediment. In clinical medicine, routine urinalysis is usually a screening test performed on a random sample without regard to time of day or prandial state. In toxicity testing, urinalyses are usually performed on samples obtained during a specified time period (eg, 12 to 24 hours), collected using an indwelling urinary catheter or a metabolism cage. Whether the collection is random or timed, evaluation of the urine may provide information regarding several organ systems. Its use in examining for lesions of renal origin is in detecting abnormal or altered components in the urine or loss of ability to concentrate urine.

Methods of Collection

To obtain interpretable results, great care must be taken in the collection and handling of the urine specimen. Unlike in humans, the collection of a urine sample in laboratory species is not simple or easily accomplished, may prove to be the most difficult part of urinalysis, and may result in artifacts that can lead to erroneous interpretation of results.

Urine should be collected in a clean, dry container and one that has been autoclaved if bacteriologic examination is to be performed. Disposable collection systems are commercially available and fully satisfactory for random samples obtained from laboratory species. If the sample will not be examined within an hour or two, it should be refrigerated at about 4°C and

then warmed to room temperature for about 1 hour before proceeding with the examination. According to Schumann (100), refrigeration up to 12 hours is satisfactory for culture of a urine specimen, and it will permit valid examination of sediment for up to 48 hours after collection of the urine sample. Chemical preservatives should be used if the urine specimen is to be transported a considerable distance. The choice of preservative depends on the tests to be performed and has previously been reviewed (34). In human medicine, probably the most popular chemical preservative is that called the Kingsbury or Metropolitan Life Insurance Co. formulation. It preserves cellular constituents well and causes minimal changes in the commonly performed physicochemical tests on urine. Toluene and mineral oil, long used as good preservatives for chemical constituents, function primarily by excluding air from the sample because they float on the surface of the specimen and prevent evaporation. Great care must be taken in aspirating urine from the container to preclude contaminating the specimen with these chemicals. However, neither of these chemicals is bacteriostatic, so frequently a crystal of thymol is added to the urine container to inhibit bacterial and fungal growth. Other preservatives may be necessary for specialized assays, such as concentrated hydrochloric acid for urinary steroid determination and sodium carbonate for porphyrin assay.

Several procedures are used for obtaining random or spot urine samples from laboratory animals. Urethral catheterization may be performed in most species and is commonly used to obtain urine samples from the larger laboratory species, such as dogs, cats, miniature swine, and nonhuman primates. The technique was previously described for use in the rabbit (73), dog, cat, and monkey (53,64,73), and the rat (60). Catheterization of female miniature swine weighing up to 90 kg is relatively easy once the technique is mastered. Restraint is by physical or chemical means (92); the urethral opening is located on the floor of the vagina and reflected dorsally to permit insertion of a catheter of appropriate size. Galitzer et al (36) described a method of collecting uncontaminated urine samples from female swine using a modified disposable pediatric urine collector.

Random urine samples may be obtained from all species by cystocentesis. This procedure obviously should be performed aseptically unless it is a terminal sample. This method may result in the urine sample being contaminated by red blood cells, but it eliminates bacterial contamination originating from the lower urinary tract, which plagues most other collection methods. Manual pressure over the bladder may be used to obtain urine in smaller laboratory species. It may also be employed successfully in larger animals if they are first anesthetized. Rats, mice, and hamsters often will urinate spontaneously when they are handled, and small quantities of urine may be collected in this manner.

Most studies evaluating the potential renal toxicity of physical or chemical insults in laboratory species use some method of collecting urine over a specific period of time. Such samples reduce some of the variability in urine constituents that may occur with a randomly collected specimen. However, other problems are evident with timed-collection specimens, not the least of which is preservation for certain assays.

The most common method of collecting timed urine samples is to use metabolic cages for most species. Several styles are commercially available; however, none totally eliminates contact between urine and feces or urine and food, and some permit drinking water to dilute the urine specimen. In most cases the animals should not have access to food during a timed urine collection. Hair and dander contamination of the urine is also a common problem. Metabolic cages are designed in various manners to trap the feces while permitting urine to flow down an incline into a collecting vessel. A disposable apparatus for collecting urine from mice was described by Smith et al (106). An apparatus for collecting urine from rodents and maintaining the specimen at a low temperature was designed by Lartigue et al (62) and should be particularly useful for urine enzyme studies. Using commercially available metabolic cages (Nalge, Kalamazoo, MI), the author and his colleagues recently developed a procedure for collecting urine samples over ice that will maintain the iced condition for 16 hours. Styrofoam shipping containers are modified to accommodate the urine collection tubes through a hole cut in the container lid. The ice is packed tightly around the collection tube and the lid placed over the container. This procedure was used successfully to collect urine from up to 60 rodents over a 16-hour collection period for urinary enzyme assays. Roerig et al (95) developed an inexpensive restraining device that permits complete separation of urine and feces from rats. Urine, uncontaminated by feces, may effectively be collected from cats using a modified plastic dishpan placed in a standard fiberglass cage (68). A unique mouse-urine collection system with a flow-through pH monitoring electrode was described by West et al (116).

Cystostomy also can be used to collect timed urine samples. Hay and Adolph (45) described a technique of creating a urinary bladder fistula in both newborn and adult rats.

The author and his colleagues used an indwelling Foley catheter to collect urine samples over periods of hours to days from female miniature swine kept in restraining cages. Prolonged catheterization resulted in moderate inflammation of the vulva, vagina, and bladder.

Physicochemical Tests

Volume

An accurate determination of urine volume for a timed-collection specimen is necessary for subsequent calculations involving some constituents. If the specimen was collected using a metabolism cage and appears to be quite dilute, it must be decided if drinking water may have contaminated the specimen. If only moderate dilution has occurred, the decision is not easily made, because it might erroneously be concluded that the dilute urine sample was the result of polydipsia on the basis of an invalid measure of water consumed.

Color

The normal yellow color of urine is primarily due to the pigment urochrome, which is a degradation product of heme (31,34). The appearance of the urine specimen, including color and transparency or turbidity, should be noted. These evaluations may provide some presumptive evidence for the presence of red or white blood cells, abnormal pigments, crystals, and/or bacteria. Normally, urine of laboratory species is varying shades of yellow depending on the degree of hydration of the animal, and it usually is quite clear. Bradley and Benson (10) tabulated the causes that may alter the normal appearance and color of human urine. These changes in gross appearance are applicable to those observed in abnormal urine specimens of laboratory species.

pH

The kidneys play a vital homeostatic role in maintaining the acid-base balance by regulation of blood bicarbonate and hydrogen ion concentrations. The pH of urine is due to many chemical constituents, primarily inorganic phosphates, sulfates, citrate, ammonium salts, bicarbonate, and carbonic acid. These result from metabolic processes that produce nonvolatile acids that are excreted by the glomerulus with cations, primarily sodium. In the renal tubules, sodium is selectively reabsorbed and exchanged for hydrogen ions which are excreted. Processes involving renal tubular excretion and reabsorption affecting urine pH are covered in detail in texts of physiology such as those of Ganong (37) and Osborne et al (80).

The pH of urine varies considerably with diet content. When animal protein intake is high, more sulfates and phosphates are produced, resulting in acidic urine. Cereal grains produce a slightly alkaline or neutral urine.

For maximum validity, urine pH should be determined on a fresh specimen. Most commonly, "old" urine becomes more alkaline because of microorganisms that produce ammonia from urea and/or because of the decomposition of carbonic acid to CO_2 with subsequent loss of CO_2 from the specimen. However, some bacteria may cause a urine specimen to become more acidic (43).

Urinary pH alone is rarely of diagnostic significance; however, it may substantiate a diagnosis of respiratory or metabolic acidosis or alkalosis if the urine pH is in the corresponding direction. Low urinary pH may result from excessive catabolic states as with fever, during starvation, or with excess ketone bodies produced in diabetes mellitus. Urinary obstruction or cystitis resulting in retention of urine in the bladder may produce an alkaline urine because of the decomposition of urea to ammonia spontaneously or by bacterial action.

Because the pH of urine is subject to relatively large and rapid fluctuations depending on physiologic processes, the precision of a pH meter is usually not required in routine urinalysis. In such cases the use of "dipstick" multiple component strips incorporating a pH segment is satisfactory. These strips permit quantitative determinations of pH in the range of 5 to 8.5. Care must be taken to remove excess urine from the strip immediately after dipping; otherwise, "runover" of acid buffer from the protein segment may contaminate the pH segment, causing an erroneous reduction in pH value. If more precise and accurate determinations of urine pH are required for special studies, a glass electrode and pH meter should be used.

By definition, pH is a measure of hydrogen ion concentration. Therefore, urine pH does not represent the amount of acid being excreted by the kidney. Total hydrogen ion excretion can be estimated and tubular function tested by determining the titratable acidity of the urine defined as the amount of base (0.1 N NaOH) required to titrate the urine back to the pH of blood. This test is performed on a timed-collection specimen and the results are usually reported in milliliters of 0.1 N NaOH required to neutralize the specific volume of urine collected,

Specific Gravity/Osmolality

The ability of the kidneys to concentrate or dilute urine is of value in diagnosing renal disease. However, specific gravity or osmolality of a random urine sample must be interpreted with caution for the same reasons that a single pH reading is of limited value, that is, the fluctuating role of the kidney in maintaining homeostasis by varying excretion and reabsorption of water and other constituents presented to the nephron. Dilution-concentration tests are used to test the functional capacity of the kidney and will be detailed later.

The three methods used to determine the total solute concentration in urine are specific gravity, refractive index, and osmolality. Because the proportions and constituents of urinary solutes are variable, these three methods do not yield equivalent information. Specific gravity is determined using a hydrometer (urinometer) and depends on both the number of particles in solution and the nature of these particles (eg, ionic bonding of solute and water molecules). Because of this, equimolar concentrations of two different solutes may result in vastly different specific gravities. The specific gravity of urine is a comparison or ratio of the density of urine to that of distilled water, which has a density of 1 g/ml at 4°C. Watts (115) described a capillary tube method in which the specific gravity of microliter quantities of urine from mice was determined.

The refractive index of a solution depends on the identity of the chemical species present as well as the number of particles. There is a high correlation between the refractive index of urine and the concentration of dissolved solutes (117). Therefore, refractometers can be calibrated to read specific gravity from a scale rather than the percentage of total solids. However, this relationship is only valid in a relatively normal urine specimen and may be variably erroneous in urine containing glucose, protein, and/or metabolic products not normally present. Refractometry has the advantages of being rapid and simple and requiring only microliter amounts of urine. It is more accurate than a urinometer and does not require the instrumentation needed for osmometry.

Determination of osmolality is the definitive method of measuring the concentration or solute-to-solvent ratios in urine and is the method of choice in toxicologic studies. Osmolality is exclusively dependent on the number of particles in solution and is not influenced by the degree of ionization nor the mass of molecules and ions contained. Osmotic pressure determinations are made by instruments measuring freezing point depression or vapor pressure, and units are expressed as milliosmoles per kilogram of water. Modern instrumentation permits osmolality determinations to be made on microliter amounts of urine both rapidly and with great accuracy and precision. Using osmometry one may easily determine a plasma-to-urine osmol ratio. This comparison also provides an indication of the glomerular filtrate-to-urine ratio because the glomerular filtrate osmolality is essentially that of plasma (102).

Chemical Constituents

Because urine is an ultrafiltrate of blood, it is a very complex mixture containing almost all of the constituents found in plasma. However, because of the homeostatic role of the kidney, concentrations of the various urine constituents are in many cases vastly different from their plasma concentrations. These concentrations are highly dependent on metabolic processes, nutritional and hydration status, and the functional integrity of the kidneys. Because of the diurnal effects of the first three of these variables, even in a normal animal, quantitation of urinary constituents is usually based on timed collection rather than random samples.

A voluminous literature is available regarding the composition of urine in man and lower animals. Values for many constituents of human urine have been tabulated by Free and Free (34), Altman and Dittmer (1), and Davidsohn and Henry (18), and for lower animals by Mitruka and Rawnsley (72), and Altman and Dittmer (1). In some cases these values must be viewed with caution because they may be based on a small sample or a select population and usually do not have information on prandial state, housing conditions, methods of collecting the urine sample, or species strain.

This section will be restricted to the urine constituents commonly used to evaluate renal function for diagnostic purposes or in toxicologic studies. For information on the more unique analytes found in urine, the current literature must be scrutinized for specific pertinent studies.

The total solids in urine can be estimated by using a factor (Long's constant) of 2.6 times the last two digits of the specific gravity determination. For example, a specimen with a specific gravity of 1.032 would contain approximately 83 g of total solids per liter of urine. The largest contribution to urine solutes is made by urea and sodium chloride.

Urea is the principal waste product of protein metabolism, so its concentration in urine varies somewhat with the amount of protein in the diet. Other nitrogenous compounds found in normal urine include creatinine and uric acid at concentrations much higher than those in plasma, and trace amounts of amino acids, proteins, glycoproteins, and enzymes. Amino acid excretion may be markedly increased in certain inborn errors of metabolism in which the plasma concentration is increased and amino acids "spill" into the urine. A primary renal tubular defect may also result in aminoaciduria. Creatinine is the result of creatine metabolism by muscle, and consequently its concentration in both plasma and urine is less dependent on diet. However, the presence of both analytes in urine is primarily due to glomerular filtration.

In normal animals, glucose only appears in trace amounts in urine because it is almost completely reabsorbed by the proximal renal tubules. However, this reabsorption is an active transport process and there is a limit, or threshold, beyond which the transport maximum is exceeded and glucose concentration in urine will increase. Glucosuria may be the result of extrarenal hyperglycemia from pancreatic disorders or inborn errors of carbohydrate metabolism or of a renal effect from damage to the tubules. Semiquantitation of urinary glucose may be accomplished using an appropriate "dipstick" strip. However, caution with strips employing glucose oxidase must be used in species excreting large amounts of ascorbic acid such as the dog and mouse. In these species the urine strip analysis for glucose should be delayed several hours to permit decomposition of the ascorbic acid.

The glomerular membrane normally serves to prevent the passage of high molecular weight proteins into the urine. Smaller proteins may be present in the glomerular filtrate, but they are reabsorbed in the proximal tubules. Proteinuria then is primarily an indicator of glomerular damage, but it may occur with renal tubular disease. However, the smaller molecular weight proteins present in the glomerular filtrate, such as the paraproteins of multiple myeloma and leukemia, may not be detected by usual analytic procedures. Extrarenal proteinuria is usually the result of inflammation, hemorrhage, or infections of the lower urinary tract; however, fever and strenuous exercise may produce transient proteinuria. In evaluating persistent proteinuria it is extremely important to conduct an exacting evaluation of the urinary sediment to determine the source of proteinuria. If casts are absent but erythrocytes and/or inflammatory cells present, it is unlikely that the proteinuria is due to renal damage. The larger weight proteins are detected semiquantitatively by dipsticks; however, highly buffered alkaline urine or urine contaminated with quaternary ammonia disinfectants may give false-positive results. Persistent proteinuria should be confirmed and quantitated using sulfosalicylic acid or comparable methods. Hoffsten et al (48) in SWR/J mice found that the dipstick method gave a high incidence of false-positive proteinuria results as compared to radial immunodiffusion. Proteinuria is common in mice and rats and is significantly higher in males than in females (personal observation).

In the rat, urine protein is primarily albumin, whereas in the mouse it is a small molecular weight protein of about 18,000 daltons (32). Urine aspirated from the urinary bladder of male mice contained as much protein as did voided urine, indicating that the proteinuria is probably of renal origin (110). Hoffsten et al (48), using radial immunodiffusion in SWR/J strain mice, found that some albuminuria was present in normal mice and that there was no sex difference. Dilena et al (22) compared six different methods of determining urine protein and found that the Ponceau-S technique had better performance characteristics than did the commonly used sulfosalicylic acid methods or the Coomassie Brilliant Blue techniques.

An increase in the urinary concentrations of the low molecular weight proteins alpha-1-microglobulin and beta-2-microglobulin has recently been shown to be a sensitive indicator of renal tubular damage in man (86,121) and in rats (84). Detection of these proteins involves radioimmunoassay procedures.

A lower molecular weight glycoprotein of renal origin, such as the Tamm-Horsfall glycoprotein, was first described in human urine and has been implicated in some disease states. It has been detected in the urine of sheep (17), hamsters (104), rat (103), and rabbits (40). Small amounts have also been detected in the serum of humans and rats (19,119).

Serum electrolytes are intimately involved in maintaining water and acid-base balances within the body, and regulation of their excretion and/or reabsorption is performed primarily by the kidney. The urinary content of electrolytes may provide some information on renal function. However, they are highly dependent on dietary intake and the general health status of the animal and must be interpreted with caution in evaluating whether an effect is due to renal or extrarenal disease.

Enzymatic Constituents

Over the past decade, increased attention has been directed toward evaluation of urinary enzymes as diagnostic indicators of renal damage. Highly sensitive tests for renal injury are needed, particularly in toxicologic testing of chemical and physical insults; because changes in common renal function tests and biochemical serum assays for kidney damage do not occur until renal insufficiency is relatively severe. Analyses of urinary enzymes have the potential added advantage of localizing the portion of the nephron that may be injured. Recently, some urine enzyme levels were validated as appropriately sensitive in detecting slight renal insufficiency. Most of these studies were conducted in man, rats, and dogs. However, there is no agreement regarding which enzyme assays are the most sensitive indicators of renal injury, and their value in appraising renal functional impairment is still somewhat controversial.

Because enzymes are intracellular or membrane-associated constituents, their extracellular presence is due to either secretion, increased permeability, or degeneration of cells. The author was unable to find evidence that enzymes found in the urine are secreted by renal cells. Therefore, their presence in urine is due to normal renal cell turnover, damage to renal cells, or serum enzymes. Because enzymes are proteins that are normally reabsorbed if they are small enough to pass the glomerular membrane (ie, those whose molecular weight is < 70,000 d), the contribution of most serum enzymes to the concentration of urine enzymes is usually negligible. In fact, the urine enzymes usually measured to evaluate renal tubular damage do not pass into the glomerular filtrate from serum because of their size; otherwise, their quantitation in urine would not be used as a measure of renal damage. Amylase and lipase levels in urine should not be used as markers of tubular injury because their levels in urine are a reflection of serum levels (34,89).

Methods for determining urine enzymes are generally similar or identical to those used for assaying serum enzymes. However, certain limitations and cautions must be observed. Attention must be paid to the collection of an uncontaminated specimen and to the preservation of the specimen. Bacteria of renal, bladder, or fecal origin may contribute enzymes, so that elevations of enzymes in urine may not be pathognomonic of renal injury. Studies of urinary enzymes in rats, recently conducted by the author, suggest that fecal contamination results in marked increases in certain enzymes, particularly glutamic oxalacetic transaminase and alkaline phosphatase. Urine may also contain enzymatic inhibitors, and preparation of the sample by gel filtration or dialysis may be necessary prior to analyses (67). However, it has not been well established which enzyme tests require such preparation of the urine. This question will be addressed in more detail when the specific enzymes are discussed.

Comprehensive reviews of enzymes in the urine have been published (23,24,69,91). Perusal of these indicates that there is no consensus regarding the use of urinary enzymes in evaluating spontaneous renal disease, drug-induced nephropathies, or rejection of kidney transplants. More than 40 enzymes, found by various investigators, have been evaluated to determine their diagnostic applicability in renal disease. However, only a few have met the necessary criteria to prove they are of renal origin. The most suitable indicators are lactic dehydrogenase (LDH), glutamic oxalacetic transaminase (GOT), glutamic pyruvic transaminase (GPT), beta-glucuronidase (β-GLU), leucine aminopeptidase (LAP), alkaline phosphatase (ALP), acid phosphatase (ACP), and N-acetyl-β-D-glucosaminidase (NAG). The muramidase level in urine is sometimes used as a sensitive indicator of tubular damage; however, because of its low molecular weight, increased urine concentrations of this enzyme must be dissociated from elevated serum concentrations for it to be of meaningful diagnostic value in renal disease. Succinate dehydrogenase is found in renal tubular epithelial cells, but it is destroyed or partially inactivated in urine and thus is of no value in diagnosing tubular lesions (91).

Most experimental studies of enzymuria use the rat as an experimental animal model, because the enzyme distribution in the kidneys of this species most closely mimics that observed in the human kidney (91). However, in investigating nephrotoxicity of drugs or other chemicals in any species, one must be certain that the compounds themselves are not acting as activators or inhibitors of enzymes found in the urine. An example of such inhibition was recently demonstrated by Fair et al (28) in which administration of methyl mercury to mice inhibited gamma glutamyl transpeptidase activity. To establish any such relationship, in vitro studies must be performed in which an effect or lack of effect of the specific chemical on urinary enzymes is demonstrated before their assay following exposure of intact animals to the chemical.

Raab (91) tabulated the many enzymes detected in the urine of man and various laboratory animals and these include oxidoreductases, transferases, hydrolases, and lysases. Isozymes of some have also been identified, and some were shown to be of value in diagnosing extrarenal disease, particularly tumors of the bladder or prostate. Hautmann (44) used ureteral catheterization to demonstrate the altered enzyme pattern of renal carcinoma in one kidney when compared to the pattern from the contralateral normal kidney.

Apparently the excretion of some urinary enzymes has a diurnal pattern (91). This coupled with the many factors that influence urine volume renders the information gained from a random urine sample almost meaningless in regard to urine enzymes. In toxicologic studies it is essential to measure urine enzymes using a timed-collection specimen.

When proteinuria is present, the significance of increased urinary enzymes must be viewed with caution. For instance, uropepsinogen levels reflect serum pepsinogen levels and are high in the presence of gastric ulcer; amylase activity correlates positively with serum activity and derives primarily from pancreatic lesions, but also from salivary and lactating mammary glands and from the small intestine.

In several species elevated urinary LDH levels were of value in diagnosing acute renal disease including tubular necrosis, acute pyelonephritis, acute glomerulonephritis, bacterial infections of the urinary tract, and rejection of a renal transplant. Urinary levels of LDH may also be elevated in chronic renal diseases, in contrast to other urinary enzymes that are elevated only in acute renal disease. Hypoxic renal damage from conditions such as myocardial infarction or vascular shock will also increase urinary LDH levels. Although many conditions may cause elevated serum LDH levels, there is no evidence that correlates LDH activities in serum with those in urine (117). Mattenheimer (69) calculated that in the worst possible case, serum LDH in urine never exceeded 1 to 2 per cent of the total urinary LDH activity. Early on, it appeared that urinary LDH levels might be of value in diagnosing malignant tumors of the urinary tract. Subsequent studies failed to confirm this because LDH is not invariably increased, there are no significant differences between increases with malignant and benign tumors, and the increases observed seemed to be nonspecific and caused by inflammation rather than primarily by tumor cells (91,117). Inhibitors of LDH are present in urine, so it is necessary to remove these by dialysis or gel filtration before assaying LDH activity.

Acid phosphatase activity is present in urine. In women and female laboratory animals it is derived only from the kidney, whereas in males some ACP activity in urine originates from prostatic secretion (91). The ACP activity is highest in the glomerular region of the human and rat kidney, but it is additionally located in the proximal tubules of the rabbit (77). The urine activity of ACP is less commonly used as a screen for renal damage than are LDH, ALP, or aminotransferase levels. However, increased ACP and ALP activities in the urine were the most sensitive indicators of renal tubular damage in the dog following injection of mercuric chloride (26).

Aspartate aminotransferase and alanine aminotransferase activities in urine are frequently assayed in tests for renal damage. The renal tubules and collecting ducts are relatively rich in these enzymes (83). Normal human urine contains very little AST or ALT activity, whereas it is present in larger amounts in normal rat urine (91,114). There is no clear evidence from the literature that inhibitors of these enzymes are present in the urine; however, most investigators routinely subject urine specimens to dialysis or gel filtration before enzyme assays.

Leucine aminopeptidase is found in high activity primarily in the proximal tubules (91). Urinary levels of this enzyme will be elevated with nephrotoxic substances that result in tubular necrosis, acute glomerulonephritis, acute pyelonephritis, or hypoxic renal vascular damage. High urinary levels of LAP activity may be seen in neoplasms of the female genital system (91). Renal tumors may also cause some increases in urinary LAP levels, but more pronounced changes in LDH activity. Some extrarenal tumors may result in elevated urinary LAP activity. However, this enzyme will not pass the glomerular membrane unless there is a defect in that part of the nephron; therefore, increased urine LAP levels with extrarenal tumors are probably due to toxic damage to the kidney (91).

N-acetyl-β-glucosaminidase is used widely as an organ-specific indicator of renal damage because it is not present in the urine or serum of clinically normal humans (88). Following toxic renal damage, NAG activity is detectable in the urine of rats (54,99). Ellis et al (38) presented evidence that the urinary and serum activity of NAG is a sensitive indicator of papillary damage in the dog. Johnston et al (51) reported that determination of urinary NAG activity is a very sensitive measure of renal disease in hypertensive patients, particularly when proteinuria is also present. Yuen et al (122) described a simplified colorimetric assay for detecting NAG in urine. The activity is stable for up to 48 hours at 4°C or for prolonged storage at −20°C.

β-glucuronidase activity is normally present in the urine of man and the rat. However, this activity does not correlate with that in the serum (91). Therefore, increases in urinary β-GLU activity are indicative of toxic renal lesions including bacteria-induced inflammation. Urinary activities of this enzyme are usually not influenced by bacterial infections of the lower urinary tract (4). Very high urinary levels have been reported in patients with renal or urinary bladder tumors (91). Inhibitors of β-GLU are found in urine, so dialysis is necessary before assaying the activity. In some species, such as the rat, secretions from the preputial gland make a significant contribution to urinary β-GLU activity (15).

In summary, elevation of certain enzymes found in urine appears to be a relatively sensitive measure of renal damage that is applicable in chemical toxicity studies and clinical medicine. It has great promise especially in toxicity studies in rats and mice as a measure of nephrotoxicity because several common renal function tests are difficult to perform in these species. However, the validity of these assays is still somewhat controversial, and the results should be interpreted with caution in attempting to specify the exact locations in the nephron that may have been damaged. In addition, the elevation of a single urinary enzyme is of limited diagnostic value; rather, the results of several urine enzymes, serum biochemical, and renal function assays should be correlated in assessing nephrotoxicity. In toxicity studies, urine enzyme assays should be conducted on timed-collection specimens along with accurate determinations of urine volume.

Urinary Sediment

General Considerations

Microscopic examination of urinary sediment should be part of any routine urinalysis because it may detect structural abnormalities of the urinary system and provide diagnostic information when compared with the resuts of physicochemical and/or renal function tests. Free and Free (34) aptly call the microscopic examination of urine sediment an "in vitro biopsy" of the kidney.

Routine examination is usually performed only with bright-field and/or phase-contrast microscopy of a stained or unstained smear of the sediment. For more in-depth or special studies, interference-contrast, fluoescence, transmission electron, or scanning electron microscopy may be used. Cytocentrifugation preparations or paraffin embedding of the sediment button with subsequent histologic sectioning may also be of value.

There are several excellent monographs, texts, and atlases on examination and constituents of urinary sediment (11,38,42,49,57,100,107,111). The techniques for examining and the descriptions of constituents in human urinary sediment are applicable in laboratory animals.

As with any microscopic examination, evaluation of urinary sediment is very subjective, imprecise, and subject to the individual variation and capabilities of the examiners. For these reasons, microscopic evaluation of urine in toxicologic studies should adhere to rigid preparatory techniques, and examinations in a specific study should be conducted by the same individual. Schumann (100) has found that cytocentrifugation and Papanicolaou staining of urinary sediment results in preparations far superior to those with conventional methods. This technique permits accurate identification of cellular constituents and tubular casts, and permanent preparations, in contrast to the temporary wet mounts more commonly used.

Concentration of the urinary sediment is necessary before microscopic examination. A well-mixed aliquot of the urine specimen is placed in a conical centrifuge tube of appropriate size and centrifuged for 10 minutes at about 700 g. For toxicity studies the urine from each animal should be concentrated to the same degree; for example, if 5 ml of urine is centrifuged and reconstituted in 0.5 ml of urine, then the proportional reconstitution of other urines should be the same regardless of the original sample volume. For more exacting studies, the use of a counting chamber to quantitate sediment constituents may be desired. For rou-

Table 14.1. Formed Elements of Urinary Sediment

Cells	Hematopoietic
	Epithelial
	Neoplastic
Casts	Hyaline
	Granular
	Red blood cell
	White blood cell
	Epithelial
	Waxy
	Fatty
	Mixed
	Renal failure (broad)
	Pseudocasts
Crystals	Phosphate
	Urate
	Oxalate
	Bilirubin
	Tyrosine
	Cystine
	Cholesterol
	Drugs
Infectious Agents	Bacteria
	Yeast
	Parasites and Ova
Miscellaneous	Lipids
	Chyle
	Mucus Threads
	Fibrin Threads
	Spermatozoa
External Contaminants	

tine wet mount preparations, a drop of resuspended sediment is placed on a clean slide and coverslipped before examination using subdued-light, bright-field, or phase-contrast microscopy. For better cellular detail, another slide should be stained with methylene blue, crystal violet-safranine, Wright stain, or a commercial stain for urinary sediment. A minimum of 10 fields should be viewed and the number of formed elements quantitated and reported as the average number per field.

Formed Elements

The formed elements of urine fall into four general types: host cells, casts, crystals, and nonhost cells such as bacteria, yeast, ova, or parasites (Table 14.1). To obtain the best results in examinations for these elements, a fresh urine specimen not more than 4 hours old should be used; alternatively, the urine specimen may be tightly capped and refrigerated.

Cells

Any of the cells of blood, including platelets, may be observed in urinary sediment and may be of diagnostic importance. The number of erythrocytes or neutrophils in "normal" urine has not been quantitatively established in man or laboratory animals. In humans less than 5 cells per high power field is considered "normal" (100). An increased number of blood cells in the urine is indicative of renal and/or lower urinary tract disease and, when combined with other urinalysis and biochemical tests, may help localize the area of disease.

According to Schumann (100), the mechanism whereby intact erythrocytes enter the urinary system is not clear. They may occur in urine without increased permeability of glomerular membranes to proteins or without evidence of kidney or urinary tract hemorrhage. Until recently, erythrocytes in urine could only be detected by macroscopic or microscopic examination of urinary sediment. Some dipstick methods are currently used to detect intact erythrocytes. Increased numbers of erythrocytes in urine may occur with acute or chronic inflammatory disease, neoplasms or calculus in the kidney or lower urinary tract.

Increased leukocytes in the urine may result from the same factor as those causing erythrocyturia. The differential leukocyte count in urine has significance similar to that in peripheral blood, that is, neutrophils are indicative of an acute inflammatory process, whereas lymphocytes, plasma cells, and macrophages are more characteristic of chronic inflammatory conditions. Plasma cells may also be seen in the urine during acute renal allograft rejection, and myeloma cells in patients with multiple myeloma (100). If blood cells are present but casts absent from the urinary sediment, then a diagnosis of cystitis or urethritis is more likely than one of renal parenchymal disease.

There is recent evidence that platelets may be found in urinary sediment in man. Small bodies with a size, shape, and appearance identical to those of platelets have been reported (56,108). If indeed these objects are platelets, their significance at present is unknown and will undoubtedly be the subject of considerable future investigations.

Epithelial cells from any segment of the urinary tract may be observed in urinary sediment.

It is important that epithelial cells of renal origin be distinguished from those of the lower urinary tract, because the presence of the former indicates active renal disease. Schumann et al (99) described the cytologic characteristics of epithelial cells from various areas of the urinary system. Schumann (100) believes that Papanicolaou staining is the method of choice in distinguishing between the various blood and epithelial cells that may be observed in urinary sediment.

Schumann (100) describes three types of epithelial fragments that may indicate the presence of renal parenchymal disease. In one type the epithelial fragments are associated with urinary casts or may actually be encased within a cast. A second configuration is a cylindrical fragment of epithelium considerably larger than a cast and not associated with casts in the urinary sediment. The third is a sheetlike configuration of epithelial cells. Comparisons of these configurations with tissue imprints suggest that the first type is from renal tubular epithelium, the second from collecting ducts, and the third from renal medullary pyramids and papillas.

Large, flattened squamous epithelial cells with a high cytoplasm-to-nucleus ratio may be seen in urinary sediment. These cells are from the urethra, vulva, or vagina.

Various benign and malignant cells may be observed in the urinary sediment. The same cytologic features used in differentiating benign from malignant cells in other exfoliative cytologic studies must be used in evaluating cells in the urine. Most tumor cells found in urine originate in the urinary tract; however, metastatic malignant cells may be observed.

The urinary tract distal from the renal pelvis is lined by transitional epithelial cells. Therefore, it is not surprising that both benign and malignant tumors of this cell type are most commonly observed, at least in man (58,100). However, because of their normal appearance, it is unlikely that transitional cell papillomas would be recognized by the characteristics of individual exfoliated cells. Most carcinomas of the urinary tract epithelium are transitional cell carcinomas and may be detected in urinary sediment with appropriate staining (100). In man the most common origin of these tumors is the urinary bladder rather than the renal pelvis or ureters. Primary squamous cell carcinomas, adenocarcinomas, and sarcomas may also occur in

the urinary system, but the spontaneous incidence is low. Metastatic tumors may occur in various portions of the urinary tract and originate from distant sites or more likely are the result of invasion from an adjacent primary site. Apparently, metastatic tumors of the urinary tract infrequently exfoliate into the urine (100). However, they may result in red and/or white blood cells in the sediment.

In some inflammations of the urinary tract in man, a peculiar type of epithelial cells observed in urine has been termed a "decoy cell" (58). These cells are relatively small with a high nuclear to cytoplasmic ratio. They appear to be necrobiotic cells with homogeneous, degenerating nuclei. However, such "decoy cells" may be confused with transitional cell carcinomas because of a superficial similarity. Highman and Wilson (47) described the cytologic features of exfoliated transitional cells observed in patients with urinary calculi, and compared these characteristics with those of differentiated transitional cell carcinomas.

Casts (cylindruria)

The search for renal casts is an extremely important aspect of examination of urinary sediment. The finding and accurate identification of casts is of considerable significance in the diagnosis and prognosis of renal disease.

Renal casts are shaped by the tubules of the nephrons and are formed when proteins gel in these tubules. The matrix of renal casts is generally the Tamm-Horsfall glycoprotein. This protein is always present in the urine, and although normally in solution, it may precipitate and gel under conditions of altered urine flow, pH, or electrolyte concentrations within the kidney. Various cellular constituents may be incorporated when the protein-gel forms. In kidney disease, blood protein may be present in the glomerular filtrate and also may become a cylindruric matrix in addition to glycoprotein. Renal casts may vary considerably in size and composition and may be of significance in detecting active renal parenchymal disease. It is important to distinguish between the various types of casts, particularly those containing cells.

Fresh urine should be examined for the presence of casts, because they may disintegrate after a few hours, particularly in alkaline urine. Casts are more readily detected with phase-contrast microscopy than with bright-field microscopy. Schumann (100) finds that permanent mounts of urinary sediment, prepared by cytocentrifugation and stained by the Papanicolaou procedure, are the most rapid and accurate preparations for the identification of casts. It has not been well established even in humans what constitutes a normal number of casts; however, a few casts per high power field are not cause for alarm if they are hyaline or granular types, which in many cases may be considered physiologic (100).

The various casts that may be observed in urine are shown in Table 14.1 and are aptly described and demonstrated in the monographs by Schumann (100), Bradley and Benson (10), and Graff (38).

Hyaline casts are basically protein casts that may form in cases of decreased urine flow, low pH, high solute concentration, or high protein concentration (100). Granular casts may be either fine or coarse. The source of the granules has not been well established; they are probably aggregated plasma proteins or the remnants of disintegrated cells. More than a few granular casts per high power field is probably indicative of renal parenchymal disease and would not be considered physiologic.

Red blood cell casts usually indicate glomerular damage sufficient to permit erythrocytes to enter the renal tubules. With glomerular damage, fibrinogen and other proteins also escape into the tubules and trap the erythrocytes in a fibrin matrix to form the cast. These casts may be made of degenerated red cells and hemosiderin, resulting in an orange-colored granular cast in unstained wet mounts of urine. In addition to acute glomerulonephritis, red cell casts may be present in acute tubular necrosis, chronic nephritis, and renal infaction.

Leukocyte casts are indicative of bacterial infections of the kidney such as pyelonephritis. Neutrophils probably gain access to the renal tubules by their own motility between and through renal epithelial cells, rather than through the glomerulus. Leukocyte casts may occur in glomerular disease, but generally are associated with tubulointerstitial disease (100).

Fatty casts are those in which lipid material is encased in a hyaline matrix. Such casts are associated primarily with acute renal diseases and tubular degeneration.

Casts of renal tubular epithelial cells may form any time there is damage to the epithelium with subsequent exfoliation of a large number of cells. Thus, tubular epithelial casts may be observed in acute tubular necrosis, interstitial nephritis, renal amyloidosis, and renal allograft rejection. Differentiation of these casts from leukocyte casts is difficult without differential staining.

Waxy casts represent the ultimate stage in cellular degeneration and are believed to be the end stage of granular casts that have been retained for a time in the tubules because of localized nephron obstruction (100). They are associated with tubular degeneration and are most commonly observed in chronic nephritis.

Broad casts, described in humans, may have the same constituents as other casts but are several times larger in diameter. They are probably due to renal tubular atrophy and dilatation. Broad waxy casts are also called renal failure cells and are considered a grave sign in cases of nephritis.

Casts that contain a combination of various cells and other material are described as mixed casts. Schumann (100) reported finding previously undescribed mixed casts with the use of Papanicolaou staining.

Bacteria or crystals may become trapped within the protein matrix of a hyaline cast. If such inclusions are numerous, the cast is described as a bacterial or crystal inclusion cast.

Pseudocasts composed of fibrin or mucous threads and aggregates of crystals or cells may be confused with casts. True casts are the result of extrusion or formation within a tube, so one would predict their characteristic shape and defined parallel sides. Pseudocasts do not have these characteristics. However, mucous threads and squamous epithelial cells that have a cylindroid shape may occasionally be confused with casts.

Crystals (crystalluria)

Various types of crystals may appear in the urinary sediment. Most are formed from normal constituents of urine and are of no specific diagnostic significance. Others are considered "pathologic" crystals and originate from exogenous compounds, defective metabolism, or abnormal excretion.

Crystals that form in normal urine are usually the result of an excessively high concentration of urine. The type of crystals formed in such cases is a function of the urine pH, and they become more abundant in refrigerated urine samples. A description of the various urine crystals, the pH at which they are most common, and the solubility characteristics have been tabulated by Bradley and Benson (10). In man, uric acid crystals may be associated with elevated serum uric acid levels and gouty arthritis or gouty nephropathy.

Abnormal or pathologic crystals may be of diagnostic significance and should always be reported. Cystine crystals in the urine may be due to a defect in renal tubular reabsorption even though plasma cystine levels are normal. Genetic defects in amino acid metabolism or severe liver disease interfering with normal amino acid metabolism may result in aminoacidemia with urinary precipitation of cystine, tyrosine, or leucine. Crystals of cholesterol can form and may be indicative of renal disease. Sulfonamide crystals may be observed in urinary sediment, but the incidence is now lower because of the introduction of more soluble sulfonamides. Use of the x-ray contrast media meglumine diatriazoate may result in crystals of this compound appearing in the urine. Ampicillin may occasionally precipitate in urine following large parenteral doses (10).

Infectious agents

Normal urine is sterile and devoid of microorganisms. However, some bacteria are present in most urine specimens unless appropriate and exacting techniques are employed to exclude contaminants present in the lower genitourinary tract. Even then, positive cultures may be obtained unless the specimen is cultured immediately or is refrigerated. Obviously, preservatives should not be used in specimens for bacteriologic evaluation.

The presence of a large number of bacteria in the sediment of a fresh urine sample may raise the suspicion of a urinary tract infection. The observance of bacteria in an uncentrifuged, fresh urine specimen is presumptive evidence of a urinary tract infection and usually indicates greater than 100,000 organisms per milliliter (100). In such cases gram stains and urine cultures are indicated.

Fungi may be observed in urinary sediment and may be either saphrophytes or pathogens.

Candida species are the most commonly observed yeast form in human urine specimens. Yeast infection may occur in animals with genetic or acquired immunodeficiency or immunsuppressive chemotherapy. Diabetes also predisposes to yeast infections of the urinary tract. A standard text on microbiology should be consulted for culture and staining methods and identification characteristics of fungi.

Only a few parasites or ova are specific to the urinary tract of laboratory animals. However, unless care is taken in obtaining the urine sample, it may contain ova and/or parasites from the gastrointestinal tract, and the ova of some may be confused with those of urinary tract parasites, such as *Capillaria* ova and *Trichuris vulpis* ova.

Diocotophyme renale is a kidney parasite that may live in the renal pelvis of the dog and mink. *Stephanurus dentatus* is a kidney worm found in swine and is relatively common in some parts of the United States. *Capillaria* species is a parasite found in the urinary bladder of dogs, cats, and rats and sometimes in the renal pelvis. This parasite is relatively nonpathogenic and rarely, if ever, occurs in laboratory-reared animals (33). *Trichosomoides crassicauda* has been reported in the urinary bladder, ureters, and renal pelvis of rats in Europe, but it usually is nonpathogenic (33). Diagnosis of urinary tract parasitism is made by detecting the characteristic ova in the urine sediment.

Miscellaneous

Lipid or fat droplets may be observed in urine specimens. They are round, highly refractile bodies that must be distinguished from erythrocytes. Under polarized microscopy they may exhibit anisotropism. Care must be taken in collecting urine specimens to be certain that contaminating fatty substances are not introduced from lubricating substances or unclean glassware. Lipid of urinary tract origin may indicate degenerative tubular disease, pyelonephritis, acute glomerulonephritis, renal carcinoma, or acute nephritis. Lipiduria may also occur in diabetes mellitus.

Chyluria may rarely occur with obstructions of the lymphatic system (100). Elevated urine protein levels and lymphocytes in the sediment along with a milky appearance of the urine specimen may be important clues in diagnosing chyluria.

Mucus or fibrin threads are commonly observed in urine. Mucus threads may form in most urine as it cools and they are composed of precipitated mucoproteins. Fibrin threads are the result of glomerular leakage or hemorrhage into the urinary tract (100).

Fibers from extraurinary sources may contaminate urine specimens and must be differentiated from casts and mucus or fibrin threads. These contaminants may be cotton, wool, or synthetic fibers, or hair.

Spermatozoa may be encountered in varying numbers in the urine of either sex. Tailless forms may be confused with bacteria, yeast, or cell nuclei.

Quality Control

Rigid quality control in the clinical pathology laboratory is as essential in toxicity testing as it is in a hospital setting. It is, in fact, dictated for certain studies by the Food and Drug Administration's Good Laboratory Practices (GLP) Regulations for the conduct of nonclinical laboratory studies (30). The GLP regulations have not changed the usual quality control practices that competent clinical laboratories have employed for years. Rather, they have defined standards of performance and markedly increased the documentation requirements in regard to procedures, protocols, instrument maintenance, and data accountability. The impact of GLP on toxicity studies has been estimated as a 15 to 25 per cent increase in cost. Clinical laboratory staff involved in studies conducted under GLP should become fully cognizant of the regulations. The text edited by Paget (81) is an excellent review of the many aspects of quality control in toxicity studies.

Quality control in urinalysis follows the same general principles applicable in hematology and clinical chemistry. The purpose is to ensure the integrity and validity of data generated. To accomplish this, a good quality control program involves two basic components: internal quality control procedures and participation in an external quality control program. An internal program involves instrument calibration and maintenance, use of reference controls and standards to assure that personnel, instruments, and reagents meet the required standards of pre-

cision and accuracy, and review of data transcriptions for accuracy. Unfortunately, there are no commercial sources of assayed species-specific reference controls for urine. An external quality control program involves participation in an interlaboratory peer comparison program. Some reagent manufacturers provide this service on a regional basis. Probably the largest program for interlaboratory comparisons is that conducted by the College of American Pathologists. A participating laboratory conducts tests on unknown specimens, reports their results, and receives reports comparing their performance with those of other laboratories using comparable instrumentation and methodology. However, these peer comparison programs are all based on materials derived from man. In spite of this they still provide the animal-oriented laboratory a valid measure of their comparative performance.

Quality control in urinalysis starts with appropriate attention and care given to collection of the specimen. Carelessness at this point may easily invalidate the benefits of a rigid quality control program in the laboratory. Quality control materials for hematology and clinical chemistry have been available for some time, but have only recently been introduced for urinalysis. Commercial lyophilized urine preparations for quantitative urinalyses are available from Hyland, Searle, Lederle, Ortho, and Dade (34). The constituents present vary from company to company, but most contain analytes common to routine urinalysis. Synthetic or simulated urine controls are also available from Ames Company and Harleco.

Establishing a good quality control program for urinalysis entails the same attention to detail given to hematology and clinical chemistry. Several quality control programs specific to urinalyses have been published (5,11,34,39).

In any quality control program it is essential to have well-trained personnel who understand the necessity of starting with quality specimens and are aware of the principle and limitations of each test to be performed. There should be a detailed written procedure for each test, which should be reviewed periodically by the laboratory supervisor and staff to be certain that the exact procedures are being followed. Daily calibrations of instruments such as osmometers, refractometers, and spectrophotometers should be made and recorded before any tests are initiated. There should also be systematic preventative maintenance performed and documented on all instruments. Positive and negative controls should be run and evaluated before any specimen assays are performed. The frequency of including controls in a run will depend on the number of samples, but at a minimum should be included at the start and completion of a run. Control values should be plotted and evaluated to detect trends in instrument drift, reagent deterioration, and/or technician-induced variability.

The use of dipsticks in routine urinalysis presents special problems in quality control because of the subjectivity and time constraints in reading the results. New staff should be thoroughly trained and their results evaluated frequently by the laboratory supervisor. It is important that the manufacturer's precautions for handling, storage, and use of reagent strips be followed precisely. Some of the subjectivity in reading dipsticks has been removed by the introduction of automated instrumentation for quantitating results.

RENAL FUNCTION TESTS

Glomerular Filtration Rate

Evaluation of the glomerular filtration rate (GFR) may be made indirectly by measuring serum levels of specific endogenous analytes or more directly by measuring the clearance of substances removed by the glomeruli and not excreted by the tubules. The most widely used indirect method is to determine serum levels of urea nitrogen and creatinine. Interpretations of these tests will be covered under "Serum Indicators of Renal Damage."

Proteinuria is a sensitive indicator of renal damage. However, it is not specific for glomerular damage, because smaller molecular weight proteins that normally pass the glomerular membrane may not be reabsorbed if tubular lesions are present, thus resulting in positive tests for urinary proteins. Dipsticks and precipitation tests for proteins do not differentiate the molecular size, so they are of no value in localizing a renal lesion. Greenhill and Gruskin (41) have described a Selective Protein Index (SPI) that may be of value in determining the significance and origin of proteinuria. The SPI is the ratio of a large molecular weight protein in serum and urine divided by the urine-to-serum ratio of albumin:

$$SPI = \frac{urine\ IgG/serum\ IgG}{urine\ albumin/serum\ albumin} \times 100$$

This ratio ignores tubular reabsorption and defines the relative glomerular permeability to proteins of different molecular weights. It would be interesting to evaluate the SPI for its potential as a specific indicator of glomerular damage, possibly using a much larger protein such as fibrinogen in the numerator.

The dipstick method is the most commonly used, but least sensitive, screening test for proteinuria. The dye, bromophenol blue, reacts fairly specifically with albumin but not with other proteins.

Clearance methods are more straightforward in estimating GFR than is determination of plasma or urine constituents; however, they are still indirect measurements. Clearances have the advantage of being much more sensitive indicators of renal damage than are serum creatinine or blood urea nitrogen levels. The ideal material to measure GFR would be one that is excreted exclusively by the glomeruli, would not be secreted or reabsorbed by renal tubules, would not be metabolized, would not be bound to proteins, and would be nontoxic. Inulin best meets these criteria and is still considered the benchmark against which the validity of other substances used to measure GFR is determined.

The clearance rate (GFR) of a substance is calculated by the formula:

$$Cx = GFR = \frac{\dfrac{Ux \cdot Uv}{Px}}{BW} = ml/m/kg$$

where Ux = urine concentration of the substance, Px = plasma concentration of the substance, Uv = minute urine volume, and BW = body weight in kilograms.

As seen from this formula, reliable clearance measurements depend on a stable plasma level of the indicator substance and on precisely timed and complete collection of urine.

Inulin is the substance of choice for reliable determinations of GFR in laboratory species, because it is cleared exclusively by glomerular filtration. However, the procedures for determining inulin clearance are complex and cannot be considered as routine tests of renal function for large-scale screening assays. Because inulin is an exogenous substance, it must be introduced by intravenous infusion to maintain a stable plasma concentration for the test period of about 30 to 60 minutes. Anesthesia or rigid restraint of the animal is required as well as complete emptying of the bladder before, during, and at the completion of the test period. Radiotracer tagging of inulin has simplified the previously demanding chemical assays for inulin (20,70,109).

Endogenous urea clearance was the first clearance test to be used widely and has a long historical background. Urea is cleared by the glomeruli but is passively reabsorbed by the renal tubules. Therefore, this clearance test is not a true measure of GFR and should not be used as such. However, urea clearance can be used as a general evaluation of the status of renal function.

The most common test used to evaluate glomerular function is the clearance of endogenous creatinine. Creatinine levels in plasma are quite constant and not greatly influenced by diet; therefore, GFR estimates using this method do not encompass the problems encountered with inulin clearance studies. Objections to using creatinine clearance to evaluate GFR are that renal tubular secretion of creatinine occurs in some species, such as rats, guinea pigs, and male dogs (21,85) and that common methods of assaying creatinine measure noncreatinine chromogens present in plasma that are not present in urine. Tubular secretion of creatinine tends to overestimate GFR, whereas the noncreatinine chromogens result in underestimation of GFR. These two opposing effects tend fortuitously to cancel each other (46). The calculation of endogenous creatinine clearance is a relatively easy test to conduct and is adaptable to screening tests for nephrotoxicity following chemical or physical insults. A plasma creatinine determination is made at the start and completion of a timed urine collection. The bladder of an adequately hydrated animal should be emptied at the start of the test (discard specimen) and again at its completion. It is necessary to accurately measure the collection period, the volume of urine, and the weight of the animal. The creatinine concentration is then determined in an aliquot of the urine and the serum samples, and the creatinine clearance per minute per kilogram of body weight may be calculated. The

clearance of exogenous creatinine, that is, injected creatinine, may also be determined but is not well suited for use in large-scale nephrotoxicity studies.

Plasma clearance of injected substances has also been used to estimate GFR without the need for urine collection. Implicit in using these substances is that plasma disappearance occurs only by renal excretion. One method is to infuse a compound at a constant rate to achieve an equilibrium between the infusion rate and the plasma clearance rate at which time this equals the excretion rate (25). Singhvi et al (105) and Aperia et al (3) described this technique in dogs and DiBona and Sawin (20) in the rat. This method is too cumbersome to use as a routine nephrotoxicity screening test. A second plasma clearance method without the need for urine collection involves the single intravenous injection of a compound and the clearance from plasma determined from collection of several blood samples. Sapirstein et al (97) developed this technique and the calculations necessary to estimate GFR using injected creatinine in the dog. More recently, radiolabeled compounds such as ^{51}Cr-EDTA, ^{125}I-sodium iothalamate, and ^{131}I-diatriazoate have been used to estimate GFR in dogs and rats (13,74,79,82). These methods are applicable for nephrotoxicity screening on a limited basis, but species differences must be evaluated to be certain the substances are cleared only by GFR and not by tubular secretion. Age-related changes in GFR and solute excretion have been described in the rat (16).

Tubular Function Tests

Nephrotoxic chemicals frequently exert their main action on the renal tubules; because of this, it is important to evaluate tubular function in toxicity studies. The renal tubules, unlike the glomeruli, have multiple functions that may be evaluated by several means. Some, like urinary concentrations of protein, amino acids, pH, glucose, and cellular constituents, have been discussed previously. Renal concentration and dilution are also a tubular function and will be discussed later. This section will address tests to evaluate the tubular functions of reabsorption or secretion using injected compounds. Such tests are not designed for large-scale nephrotoxicity screening and will not be covered in detail.

These tests determine the maximum ability of the renal tubule to reabsorb substances such as glucose or to secrete substances such as para-aminohippurate (PAH). This ability is referred to as the tubular maximum (Tm) for the substances. However, renal clearances of these substances depend on glomerular as well as tubular function, so that it is necessary to determine GFR concurrent with the tubular functions. It is also necessary to infuse the test material, such as glucose or PAH, to saturate the Tm for the substance and then to maintain that level for some time by continued infusion. The procedure for conducting these tests and the necessary calculations to determine reabsorption or secretion have been described for man (46,71,86), dog (79,82,87,105), rats (101), and rabbits (77,78).

Concentration/Dilution Tests

The ability of the kidney to concentrate urine above that of the glomerular filtrate is primarily a function of the loop of Henle and the distal tubule (46,71). However, these functions are highly dependent on the production of and responsiveness to antidiuretic hormone and a normal or near normal GFR. The basis of the test is that water deprivation results in plasma hyperosmolality triggering the release of anti-diuretic hormone which in turn acts on the renal tubule cells causing reabsorption of water and an increase in urine specific gravity and osmolality. The volume of urine and consequently the concentration may also be influenced by extra-renal effects; for example, Sharratt and Frazer (101) found that diarrhea in rats reduced the volume of urine excreted during a concentration test.

Urine concentration tests are generally considered a moderately sensitive measure of renal function. Sharratt and Frazer (101) found functional impairment using the concentration test in rats when renal injury was not severe. However, Osborne et al (80) report that in the dog, urine concentrating ability is not impaired until at least 66 per cent of the renal parenchyma has been damaged. A concentration test (water deprivation test) is relatively readily adaptable for use in large-scale screening studies for nephrotoxicity.

To use the concentration test for nephrotoxicity screening on a large-scale basis, it should be modified to delete bladder catheterization typically used in the clinical setting in which only an individual animal is being examined. A practical approach is to place the animals in metabolism cages with free access to water and collection of a 16- to 24-hour urine sample for urinalysis. At the end of this collection period, the source of water is removed and the water deprivation test begun. After 12 hours the voided urine is discarded and an additional urine collection made for another 12 to 16 hours. The urine sample should be collected under mineral oil to prevent evaporation. The specific gravity, or preferably the osmolality, of the urine sample is determined and compared with that obtained when the animal was well hydrated. The urine-concentrating ability of the experimental groups is compared with the mean values from the control animals to assess renal function. Following renal tubular damage the ability to concentrate urine is variably reduced.

The ability of the kidney to dilute the urine is also a tubular function. However, urine dilution tests are cumbersome because they entail the administration of a water load by gavage and thus are not very practical for large-scale screening tests for nephrotoxicity. Extrarenal effects such as vomiting, diarrhea, delayed absorption from the gastrointestinal tract, and hypoadrenocorticism influence the results (71). In man, this test is conducted by administering (drinking) 20 ml of water per kilogram of body weight over a 10- to 20-minute period and collecting urine hourly for 4 hours. With normal renal function, 75 per cent of the ingested dose is excreted during the 4-hour period, and the specific gravity of at least one specimen should be 1.004 (71). Sharratt and Fraser (101) used this test in rats by gavaging them with water at 5 per cent of their body weight and collecting urine every 30 minutes for 2 hours. They determined the volume and specific gravity of each sample and calculated the percentage of the administered dose that was excreted over the 2-hour collection period. These workers reported the dilution test to be a less sensitive indicator of renal damage than the urine concentration test.

The osmolar clearance and freewater clearance are a valuable indication of whether the kidney is excreting water in excess of solute excretion. To determine solute (osmolar) excretion, urine osmolality is compared with plasma osmolality which is equivalent to the osmolality of the glomerular filtrate. Urine volume is measured over a specific interval and the osmolar clearance calculated from a typical clearance formula:

$$C_{osm} = \frac{U_{osm}V}{P_{osm}}$$

where U_{osm} is the urine osmolality (mosm/kg of water), P_{osm} the plasma osmolality (mosm/kg of water), and V the urine flow (ml/m).

A U_{osm} to P_{osm} ratio greater than 1 indicates the kidney is excreting a concentrated urine, whereas a ratio less than 1 means excess water is being excreted. A more quantitative estimate of renal handling of water may be calculated as the freewater clearance, or the amount of urine excretion in excess of that needed to excrete solutes at an osmolality equal to that of plasma (71).

Freewater clearance $(C_{H_2O}) = C_{osm}$ or

$$C_{H_2O} = V\left[1 - \frac{U_{osm}}{P_{osm}}\right]$$

Renal Blood Flow

Several techniques are available for the determination of renal blood flow in laboratory animals. However, none are suitable for routine nephrotoxicity screening and they will not be covered in any depth in this section. The techniques are used primarily in laboratories conducting in-depth studies of renal physiology.

Direct measures of renal blood flow involve the use of sensors such as electromagnetic or Doppler flowmeters around a renal artery. Renal blood flow may be determined indirectly by determining the clearance from plasma of a substance infused at a constant rate. This technique involves collection of arterial blood samples and renal vein samples and assays for the injected substance which must be removed from the circulation only via the kidney. Because any such substance is removed primarily from the plasma, this method estimates renal plasma flow (RPF) rather than renal blood flow and is calculated as follows:

$$RPF = \frac{U_x \cdot V}{RA_x \cdot RV_x}$$

where U_x is the concentration of substance in urine, V the urine volume in ml/m, RA_x the concentration of substance in renal artery, and RV_x the concentration of substance in renal vein.

Renal blood flow (RBF) may then be calculated as follows:

$$RBF = \frac{RPF}{1 - VPRC}$$

where VPRC is the volume of packed red cells.

If a substance were removed from renal arterial blood in a single pass through the kidney, it would be unnecessary to sample renal venous blood to arrive at renal blood flow. If the substance were not metabolized by the tissues, the concentration in peripheral venous blood would equal the concentration in the renal artery and would preclude the need to sample renal artery blood. A substance meeting these criteria, and one to which other substances are compared, is *para*-aminohippurate (PAH). This compound and ortho-iodohippurate (OIH) are filtered completely by the glomerulus and are secreted by the renal tubules. Therefore, their extraction ratio (E), that is, the fraction removed from the plasma in a single pass through the kidney, is near 100 per cent. E is determined by measuring the concentration of the indicator substance in renal artery and vein, and for PAH and OIH is actually only 80 to 90 per cent, because some of the blood entering the kidney will perfuse nontubular tissues such as the medulla and capsular areas (21). Thus, PAH and OIH correspond to cortical plasma flow rather than RPF and are known as the effective renal plasma flow (ERPF). True RPF may then be calculated as follows:

$$RPF = \frac{ERPF}{E}$$

The ERPF may be determined by measuring the plasma disappearance of the indicator. However, calculation of RPF may be in serious error unless E is actually determined, because renal parenchymal lesions can markedly change the ability of the kidney to extract the indicator.

The dog has been the most common experimental animal for studies of RPF. Representative publications describing techniques in the dog include those of Oester et al (79), Aperia et al (3), and Binnion and Cummings (8), and in the rat Sharratt and Frazer (101).

Studies to evaluate the internal blood flow have been conducted using "washout" techniques. These methods use injection of inert gases, such as radiolabeled xenon or krypton, or microspheres into a renal artery. These are used for specific renal physiologic studies and are not applicable in large-scale nephrotoxicity screening assays.

Serum Indicators of Renal Damage

Serum (blood) levels of urea nitrogen (BUN) and creatinine are traditionally the most widely used screening tests to evaluate renal function in all species. Urea is an end product of nitrogen metabolism, and serum levels are significantly influenced by diet, liver function, gastrointestinal absorption of nitrogen, and the state of hydration. Creatinine, however, is a product of muscle metabolism, and although serum levels tend to remain relatively constant, they may be influenced by diet and nitrogen balance (8). Both substances are excreted primarily by glomerular filtration.

Blood urea nitrogen is not a good indicator of mild to moderate renal damage because serum levels may remain within a normal range until renal function has been reduced more than 50 per cent (29). In addition to glomerular lesions, renal tubular necrosis may result in decreased urea clearance, thus causing elevated BUN levels. Postrenal obstructions caused by tumors or stones in the urinary tract may result in elevated BUN concentrations. Gastrointestinal hemorrhage may result in elevated BUN levels because of the bacterial degradation of hemoglobin to ammonia and subsequent incorporation into urea. Despite these constraints, BUN is a valuable test in nephrotoxicity screening of a large number of animals, provided the control and treated groups are fasted at least 12 hours before the blood sample is obtained.

Serum creatinine levels are less influenced by extrarenal factors than are BUN levels and generally are considered more sensitive than BUN in detecting nephropathy. A doubling of serum creatinine concentration indicates that creatinine clearance has been at least halved (2). The noncreatinine chromogens in plasma, which

are assayed by the usual creatinine methods, decrease proportionately as creatinine levels increase following a renal insult. The BUN to creatinine ration may be calculated in an attempt to differentiate more precisely pre- or postrenal disease from renal parenchymal disease. Elevations in this ratio in a treated group of animals as compared with their controls would theoretically indicate an extrarenal rather than a renal effect.

Serum electrolytes may be of value in nephrotoxicity screening tests; however, sodium and chloride levels are subject to so many prerenal influences that serum levels are of limited value in renal toxicity studies. Acute renal insufficiency markedly influences potassium balance, and serum levels are characteristically elevated. Phosphate excretion is primarily a function of glomerular filtration and tubular reabsorption, and serum levels may be elevated in acute nephropathies. In chronic renal disease compensatory homeostatic mechanisms tend to result in normal serum levels of both potassium and phosphorus. Serum calcium may be significantly reduced with severe, acute renal failure depending on the degree of hyperphosphatemia. Acute renal toxicity may result in metabolic acidosis due to reduced serum bicarbonate levels. More recent evidence suggests that a specific defect in hydrogen ion excretion is also operative in acute renal failure and also contributes to metabolic acidosis (118). As renal disease progresses and, if uncompensated, hydrogen ion retention increases and serum pH falls.

Some serum enzymes may be elevated in renal disease. It is important to remember that serum levels of enzymes may be due to cell destruction, increased cell turnover, enhanced production of an enzyme, or reduced clearance from the serum. In addition, elevations of serum enzymes generally occur during acute disease processes rather than chronic phases. Boyd (9) reviewed the relative concentration of several enzymes in numerous tissues of 10 species including man. Unfortunately, most of the enzymes with relatively high renal concentrations are found in high concentrations in other tissues, particularly liver. Gamma glutamyl transferase and alkaline phosphatase are two exceptions and should be of some value in evaluating acute renal damage. Serum amylase and lipase may be elevated in renal disease, probably because of decreased renal clearance of these enzymes which are excreted by the kidney. Raab (89,90) induced renal damage in rats by injection of sodium tetrathionate and found serum elevations of isocitrate dehydrogenase and cholinesterase to an extent that he thought these enzymes might be of value in assessing acute renal damage.

Hypoproteinemia may be present following renal damage, with resultant loss of protein at the glomerular membrane and/or failure of tubular reabsorption. The concomitant hypercholesterolemia has been theorized to result from the compensatory hepatic synthesis of all plasma proteins including the lipoproteins (66).

REFERENCES

1. Altman PL, Dittmer DS (1969) Biological Handbook of Metabolism. Fed Am Soc Exp Biol Med, Bethesda, p 523
2. Anderson CF (1978) Renal Failure. In Knox FG (ed) Renal Pathophysiology, Ch 13. Harper & Row, New York
3. Aperia A, Herin P, Josephson S, Lannergren K (1982) Renal functions in dogs with chronic moderate unilateral ureteral obstruction. Scand J Clin Lab Invest 42: 1–8
4. Banks N, Bailine SH (1965) Urinary β-glucuronidase activity in patients with urinary tract infections. N Engl J Med 272: 70–75
5. Becker SM, Ramirez C, Pribor HC, Gillen AL (1973) A quality control product for urinalysis. Am J Clin Path 59: 185–191
6. Berndt WO (1981) Use of renal function tests in evaluation of nephrotoxic effects. In Hook JB (ed), Toxicology of the Kidney. Raven Press, New York, pp 1–29
7. Binnion PF, Cumming JK (1967) A study of ^{131}I-hippuran excretion in dogs as a measure of renal plasma flow. Clin Sci 33: 313–318
8. Bleiler RE, Schedl HP (1962) Creatinine excretion: Variability and relationships to diet. J Lab Clin Med 59: 945–955
9. Boyd JW (1983) The mechanisms relating to increases in plasma enzymes and isoenzymes in diseases of animals. Vet Clin Pathol 12: 9–24
10. Bradley GM, Benson ES (1974) Examination of the urine. In Davidsohn I, Henry JB (eds), Todd-Sanford Clinical Diagnosis, 1st ed. WB Saunders, Philadelphia
11. Bradley M, Schumann GB, Ward PC (1979) Examination of Urine. In Henry JB, Todd-Sanford-Davidsohn; Clinical Diagnosis and Management, 16th ed. WB Saunders, Philadelphia, pp 559–634
12. Brenner BM, Rector FC (eds) (1986) The Kidney, 3rd ed. WB Saunders, Philadelphia.
13. Bryan C, Jarchow R, Maher J (1972) Measurement of glomerular filtration rate in small animals without urine collection. Clin Res 20: 62
14. Burkhardt AE, Johnston KG, Waszak CE (1982) A reagent strip for measuring the specific gravity of urine. Clin Chem 28: 2068–2072
15. Coonrad D, Paterson PY (1969) Urinary beta-glucuronidase in renal injury. I. Enzyme assay conditions and response to mercuric chloride in rats. J Lab Clin Med 73: 6–16
16. Corman B, Pratz J, Poujeol P (1985) Changes in anatomy, glomerular filtration rate, and solute excretion in aging rat kidney. Am J Physiol 248: R282–R287
17. Cornelius CE, Mia AS, Rosenfeld S (1965) Ruminant urolithiasis: Studies on the origin of Tamm-Horsfall urinary microprotein and its presence in ovine calculus matrix. Invest Urol 2: 452–457
18. Davidsohn I, Henry JB (1974) Todd and Sanford Clinical Diagnosis by Laboratory Methods. WB Saunders, Philadelphia, Appendix 3
19. Dawnay ABSJ, Cattell WR (1981) Serum Tamm-Horsfall glycoprotein in levels in health and renal disease. Clin Nephrol 15: 5–8
20. DeWardener HE (1985) The Kidney: An Outline of Normal and Abnormal Function. Churchill Livingstone, New York
21. Diezi J, Biollaz J (1979) Renal function tests in experimental toxicity studies. Pharmac Ther 5: 135–145
22. Dilena BA, Penberthy LA, Fraser CG (1983) Six methods for determining urinary protein compared. Clin Chem 29: 553–557
23. Dubach UC (1968) Enzymes in urine and kidney. Hans Huber, Stuttgart
24. Dubach UC, Schmidt U (eds) (1979) Diagnostic Significance of Enzymes and Proteins in Urine. Hans Huber, Stuttgart
25. Earle DP, Berliner RW (1946) A simplified clinical procedure for measurements of glomerular filtration rate and renal plasma flow. Proc Soc Exp Biol Med 62: 262–264
26. Ellis BG, Price RG, Topham JC (1973a) The effect of tubular damage by mercuric chloride on kidney function and some urinary enzymes in the dog. Chem Biol Interactions 7: 101–113
27. Ellis BG, Price RG, and Topham JC (1973b) The effect of papillary damage by ethyleneimine on kidney function and some urinary enzymes in the dog. Chem Biol Interactions 7: 131–142
28. Fair PH, Daugherty WJ, Braddon SA (1985) Methyl mercury and selenium interaction in relation to mouse kidney α-blutamyltranspeptidase, ultrastructure and function. Toxicol Appl Pharmacol 80: 78–96
29. Faulkner WR, King JW (1976) Renal function. In Tietz NW (ed), Clinical Chemistry, Chap 17. WB Saunders, Philadelphia
30. Federal Register: Food and Drug Administration, Nonclinical Laboratory Studies; Good Laboratory Practice Regulations. 43: 59986–60025 (Dec. 22, 1978; Part II)
31. Finco DR (1980) Kidney Function. In Kaneko JJ (ed) Clinical Biochemistry of Domestic Animals. Academic Press, New York, p 367
32. Finlayson JS, Baumann CA (1958) Mouse proteinuria. Am J Physiol 192: 69–72
33. Flynn RJ (1973) Parasites of laboratory animals. Iowa State University, Ames

34. Free AH, Free HM (1975) Urinalysis in clinical laboratory practice. CRC Press, West Palm Beach

35. Gabizon D, Goren E, Shaked U, Averbukh Z, Rosenmann E, Modai D (1985) Induction of chronic renal failure in the mouse: A new model. Nephron 40: 349–352

36. Galitzer SJ, Hayes RH, Oehme FW (1979) A simple urine collection method for female swine. Lab An Sci 29: 404–405

37. Ganong WF (1979) Renal function. In: Review of Medical Physiology, 9th Ed. Lange Medical Publications, Los Altos, CA

38. Graff L (1983) A Handbook of Routine Urinalysis. JB Lippincott, Philadelphia

39. Grannis GF, Statland BE (1979) Monitoring the quality of laboratory measurements. In Henry JB (ed), Todd-Sanford-Davidsohn, Clinical Diagnosis and Management by Laboratory Methods. WB Saunders, Philadelphia, pp 2049–2068

40. Grant AMS, Neuberger A (1973) The turnover rate of rabbit urinary Tamm-Horsfall glycoprotein. Biochem J 136: 659–668

41. Greenhill A, Gruskin AB (1976) Laboratory evaluation of renal function. Pediat Chemics NA 23: 661–679

42. Haber MH (1981) Urinary Sediment: A Textbook Atlas. American Society of Clinical Pathologists, Chicago, IL

43. Hansen S, Perry TL, Lesk D (1972) Urinary bacteria: A potential source of some organic acidurias. Clin Chim Acta 39: 71

44. Hautmann R (1979) Diagnosis of renal disorders: Comparison of urinary enzyme patterns with corresponding tissue patterns. In Dubach UC, Schmidt U (eds), Diagnostic Significance of Enzymes and Proteins in Urine. Hans Huber, Stuttgart, pp 58–70

45. Hay PA, Adolph EF (1956) Diuresis in response to hypoxia and epinephrine in infant rats. Am J Physiol 187: 32–40

46. Haycock GB (1981) Old and new tests of renal function. J Clin Pathol 34: 1226–1281

47. Highman W, Wilson E (1982) Urine cytology in patients with calculi. J Clin Pathol 35: 350–356

48. Hoffsten PE, Hill CL, Klahr S (1975) Studies of albuminuria and proteinuria in normal mice and mice with immune complex glomerulonephritis. J Lab Clin Med 86: 920–930

49. Holmquist ND (1977) Diagnostic Cytology of the Urinary Tract. Monographs in Clinical Cytology. S Karger, New York

50. Hook JB (1981) Toxicology of the Kidney. Raven Press, New York

51. Johnston IDA, Jones NF, Scoble JE, Yuen CT, Price RG (1983) The diagnostic value of urinary enzyme measurements in hypertension. Clin Chem Acta 133: 317–325

52. Kinne RKH (ed) (1985) Renal Biochemistry, Cells, Membranes, Molecules. Elsevier, New York

53. Kirk RW, Bistner SI (1969) Handbook of Veterinary Procedures and Emergency Treatment. WB Saunders, Philadelphia, PA, p 205

54. Kluwe WM (1981) Renal Function Tests as Indicators of Kidney Injury in Subacute Toxicity Studies. Toxicol Appl Pharmacol 57: 414–424

55. Knox FG (1978) Renal Pathophysiology. Harper & Row, New York

56. Kono N, Sasaki N (1975) Platelets in human urine. N Engl J Med 293: 44–45

57. Koss LG (1974) Tumors of the Urinary Bladder. Atlas of Tumor Pathology, Fascicle II. AFIP, Washington, DC

58. Koss LG (1968) Diagnostic Cytology. Chapter 19. The Urinary Tract, JB Lippincott, Philadelphia, pp 404–451

59. Koushanpour E (1976) Renal Physiology: Principles and Function. WB Saunders, Philadelphia

60. Kraus AL (1980) Research Methodology. In Baker HJ, Lindsey JR, Weisbroth SH (eds), The Laboratory Rat. Vol II. Research Applications. Academic Press, New York, p 11

61. Kurtzman NA, Martinez-Maldonado M (eds) (1977) Pathophysiology of the Kidney. Charles C Thomas, Springfield, IL

62. Lartigue CW, Driscoll TB, Johnson PC (1978) Low-temperature urine collection apparatus for laboratory rodents. Lab An Sci 28: 594–597

63. Leaf A, Cotran RS (1985) Renal Pathophysiology, 3rd ed. Oxford University Press, New York

64. Loeb WF (1964) The clinical examination : Laboratory procedures. In Catcott EJ (ed), Feline Medicine and Surgery. American Veterinary, Santa Barbara, p 25–26

65. MacKenzie R, Asscher AW (1986) Progression of chronic pyelonephritis in the rat. Nephron 42: 171–176

66. March GB, Drablein DL (1960) Experimental reconstruction of metabolic patterns of lipids nephrosis: Key role of hepatic protein synthesis in hyperlipemia. Metab 9: 946–955

67. Maruhn D (1979) Preparation of urine for enzyme determinations by gel filtration. In Dubach UC, Schwedt U (eds), Diagnostic Significance of Enzymes and Proteins in Urine. Hans Huber, Stuttgart

68. Matandos CK, Franz DR (1980) Collection of urine from caged cats. Lab An Sci 30: 562–564

69. Mattenheimer H (1971) Enzymes in the urine. Med Clin 55: 1493–1508

70. McCormack KM, Kluwe WM, Rickert DE, Singer UL, Hook JB (1978) Renal and hepatic microsomal enzyme stimulation and renal function following three months of dietary exposure to polybrominated biphenyls. Toxicol Appl Pharmacol 44: 539–553

71. Mitchell FL, Veall N, Watts RWE (1979) Renal function tests suitable for clinical practice. Scientific Review No. 2. Ann Clin Biochem 9: 1–20

72. Mitruka BM, Rawnsley HM (1977) Clinical Biochemical and Hematological Reference Values in Normal Experimental Animals. Masson, New York

73. Moreland AF (1965) In Gay WI (ed) Methods of Animal Experimentation, Vol 1. Academic Press, New York, p 19

74. Mudge GH, Berndt WO, Saunders A, Beattie B (1971) Renal transport of diatriazoate in the rabbit, dog, and rat. Nephron 8: 156–172

75. Nakamura T, Oite T, Shimizu F, Matsuyama M, Kazama T, Koda Y, Arakawa M (1986) Sclerotic

lesions in the glomeruli of Buffalo-Mna rats. Nephron 43: 50–55

76. Newton JF, Yoshimoto M, Bernstein J, Rush GF, Hook JB (1983). Acetominophen nephrotoxicity in the rat. 1. Strain difference in nephrotoxicity and metabolism. Toxicol Appl Pharmacol 69: 291–306

77. Nomiyama K, Sato C, Yamamoto A (1973) Early signs of cadmium intoxication in rabbits. Toxicol Appl Pharmacol 24: 625–635

78. Nomiyama K, Yamamoto A, Sato C (1974) Assay of urinary enzymes in toxic nephropathy. Toxicol Appl Pharmacol 27: 484–490

79. Oester A, Wolf H, Madsen PO (1969) Measurement of glomerular filtration rate using ^{131}I-diatriazoate. Lancet 1: 397–399

80. Osborne CA, Finco DR, Low DG (1983) Pathophysiology of Renal Disease, Renal Failure and Uremia. In Ettinger SJ (ed), Textbook of Veterinary Internal Medicine. WB Saunder, Philadelphia, p 1733

81. Paget GE (ed) (1979) Quality Control in Toxicology. University Park Press, Baltimore

82. Pihl B, Nosslin B (1974) Single injection technique for determination of renal clearance: I. Clearance of iothalamate and iodohippurate in dogs. Scand J Urol Nephrol 8: 138–146

83. Piperno E (1981) Detection of drug induced nephrotoxicity with urinalysis and enzymuria assessment. In Hook JB (ed), Toxicology of the Kidney. Raven Press, New York, pp 31–55

84. Piscator M, Bjorek L, Nordberg M (1981) β_2-microglobulin levels in serum and urine of cadmium exposed rabbits. Acta Pharmacol Toxical 49: 1–7

85. Pitts RF (1974) Physiology of the Kidney and Body Fluids. Yearbook Medical Publishers, Chicago

86. Plesner T, Pederson B, Boenisch T (1975) Radioimmunoassay of β_2-microglobulin. Scand J Clin Lab Invest 35: 729–735

87. Powers TE, Powers JD, Garg RC (1977) Study of the double isotope single-injection method for estimating renal function in purebred beagle dogs. Am J Vet Res 38: 1933–1936

88. Price R, Dance N, Richards B, Catell WR (1970) The excretion of N-acetyl-glucosaminidase and -galatosidase following surgery to kidneys. Clin Chem Acta 27: 65–68

89. Raab WP (1969a) Isocitrate dehydrogenase activity of serum in experimental kidney damage. Enzymologia 37: 179–183

90. Raab W (1969b) Cholinesterase activity of rat serum following renal damage. Clin Chem Acta 24: 135–138

91. Raab WP (1972) Diagnostic value of urinary enzyme determinations. Clin Chem 18: 5–25

92. Ragan HA, Gillis MF (1975) Restraint, venipuncture, endotracheal intubation and anesthesia of miniature swine. Lab An Sci 25: 409–419

93. Robertson JL, Goldschmidt M, Kronfeld DS, Tomaszewski JE, Hill GS, Bovee KC (1986) Long-term renal responses to high dietary protein in dogs with 75 per cent nephrectomy. Kidney Int 29: 511–519

94. Robinson D, Price RG, Dance N (1967) Rat urine glycosidases and kidney damage. Biochem J 102: 533–538

95. Roerig DL, Hasegawa AT, Wang RIH (1980) Rat restrainer for separation and collection of urine and feces. Lab An Sci 30: 549–551

96. Rubini ME, Wolf AV (1975) Refactrometric determination of total solids and water of serum and urine. J Biol Chem 225: 869

97. Sapirstein LG, Vidt DC, Mandel MJ, Hanusek G (1955) Volumes of distribution and clearances of intravenously injected creatinine in the dog. Am J Physiol 181: 330–336

98. Schrier RW (ed), (1986) Renal and Electrolyte Disorders, 3rd ed. Little Brown, Boston

99. Schumann GB, Palmieri LJ, Jones DB (1977) Differentiation of renal tubular epithelium in renal transplantation cytology. Am J Clin Pathol 67: 580

100. Schumann GB (1980) Urine Sediment Examination. Williams & Wilkins, Baltimore

101. Sharratt M, Frazer AC (1963) The sensitivity of function tests in detecting renal damage in the rat. Toxicol Appl Pharmacol 5: 36–48

102. Shaw ST, Benson ES (1974) Renal function and its evaluation. In Davidsohn I, Henry JB (eds), Todd-Sanford Clinical Diagnosis, 15th ed, WB Saunders, Philadelphia

103. Sikri KL, Alexander DP, Foster CL (1982) Localization of Tamm-Horsfall glycoprotein in the normal rat kidney and the effects of adrenalectomy on its localization in the hamster and rat kidney. J Anat 135: 29–45

104. Sikri KL, Foster CL, Alexander DP, Marshall RD (1981) Localization of Tamm-Horsfall glycoprotein in the fetal and neonatal hamster kidney as demonstrated by immunofluorescence and immuno-electron microscopic techniques. Biol Neonate 39: 305–312

105. Singhvi SM, Heald AF, Murphy BF, Difazio LT, Schreiber EC, Poutsiaka JW (1978) Disposition of $^{[14]}$Nadolol in dogs with reversible renal impairment induced by uranyl nitrate. Toxicol Appl Pharmacol 43: 99–109

106. Smith CR, Felton JS, Taulor RT (1981) Description of a disposable individual-mouse urine collection apparatus. Lab An Sci 31: 80–82

107. Spencer ES, Pedersen I (1976) Hand Atlas of Urinary Sediment. Bright-Field, Phase-Contrast, and Polarized-Light. University Park Press, Baltimore

108. Sutor AH (1973) Thrombocyturia after aspirin. N Engl J Med 288: 794–795

109. Thomsen K, Olesen OV (1981) Effect of anaesthesia and surgery on urine flow and electrolyte excretion in different rat strains. Renal Physiol 4: 165–172

110. Thung PJ (1962) Physiologic proteinuria in mice. Acta Physiol Pharmacol Nrl 10: 248–261

111. Tweeddale DN (1977) Urinary Cytology. Little, Brown, Boston

112. Vander AJ (1985) Renal Physiology, 3rd ed. McGraw-Hill, New York

113. Walker RG, Escott M, Buchall I, Dowling JP, Kincaid-Smith P (1986) Chronic progressive renal lesions induced by lithium. Kidney Int 29: 875–881

114. Watanabe M, Nomura G, Hirata H, Imai K,

Koizumi H (1980) Studies on the validity of urine enzyme assay in the diagnosis of drug-induced renal lesions in rats. Toxicol Pathol 8: 22–23

115. Watts RH (1971) A simple capillary tube method for the determination of the specific gravity of 25 and 50 μl quantities of urine. J Clin Pathol 24: 667–668

116. West RW, Stanley JW, Newport GD (1978) Single-mouse urine collection and pH monitoring system. Lab An Sci 28: 343–345

117. Wilkinson JH (1968) Diagnostic significance of enzyme determinations in urine. In Dubach UC (ed), Enzymes in Urine and Kidney. Hans Huber, Stuttgart

118. Winaver J, Agmon D, Harari R, Better OS (1986) Impaired renal acidification following acute renal ischemia in the dog. Kidney Int 30: 906–913

119. Wirdnam PK, Milner RDG (1985) Radioimmunoassay for serum and urinary Tamm-Horsfall glycoprotein in the rat. Nephron 40: 362–367

120. Yokazawa T, Zheng PD, Oura H, Koizumi F (1986) Animal model of adenine-induced chronic renal failure in rats. Nephron 44: 230–234

121. Yu H, Yanagisawa Y, Forbes MA, Cooper EH, Crockson RA, MacLennan ICM (1983) Alpha 1 microglobulin: An indicator protein for renal tubular function. J Clin Pathol 36: 253–259

122. Yuen CT, Price RG, Chattagoon L, Richardson AC, Praill PFG (1982) Colorimetric assays for N-acetyl-β-D-glucosaminidase and β-D-Galactosidase in human urine using newly developed nitrostyryl substrates. Clin Chim Acta 124: 195–204

15

Electrolytes, Blood Gases, and Acid Base Balance

JULIA H. RILEY, BVSc, MS and LARRY M. CORNELIUS, DVM, PhD

Laboratory animals species, especially dogs, cats, and rodents, have been used extensively by investigators studying electrolytes, blood gases, and acid base balance. In the clinical treatment of disease, knowledge gained from these endeavors has been applied to man and other species. In particular, various forms of fluid, electrolyte, respiratory, and drug therapy rely for their success on accurate quantification of electrolytes, acid base, and blood gas parameters.

The following text will stress mechanisms responsible for changes in the analyte (cause), the change itself (pathology), and the recovery or compensatory mechanisms (effect). Species differences, where they exist, will be addressed. Laboratory data interpretation emphasizes the manner in which components of the acid base system modify chemical reaction rates, distribution and partition of substances, and electrical activity.

The absolute and relative amounts of extracellular fluid analytes (variables), and their interrelationships, determine the osmolality, state of hydration, and membrane potentials for the organism, and fix its acid base balance. Metabolic functions are affected by a change in any variable and alterations in a variable pro-

duce a response in the animal's homeostatic mechanisms (250).

Analytes are measured in terms of the quantity present (stoichiometry) and the degree to which they exert their effect (chemical activity). Both the amount of analyte present and its activity are under close metabolic control. Survival is jeopardized if control is lost.

Each variable or analyte will be addressed in the following order:

(1) *Introduction*: The analyte, its biochemistry, intake, distribution, excretion, and control mechanisms are discussed. The suitability of analytes for measurement in the various species is discussed.

(2) *Hyper-, Hypo- Analyte Conditions*: The severity of changes is addressed. Disease mechanisms and laboratory errors that produce the change follow. Next, the effect of alterations of an analyte on the biochemical and physiologic profile is described. Discussion of the analytes is followed by sections on Anion Gap and Osmolality. Alterations in these are reviewed. Buffers are considered next and their action and sites of action are described. The final section is devoted to respiratory and metabolic acid base disturbances.

345

UNITS SYMBOLS AND ABBREVIATIONS

The metric system is used. Application of the System International (SI) is briefly outlined as its general use seems very desirable. A brief outline of the rules governing use of the SI follows (27):

1. No space is left between a symbol for a prefix and its unit, for example, μl.
2. Derived units are separated and a point above the line is used to indicate the division, for example, g·s is grams per second.
3. A symbol and prefix are read as a new unit, for example, μl.
4. Prefixes are simple and not compound, for example, picogram and not micromicrogram.
5. Prefixes, using 10 to the power of 3, are preferred, for example, kilo-, milli-, and micro-.
6. Units are not pluralized and are not followed by a period, for example, 90 g.
7. A period is used to indicate a decimal point and every three digits are separated by a space. A decimal point is preceded by zero.
8. A whole number is preferred to a fraction of a unit; this is achieved by changing to a smaller unit.
9. A solidus, or / (per), is used only once for each expression, for example, 5 mg/ml.

Symbols are used to specify and qualify either the amount or activity of an analyte. Each analyte has (a) an appropriate name, (b) body site from whence the sample was derived, (c) dimension in the form of mass, volume, and length, (d) numerical value, and (e) unit of measurement. The name of each analyte is specific and explicit, for example, total plasma protein, free plasma cortisol, and unconjugated bilirubin.

Abbreviations used to indicate sample site in the SI are as follows (27,282):

B = whole blood;
S = serum;
P = plasma;
a = arterial;
v = venous;
F = feces;
U = urine;
Csf = cerebrospinal fluid;
Erc = erythrocyte;
Lkc = leukocyte.

The term for the maximally ionized form is used for plasma acids and bases such as lactate, pyruvate, and oxalate. This term expresses the most common species present but also includes other forms. For example, the plasma sulfate concentration includes the small amount of sulfuric acid.

Concentration—when the molecular weight of the substance is known, it is expressed as a molar concentration (mol/l); the amount of a substance present, or as a mass concentration (g/l), when the precise composition is not known (hemoglobin). Immunoglobulins are defined in terms of International Units. The SI uses the mole unit. Because variables in acid base chemistry are still defined in terms of equivalents, this term is used in this chapter.

Volume is expressed in liters because it is the most convenient form.

Pressure is expressed in many ways. The SI unit is the kiloPascal (kPa), but as yet no analyzer reports values in this unit. A Pascal is 1 N/m^2. Millimeters of mercury (mmHg) is used here. To convert mmHg to kPa a multiplication factor of 0.1333 is used (282).

Time is recorded in seconds, minutes, hours, and days. Prefixes are necessary for seconds only (27):

a = year;
d = day;
h = hour;
min = minute;
s = second.

Temperature is stated in centigrade units (C).

Osmolality is expressed as millimoles per kilogram of water.

The terminology for radiation is under review. The current units of radiation used are: curie, rem, roentgen, and rad.

ABBREVIATIONS FOR CHEMICAL AND PHYSICAL TERMS (7,110,172)

The abbreviations and definitions of terms presented below are the recommendations of an international steering committee (172) and a panel of physiologists (7):

Hb = hemoglobin;
pH = negative logarithm of the hydrogen ion activity;
PCO_2 = partial pressure of carbon dioxide;
PO_2 = partial pressure of oxygen;
BTPS = body temperature, barometic pressure, and saturated with water vapor, the conditions existing in the gas phase of the lungs.

Usually calculations are based on values derived from man, in whom the rectal temperature is taken at 38°C and the partial pressure of water vapor is 47 mmHg. For accurate work in animals a table of vapor pressures can be consulted (CRC Handbook of Chemistry and Physics), and appropriate adjustments based on the actual body temperature are made to the calibration of the pH and blood gas analyzer.

ATPS = ambient temperature and pressure, saturated with water vapor;

STPD = standard temperature and pressure, dry;

cCO_2 = concentration of carbon dioxide;

HbCO = carboxyhemoglobin;

cO_2 = concentration of oxygen;

Pa = Pascal;

c = concentration of substance;

P50 = the pressure of oxygen at which 50 per cent of the hemoglobin is saturated;

eV = electron volt;

F = farad;

V = volt;

W = watt;

C = coulomb;

A = Ampere;

Eq = equivalent;

Hz = Hertz;

rpm = revolutions per minute;

mol = mole;

M = molar;

L/l = liter;

m = meter;

IU = international unit;

cd = candela;

cpm = counts per minute;

dpm = disintegrations per minute;

Ci = curie.

Additional abbreviations and symbols used in this chapter are:

^ = used to indicate exponentiation;

Δ/S = (delta) change in a variable;

~ = approximately equal to;

K = absolute temperature;

T = temperature in degrees centigrade;

k = kilo (10 to the 3rd power);

N = Newton (unit of force [SI]).

GLOSSARY OF TERMS

The following terms are taken from a list compiled by a committee that attempted to standardize nomenclature on respiration and gas exchange (29). The numerical values are for man unless otherwise stated.

Acidemia: Any state of systemic arterial plasma in which the pH is significantly less than the normal value.

Acidosis: The result of any process which by itself adds excess CO_2 (respiratory acidosis) or nonvolatile acids (metabolic acidosis) to arterial blood. Acidemia does not necessarily result since compensating mechanisms (increase of HCO_3^- in respiratory acidosis, increase of ventilation and consequently decrease of arterial CO_2 in metabolic acidosis) may intervene to restore plasma pH to normal.

Alkalemia: Any state of systemic arterial plasma in which the pH is significantly greater than the normal value.

Alkalosis: The result of any process which, by itself, diminishes acids (respiratory alkalosis) or increases bases (metabolic alkalosis) in arterial blood.

Apnea: Cessation of breathing.

Base Excess: Measure of metabolic alkalosis or metabolic acidosis expressed as the mEq of strong acid or alkali required to titrate a sample of 1 liter of the blood to a pH of 7.40. The titration is made with the blood kept at 37°C, oxygenated, and equilibrated at PCO_2 of 45 torr (mmHg).

Base excess is measured in vitro. A derived value for base excess is calculated by most blood gas machines from the bicarbonate, hemoglobin, and pH measurements. Different values for base excess are obtained from different analyzer manufacturers because base excess is a derived quantity and depends on the algorithm the instrument uses (33,50). It is important to know how the instrument obtains the value for hemoglobin before any valid interpretation can be placed on base excess. The hemoglobin concentration may be assumed to be normal, determined, usually poorly by the instrument, entered by the operator from a standard method or assumed to be 30 g/l (33). The weighting value on hemoglobin must be checked to ensure that valid changes occur with real changes in hemoglobin concentration.

Blood Buffering Capacity: The maximum mEq of acid that can be made to combine with the solutes in 1 liter of blood. The normal capacity is 45 to 53 mEq/l and in practice it is estimated as the sum of bicarbonate ions and the anionic charges on the hemoglobin and plasma proteins. To a much lesser extent phosphate and other buffers are included.

Bohr Effect: Dependency of oxygen saturation of hemoglobin on H^+ concentration. An increase in H^+ concentration decreases oxygen saturation of hemoglobin.

Carbaminohemoglobin: Hemoglobin in which ionized amino groups ($Hb-NH_2$) are combined with carbon dioxide to form carbamino compound $Hb-NH-COO^-$ plus H^+). The carbon dioxide content of blood is partly dependent on the hematocrit.

Carbon Dioxide Concentration: The amount of carbon dioxide that can be extracted by evacuation from an acidified sample of a liquid, including, in the case of blood, the physically dissolved CO_2, the bicarbonate, and the CO_2 bound to hemoglobin.

Carboxyhemoglobin: Hemoglobin in which the iron is associated with carbon monoxide. The affinity of hemoglobin for CO is 300 times greater than for O_2.

Chloride Shift: Increase of red cell HCO_3^- concentration during CO_2 uptake by the blood in peripheral capillaries results in a concentration gradient for HCO_3^- which favors diffusion of HCO_3^- from the red cells into the plasma. In exchange, Cl^- diffuses from the plasma into the red cells to maintain electroneutrality. This is known as the chloride shift. Because the amount of intracellular solute is increased by entrance of CO_2 to form the HCO_3^- in the cell and is not further changed by the HCO_3^-/Cl- exchange, water also diffuses into the cell, which consequently swells very slightly.

Christiansen-Douglas-Haldane Effect: Dependence of the carbon dioxide binding capability of the blood on the oxygen saturation of hemoglobin. An increase of oxygen saturation decreases the carbon dioxide binding capability.

Cyanosis: Cyanosis is a condition characterized by a blue-purple color of the skin and mucosae. It is due to an abnormally high amount of deoxygenated hemoglobin in the capillaries of the skin and mucosae.

(In laboratory animals the amount of pigment in the skin and coat may interfere with the expression of cyanosis. Both skin thickness and its degree of vascularity must be considered when cyanosis is evaluated. The mucosae are preferred for the evaluation of cyanosis in animals. Cyanosis in humans appears when the capillary blood contains about 5 g of deoxygenated hemoglobin/100 ml of blood.)

Dypsnea: An unpleasant subjective feeling of difficult or labored breathing.

This term is used in the following text to describe labored breathing, as subjective feelings are not recognized in animals.

Henderson-Hasselbalch Equation: This equation relates the forms of carbon dioxide in the plasma:

$$pH = pK' + \frac{log\,[total\,CO_2] - S \times PCO_2}{S \times PCO_2}$$

$$= pK' + \frac{log\,[HCO_3^-]}{S \times PCO_2}$$

pK' is the negative logarithm of the apparent first ionization constant of H_2CO_3 corrected for the ratio of CO_2 to H_2CO_3. S is the factor relating the partial pressure of carbon dioxide and the sum of the millimolar concentrations of dissolved carbon dioxide and carbonic acid in plasma (0.0301). [HCO_3^-] is expressed in millimoles per liter, PCO_2 in millimeters of mercury,

S in millimoles per liter of plasma per millimeter of mercury (243). Calculation of one of the three variables, pH, HCO_3^- and PCO_2, from the other two is only valid for a single phase, such as plasma or serum, when separated from whole blood.

There is no simple procedure for applying the Henderson-Hasselbalch equation to whole blood (29,51). Recently the validity of using a pK of 6.1 especially in pathologic plasma was addressed by Flear (96) and others.

Hyperbaric Oxygenation: The condition produced by breathing a gas in which the partial pressure of oxygen is greater than that of 100 per cent oxygen at sea level.

Hypercapnia: Any state in which the systemic arterial carbon dioxide pressure is significantly above 40 torr (mmHg) (30 torr in the dog, LC). May occur when alveolar ventilation is inadequate for a given metabolic rate or during CO_2 inhalation (also *Hypercarbia*).

Hyperoxia: A condition in which the inspired oxygen pressure is greater than that of air at sea level but not more than 1 atmosphere.

Hyperventilation: An alveolar ventilation which is excessive relative to the simultaneous metabolic rate. As a result, the alveolar PCO_2 is significantly reduced below the normal 40 torr (mmHg) (also *Hypocapnia*).

Hypocapnia: Any state in which the systemic arterial carbon dioxide pressure is significantly below 40 torr (mmHg) (man), as in hyperventilation (also *Hypocarbia*).

Hypopnea: Decreased breathing in comparison with breathing at rest (less than and not to be confused with hypoventilation).

Hypoventilation: An alveolar ventilation which is small relative to the simultaneous metabolic rate, so that alveolar PCO_2 rises significantly above the normal 40 torr (mmHg).

Hypoxemia: A state in which the oxygen pressure and/or concentration in arterial and/or venous blood is lower than its normal value at sea level.

Hypoxia: Any state in which the oxygen in the lung, blood, and/or tissues is abnormally low compared with that of normal resting man breathing air at sea level. If the PO_2 is low in the environment, whether because of decreased barometric pressure or decreased fractional concentration of O_2, the condition is termed environmental hypoxia. Hypoxia, when referring to the blood, is termed hypoxemia. Tissues are said to be hypoxic when their PO_2 is low, even if there is no arterial hypoxemia, as in "stagnant hypoxia" which occurs when the local circulation is low compared to the local metabolism.

Methemoglobin: Hemoglobin in which iron is in the ferric state. Because the iron is oxidized, methemoglobin is incapable of oxygen transport. Methemoglobins are formed by various drugs and occur under pathological conditions.

Mixed Venous Blood: Blood composed of a mixture of the venous blood from all systemic tissues in proportion to their venous returns. In the absence of abnormalities of the heart and great vessels, mixed venous blood is present in the main pulmonary artery.

Blood samples drawn from right atrium or even right ventricle may be inadequately mixed.

Myoglobin: A hemoprotein naturally occurring in muscle cells, consisting of one polypeptide chain to which a heme group is attached. The heme is made of four pyrrole rings and a divalent iron (Fe^{++}—protoporphyrin) which combines reversibly with molecular oxygen.

Normoventilation: Normoventilation is characterized by an adequate ventilation that produces an alveolar carbon dioxide pressure of about 40 torr (mmHg) at any metabolic rate.

Normoxia: A state in which the ambient oxygen pressure is approximately 150 torr (ie, the partial pressure of oxygen in air at sea level).

Oxygen Capacity: The maximum amount of oxygen that can be made to combine chemically with the hemoglobin in a fixed volume of blood. (Physically dissolved oxygen is not included).

Oxygen Concentration: The concentration of oxygen in a blood sample, including both oxygen combined with hemoglobin and physically dissolved oxygen, ordinarily expressed as milliliters of O_2 (STPD) per 100 ml blood or millimoles of O_2 per liter (also oxygen content).

Oxygen Half Saturation Pressure of Hemoglobin: Oxygen pressure necessary to saturate hemoglobin 50 per cent with oxygen (at pH 7.4 or 40 torr [mmHg] CO_2 pressure and body temperature).

Oxygen Hemoglobin Equilibrium Curve: Relation of the amount of oxygen chemically bound to hemoglobin as a function of the oxygen pressure in torr (pH or PCO_2 and temperature should be stated).

Oxygen Saturation: The amount of oxygen combined with hemoglobin, expressed as a percentage of the oxygen capacity of that hemoglobin.

Solubility Coefficient for Gases: The milliliters of gas physically dissolved (STPD) in 1 ml of fluid at 1 atmosphere test gas pressure at a given temperature.

Standard Bicarbonate: Bicarbonate concentration in plasma separated anaerobically from whole blood that has been saturated with oxygen and equilibrated at PCO_2 equal to 40 torr (mmHg) at 37C. A measure of the metabolic disturbance of acid base balance in a sample of blood after any respiratory disturbance has been corrected.

STPD Conditions: These are the conditions of a volume of gas at 0°C at 760 torr (mmHg) without water vapor. A STPD volume of a given gas contains a known number of moles of that gas.

ANALYSIS, PRECISION, AND ACCURACY

Analyses of electrolytes, blood gas, and pH are complex operations in which quality control is most dependent on control of the sample collection procedure, method of transport of the sample, and strict handling criteria for the sample once it reaches the laboratory. Some workers (182) (including JHR) believe anaerobic samples are best collected by staff from the laboratory. A full understanding of clinical and chemical changes involved is imperative to production of valid data. Interpretation of numerical values by the pathologist requires a full knowledge and understanding of the following areas:

1. Sample collection.
2. Sample transport to the laboratory.
3. Sample storage before analysis.
4. Separations, dilutions, and other steps samples undergo before analysis.
5. Laboratory environment: light, temperature, humidity, and air movements.
6. The sample container: type of vessel, chemical composition of vessel, size of vessel, air space, preservatives, and anticoagulants.
7. Equipment, methods, and reagents used.
8. Animals: Although laboratory animals are bred and housed in a uniform fashion, there are unexpected variations, some iatrogenic in the form of handling induced changes (26,28,55,170). Knowledge of such occurrences is essential to the pathologist. Altitude, seasonal and diurnal changes, and breeding cycles need to be carefully assessed during the process of data interpretation. For instance, in the squirrel monkey and man in both their natural environment and housed under laboratory conditions, the circadian rhythm affects the rate of potassium, sodium, and water excretion. In the rat and dog, urinary excretion of electrolytes is almost constant throughout the entire 24-hour period if food and water are given ad libitum (163). Significant changes take place in the plasma electrolytes in the animal over a 2-hour period; therefore, delays in sampling must be documented to avoid erroneous conclusions (283). Potassium and bicarbonate are influenced by diurnal variation and intake of food (37,138). Because struggling and excitement produce a pronounced effect on acid base parameters, such activity should be recorded for each animal (26,55,170).

Blood for analysis is taken from arteries, veins, and capillaries. It is used whole or separated into serum or plasma. Two major obstacles are associated with collecting blood from small animals; (1) adequate sample size, and (2) hemolysis. Small volumes limit proper use of analyzers. Extracting life-threatening amounts of blood from the animal produces unphysiologic results and may possibly obscure treatment effects (13,124). Hemolysis releases intracellular electrolytes into the plasma or serum (37), altering its composition (46). Multiple interferences in analyte measurements including a falsely lowered pH are caused by hemolysis. The serum electrolytes, potassium and magnesium, are increased by leakage of cellular constituents into the serum. Dog red cells (and possibly those of the cat) do not cause interference with respect to potassium, but good collection technique is best adhered to for all species as potassium is not usually the only analyte measured. If a tourniquet is used, pressure should be sufficient to occlude only superficial vessels and should be released 1 to 2 minutes before the sample is collected (37). Prolonged occlusion is undesirable as it leads to spurious hyperproteinemia. Muscular activity, fist clenching or pumping of the foot, erroneously increases plasma or serum potassium (37). The flow of blood into a syringe or capillary tube must be uniform and steady. Excessive negative pressure in vacuum tubes or that produced by withdrawing the syringe plunger rapidly causes hemolysis. Blood must be transferred gently between vessels and a drop-by-drop collection avoided. The sample container is filled, capped, and cooled to halt metabolic activity and prevent loss of carbon dioxide. Elevation of pH resulting from loss of carbon dioxide causes hemolysis. Accurate potassium measurements require lithium heparin as an anticoagulant. Clot formation produces hemolysis (37) and potassium is released from the cell. In humans, leakage of potassium from cells left standing on a clot is significant at 30 minutes (37). Clot adherence to the container wall may be prevented by using a siliconized tube. Ringing the tube before centrifugation causes hemolysis. Double centrifugation of plasma and serum samples is preferred. Capillary samples for electrolyte, blood gas, and pH measurements require extreme care in collection for truly representative samples to be obtained (21,218). The sample site must be clean and preferably coated with a thin film of silicone grease. A clean stab wound of the correct depth is made so larger vessels are not tapped. Heat, friction, tetrahydrofurfuryl nicotinate, or ethylene chloride can be used to increase the size of the capillary bed for this type of sample. The first drop of blood is removed as it contains intracellular fluid. For anaerobic samples the tip of the sampling tube is not withdrawn from the drop until collection is complete.

Arterial and venous blood destined for respiratory gas and pH measurement must be collected in special syringes.

The blood gas sample is collected using anaerobic technique and is maintained anaerobically (33) by eliminating all possible dead space in the sample container while the needle and hub of the collection syringe are filled with "neutral" heparin to prevent coagulation. Although this step introduces a small error as the heparin is in equilibrium with air, it is unavoidable. (Too much heparin produces serious errors [44].) For arterial samples, a syringe containing lyophilized heparin is available. It vents air as the blood pressure forces out the plunger.

Blood samples must be free of bubbles (167) and contained in capped, small bore syringes. These are placed in "iced" water immediately and analyzed promptly (263). Blood must not contact ice as it is liable to hemolyze.

Unreliable results for pH will be produced by (1) inaccurate calibration buffers (248), (2) unregulated sample chamber and salt bridge temperature (19), (3) improper adjustment on the readout device, allowing the sample to be measured before it reaches equilibrium with the chamber temperature, (4) electrode drift (worsened by protein coating of the electrode) (263), (5) memory effect (also increased by protein), (6) bubbles in the test specimen, (7) potassium chloride contamination (148), (8) loss of the salt bridge contact with the reference electrode, and (9) dilution of the potassium chloride solution.

As the PCO_2 electrode is really a modified pH electrode, the operational errors described for a pH electrode also pertain to the PCO_2 electrode in addition to the following: (1) an incorrect concentration of bicarbonate in the electrode, (2) variations in the membrane thickness (affects response time) and integrity, (3) unreliable barometric pressure readings (148) and inaccurate calibration materials (101,148,217).

Special operational problems are associated with the oxygen electrode. It is temperature dependent and unstable and requires frequent calibration (219). The thickness of the membranes used may vary and membrane integrity may be lost when protein is deposited on its surface or cracks occur in it. Silver deposition and microbial contamination interfere with the proper functioning of this electrode. Oxygen delivery tubing should be flushed frequently to avoid equilibration of the calibration gas with ambient air (263).

To maintain adequate quality control of a blood gas and pH analyzer the following items need to be addressed regularly (83,115,168, 184,239,263,273):

1. The validity of the readout devices must be checked.
2. Chamber temperatures must be recorded.

3. Samples must be at the required temperature before the value is recorded (16).

4. The local barometric presssure must be known accurately at the time the samples are read.

5. Calibration gases must be saturated with the appropriate amount of water vapor for the body temperature of the animal.

6. Two or three sets of calibrants need to be used.

7. Electrode responses must be standardized after any maintenance procedure. This should include a linearity check.

8. The confidence limits for each analyzer must be known.

9. Repairs, maintenance, and aberrant results must be documented adequately.

10. Maintenance and quality control values must be reviewed together.

The accuracy of electrolyte measurements is readily checked as stable certified sources exist. Blood substitute standards and controls for respiratory gas and pH measurements have not been developed (148). They should be free from the variations in protein content, viscosity, ionic strength, and cellularity. Then the problem of temperature dependence of pH, PCO_2, and PO_2 must be overcome (33). A limited number of materials are available for accuracy testing and they are expensive and difficult to use (33,83, 168,184,238,263,273). Precision determinations in electrolyte analysis are not associated with any special problems and are part of the "in-house" quality control program of each laboratory (148).

To produce accurate and reliable measurements, checking and calibration procedures must be strictly followed. For pH measurements both buffers are checked every 2 hours and the pH 7.4 buffer is checked before each sample is measured. The latter step produces a constant memory effect for each sample. The carbon dioxide electrode is calibrated between samples and before each sample with one gas to avoid an inconsistent memory effect (263). The memory effect is most severe when an attempt is made to read a low value following a high one. Both halothane and nitrous oxide interfere with oxygen measurement (236). Oxygen electrodes are not linear and require calibration for the range used (131,219,263). For accurate work tonometered blood is used as the calibrant.

An approximate check on the accuracy of sodium, chloride, and carbon dioxide values is made by calculating the difference between sodium, and chloride and carbon dioxide to give the value of the unmeasured cations:

$$Na - [Cl + CO_2] = 5 - 14 \ mmol/l \ (human).$$

To check the accuracy of blood gas and pH measurements the following calculation is made using measured values for PCO_2 and HCO_3^- (23,126):

$$[H^+] = 24(pCO_2)/[HCO_3^-].$$

The $[H^+]$ is calculated in nanomoles per liter from the pH value. For example, when the pH is 7.4, the $[H^+]$ is 40 nmol/L and for a pH of 7.39 it is 4 nmol/L. Each deviation in pH of 0.01 units from normal is matched by a deviation in $[H^+]$ of 1 nmol/L. The two hydrogen ion concentrations should closely match each other. The accuracy of this pH approximation is invalid in extreme pH ranges; however, between pH 7.28 to 7.10 and 7.45 to 7.50 only small inaccuracies occur (126).

ELECTROLYTES

Sodium

Sodium is the major cation of extracellular fluid. Its two principal plasma anions are chloride and bicarbonate. A small amount is bound to albumin and about 7 per cent is undissociated. The sodium concentration of cellular fluid is about 5 mEq/l. Sodium is mainly responsible for the osmotic pressure of body fluid and control of fluid balance. Sodium, like glucose and mannitol, is an effective osmole moving water across cell membranes. Membrane irritability and permeability are sodium dependent.

Filtered sodium is actively resorbed with chloride by the renal tubules (269). Some is exchanged for hydrogen and potassium. Sodium has a renal threshold and is excreted mainly in the urine, but considerable loss can occur in sweat (human) or feces under abnormal conditions.

Atrial natriuric factor is intimately involved in sodium homeostasis. It produces natriuresis, inhibits aldosterone release, helps release vasopressin (in vitro), and causes vasodilation in dogs, rats, and humans (1,195). The exact mechanisms of action of atrial natriuric factors are still controversial (1,62,129,195,260).

Aldosterone controls sodium through the kidney, digestive tract, and skin. Control in terrestrial animals is very tight because maintenance of the circulating fluid volume is crucial to survival.

Sodium is almost completely absorbed in the ileum. Diffusion is contingent upon its concentration in the intestinal contents. Active absorption is coupled with that of other substances. It is pumped out of the colon lumen with water following it. Sodium is chiefly regulated in the kidney by aldosterone and to a minor degree other mineralocorticoids. Aldosterone, acting on the distal convoluted tubule, sweat and salivary glands, and gastrointestinal mucosae, conserves sodium. Release of aldosterone is controlled by potassium, ACTH, and the renin-angiotensin system (3). A drop of 20 mEq/1 of P-sodium or rise of 1 mEq/l of P-potassium in the dog increases secretion (3).

Sodium is measured in all laboratory animal species by instruments requiring a relatively large sample volume (emission flame photometer, atomic absorption spectrophotometer, and specific ion electrode) (115). Measured as part of a profile, with other electrolytes having similar volume requirements, it limits the profile choices. Fasted mice, young rats, and other very small laboratory animals do not yield a large volume of blood. Therefore, extra animals must be assigned to studies specifically for electrolye measurements or measurements must be taken from pooled serum samples. The latter choice is less desirable. Samples must not be diluted beyond the range specified for the analytic instrument as many of the reactions are not linear outside the prescribed analytic range.

The practice of fasting rodents and removing drinking water during their activity period produces dehydration and thus restricts the sample volume obtained (133,209). Interpretation of results from these animals must encompass the effects of increased plasma viscosity on the analytic procedures and the metabolic disturbances caused by dehydration.

Hypernatremia

Levels of biologic significance

The severity of hypernatremia depends on the speed of its development; acute hypernatremias are serious (133). In man normal serum sodium is 135 to 148 mEq/l (134). Sodium greater than 160 mEq/l represents severe hypernatremia (133,134).

Mechanisms

Hypernatremia arises when water and/or sodium are lost, with the former always predominating. Both losses are exacerbated by a high protein diet (1 g of protein produces 6 mmol of urea) (100). The mechanisms altering plasma sodium concentration operate mainly in the digestive tract, kidney, and sweat glands. Changes in plasma sodium are affected by changes in the total body water, total exchangeable body sodium, and total exchangeable body potassium.

Considering the disease processes leading to the development of hypernatremia and their sequelae, the following statement by Narins et al (177) should be kept in mind: "Hypernatremia is always associated with hypertonicity, thus eliminating need for measurements of serum osmolality."

Disease states

Diabetes insipidus: The condition is "neurogenic (central)" or "nephrogenic" in origin (133). Neurogenic diabetes insipidus is due to secretion of inadequate amounts of vasopressin. Nephrogenic diabetes insipidus is characterized by the inability of the tubule to respond appropriately to vasopressin (water transport defect). Both types of diabetes are expressed in varying degrees of severity. In both forms pure water is first lost from the extracellular compartment. This loss is borne most by the cells (two thirds) and to a lesser extent by the interstitial and extracellular fluid (one third). Animals frequently are able to drink sufficient quantities of water to minimize the dehydrating effect of water loss (thirst is stimulated by increased effective plasma osmotic pressure and decreased extracellular fluid volume). Diabetes insipidus causes hypovolemic hypernatremia because pure water is lost. The response to ADH differentiates the foregoing two conditions.

Lesions of the posterior pituitary gland (especially leukemic cell infiltrates) interfere with arginine vasopressin release (swine are the only mammals with lysine vasopressin). Lesions in the lateral hypothalamus behind the feeding center in the rat and in the dorsal area lateral to the paraventricular nuclei in the dog abolish the thirst center. Rats, with the center removed, continue drinking small amounts due to stimulation from dry pharyngeal mucosa. Hereditary neurogenic diabetes insipidus occurs in the Brattleboro strain of Long-Evans rats (165) and nephrogenic diabetes is seen in mice (174).

Primary hyperaldosteronism (Conn's Syndrome): This condition is due to excess aldosterone (133). Tumors in the adrenal cortex secrete aldosterone which increases sodium resorption from the renal tubular lumen. As excess mineralocorticoids are produced in hyperaldosteronism, the ADH release threshold is increased; a higher osmolality is needed before ADH is released. Sodium is increased only slightly in hyperaldosteronism, firstly, because water is retained, and secondly, because an "escape" phenomenon occurs once the extracellular fluid has reached a certain level.

Hyperaldosteronism produces hypernatremic hypervolemia as both water and sodium are retained, with the latter predominating. Primary aldosteronism and its attendant hypokalemia may produce a diabetic glucose tolerance curve that is restored to normal by administration of potassium.

Secondary hyperaldosteronism: Aldosterone concentration is elevated when its catabolism is decreased, as seen in chronic liver disease and venous congestion. Aldosterone is also increased in the nephrotic syndrome by the reduced renal blood flow that causes an increased output of renin.

Hyperadrenalism (Cushing's syndrome): Excessive levels of glucocorticoids are produced by (1) an adrenal tumor, or (2) adrenal hyperplasia by abnormal ACTH stimulation of the gland. The ACTH arises from a pituitary or hypothalamic lesion or from carcinomas of the lung, pancreas, thymus, or other tissue. "Hypervolemic hypernatremia" is seen in Cushing's syndrome when hormonal conditions are adjusted so both sodium and water are retained with excess retention of sodium over water. Dogs and cats usually do not exhibit this feature of hyperadrenalism (LMC).

Iatrogenic: Hypernatremic hypervolemia follows the parenteral use of sodium bicarbonate (if unaccompanied by appropriate water). Other sodium-containing parenteral compounds have the propensity to act similarly.

Diabetes mellitus: Two sets of conditions operate to produce hypernatremia in diabetes. Glucose is removed from the serum when insulin is given and is replaced by cellular sodium (maintaining osmotic equilibrium). Water is removed from plasma by the osmotic effects of glucose. "Hypovolemic hypernatremia" ensues as sodium is retained and water lost. For older dogs in oral contraceptive studies diabetes mellitus is likely to develop as progestins stimulate growth hormone output and growth hormone is diabetogenic. Frequently, hyponatremia is seen in diabetes mellitus (vide infra).

Renal disease: A number of renal diseases cause retention of sodium (133). In nephrosis, an increase in aldosterone is responsible for sodium retention and in glomerulonephritis, the amount of sodium filtered is disproportionate to that resorbed; consequently, plasma sodium is increased.

A complication of renal disease is heart failure. Both mineralization and myocarditis occur. Heart failure results in abnormal salt retention. In laboratory rats myocarditis is commonly associated with chronic rat nephropathy. These conditions, in which urine sodium is lower than that of the plasma produce "hypovolemic hypernatremia."

Digestive disorders: Ptyalism and diarrhea both result in hypotonic fluid losses. Dehydration and increased sodium occur in these disorders. In the dog and cat salivary and digestive losses are more isotonic than they are in man and other species, so they are less prone to develop hypernatremia.

Uremia: Feeding cachectic animals a high protein diet results in urea diuresis with loss of water over sodium and resultant hypovolemic hypernatremia. Nephrogenic diabetes insipidus is produced.

Amyloidosis: The laboratory mouse commonly acquires renal amyloidosis. Renal water losses exceed those for sodium and a state of nephrogenic diabetes insipidus results.

Hypokalemia and potassium deficiency: In all species hypokalemia produces nephropathy that interferes with the concentrating mechanism of the kidney and produces nephrogenic diabetes insipidus.

Hypercalcemia and hypothyroidism: Hypercalcemia and hypothyroidism produce nephrogenic diabetes insipidus. In both, deficient formation of cyclic AMP interferes with free water resorption in the renal tubules and excess water is lost.

Evaporative water loss: Evaporative skin loss of water in animals not acclimated to heat and dryness causes dehydration and hypernatremia. Large areas of the body, devoid of normal epithelium (burns, excoriation, and ulcerated tumors), lose hypotonic fluid and hypernatremia is produced. Water is constantly lost from the respiratory tract. Dry inspired air aggravates this loss.

Feeding accidents: Frank salt poisoning occurs when mistakes are made in ration preparations. There is a gain of both salt and water; salt gain predominates and causes hypervolemic hypernatremia (133).

Laboratory error

Dilution errors: Instruments measuring sodium usually require samples to be diluted. Incorrect dilution may produce spurious hypernatremia.

Most dilution devices are designed to operate in a fixed temperature range. Operation outside this range produces errors. These arise because the relative coefficients of expansion of the sample and instrument will be different from those calculated by the manufacturer.

Evaporation: Small plasma or serum samples are especially prone to large errors in sodium values because of evaporative water losses. Samples exposed to air, particularly rapidly moving, in wide-mouthed open containers or capped containers with large air spaces lose water (176).

Lithium: Lithium interferes with determination of sodium by the flame photometer, atomic absorption, or specific ion electrode. Most instruments are adjusted to account for these errors, but the possibility of error exists in lithium anticoagulated samples.

Accompanying changes

Biochemical: *Hyperosmolality.* Hyperosmolality follows hypernatremia because sodium contributes almost exclusively to fluid osmolality (133).

Hyperproteinemia. When hypovolemia accompanies hypernatremia, serum protein not lost or catabolized as a result of the disease process causing hypovolemic hypernatremia, will be elevated. The albumin elevation will be proportional to the degree of hypovolemic hypernatremia. Globulin increases may be disproportionate, antigenic stimulation accounting for the difference. Catabolism of albumin or

reduced intake of protein in hypovolemic states produces situations in which albumin appears normal or decreased (133).

Azotemia, creatininemia. When hypovolemia accompanies hypernatremia, plasma urea nitrogen and creatinine increase because of decreased renal blood flow and solute clearance.

Other electrolytes. Alterations may occur in other electrolytes when hypernatremia is present. If hypovolemia occurs or glomerular filtration is decreased, most electrolytes will increase. Kaliuresis and hypokalemia are features of mineralocorticoid and glucocorticoid excess in man but are unusual findings in dogs and cats (LMC).

Polycythemia. If erythropoiesis is normal, polycythemia is usually seen when hypovolemic hypernatremia occurs. Failure of renal function is frequently tied to anemia by the renal hormone erythropoietin.

Urine electrolytes. In hypovolemic hypernatremia of renal origin urinary output of sodium rises.

Physiological: *Central nervous system depression.* The main effect of hypernatremia is dehydration of the central nervous system (133)

Edema, ascites. Hypervolemic hypernatremia produces edema and ascites.

Shock. Shock occurs in hypovolemic hypernatremia because of the fluid deficits.

Hyponatremia

Levels of biologic significance

Serious hyponatremia occurs when the plasma sodium is less then 120 mEq/l and profound hyponatremia is seen at 100 mEq/l. In man signs of slowly induced hyponatremia do not occur until sodium falls to less than 100 mEq/l.

Mechanisms

Failure to respond to dilution of sodium in the extracellular fluid produces hyponatremia. This occurs when there is loss of control over sodium and water intake or there is an inability to generate dilute urine and sodium loss or water gain is favored. Sodium loss and water gain can occur together, but water gain must predominate to produce hyponatremia. Hyponatremia does not necessarily follow the sodium loss. Hyponatremia may be relieved by diuresis when the action of ADH is blocked and renal blood flow adequate. Theoretically, hyponatremia may be hypertonic, isotonic, or hypotonic.

Disease states

Hyperglycemia: Hyponatremia is produced by dilution in hyperglycemia. Water leaves cells and moves into the plasma in response to the osmotic pull created by high extracellular glucose or other impermeating solutes (222). Serum sodium becomes diluted and falls by 1.6 mEq/l for each 100 mg/dl increase in glucose, or mannitol, and by 3.8 mEq/l for glycine (177). Hyponatremia created by these circumstances presents with hypertonic extracellular fluid. Hyponatremia is also produced by hyperglycemic osmotic diuresis; the solute load causes both excess water and sodium loss (133).

Fluid loss: Loss of sodium-rich fluid and replacement by sodium-poor fluid produces hyponatremic hypovolemia. Hyponatremia follows fluid loss from the gastrointestinal tract, skin, lung, and kidney and the sequestration of plasma volume. The sodium-rich fluid deficit is repaired when the animal drinks water in response to the stimulus of thirst: dilution of extracellular fluid is the short-term consequence. In time renal mechanisms operate to retain sodium and restore osmolality to normal.

Congestive heart failure: Conditions causing hyponatremia and hypervolemia in heart failure are: decreased effective arterial blood volume and renal retention of sodium and water with disproportionate retention of imbibed water (133).

Hypoalbuminemia: This condition, when it is associated with severe liver disease and nephrosis, is characterized by renal retention of water in disproportionate amounts to sodium.

Severe chronic disease: A resetting of the mechanisms controlling osmolality involving antidiuretic hormone (ADH), renal mechanisms and thirst sensitivity that occur, for example, in cirrhosis cause this condition. Osmolality is maintained at a lower level and consequently hyponatremia (isovolemic) is produced.

Syndrome of inappropriate ADH secretion (SIADH): In SIADH, secretion of ADH is not turned off by extracellular fluid hypotonicity, and hyponatremia follows. Hyponatremia is mostly due to water retention, but sodium also

continues to be lost in the urine, creating a negative balance. Serum sodium may fall as low as 100 to 110 mEq/l (231). Inappropriate ADH secretion is seen with a variety of neoplasms and in other diseases such as hypothyroidism, pneumonia, heartworm disease, and lesions of the CNS (188). The plasma is isotonic.

Adrenal insufficiency ("Addison's disease"): Hyponatremia is produced by renal loss of sodium chloride. Concomitant potassium retention and limited water diuresis occur. The sequence of events begins with a deficit of mineralocorticoid hormones that leads to a decline in sodium followed by a reduction in extracellular fluid volume. Subsequently, glomerular filtration is reduced. The hypoaldosteronism is responsible for sodium wasting and the loss of glucocorticoids for failure to maintain water impermeability of the nephron as well as part of the reduction in filtration.

Renal disease: In severe renal disease, a high sodium isotonic urine is excreted. Hypovolemic, hypotonic hyponatremia is produced (177).

Loss of intracellular potassuim: Isovolemic hyponatremia results from loss of intracellular potassium that accompanies fluid loss from the gastrointestinal tract. Potassium depletion causes ADH release and the subsequent transfer of some extracellular sodium into cells. Retained water approximates that lost. Potassuim depletion heightens the sensitivity of the ADH secretory mechanism so that it responds to lesser degrees of hypovolemia than it normally does (177).

Sick cell syndrome: Chronic illness or severe trauma causes renal sodium retention and hyponatremia. These conditions arise when intracellular sodium is elevated from (1) the effects of trauma, (2) water overload, (3) impaired renal dilution, (4) increased permeability in the areas sensitive to ADH (ADH normal), (5) loss of control of membrane permeability, allowing potassium to leave the cell and sodium and water to enter, and/or (6) inappropriate ADH secretion. (Also, see Sick Cell Syndrome under Hypoosmolality.)

Psychogenic polydipsia: Occasionally an animal will voluntarily imbibe sufficient quantities of water to cause hyponatremia. This process becomes self-perpetuating as the expanded plasma volume activates natriuretic mechanisms that cause an increase in sodium excretion despite the existing dilutional hyponatremia.

Laboratory error

Hyperlipemia, hyperproteinemia: Sodium concentration is measured per unit volume of fluid. If part of the reference volume does not contain sodium, it will appear that the amount of sodium is reduced. The hyponatremia is false and it is accompanied by an isotonic plasma. The plasma sodium remains unknown until measured by another method or a correction factor applied. For man, multiplication of the plasma lipid value by 0.0002 and the plasma protein in excess of 8.0 g/dl by 0.25 will give an approximation of the reduction in plasma sodium due to interfering excesses of these analytes (275). Acute reductions in plasma sodium may be caused by isotonic infusions of glucose, mannitol, and glycine.

Dilution error: Sample dilution is a source of error. Increased plasma viscosity predisposes the sample to dilutional error.

Accompanying changes

Biochemical: *Disproportionate elevation of serum urea nitrogen over creatinine.* This anomaly accompaning hypovolemic hyponatremia is created by "third spacing" (sequestration of plasma volume), with reduced rates of urine formation (normal glomerular filtration), and back-diffusion of urea, but not creatinine. The response to a perceived loss of the plasma volume is both hormonal and hemodynamic and results in a net effort to retain and conserve water. The lost, sodium-rich plasma is replaced by sodium-poor water (177).

Hyperkalemia. Adrenal insufficiency is characterized by both hyponatremia and hyperkalemia. The kidney retains potassium and wastes sodium as it lacks the influence of aldosterone.

Hypokalemia. Hypokalemia, hypertonic urine, low urine sodium, and low urine volume are features of hyponatremia caused by gastrointestinal fluid loss. The former features differentiate this condition from isovolemic hyponatremia due to inappropriate ADH secretion. Hypokalemia arises directly from potassium losses in the gastrointestinal tract and indirectly from loss of potassium by the kidney. Potassium is lost because volume depletion stimulates sodium retention and urine potassium excretion. Loss of intracellular pot-

assium activates two systems whereby sodium is moved to intracellular sites and the ADH secretory mechanism is supersensitized to small changes in plasma volume.

Urine osmolality. Excess ADH secretion produces abnormal water retention, and urine that is hypertonic to the plasma. Urine sodium is high. Renal disease and partial urinary tract obstruction are examples of hypovolemic hypotonic hyponatremias that are characterized by isotonic sodium-rich urine.

Low serum urea nitrogen and creatinine. Characteristics of SIADH are low plasma creatinine and urea nitrogen. Urine concentration is disproportionately high relative to the plasma osmolality (plasma osmolality is low).

Natriuresis. Hyponatremia occurs in diabetes mellitus. Hyponatremia results from excessive sodium loss in the urine caused by the osmotic effect of glucose and the obligatory excretion of sodium with ketone bodies (136).

Physiologic: *Neurologic dysfunction.* The neurologic signs of hyponatremia vary and depend on its severity and rapidity of onset. Initially weakness, lethargy, and confusion are seen and these are followed by coma and convulsions. The signs are due to inhibition of neurotransmitter amino acid transport in the brain and spinal cord. These transmitter systems are sodium dependent (144).

Polyuria. Hyponatremia and associated polyuria are found in hyperglycemia, diabetes insipidus, renal failure, and psychogenic polydipsia.

Dehydration. Both hyponatremia and dehydration are produced by fluid loss from the digestive tract, skin, and kidney. They also occur in adrenal insufficiency and in "third spacing" in which fluid accumulates outside the vascular system but inside the body.

Protein dissociation. Changes in plasma sodium are counteracted by changes in the degree of dissociation of plasma proteins as they act as a zwitterion; able to donate or accept hydrogen ions.

Chloride

Chloride exists in the body principally in combination with sodium. Chloride shares with sodium the functions of maintenance of osmotic pressure, water distribution, and acid base equilibrium.

Chloride is involved in a unique exchange in the erythrocyte. Here, it is exchanged for bicarbonate, formed from CO_2 taken on in the tissues. This exchange of chloride for bicarbonate is reversed in the lungs: as the erythrocyte releases CO_2, chloride moves into the plasma. A consequence of the exchange is a higher chloride value in arterial blood than in venous blood.

Hydrogen ions are buffered in erythrocytes, increasing the number of intracellular osmotically active particles. This increase in solute draws water into the cell, causing it to swell. Cell swelling, caused by the buffering of hydrogen ions in erythrocytes, accounts for venous blood hematocrits being higher than those of arterial blood.

The concentration of chloride in plasma is about half that in the erythrocyte. About 2 mEq/l are bound to albumin. Tissue levels are almost negligible in normal circumstances; however, chloride does enter damaged cells (37). Chloride leaves the body in saliva, vomitus, sweat, urine, and feces.

Chloride is almost completely absorbed in the intestine. It is filtered by the kidney and passively resorbed with sodium by the proximal tubules. Active resorption of chloride occurs in the ascending loop of Henle.

Determination of the chloride in the extracellular fluid is useful because it gives an indication of the acid base status of the animal. If chloride is high, the bicarbonate is likely to be low, suggesting a metabolic acidemia. The reverse situation suggests metabolic alkalemia, but strict interpretation of these changes is invalid as the normal range for chloride is rather wide.

Hyperchloremia

Levels of biologic significance

As stated, the normal variation in chloride is rather large, which make judgments of the severity of changes difficult.

Mechanisms

Hyperchloremia is produced by contraction of the extracellular fluid, loss of bicarbonate from the extracellular fluid, and excessive intake of chloride. Many changes affecting sodium are reflected by changes in chloride because it is sodium's passive partner. There is no chloride hormone.

Disease states

Hypotonic sodium and water losses: Fluid lost in sweat, feces, vomitus, wound drainage, third spacing, and saliva or via the urinary tract is hypotonic to the plasma and causes hyperchloremia.

Pure water depletion: Restriction of water intake and administration of hypertonic saline both produce hyperchloremia.

Diabetes insipidus: Neurogenic (central) and nephrogenic (renal) diabetes insipidus cause hyperchloremia when the oral intake of water is less than the renal loss. In neurogenic diabetes insipidus the defect is a lack of sufficient quantities of ADH. In nephrogenic diabetes insipidus there is an inability of the hormone to act effectively on the tubule. Both forms are expressed to varying degrees and may be congenital or acquired. Acquired neurogenic diabetes is mostly due to neoplasms.

Osmotic diuresis: In urea and glucose diuresis, water is lost in excess of either sodium or chloride. Hyperchloremia is produced. A state of nephrogenic diabetes insipidus ensues.

Hypokalemia and potassium deficiency: Hypokalemia causes renal damage, the kidney loses its concentrating ability, water is lost, and hyperchloremia is manifested. Nephrogenic diabetes insipidus is acquired as a result of hypokalemia (252).

Hypercalcemia: Acute hypercalcemia interferes with the action of cAMP and as a consequence water is lost. Hyperchloremia is created by the water deficit.

A state of renal diabetes insipidus is produced when hypercalcemia is present by the failure of cAMP to act at the tubule. Renal diabetes insipidus exists until the process of renal calcification becomes severe enough to cause an intolerable loss of renal tissue that terminates in renal failure.

Primary hyperparathyroidism, pseudohyperparathyroidism, vitamin D intoxication, and occasionally secondary hyperparathyroidism can cause hypercalcemia.

Renal amyloidosis: The permeability of renal tubules to water is altered by the presence of amyloid in the kidney. Hyperchloremia of renal amyloidosis is due to a shrunken extracellular fluid volume, incurred as a result of water loss. Amyloid is commonly deposited in the kidney of certain strains of mice and Syrian hamsters as they age. An acquired form of renal diabetes insipidus is created by deposition of amyloid.

Renal tubular acidosis (RTA): In RTA plasma chloride concentration is high, and sodium, potassium, and bicarbonate concentration low. Tubular damage results in a loss of water, sodium, and potassium in the urine.

Respiratory alkalosis: Reduction of plasma carbon dioxide subsequently lowers plasma bicarbonate concentration. Plasma chloride increases to replace the lost bicarbonate, balancing the ion charges. Electrical neutrality of the plasma is maintained.

Metabolic acidosis: The mechanism for hyperchloremia is the same as the foregoing except the bicarbonate ion itself is directly reduced.

Decreased renal blood flow: Abnormal sodium chloride retention results from decreased renal blood flow.

Laboratory error

Titration error: The determination of chloride by certain methods of titration is affected by pigmented samples. Pigment in the sample causes a positive error.

Other ions: Mercury ions react with Br-, CN-, CNS-, and -SH groups as if these anions were chloride anions. Some substances administered to test animals contain free Br-; values for chloride can approach 200 mEq/l because of this interference.

Deproteinization error: For analytic methods requiring deproteinization, failure to deproteinize a sample allows the protein -SH groups to react with mercury ions. The size of the chloride error produced by failure to deproteinize depends on the amount of protein present. Consideration must be given to this form of error in diseases in which there is volume contraction or hyperglobulinemia.

Accompanying changes

Biochemical: *Hyperproteinemia.* Fluid loss from the vascular space usually produces hyperproteinemia. Almost always, albumin is increased in proportion to the degree of dehydration. This relationship may be altered by (1)

catabolism of albumin, (2) loss of albumin from the kidney or (3) digestive tract, (4) decreased protein intake, and (5) decreased liver function. Globulin may be increased in dehydration. However, its response is unpredictable as antigenic stimulation may increase this analyte irrespective of the presence of dehydration.

Hypernatremia. Except in renal tubular acidosis, in which sodium concentration is low, hypernatremia will accompany hyperchloremia.

Physiologic: *Dehydration.* Severe fluid loss produces dry mucous membranes and loss of skin turgor.

Central nervous system. Both excitement and/or depression occur as the brain dehydrates; the latter is seen terminally in severe dehydration.

Hypochloremia

Levels of biologic significance

Wide variation in the normal range for chloride makes it difficult to attach biologic significance to any changes except those at the extreme end of the range.

Mechanisms

Hypochloremia is produced by excessive chloride loss from the digestive tract and kidney. Loss from the gut occurs when chloride leaves either the cranial or caudal end or when it is sequestered in the lumen. Renal loss is due to renal disease and ion exchanges in the tubule. Chloride may be decreased by excess of a competing ion.

The movement of chloride in the body is closely tied to that of sodium, and conditions affecting sodium will influence chloride.

Disease states

Hyperglycemia: Hyperglycemia of endogenous or exogenous origin has the effect of diluting all extracellular electrolytes, including chloride. Hyperglycemia produces mild hypochloremia.

Diarrhea: Mild hypochloremia is produced when chloride is lost with other electrolytes and water in the feces; chloride is actively secreted into the intestinal lumen in secretory diarrheas. Water replacement of these losses further dilutes the electrolyte.

Vomiting: The chloride concentration of gastric fluid is high. Chloride is lost from the stomach in vomitus and hypochloremia follows.

Sequestration of chloride in the gut caused by stasis or obstruction effectively removes chloride from the plasma. Hypochloremia results from such a loss.

Nephritis: In severe renal tubular disease the kidney loses control of sodium and chloride and they are lost in the urine. Both hypochloremia and hyponatremia are produced as a result of nephritis.

Hyperadrenocorticism (Cushing's syndrome): Excess cortical steroids cause renal tubular potassium chloride wasting. A slight increase in glucose may also be found in hyperadrenocorticism. The extra glucose dilutes all plasma electrolytes and further exacerbates the hypochloremia produced by the steroids. In the dog and cat a slight decrease in chloride is more usual when they are vomiting; however, vomiting of pure gastric fluid, as may occur in pyloric outlet obstruction, will severely depress chloride concentration. Pathologic lesions associated with hyperadrenocorticism are pituitary adenoma, adrenal adenoma or carcinoma, adrenal hyperplasia, and lung tumors producing an ACTH-like peptide.

Hyperaldosteronism (Conn's syndrome): Aldosterone, acting on the tubule, produces sodium retention while potassium and chloride are lost. These actions, when aldosterone is in excess, lead to hypochloremia.

Secondary aldosteronism: Secondary aldosteronism is the result of pathologic processes that cause abnormal aldosterone secretion. In these conditions (congestive heart failure and nephrosis) in which the stimuli of (1) decreased arterial volume, (2) decreased sodium presentation to the renal tubules, and (3) hypokalemia are present, excessive aldosterone secretion produces hypochloremia.

In congestive heart failure, a second factor operates to lower chloride concentration. Increased intravascular volume, the result of heart failure, effectively dilutes chloride in the extracellular fluid.

Aldosterone is increased in conditions in which its degradation is decreased (cirrhosis of the liver). Hypochloremia is likely to occur when there is excessive aldosterone action. This condition is often accompanied by hypokalemia.

Metabolic acidosis: Organic acid anions will partially replace chloride and in doing so cause hypochloremia. Such anions include lactate, B-hydroxybutyrate, acetoacetate, phosphate, and sulfate. These anions accompany acidosis caused by anaerobic respiration, ketosis, and renal insufficiency.

Respiratory acidosis: As increments of carbon dioxide are added to the plasma, some increase in bicarbonate is produced. The increase in bicarbonate causes a reciprocal decrease in chloride.

Inappropriate ADH secretion: Retention of water due to the inappropiate secretion of ADH dilutes chloride and the electrolytes.

Hypothyroidism: Both sodium and chloride are decreased by the inappropriate secretion of ADH that is associated with hypothyroidism. All electrolytes are further artifactually decreased by the lipemia that sometimes accompanies hypothyroidism. The lipemia produces pseudohypochloremia.

Hypoaldosteronism (Addison's disease): In this desease lack of aldosterone causes the renal tubules to lose their ability to retain sodium and chloride. The urine loss produces hypochloremia.

Chronic hypercarbia: An increase in the atmospheric concentration of carbon dioxide causes both hypochloremia and hypobicarbonatemia. In the rat chronic hypercarbia produces an increase in the urinary excretion of chloride, potassium, ammonium, phosphorus, and titratable acid with little change in sodium excretion (133).

Laboratory error

Hyperlipemia and hyperproteinemia: Pseudohypochloremia can be produced by instruments that measure the amount of chloride present in a reference volume of fluid. The error occurs because both lipid and protein, although occupying part of the measured volume, do not contain chloride.

Masked hypochloremia: Other ions (Br-, -SH, CN- and CNS-) are not differentiated from chloride in most laboratory titrations of chloride and they may make up a chloride deficit. This gives a false picture of the status of chloride.

Postprandial hypochloremia: Two potential mechanismas operate to cause postprandial hypochloremia: (1) Chloride is secreted into the stomach lumen after eating. An acute decrease in chloride, which corrects itself after a short time, may be seen. (2) Postprandial hyperlipemia is also capable of causing a spurious hypochloremia.

Accompanying changes

Biochemical: *Hyponatremia*. Plasma solutes are diluted when excess water is retained.

Hypobicarbonatemia. Hypobicarbonatemia and hypochloridemia may arise simultaneously as a result of diarrhea or renal failure. Abnormal chloride losses from the digestive tract are due to rapid passage of ingesta, or active secretion of chloride into the lumen, as a result of deranged function (diarrhea). Chloride is lost in renal disease when the functions of the kidney fail, while at the same time bicarbonate is decreased as it buffers excess hydrogen ions.

In diarrhea and renal failure bicarbonate losses are abnormal because of the need to buffer sulfuric, phosphoric, and lactic acids that accumulate. In renal failure a further loss of bicarbonate occurs as it is needed to replace ammonium ions that are no longer produced at a sufficient level by the failed kidney. Frequently, metabolic acidosis accompanies both renal failure and diarrhea.

Hyperbicarbonatemia. The loss of chloride in vomited gastric contents produces a compensatory increase in bicarbonate. To replace the lost anion the kidney increases bicarbonate retention (and maintains electrical neutrality). Hyperbicarbonatemia arises in hyperadrenocorticism (hyperaldosteronism). In an effort to retain potassium, the tubule secretes hydrogen ion. Compensatory metabolic alkalosis ensues.

Acidosis. Nephritis, diarrhea, ketosis, diabetes mellitus, and other conditions add excess acid to the plasma, and the anions accompanying these acids replace chloride.

Physiologic: *Central nervous disturbance*. Hypoosmolality, if it accompanies hypochloremia, causes both excitatory and inhibitory reactions in the central nervous system.

Potassium

Potassium is the chief intracellular cation. Small amounts are found in the serum and even smaller amounts in the plasma; cellular damage releases potassium. About 20 per cent is undissociated in the plasma and some is bound to albumin.

The part played by this analyte in its interactions and exchanges with sodium, chloride, bicarbonate, and hydrogen ions is important, regardless of the actual amount of potassium present. In its intracellular environment, potassium regulates osmotic pressure and here and in the plasma it has an important influence on acid base relationships. With sodium, potassium maintains membrane potentials. Potassium is also needed by certain enzymes, such as pyruvic kinase, for their proper activity.

Potassium is absorbed from the gut. About 10 per cent of the intake escapes in the feces normally (63). Its excretion by the colon increases in chronic renal disease (137). In the kidney and intestine, potassium is both secreted and resorbed. Unlike sodium and chloride, it is reexcreted by the distal tubules and collecting ducts. The kidney, the main excretory and regulatory site, has almost unlimited ability to remove this ion if renal function is normal (63). No renal threshold level exists for potassium. Excretion depends on the glomerular filtration rate and the amount of potassium filtered (63).

Small amounts of potassium are lost in the saliva, gastrointestinal tract, and sweat. No relationship between plasma potassium and the total body content of potassium exists.

The adrenal hormones, insulin, and adrenergic nervous system regulate potassium in the body (63,79,88,258). Aldosterone, epinephrine, and insulin drive potassium into cells (177). Acid base alterations affect potassium's transcellular movements and modulate renal potassium excretion. Acute alterations in potassium are curbed by the catecholamines, glucagon and insulin (70,88).

Hyperkalemia directly stimulates the adrenal cortex (63). When the renin-angiotensin system fails, the adrenal mechanism protects the organism from certain death. The adrenal steroid aldosterone enables animals to adapt to extremely high dietary potassium levels. Rats can tolerate 33 mEq/100 g of body weight daily intake.

Potassium values are affected by blood pH, and it is higher in acidotic animals and lower in alkalotic animals.

Hyperkalemia

Levels of biologic significance

The severity of hyperkalemia depends on how rapidly it develops. A higher potassium level will be better tolerated if the disturbance develops slowly. In humans, cardiotoxicity is seen in rapidly developing hyperkalemia when the potassium is 6 to 7 mEq/l. Minimal toxicity occurs at 8 to 9 mEq/l if the hyperkalemia arose slowly (63). The mechanisms controlling potassium are sensitive and respond to 0.2 to 0.4 mEq/l increases. Measurements of potassium must therefore be extremely accurate.

Mechanisms

The kidney exercises sole control over excretion of potassium, and any process reducing delivery, filtration, or removal of potassium from the body poses a hyperkalemic threat (63). Injury to the distal tubules and collecting ducts, potassium's excretory sites, produces hyperkalemia. Competition with another ion at the kidney for secretion increases plasma potassium. Under normal circumstances transient hyperkalemia is seen in the postprandial period and following exercise. Transcellular redistribution of potassium in acid base distrubances causes acute critical hyperkalemia. Excess dietary intake usually only causes a slight transient increase in potassium.

Disease states

Hypoaldosteronism: Hyperkalemia results from either a lack of or improper action of aldosterone. In hypoaldosteronism, hyperkalemia is produced by renal wastage of sodium chloride with retention of potassium. Normally, increased levels of potassium stimulate the release of aldosterone (70,108).

Failure of the renin-angiotensin system alone produces only small increases in potassium.

Increased inspired oxygen: Increased inspired oxygen, as may occur in acute hypercapnia, increases potassium concentration.

Acidosis: In acute metabolic acidosis the hydrogen ion from hydrochloric acid displaces intracellular potassium; extracellular potassium is increased (43). This exchange only occurs in acidosis accompanied by hypobicarbonatemia.

Organic acidoses do not change potassium concentrations.

Many modifying factors need to be considered in the response of potassium to acidosis. The reader is advised to consult an excellent review of the current knowledge on this subject by Adrogué and Madias (3).

Respiratory acidosis increases plasma potassium. Such increases are of smaller magnitude per unit pH change than are those due to metabolic acidosis. Acute respiratory acidosis moves potassium out of muscle and liver cells and into osseous, cardiac, and renal tubule tissue (3). In acute respiratory acidosis increases in osmolality account for hyperkalemia. Respiratory acidosis is accompanied by hyperbicarbonatemia.

Cationic amino acids: Cationic amino acids shift potassium into the plasma (177).

Hyperosmolality, hyperglycemia: Potassium accompanies water, leaving cells in conditions in which the plasma glucose or osmolality are high. The osmotic gradient between the cells and plasma is responsible for the hyperkalemia (70,108).

Diabetes mellitus: In addition to the foregoing osmotic effect, insulin, required to drive potassium into cells, is absent, low, or ineffective in diabetes mellitus. Slight hyperkalemia may result from the insulin deficiency. Only a small amount of insulin is required to shift potassium intracellularly (3,70,177).

Cellular damage: Tissue damage releases intracellular potassium (150 mEq/l) into the plasma (63). Excessive bruising, burns, surgery, and rhabdomyolysis as well as fist (paw) clenching will increase plasma potassium.

Renal insufficiency: Ingested potassium must be removed by the kidney, otherwise hyperkalemia results. Decreased clearance by the kidney or urinary tract invariably causes hyperkalemia. Oliguria, urinary obstruction, decreased glomerular filtration, and interference with the sodium-hydrogen-potassium exchange all produce hyperkalemia. Potassium filtration and excretion are loosely coupled processes; the effect of decreased filtration is not as severe as it is for sodium.

The colon actively secretes potassium in chronic renal failure. Constipation can cause decompensation in a patient in chronic renal failure (137).

Dietary excess: It is rare for a normal animal

to be able to ingest a sufficient load of potassium to cause hyperkalemia.

Iatrogenic: Treatment with large doses of potassium penicillin (1.7 mEq/million units) may cause hyperkalemia (63).

Hyporeninemic hypoaldosteronism: This syndrome often occurs with chronic interstitial renal disease and/or diabetes mellitus and produces hyperkalemia (3,63).

Alpha adrenergic stimulation: Hyperkalemia caused by sympathetic stimulation is most likely due to stimulation of the liver and subsequent release of potassium (3,52,88). Catecholamines are secreted in response to acute hypercapnia. They cause release of liver glucose and potassium and uptake of potassium by cardiac muscle (3).

Laboratory error

Thrombocytosis and leukocytosis: Intravascular cytosis increases serum potassium as a result of a release of potassium during clot formation from a greater number of cells (37). Measurement of the plasma potassium (using lithium heparin) will avoid this spurious hyperkalemia when the cells are normal (63) but may not prevent it when the cells are neoplastic (191).

Muscular activity: Squeezing, clenching, and similar types of muscular activity before blood collection increase plasma potassium (37). Animals must be taken quietly from their cages to prevent overzealous muscular activity.

Penicillin: Penicillin preparations contain considerable amounts of potassium; their effect is especially noticeable if large doses are given (63).

Hemolysis: Hemolyzed samples are invalid for measurement of potassium because potassium is released in extremely large amounts from the erythrocytes except in dogs and cats (3,37,63).

Refrigeration: Refrigeration inhibits phosphorylation, which is necessary for active transport of potassium into cells and is dependent on a supply of glucose. Potassium leaks from cells when glucose is low or its phosphorylation is prevented by refrigeration.

Evaporation: Unprotected, standing samples lose water while awaiting analysis; increases in potassium occur (176).

Dilution: Whenever a sample is concentrated or diluted, errors may occur.

Deproteinization: Deproteinized serum or plasma samples have higher potassium concentration when values are determined by flame photometry.

Accompanying changes

Biochemical: *Azotemia, hypochloremia, hyponatremia, and hypoglycemia.* Azotemia, the result of hypovolemia, accompanies hyperkalemia in Addison's disease. In this disease also, sodium chloride, and bicarbonate are lost in the urine. Glucose is low in Addison's disease and high in Cushing's disease.

Hypobicarbonatemia and hyperbicarbonatemia. Hyperkalemia of metabolic acidosis is accompanied by low bicarbonate concentration; with respiratory acidosis bicarbonate concentration will be high.

Hyperphosphatemia. Hyperphosphatemia accompanies hyperkalemia when renal filtration is impaired or phosphorylation of glucose decreased.

pH. Plasma potassium concentration is related to pH in acute disturbances by the following (243):

$$\Delta cK/\Delta pH = -1 \text{ to } -3 \text{ mmol}/l.$$

Physiologic: *Cardiac toxicity.* Cardiac arrhythmias arise in hyperkalemia and, if untreated, lead to ventricular fibrillation terminally.

Muscle weakness. Muscle weakness is a subjective feature of mild hyperkalemia in man. When hyperkalemia is severe, paralysis ensues.

Adaptation. Hyperkalemia causes adaptive increases in renal potassium excretion and movement of potassium into cells. Both responses are dependent on aldosterone (63).

Hypokalemia

Levels of biologic significance

A 5- to 10-per-cent loss of total body potassium is considered a moderate loss for a person and is usually not symptomatic (63). Hypokalemia is as serious as hyperkalemia. Small changes in plasma potassium must be detected by the testing system.

Mechanisms

Hypokalemia may arise in any of the following situations: (1) decreased intake of potassium, (2) excess potassium lost from the digestive tract, (3) potassium movement out of the plasma, and (4) excess renal excretion.

Disease states

Reduced intake: Potassium is not stored in the body. A constant intake is necessary to prevent hypokalemia.

Antibiotic therapy: Carbenicillin and others contain sodium and a slowly metabolizable, poorly resorbed anion. The kidney retains the sodium, while the anion is allowed to pass in the urine where it produces a negative charge in the tubular lumen. The charge difference created by the anion increases urinary loss of potassium and hydrogen and results in hypokalemia and metabolic alkalosis (177).

Vomiting: Loss of gastric juice depletes plasma potassium mainly by a mechanism that is chloride dependent. Small amounts of potassium are lost in the vomitus, and a chloride deficit is produced by vomiting. It is the chloride deficit that causes the hypokalemia by producing a reciprocal increase in bicarbonate. The excess bicarbonate is presented to the proximal tubule, exceeding its capacity to resorb bicarbonate, so that bicarbonate along with sodium passes to the distal tubule. Sodium is now forced to compete for potassium-resorbing sites on the distal tubule. This competition favors sodium, and potassium is lost in the urine (117).

Diarrhea: Diarrhea, especially mucoid, produces hypokalemia (63). Mucus is rich in potassium (10 to 110 mEq/l in man).

Sweat: Sweat contains almost no potassium, so exceptionally large volumes have to be lost to deplete the plasma potassium (63,177).

Metabolic alkalosis: Chronic metabolic alkalosis has traditionally been associated with movement of potassium caused by changes in bicarbonate. Now, the role of potassium is in dispute and its influence, if any, on bicarbonate redistribution between cells and plasma is undecided. However, it is true that acute metabolic alkalosis is mostly seen with reduced plasma potassium and for humans the plasma potassium has been calculated to fall 0.6 mEq/0.1 pH unit rise. Less severe hypokalemia occurs with respiratory alkalosis (243).

Chronic metabolic alkalosis is seen when plasma chloride deficits created by gastric loss

are replaced by bicarbonate; the kidney increases bicarbonate retention in response to the chloride deficit. The proximal tubule receives the excess filtered bicarbonate, exceeding its transport maximum and allowing bicarbonate to spill over into the distal tubular filtrate. Some sodium along with the excess bicarbonate is lost into the distal tubular filtrate, and there is an exchange of sodium for potassium, thus stimulating potassium excretion. The volume deficit created by vomiting stimulates sodium resorption with the resultant loss of hydrogen ion and potassium.

Hyperthyroidism: The hyperkalemia of hyperthyroidism is probably due to beta sympathetic stimulation (88).

Osmotic diuresis: Increases in nonabsorbable solute delivered to the tubules causes kaliuresis. Kaliuresis of this type is a feature of diabetes mellitus because of its attendant glycosuria.

Diabetes mellitus: Hypokalemia in diabetes mellitus is partly due to the excretion of potassium with nonresorbable keto anions (63). Furthermore, shifts of potassium occur in diabetes mellitus. Potassium shifts out of cells because of the accompanying metabolic acidosis and may produce temporary hyperkalemia. Hyperosmolality of the plasma causes potassium and water to leave the cells. Hypoinsulinemia impairs potassium entry into cells and potassium is lost in the vomitus.

Distal renal tubular acidosis: Potassium may be severely depleted in this condition by loss into the urine. In proximal tubular acidosis, potassiumm levels are usually normal (63).

Edema-forming states: The mechanism for hypokalemia and potassium depletion is not known in congestive heart failure, the nephrotic syndrome, and hepatic cirrhosis (117).

Hyperaldosteronism (Conn's syndrome): In this condition aldosterone causes the renal tubules to retain sodium and excrete potassium chloride. Some potassium is conserved by exchange with hydrogen ions, but not enough, and compensatory metabolic alkalosis and hypokalemia ensue.

Hyperadrenocorticism (Cushing's syndrome): The mechanism and consequences are described above; however, in this case the lesion if different. Pituitary or adrenal tumors, or hyperplasia of the adrenal gland due to ectopic hormone production may cause the syndrome.

Leukemia: Leukemia in man and rat and

probably others produces hypokalemia. The cause is unknown (191).

Catecholamines: Increased sympathetic tone as seen in acute illness produces hypokalemia, probably as a result of movement of potassium into cells.

Barium toxicity: Potassium moves into cells in barium toxicities (77).

Laboratory error

Dilution: Errors in dilution lead to false values for potassium. Examples of some factors leading to these errors are (1) hyperviscosity of the blood sample, (2) room temperature variations, and (3) incomplete defibrination.

Hyperlipemia/hyperproteinemia: Spurious hypokalemia as described for sodium may arise with these two conditions.

B_{12} therapy: Potassium decreases suddenly following administration of vitamin B_{12} as a result of the rapid erythropoiesis that takes place after treatment of B_{12} deficiency (121).

Hypomagnesemia: Magnesium deficiency stimulates aldosterone secretion. Sodium is conserved and potassium lost when the tubules are under the influence of aldosterone.

Accompanying changes

Biochemical: *Renal ammonia.* Potassium depletion and hypokalemia may result in decreased activity of renal glutaminase and increased excretion of ammonium ions in the rat (144).

Hypobicarbonatemia. Hypobicarbonatemia accompanies hypokalemia in diarrhea, diabetes mellitus, and renal tubular acidosis. In diabetes mellitus the elevated keto anions and hyperglycemia are characteristics that help to distinguish this from other diseases. In diarrhea and renal tubules acidosis, sodium is likely to be decreased. Hyperchloremia is usually a feature of hypobicarbonatemia.

Hyperbicarbonatemia. Hypokalemia usually occurs with an increase in pH and hypochloremia when bicarbonate is increased.

Hypernatremia. Hypernatremia may be seen in dehydration and in hyperadrenal syndromes along with their attendant hypokalemia.

Decreased hormone secretion. Potassium is needed for insulin and aldosterone release, and when it is not present, secretion is inadequate.

Diabetic glucose tolerance curves are seen when hypokalemia accompanies hyperaldosteronism (63).

Low urine potassium. During renal potassium conservation, its urine value is usually low.

Physiologic: *Nephrosis.* Hypokalemia produces nephrosis. The mechanism has not been explained (63).

Muscle weakness. In severe cases of hypokalemia paralysis and respiratory failure occur. Smooth muscle also ceases to function normally when potassium is deficient. Gastric dilatation (seen commonly in rabbits with mucoid enteritis and monkeys as a result of overeating), and paralytic ileus are the result of hypokalemia (63).

Histologic evidence of hypokalemia is nonspecific in the form of cytoplasmic degeneration and reduced myofibrillar content (63).

Rhabdomyolysis. Severe hypokalemia produces lysis of muscle. This response is probably a desperate attempt to normalize plasma potassium by releasing it from intracellular sites. Unfortunately such a measure is not always lifesaving (63).

Cardiac arrest. Severe hypokalemia causes cardiac muscle membrane instability and produces arrest.

Dilute urine. Hypokalemia interferes with the action of ADH; maximal urine concentration is not attained (63).

Calcium

Calcium is present in both free ionized and bound ionized forms in the cytosol ($10-5$ to $10-8$ mol/l total ionized) and plasma ($10-3$ mol/l total ionized) (212). There is an interchange of the two forms within each compartment and between compartments. Calcium biochemistry is linked to its structural role in osseous tissues, activation of excitable cells, and its role as an enzyme activator in all tissues. Plasma calcium decreases with age (25). Human adult levels are reached at 16 years of age (25).

In the plasma, 30 to 40 per cent of the total calcium is bound to proteins. Albumin serves as the major calcium binding protein with glutamic and aspartic acid residues binding calcium through electrostatic attraction (25). Globulins also serve as calcium binding proteins. Fourteen per cent is diffusible, that is complexed with anions such as bicarbonate, citrate, phosphate, and sulfate. About 40 per cent is in the active or free form. Ionized calcium (free and bound) is the functional and physiologically active form.

Calcium is mainly absorbed in the duodenum, where an acid pH favors absorption. Intestinal absorption decreases with age (20). Calcium is excreted in urine and feces and is present in all gastrointestinal secretions.

Plasma calcium is controlled by the parathyroid hormone, calcitonin, vitamin D, magnesium, and the concentration of hydrogen ion. Parathyroid hormone or PTH acts by causing (1) increases in intestinal absorption, (2) increases in the active form of vitamin D, (3) increases in renal tubular resorption, and (4) release of calcium from osseous tissue. A negative feedback of calcium on parathormone secretion is the principal control mechanism; however, magnesium is also important in this respect and has actions similar to calcium with half to one third the potency. Parathormone is activated and degraded by the liver and in man and dog the kidney. It is excreted in the urine. Another hormone, calcitonin or thyrocalcitonin, with as yet an uncertain role in man, acts in animals by producing (1) a block on bone resorption, and (2) decreases in renal tubular resorption. Thyrocalcitonin is responsible for preventing acute increases in calcium by acting on bone, the intestinal tract, and kidney (208). Thyrocalcitonin depresses gastrin and pepsin secretion. Vitamin D acts on plasma calcium to cause (1) increases in intestinal absorption, and (2) release of calcium from osseous tissue. Hydrogen ion changes the dissociation and protein binding of calcium. The plasma proteins control calcium indirectly by binding to it.

In older rats thyrocalcitonin exerts tonic physiologic control over calcium and is active in many species in the regulation of calcium in pregnancy, egg laying, growth, and lactation (208). In the rat the physiologic effect of PTH on intestinal absorption is small, whereas renal calcium regulation by PTH in hamsters is important (41).

Although ionized calcium provides a better assessment of clinical conditions, it is often useful to measure total calcium as well (48,139, 151,200,226). Total calcium values provide a more valid estimate of their physiologic effect if they are corrected for variations in albumin concentration. For lowered albumin levels in man the formula is (197):

$$\text{adjusted calcium} = \text{plasma calcium} - \text{serum albumin} + 4.$$

Serum or plasma samples are used for determination of total calcium. Whole blood is preferable for measurement of ionized calcium (139,151). Using whole blood for estimations of rodent calcium overcomes the problems of obtaining a large enough sample for analysis and the tedious task of separating cells and plasma anaerobically. Whole blood calcium is justifiable biochemically because of the very low levels of calcium in cells. Recently a new method, inductively coupled plasma emission spectroscopy, has been developed for measuring calcium, magnesium, zinc, copper, and iron in one serum or urine sample simultaneously. No preparative procedures are necessary before measurement (183).

Hypercalcemia

Mechanisms

The mechanisms elevating total plasma calcium operate through increases in the hormones controlling calcium uptake, mobilization and resorption, increases in the calcium carrying plasma proteins, and shrinkage of the plasma volume (25). Free calcium is elevated by thyroxin, parathormone, and acidosis (25).

Disease states

Primary hyperparathyroidism: Increased circulating levels of parathormone mostly cause a direct increase in free calcium and only a small increase in total serum calcium. Hyperplasia and adenomas of the parathyroid give rise to increased hormone levels. The condition of hypercalcemia in pseudohyperparathyroidism is due to tumor proteins that spuriously elevate the value for parathormone (see below).

Ectopic PTH secretion: Many neoplastic diseases are associated with production of a peptide with actions similar to PTH. Lymphoid tumors, tumors of osseous tissue, and tumors of the lung are commonly seen with manifestations of PTH-like activity and hypercalcemia (191).

Hypervitaminosis D: Excessive amounts of vitamin D cause increased plasma calcium levels. The mechanism involves an increase in calcium absorption from the gut and increased mobilization from bone.

Hypervitaminosis A: Large amounts of

ingested vitamin A can produce hypercalcemia (100).

Paraproteinemia: Elevated total plasma calcium is due to increases in the plasma proteins, especially abnormal globulins, that bind calcium. Free calcium is not elevated in these conditions and there is a discrepancy between the amount of protein determined by refractometry and that measured by binding methods (higher).

Hemoconcentration: Each gram elevation of albumin increases the serum calcium by 0.8 mg/dl (177). Hypoalbuminemia with a normal serum calcium is interpreted as hypercalcemia.

Acidosis: Free calcium is increased by acidosis. For man, an increase of 5 per cent for each decrease of 0.1 units of pH is expected (106,257).

Familial hypercalciuric hypercalcemia: This disease is due to an autosomal defect in humans (25).

Renal insufficiency: See Secondary hyperparathyroidism.

Secondary hyperparathyroidism: In renal insufficiency and in recovery from acute renal failure hypercalcemia may be seen (177). Initially in both diseases hypocalcemia is responsible for stimulating PTH secretion. Prolonged PTH secretion blocks the calcium feedback mechanism and the parathyroids secrete independently of the serum calcium concentration (25).

In renal failure in dogs and humans, both renal and extrarenal clearance of PTH is decreased. This has the effect of prolonging the action of PTH and maintaining a higher level of active hormone (208).

Neoplasia: Two main mechanisms operate to produce hypercalcemia in neoplasia: (1) invasion and lysis of bone by the tumor cells, and (2) tumor secretion of sterols with vitamin D-like activity and or ectopic PTH or a PTH-like peptide. A third mechanism has been proven in animals but not man: increased prostaglandin synthesis (191,208,237,256). Carcinomas and lymphomas are common tumors that produce hypercalcemia. Lymposarcoma and circumanal gland tumors in the dog may be associated with hypercalcemia. The mechanism producing hypercalcemia is not yet determined and the mechanism producing hypercalcemia in pheochromocytoma in animals is postulated to be epinephrine stimulation of PTH.

Lithium: Lithium acts to produce hypercalcemia by decreasing the responsiveness of the parathyroid to plasma calcium levels.

Steroids: Estrogens and glucocorticoids produce hypercalcemia. The glucocorticoids produce hypercalcemia by decreasing vitamin D catabolism, thus causing hypervitaminosis D (25). The effect of glucocorticoids on the bone receptor site is dose dependent (208). Glucocorticoids are used in hypercalcemic dogs and cats because of their calciuric effect. Androgens cause hypercalcemia by stimulating the growth of hormone-responsive tumors, especially those of bone.

Granulomatous disease: In granulomatous disease an increase in intestinal absorption of calcium leads to hypercalcemia. The effect is more severe if calcium clearance is blocked (25).

Hyperthyroidism: Hypercalcemia may be seen with elevations in thyroxin (25).

Acute adrenal insufficiency: Infrequently, hypercalcemia is found in this disease. It is probably due to decreased calcium excretion in the urine.

Hypomagnesemia: In rats, calves, pigs, and humans "moderate" degrees of hypomagnesemia stimulate the parathyroid gland in a way similar to that of calcium giving rise to hypercalcemia (208). Severe hypomagnesemia impairs PTH secretion and the action of PTH on bone.

Inactivity: Prolonged inactivity may cause hypercalcemia.

Laboratory error

pH, temperature: Ionized calcium is altered by changes in pH. Any decrease in the pH of an anaerobic sample awaiting calcium analysis, as in increased glycolysis, increases the ionized calcium portion (182). The degree of calcium dissociation increases as the temperature rises (160,182).

Plasma: Plasma calcium is higher than serum calcium because it contains protein bound calcium that is removed from serum in the clot.

Venous stasis: Hemoconcentration is caused by stasis. Stasis increases calcium, mainly protein bound calcium.

Deproteinization: Methods of calcium analysis employing precipitation of proteins give higher values for calcium than do those not removing protein, because the reference sample volume is reduced by removal of the protein portion.

Accompanying changes

Biochemical: *Alkaline phosphatase.* Elevated serum alkaline phosphatase of osseous origin may accompany hypercalcemia. Alkaline phosphatase is elevated because of increases in osteoblastic activity. Decreased alkaline phosphatase levels occur in hypervitaminosis D. Because serum phosphate is elevated in hypervitaminosis D, osteoblastic activity shuts off.

Hyperphosphatemia. Excess vitamin D increases absorption of both calcium and phosphate from the gut; plasma levels of both increase. Osteolytic lesions producing hypercalcemia do not uniformly give rise to hyperphosphatemia; when they do, the increase in phosphorus is slight.

Hyperproteinemia. Increases in protein produce increased protein bound calcium. Proteins are increased by hemoconcentration and paraproteinemia.

Hypophosphatemia. An increase in PTH resets the renal threshold for phosphate; hyperphosphaturia is produced.

Hypobicarbonatemia. When hyperparathyroidism is accompanied by renal tubular acidosis, hyperchloremic acidosis is produced.

Metabolic alkalosis. In rats, an experimentally induced chronic hypercalcemia (primary hyperparathyroidism of chronic vitamin D administration) results in metabolic alkalosis. The alkalosis is due to a change in tubular hydrogen ion handling. Serum calcium changes are highly correlated with serum bicarbonate (162).

Hyperchloremic acidosis. Primary hyperparathyroidism in adult animals is associated with decreased hydrogen ion secretion and increased bicarbonate resorption (208).

Physiologic: Hypotonia, weakness, anorexia, vomiting, constipation, depression, and coma are pathophysiologic signs generally found with hypercalcemia.

Calcification. High levels of calcium in the serum eventually lead to deposition in the tissues and organ failure because of mineralization (61).

Parathormone. Hypercalcemia blocks the action of PTH on renal phosphate excretion (208).

Hypocalcemia

Levels of biologic significance

The biologic activity of calcium is determined by the degree to which it is ionized, and decreases in serum ionized calcium of 1 per cent cause a rise in PTH in a few seconds (208). Low serum calcium rarely causes any detrimental changes in the coagulation system. The main effect is seen in the contractility of muscles.

Mechanisms

The mechanisms producing hypocalcemia center around reduction in: (1) plasma protein, (2) calcium absorption, (3) calcium mobilization from bone, (4) calcium resorption at the kidney, (5) magnesium concentration, (6) the active form of vitamin D, and (7) increases in phosphate concentration.

Disease states

Hypoparathyroidism: Deficiency of parathormone decreases free calcium in the plasma by reducing (1) its absorption from the gut, (2) its mobilization from bone, (3) the formation of active vitamin D, and (4) calcium resorption at the kidney.

Steatorrhea: Calcium is low in this condition because of decreased absorption from the gut; it is lost as soaps.

Nephrosis: Calcium is decreased in nephrosis as loss of its plasma binding proteins occur through the kidney.

Nephritis: In nephritis calcium absorption from the gut is decreased. The decrease in absorption arises from aberrant hydroxylation of vitamin D by the malfunctioning kidneys (20). In chronic renal failure increased phosphate, decreased absorption, and decreased albumin all contribute toward lowering the calcium concentration (191).

Pancreatitis: Calcium may be lost in pancreatitis as a result of the formation of calcium soaps by combination of calcium with fatty acids in the peritoneal cavity. Other mechanisms have been suggested to account for the hypocalcemia of pancreatitis. An increase in thyrocalcitonin and a decrease in parathormone probably occur. Also, there is decreased albumin because of reduced intake, and this may further decrease calcium by lowering the protein bound portion. Concurrent acidosis will reduce the amount of bound calcium and increase its ionized form. Commonly, metabolic alkalosis occurs in pancreatitis as a result of vomiting.

Alkalosis: Ionized calcium is reduced when the pH is increased.

Pseudohypoparathyroidism: In man this disease is rare and inherited. It is characterized by increased parathormone, hyperphosphatemia, hypocalcemia, and an ineffective end organ response.

Malabsorption: The causes of hypocalcemia in malabsorption conditions are: (1) decreased calcium absorption from a damaged gut, (2) decreased absorption caused by formation of calcium soaps with free fatty acids in the gut, (3) decreased absorption of calcium's binding protein albumin, and (4) decreased absorption of fat-souble vitamin D.

Dietary interference: Calcium absorption from the gut is decreased by the presence of excess phosphate, oxalate, and phytate. These compounds form insoluble complexes with calcium and prevent its absorption.

Hypovitaminosis D: Dietary deficiency, decreased intestinal absorption, or decreased formation of the active vitamin cause hypovitaminosis D. The proper functioning of both kidney and liver is required to produce active hormone. Vitamin D is converted in the liver to 25-hydroxyvitamin D which is transported to the kidney where it is converted to 1,25-dihydroxyvitamin D, the biologically active form. (See Endocrine Hormones in Laboratory Animals.) Vitamin D is oxidized to inactive metabolites by the hepatic microsomal system. Renal disease, liver disease, and stimulation of the liver microsomal system result in vitamin D deficiency. Loss of vitamin D activity results in inadequate calcium absorption from the gut and hypocalcemia (20).

Hypoproteinemia: For every gram decrease in albumin there is an approximate 0.8 mg/dl decrease in total serum calcium.

Chelation: Ingestion of ethylene glycol leads to binding of calcium by the products of ethylene glycol metabolism (citrate, oxalate). Chelated calcium is unavailable for analysis by most methods.

Food: Plasma calcium decreases during intake of food probably by stimulation of gastrin with subsequent release of calcitonin.

Laboratory error

Anticoagulant: Oxalate, EDTA, and to a slight extent heparin all decrease calcium available for analysis by most methods, because they bind calcium.

Accompanying changes

Biochemical: *Hypophosphatemia.* Hypophosphatemia accompanies hypocalcemia in disorders that result in decreased calcium absorption.

Hyperphosphatemia. Plasma phosphate is usually high in hypoparathyroidism, pseudohypoparathyroidism, and hypocalcemia caused by renal failure.

Serum alkaline phosphatase. This enzyme is elevated in conditions in which active remodeling of bone (with osteoblast activity) occurs. Alkaline phosphatase (osseous) is not elevated in hypoparathyroidism, pseudohypoparathyroidism, or hypomagnesemia.

Hypomagnesemia. Hypomagnesemia may exist alongside hypocalcemia. Correction of the magnesium defect will also correct the hypocalcemia. The reason for this is that in severe hypomagnesemia the secretion of PTH is inhibited and there is interference with its actions. When conditions are reversed and severe hypermagnesemia exists, hypocalcemia is seen, again as a result of direct inhibition of the parathyroid.

Physiologic: *Tetany.* Lowering the level of free unbound calcium causes tetany. The associated laryngospasm can cause death.

Lactation. Calcium is lost in large amounts in milk. Lactation may produce hypocalcemia.

Phosphorus

Phosphorus is ubiquitous in organisms. It is concerned with intermediary metabolism and energy production and is a structural component of bone and cell membranes. Phosphorus is contained in a large number of compounds —nucleic acids, phosphate esters, and nucleotides (ATP) (194). About 12 to 15 per cent of blood phosphorus is bound to plasma proteins. The free forms are $HPO_4^=$, $NaHPO_4^-$ (75 per cent), and $H_2PO_4^-$ (10 per cent). The species present is dependent on pH and other factors.

Intestinal absorption varies, depending on the

amount present, and it may range from 70 to 90 per cent. Phosphorus, like potassium, is concentrated intracellularly where uptake is enhanced by insulin, glucose, and alkalosis. It is lost in urine, feces, and mucous secretions. Parathormone and the active forms of vitamin D control phosphorus absorption and excretion. Other analytes, estrogens, androgens, thyroxin, and growth hormone affect metabolism of phosphorus in the kidney. Hydrogen ions modulate hormonal control.

The application of phosphorus measurements to the interpretation of biochemical profiles is very important because of the widespread effects of phosphorus on metabolism.

Hyperphosphatemia

Levels of biologic significance

Unlike that of other metabolites, increases in phosphate per se are not extremely detrimental. It is important to know the mechanism producing the hyperphosphatemia. Usually the severity of the defect is correlated with the incremental phosphate change. Young animals have a higher phosphate level than do old animals (208).

Mechanisms

Hyperphosphatemia develops when (1) renal clearance fails, (2) intestinal absorption is increased, and (3) intracelular release occurs.

Disease states

Renal failure: Decreased renal clearance of phosphate in severe renal diseases produces hyperphosphatemia (95).

Hypervitaminosis D: Excessive vitamin D increases intestinal phosphate uptake and stimulates bone resorption. Excessive intake or decreased liver degradation of vitamin D produce hyperphosphatemia.

Pseudohyperparathyroidism: In this disease PTH is increased, but the renal tubules are unresponsive and phosphate diuresis is decreased.

Glucose intolerance: Hyperphosphatemia results from decreased glucose phosphorylation. Diabetes mellitus and Cushing's disease are glucose-intolerant states and may often be seen with hyperphosphatemia in man.

Dehydration: Reduction of plasma water concentrates both protein-bound and other forms of plasma phosphate.

Hypoparathyroidism: Loss of PTH activity causes renal calcium wasting and phosphate retention.

Rhabdomyolysis: Muscle lysis releases large amounts of intracellular phosphate (194).

Muscle trauma: Any surgical or other interference traumatizing sufficient amounts of muscle produces hyperphosphatemia.

Laboratory error

Cell lysis: Cellular damage releases intracellular phosphate and causes spurious hyperphosphatemia. The spurious hyperphosphatemia occurring in whole blood on standing originates from platelets and leukocytes rather than from erythrocytes that contain less phosphate than does plasma.

Contamination: Collection apparatus, water, and the like contaminate samples and cause false hyperphosphatemia.

Evaporation: Loss of sample water raises the phosphate value (176).

Accompanying changes

Biochemical: *Azotemia.* Azotemia occurs with hyperphosphatemia in renal failure and in dehydration.

Hypercalcemia. Calcium and phosphate are elevated in young animals and in hypervitaminosis D.

Hypocalcemia. Pseudohypoparathyroidism and hypoparathyroidism are characterized by phosphate retention and calcium loss (hypocalcemia with low total and ionized calcium).

Phosphorylation. Reduced glucose phosphorylation allows plasma phosphate levels to rise.

Creatine kinase. Damaged muscle releases creatine kinase into the plasma.

Physiologic: Young animals have high phosphate values because growth hormone raises vitamin D levels, which in turn increases calcium and phosphorus absorption from the gut (95).

Calcification. Prolonged hyperphosphatemia is likely to produce tissue calcification.

Hypophosphatemia

Levels of biologic significance

When serum phosphate falls to 2 mg/dl or less, symptoms of hypophosphatemia become evident in man, and severe effects on tissue metabolism and organ function are noted at 0.2 mg/dl (95). In normal man the serum phosphate may very by 2 mg/dl because of its diurnal intercellular movement (135,194).

Mechanisms

Hypophosphatemia is caused by: (1) decreased intake of phosphorus, (2) transcellular shifts of phosphorus, and (3) increased loss of phosphorus from either the gut or kidney.

Disease states

Starvation, malabsorption, and vomiting: In these three disease states phosphorus intake is reduced. Hypophosphatemia results when they become chronic or severe.

Vitamin D deficiency: Hypovitaminosis D decreases gut absorption of calcium and phosphorus while increasing renal excretion of phosphate as well as decreasing bone resorption. Hypophosphatemia and hypocalcemia result from hypovitaminosis D.

Insulin: Insulin facilitates the transport of glucose and phosphorus into cells.

Alkalosis: Alkalosis accelerates glycolysis. It acts on phosphofructokinase and increases the use of phosphate by intermediate compounds, causing a decline in plasma phosphate. In respiratory alkalosis, the pH change is rapidly transmitted to cells and is more likely to cause hypophosphatemia than is metabolic alkalosis. Hypophosphatemia occurs infrequently in metabolic alkalosis despite accelerated renal loss of phosphate (135).

Osmotic diuresis: Diuresis depletes phosphate by increasing its renal clearance.

Hypomagnesemia: Hypomagnesemia releases PTH. Parathormone increases urinary excretion of phosphate, resulting in hypophosphatemia.

Acidosis: In acidosis phosphate is removed from cells and presented to the renal tubule where its excretion is enhanced. Acidosis switches off synthesis of 2,3-DPG in the erythrocyte. Phosphate incorporation in 2,3-DPG is reduced by hypophosphatemia.

Hyperparathyroidism: Parathormone acts on the kidney to produce calcium retention and phosphate loss. This activity causes a moderate phosphate reduction.

Secondary hyperparathyroidism: Phosphorus is lost in the urine in this condition, the result of increased PTH activity.

Vitamin B_{12} deficiency: Diarrhea of vitamin B_{12} deficiency causes hypokalemia. Hypokalemia causes a decrease in the plasma phosphate by allowing phosphate to pass out in the urine. Both conditions, hypokalemia and hypophosphatemia, are further accentuated if treatment with vitamin B_{12} is given. Phosphate and potassium move into nucleated erythrocytes. Here phosphorus is required to maintain the three-dimensional structure of the new protein molecules, is incorporated in nucleic acid sysnthesis, is needed for synthesis of biochemical intermediates, and is an integral part of ATP and 2,3-DPG (194). The relationship of vitamin B_{12} to this complex in species other than man remains to be defined.

Hypokalemia: Hypokalemia produces a vacuolar nephropathy and thus causes loss of phosphate.

Renal tubular acidosis: In renal tubular acidosis phosphate is lost in urine.

De Toni Fanconi syndrome: In this syndrome a renal tubular defect characterized by failure to resorb amino acids, glucose, and phosphate produces hypophosphatemia.

Hypothyroidism: Phosphate is decreased in hypothyroidism.

Diabetes mellitus: The plasma concentration of organic phosphate is decreased and that of inorganic phosphate increased by diabetes mellitus.

Laboratory error

See Hyperphosphatemia.

Accompanying changes

Biochemical: *Adenosine triphosphate and 2,3-DPG.* Hypophosphatemia directly effects synthesis of both these compounds. All energy and oxygenation reactions are affected by this change (135).

Creatine kinase. Severe hypophosphatemia damages muscle releasing creatine kinase (135).

Hypercalciuria. Hypophosphatemia causes decalcification and calciuria. The mechanism is unknown (135).

Hemolytic anemia. Adenosine triphosphate is required to maintain the erythrocyte's biconcavity, an energy-dependent process. The erythrocytic membrane is predominately phospholipid. Lack of ATP (energy) and structural materials (phospholipid) causes spherocytosis and its natural sequelae—hemolytic anemia (135).

Coagulopathy. Hypophosphatemia in animals produces platelet defects, probably all related to decreased levels of ATP. Clot retraction is abnormal, platelet survival is decreased, and thrombocytopenia and hemorrhages occur (281). The defects in man have not been proven; however, hemorrhages have been reported (135).

Leukocytes. The energy-dependent processes of phagocytosis, killing, and chemotaxis are decreased in hypophosphatemic animals (135).

Renal ammoniogenesis. In rabbits renal ammonia formation and excretion are decreased by hypophosphatemia (135).

Renal glucose transport. Hypophosphatemia in dogs produces a defect in renal glucose transport and glucose intolerance (135).

pH. The renal excretion of bicarbonate is increased in phosphate-depleted dogs (84,229). The mechanism for the resultant acidosis is the action of PTH. (See Hypophosphatemia under Hypobicarbonatemia for mechanism.)

Urine calcium and phosphate. Hypophosphatemia increases urine calcium excretion and decreases phosphate excretion.

Tissue hypoxia. Decreases in erythrocyte 2,3-DPG due to hypophosphatemia produce a shift in the oxygen dissociation curve that results in decreased oxygen delivery to the tissues (194).

Physiologic: Sepsis. Hypophosphatemic animals have increased susceptibility to infectious agents. The neutrophilic, chemotactic, and phagocytic functions are depressed by low phosphate levels (194).

Impaired acid excretion. Insufficient phosphate buffer formation impairs renal acid excretion.

Insulin resistance. Hypophosphatemia causes insulin resistance because phosphorus is required for glucose metabolism.

Neuromuscular changes. A multitude of changes occur in hypophosphatemia. These range from muscle weakness to paralysis, and from tremor to coma. The severity of the hypophosphatemia governs the degree to which signs are expressed.

Skeletal system. Bone pain, probably related to osteomalacia, and joint pain due to arthritis are features of hypophosphatemia.

Insoluble complexes. Phosphate in the gut is complexed with aluminum, magnesium hydroxide, and others, rendering it unavailable for absorption.

Postcibal decline. Phosphorus and glucose enter cells together. Phosphorus falls about 0.25 mg/dl in mature humans after eating. The postcibal decline in a starved animal fed carbohydrate is much larger (194).

Magnesium

Magnesium ions are important enzyme activators, activating ATP (243). They regulate PTH secretion similarly to the way it is regulated by calcium in both man and animals, but their potency is one half to one third that of calcium. Interrelationships with calcium and phosphorus are not fully understood. Elevated pH decreases the ionized magnesium. Magnesium, like calcium and phosphorus, is partitioned into a relatively fixed osseous form and mobile cellular and plasma forms. About 70 per cent of the plasma magnesium is diffusible; the rest is bound to plasma proteins. Magnesium is the second most prevalent intracellular cation and is 3 times more abundant in erythrocytes and 10 times more abundant in other cells than it is in plasma.

The absorption of ingested magnesium appears to be unregulated, that is, not responsive to the status of magnesium stores in the body. Plasma levels are influenced by PTH and aldosterone. Parathormone enhances resorption and elevated calcium inhibits resorption. Filtered magnesium is almost completely resorbed. A transport maximum is present. Renal regulation is responsible for maintenance of body stores. Plasma and serum magnesium levels differ because although a small amount of protein-bound magnesium is removed in the clot, more is released into the serum by the activated platelets.

Measurement of ionized magnesium in the plasma is not a good indicator of cellular magnesium levels. High values are always diagnostic.

Hypermagnesemia

Levels of biologic significance

The serum and plasma levels of magnesium act only as a guide to the cellular level of magnesium. A more accurate assessment of the status of the physiologically important cellular level can be obtained by measuring magnesium contained in erythrocytes and in a 24-hour urine sample. Decreased intracellular magnesium corresponds to reduced excretion. Increased plasma magnesium is evidence of hypermagnesemia.

Mechanisms

Hypermagnesemia is produced by contraction of the extracellular fluid volume and by decreased excretion.

Disease states

Dehydration: Fluid lost from all body routes causes hypermagnesemia, as it shrinks the fluid volume in which the magnesium is distributed.

Addison's disease: Decreased renal clearance of magnesium, a direct result of aldosterone deficiency, produces hypermagnesemia.

Hyperparathyroidism: Hypermagnesemia develops if the effect of PTH in causing magnesium retention is greater than the calcium-inhibiting effect on magnesium. Calcium and magnesium compete for resorption in the loop of Henle.

Hypothyroidism: Magnesium may be increased when thyroxin is deficient.

Decreased glomerular filtration and renal failure: Magnesium is cleared from the body in urine; therefore, a decrease in urine formation leads to accumulation of magnesium in the plasma.

Laboratory error

Venous stasis: Magnesium leaks from erythrocytes and other cells under hypoxic conditions, increasing the plasma level. The plasma proteins increase in venous congestion and so do the ions they carry.

Thrombolysis: The serum level of magnesium is usually higher than that of plasma because of magnesium leaked from platelets. Serum magnesium is elevated in thrombocytotic states. Protein-bound magnesium is removed from the serum in the clot. Only a small amount is removed, as only 20 per cent of magnesium is protein bound.

Evaporation: Evaporative water losses will produce an erroneously high magnesium concentration.

Accompanying changes

Biochemical: *Calcium.* There is a reciprocal relationship between plasma magnesium and calcium levels. Both ions compete in the loop of Henle for resorption. Hypermagnesemia inhibits PTH secretion, causing renal loss of calcium and hypocalcemia in man and animals.

Physiologic: *Anesthesia.* By depressing activity of the nervous system hypermagnesemia produces a state akin to anesthesia. Hypermagnesemia depresses skeletal muscle activity.

Vasodilation. An increase in magnesium ion causes vasodilation.

Hypomagnesemia

Levels of biologic significance

The plasma level of magnesium should be used only as a guide in making decisions on the status of magnesium. To determine the actual level of magnesium, intracellular fluid is sampled (243).

Mechanisms

Hypomagnesemia results from decreased magnesium intake and/or increased loss from the gastrointestinal and renal system or through lactiferous secretions. Extrarenal losses are characterized by renal retention of magnesium.

Disease states

Malabsorption and chronic pancreatitis: Hypomagnesemia is due to decreased absorption from the gut. In steatorrhea magnesium forms insoluble soaps.

Hyperparathyroidism: Hyperparathyroidism depletes magnesium by favoring calcium retention in the loop of Henle. Parathormone is responsible for the increase in calcium retention.

Diabetes mellitus: Glycosuria produces osmotic diuresis resulting in hypermagnesuria and hypomagnesemia.

Renal disease: Pathologic processes affecting

the proximal tubule or thick ascending limb of Henle's loop will compromise magnesium resorption because more than 90 per cent of filtered magnesium is resorbed by the kidney.

Hyperaldosteronism: Aldosterone acts to conserve sodium and waste potassium and magnesium. Also, extracellular fluid volume is increased when sodium is retained and plasma magnesium is diluted.

Protein deficiency: Decreased gut absorption is the probable cause of hypomagnesemia in protein deficiency.

Laboratory error

Dilutional errors: Incorrect dilution of plasma samples results in erroneous magnesium levels.

Sample site: For erythrocyte magnesium levels the same site is always used to collect blood because of erythrocyte volume differences (between arterial and venous blood). This restriction usually presents no problem to the phlebotomist except in nonhuman primates when the blood samples are drawn from the femoral artery or vein. Entry of either one from the other contamination of arterial with venous blood must be avoided.

Accompanying changes

Biochemical: *Parathormone.* Severe hypomagnesemia inhibits secretion of PTH and impairs its peripheral action.

Urine phosphate. An increase in urine phosphate excretion is seen in hypomagnesemia.

Physiologic: *Neuromuscular dysfunction.* Hypomagnesemia is accompanied by hyperexcitabiltiy, muscle tremor, convulsions, and, if severe, death. Lowered magnesium concentrations destabilize the granules of Kühn (synaptic vesicles).

Mean corpuscular volume. The mean corpuscular volume in man is decreased in hypomagnesemia.

Proteinate

Proteins are amphoteric, having both positive and negative groups on the same molecule. In the physiologic pH range plasma proteins have an excess of negative charge and behave as anions (187). The net protein cation equivalency (base binding power) of the plasma proteins is said to be 16 to 19.0 mEq/l (16.4 mEq/l in the dog [285]). The former value was calculated almost 60 years ago, using serum from two horses and one man (265). Published values for laboratory animal species, other than the dog, are not available.

Measurement of the base binding power (net cation equivalency) entails summing the individual anions and cations and subtracting one from the other. The value contributed by protein anions, that are never measured is the difference (264).

The net effect of plasma proteins is that of an anion, because proteins bind more cations than anions. The fully dissociated albumin molecule, the main proteinate, has 200 hydrogen ion binding sites of various strengths.

Other cations compete unfavorably with hydrogen ions for albumin binding sites (264). To compete they have to be present in greater numbers. A decrease in hydrogen ion numbers or an increase in competing cations means that more of the latter are bound. The strongest of these competitors are copper, zinc, iron, and cobalt. Calcium and magnesium are partially complex bound, whereas sodium and potassium are bound in a salt type manner up to pH 8.0. Chloride is complex bound to albumin at physiologic pH, but little is known about bicarbonate binding. Abnormal binding is possible in disease states. Unless there is a specific reason to quantify the contributions of plasma proteins to the acid base balance (contribution to an anion gap), they are usually not measured. This does not mean they do not contribute significantly to acid base disturbances. Their effects should always be considered.

Many substances, aside from hydrogen ions and electrolytes, bind to albumin. The effects of changes in the net cation eqivalency on the binding of these are an important consideration.

Increased Net Protein Cation Equivalency or Base Binding Power

Levels of biologic significance

Increased levels of anionic proteins have rarely been reported. The reason is not entirely obvious, but it may be the difficulty in recognition of the disorder. Human IgA levels of 2 to 8 g/dl, and bovine IgG levels of 4 g/dl (JHR, unpublished data) have been noted to cause an increase in anionic protein.

The contribution of proteinate is assessed using the technique for measurement of the charge density on a protein molecule or by analytic isoelectric focusing. It can usually only be inferred that an increased anion gap associated with increased total protein is due to anionic protein unless either of the two techniques mentioned is used. (Isoelectric focusing data from the cow already mentioned revealed that both cationic and anionic proteins were elevated but anionic proteins predominated.)

Mechanisms

Plasma protein net cation equivalency is increased by (1) concentration of normal proteins (dehydration), (2) addition of new anionic proteins (paraproteins), and (3) alkalemia-induced elevations in the net negative charge of plasma proteins.

Disease states

Extracellular fluid volume depletion: Plasma proteins are increased when protein-free fluid leaves the vascular system. Albumin contributes most to net negative charge of protein; however, most other normal proteins act as anions too.

Alkalosis: Alkalemia causes plasma proteins to take on a more negative net charge because of their titration with plasma. Volume deficits and alkalosis often occur together (152).

The possible contribution of proteinate to the anion gap should be considered whenever the anion gap is interpreted.

Polyclonal gammopathy: Increases in both anionic and cationic proteins, with the former predominating, have been observed in a cow (JHR, unpublished data). The bovine gamma globulins and an excessively negatively charged prealbumin were increased.

Paraproteins: Multiple myeloma in man causes an increase in net plasma protein cation equivalency. The paraproteins IGG and IGA are responsible for this increase.

Laboratory error

Because net cation equivalency is a derived value, errors in measurement or calculation may produce spurious increases in the net cation

equivalency. Such errors should always be considered in interpretation of acid base disorders.

Accompanying changes

The anion gap is increased by a "hidden acidosis" that may be accompanied by hypochloremia. The spurious acidosis is due to the increased negative net charge of protein that results from an increase in the contribution of protein to the "unmeasured anions." The increased protein net negative charge balances the anion deficit (hypobicarbonatemia or hypochloremia).

Decreased Net Protein Cation Equivalency

Mechanisms

Two mechanisms that lead to a decrease in net protein cation equivalency have been identified: (1) absolute reduction in protein level, and (2) abnormal proteins carrying a cation excess rather than the normal anion excess.

Disease states

Hypoalbuminemia: Reductions in total albumin levels by absolute or relative means (dilution) produce a decrease in net cation equivalency. (Albumin contributes most to plasma anions because it is present in the greatest amount and carries the highest charge density on its molecule.)

Paraproteins: In man, both muliple myeloma and monoclonal gammopathy may cause decreases in the net cation equivalency of protein. In both diseases this is due to increases in cationic proteins.

Laboratory error

Errors in measurement or calculation cause spurious results.

Accompanying changes

The anion gap is directly decreased by reductions in the net cation equivalency of proteins.

Sulfate

The normal plasma sulfate concentration in man is 0.7 mEq/l. It is actively resorbed in the renal tubule and has a high transport maximum. Its plasma level is increased when its renal excretion is decreased or when sulfur containing amino acids are catabolized.

Bicarbonate

Bicarbonate is the second largest fraction of the extracellular anions. With carbonic acid it forms an important open buffer system. By interaction with hydrogen ions and bases it prevents large pH shifts. Bicarbonate is mainly concentrated in plasma; smaller amounts are present in erythrocytes.

Bicarbonate is a dependent variable, being dependent of PCO_2 and pH. Essentially all acids, bases, and electolytes including protein interact with bicarbonate. Bicarbonate is absorbed by and secreted into the gut. Pancreatic secretions are high in bicarbonate as is the saliva of herbivores. Bicarbonate is formed from the reaction of carbon dioxide and water. This reaction is important in the reclamation of bicarbonate by the kidney.

Organic anions, citrate and lactate, are catabolized to carbon dioxide and water with the subsequent formation of bicarbonate. Herbivores' intake of bases, in the form of sodium or potassium salts, guarantees an alkaline urine in these species and in others in which there is a high intake of vegetable matter.

Bicarbonate has an apparent transport maximum in the kidney. If this is exceeded, bicarbonate spills into the urine where a maximal pH of 8 is possible in humans. This is equivalent to a maximal plasma bicarbonate concentration of 28 mEq/l.

Metabolic disturbances cause the greatest changes in bicarbonate concentration. Bicarbonate concentration usually reflects hydrogen ion concentration, but it is upset by changes in other anions and concomitant changes in PCO_2.

Bicarbonate concentration is usually calculated from PCO_2 and pH. A small error may occur because the ionic strength of samples varies. An indirect titrimetric method, determining total CO_2, is used; however, it must be corrected for carbamate and carbonate. An altered bicarbonate value must be accompanied by other data for proper interpretation.

Obtaining a satisfactory arterial sample from dogs, cats, rabbits, pigs, horses, cows, goats, sheep, and primates is not difficult. In rodents it can probably best be obtained by permanent surgical exteriorization of the carotid artery.

Hyperbicarbonatemia

Levels of biologic significance

Very few values have been accurately determined for bicarbonate in animals. In one study the normal bicarbonate level for the female dog was determined as 19.8 mEq/l, and a high value of 30 mEq/l was produced by acute hypercapnia with PCO_2 levels of 130 to 140 mmHg (64).

Mechanisms

Bicarbonate is indirectly elevated by increased PCO_2 and decreased titratable hydrogen ion concentration and is directly elevated by the conversion of lactate (and other bases) to bicarbonate. Increased PCO_2 raises the carbonic acid level, and the subsequent dissociation of the acid produces bicarbonate. The increase in bicarbonate is slight in acute and larger in chronic disorders.

Disease states

Vomiting: Two main mechanisms operate when gastric contents are lost. Hydrochloric acid is lost in the vomitus and at the same time there is diuresis of alkali and a slight loss of sodium. Other changes that occur are: increased renal potassium excretion, a rise in the renal threshold for bicarbonate, and increased sodium-hydrogen ion exchange (128,231).

The kidney resorbs sodium (without chloride) by an accelerated sodium-cation exchange, producing hyperbicarbonatemia and potassium depletion (231). The sodium loss is small and volume is conserved (128). Volume conservation is considered to be more important than maintenance of normal acid base and potassium balance. Bicarbonate is increased directly by increased resorption at the kidney and indirectly by reduced consumption as there are fewer hydrogen ions.

Active secretion of hydrogen ions by the gastric or abomasal mucosa following a meal decreases the plasma concentration. Alkalinuria follows food ingestion.

Gastric fluid becomes sequestered by dilatation of the stomach or abomasum. The sequestered hydrochloric acid results in a lower plasma hydrogen ion concentration (161).

Ingestion of alkali: Ingestion of bicarbonate and other bases (lactate, citrate, and isocitrate), metabolizable into bicarbonate, directly raises plasma bicarbonate concentration. Vegetarians and herbivores have a high plasma bicarbonate concentration because their diet has a high base component of weak organic acids that are metabolized into bicarbonate.

Hyperadrenocorticism: In hyperadrenocorticism the renal tubule is controlled by sodium-retaining aldosterone. Sodium is retained and hydrogen ions are inappropriately excreted. A detailed description of how the alkalosis is achieved in the rat is given by Wamberg et al (268).

Hypoparathyroidism: Bicarbonate is retained by the kidney in hypoparathyroidism.

Cushing's disease: Hydrocorisone is responsible for elevating plasma bicarbonate concentration and increasing secretion of hydrogen ions.

Hypercapnia: Experimentally induced chronic hypercapnia in dogs produces a rise in acid, ammonium, sodium and potassium excretion, increased renal bicarbonate production, and chloriuresis. The elevated PCO_2 is now believed to exert its effect on chloride resorption and not by stimulation of tubular acid excretion with retention of bicarbonate, as once was believed. Chronic hypercapnia causes both hyperbicarbonatemia and hypochloremia (231).

Adaptive processes take place slowly over several weeks, resulting in higher bicarbonate values than those found in acute respiratory acidosis. With adaptation the loss of sodium and potassium in the urine ceases as their function is replaced by newly generated ammonium ion.

Alkalosis may be prolonged by feeding a low chloride diet. The kidney needs chloride to excrete bicarbonate and a cation. To achieve this, chloride is resorbed in place of bicarbonate, permitting the latter to pass into the urine. Sodium and potassium are now retained by the body. To prevent a negative cation balance the kidney conserves both cations with bicarbonate. Therefore, the chloride deficit, and not the hypokalemia as popularly believed, prolongs the alkalosis (231).

In acute respiratory acidosis the increase in plasma bicarbonate is due to the reaction between CO_2 and the nonbicarbonate buffer system. The change in bicarbonate is less than that produced by chronic respiratory acidosis.

Preexisting chronic metabolic acid base disturbances have been found to influence the whole body response to acute hypercapnia. In dogs the hydrogen ion concentration is progressively more easily maintained as the chronic level of bicarbonate increases (154).

Contraction alkalosis: Hyperbicarbonatemia arises in contraction alkalosis because physiologic forces prevent bicarbonaturia. Loss of both sodium and chloride without the concomitant loss of bicarbonate from the extracellular fluid causes contraction of the extracellular fluid volume. If the bicarbonate concentration is normal before saline diuresis, the elevation in bicarbonate is small. Preexisting edema and ascites accentuate the effect of contraction alkalosis (177).

Chronic hypercalcemia: Experimental primary hyperparathyroidism and chronic hypervitaminosis D cause hypercalcemia and metabolic alkalosis in the rat. Acute hypercalcemia in the rat stimulates bicarbonate resorption and hydrogen ion secretion (162). The effect is linear. Parathormone inhibits bicarbonate resorption in the proximal nephron in the acute situation but has little effect in the long term (162).

Laboratory error

Temperature: Blood gas determinations with the analyzer set at a lower temperature than that of the animal are erroneous (33). The pH is higher and the hydrogen ion concentration lower than the real value. The PCO_2 reading is also erroneous as it decreases 4 to 5 per cent for every degree centigrade drop in temperature (33). The calculated value for bicarbonate will be severely affected as both the pH and the PCO_2 errors are additive.

The solubility of gases and the hydrogen ion concentration of the buffers used in calibration vary with temperature. Resetting the analyzer necessitates recalculation of these values for calibration.

The glass and reference electrode, liquid junction, and blood sample are held at the same temperature. If a discrepancy is present, the readings will be erroneous (33).

Loss of carbon dioxide: Exposure of blood samples to air or plastic containers that absorb carbon dioxide produces a loss of the volatile acid carbon dioxide. Air bubbles erroneously lower PCO_2 by dilution (33).

Heparin: Acidic heparin causes a pH error. Heparin should be sterile, isotonic, and have a neutral pH (33,44).

Calibration: Careful calibration and cleaning of blood gas equipment is essential for accurate and reliable measurements. The response time of electrodes is prolonged by protein coating. Instruments reading in a fixed time frame are especially affected (33).

Adjusting the temperature setting on an analyzer changes the values on calibration gases because the vapor pressure of water is altered by the new temperature. These new values must be taken into account and the gases assigned corrected values. Calibration buffers are also subject to temperature changes.

Although the newest generation of blood gas analyzers are easy to operate, they are prone to give results that appear correct and yet are in error. This happens because operations are automatic and algorithms are used. Neither of the aforementioned are inconsistent with proper and accurate measurements, but stricter quality control and an understanding of the machine's algorithms and operational characteristics are needed to use this equipment.

Grounding: Analyzers need to be grounded. Synthetic clothing and insulating footwear are to be avoided as they predispose to build up of static electricity (22).

Ice: Cells are ruptured by direct contact with ice. The released intracellular ions and protein and loss of red cell negative charge cause spurious results (33).

Venous contamination: Some arterial sampling sites, such as the posterior auricular branch of the posterior auricular artery of a cow, and the equivalent vessel in the rabbit are almost entirely free from the possibility of venous contamination, since the artery is visible and separate from the vein. In other sampling sites the artery (carotid, femoral, and metacarpal) lies close to the vein and is only definable by palpation. Here venous contamination is a hazard but can be avoided if the arterial pressure is allowed to fill the syringe.

Inadequate mixing: The pH of whole blood is about 0.01 units lower than that of plasma because of the effects of the negatively charged and hemolyzed and precipitated erythrocytes at the potassium chloride junction (240,244).

Accompanying changes

Biochemical: *Ionized calcium.* Elevated bicarbonate causes a decrease in ionized calcium, a direct effect of hyperbicarbonatemia. Secondary effects are due to changes in the concentration of hydrogen ion or PCO_2.

Hypochloremia. Loss or sequestration of gastric juice produces hypochloremia.

Hypokalemia. Hypokalemia develops when the tubules, under the influence of aldosterone, cause sodium retention and potassium excretion. Aldosterone is secreted in response to volume depletion or autonomously by adrenal neoplasms. Hypercarbia accelerates exchange of hydrogen and cations and increases kaliuresis.

Aciduria. In hyperbicarbonatemia, hydrogen ions are paired with poorly resorbable anions such as phosphate, sulfate, and organic acid ions and excreted. The kidney does this because suitable cations are limited—sodium is retained by aldosterone, potassium is deficient, and hydrogen ions, although unsuitable, are available. Thus, sodium-hydrogen ion exchange is accelerated and aciduria results (65).

Physiologic: *Tissue oxygenation.* Increased bicarbonate (hydrogen ion decrease) shifts the oxygen dissociation curve in favor of oxygen uptake. Oxygen delivered to tissues is compromised by alkalosis (hyperbicarbonatemia).

Tetany. Ionized calcium and ionized magnesium are directly decreased by hyperbicarbonatemia (alkalosis). Tetany is due to decreases in the ionized forms of either cation.

Glycolysis. The glycolytic rate is increased by increased activity of phosphofructokinase. Other pH-sensitive enzymes are probably also affected.

Hypobicarbonatemia

Levels of biologic significance

Bicarbonate levels of 8 to 10 mEq/l are incompatible with life in man if they are maintained for more than a short time (179).

Mechanisms

Primary hypobicarbonatemia occurs as a direct result of loss from the body and indirectly as a consequence of consumption in buffer action and as a complication of renal failure when the mechanism for its replacement fails. Other buffers and bases are used or lost concomitantly with bicarbonate, but they are not routinely measured. The lost bicarbonate is replaced by the conjugate base of the acid. These bases are metabolized organic (lactate and citrate) or excreted inorganic (sulfate).

Disease states

Tubular dysfunction: Renal tubular failure leads to failure of (1) the hydrogen-sodium exchange so the normal acid load is not excreted, (2) ammonia synthesis that normally buffers free hydrogen ions (see loss of renal ammoniagenesis under Hypocarbonatemia for mechanism), and (3) bicarbonate resorption, the normal regenerative reclamation mechanism for bicarbonate. These failures result in retained acid and depletion of bicarbonate because bicarbonate has an obligatory buffering action and is unable to replenish itself.

Lactic acidosis: The biochemical pathways leading to lactic acidosis have been reviewed (66,109,157,173,190,193,251). Lactic acid production is enhanced in severe acidemia. Acidemia is offset by inhibition of phosphofructokinase by the acidosis itself.

Early in lactacidemia protons are added to the plasma, and bicarbonate is used. Later, if the cause is removed, the liver, kidney, and muscle convert the added lactate to bicarbonate. Conversion to bicarbonate occurs slowly and only if organ perfusion and energy metabolism are normal. The increase in lactic acid is equivalent to the decrease in bicarbonate.

Lactic acidosis occurs in hypoxia (L-lactate), in abnormal bacterial rumen fermentation of cattle with "grain overload" (D-lactate), and in abnormal colon fermentation in man with short bowel syndrome (D-lactate) in which excess carbohydrate precipitates the D-lactic acidoses (189). D-lactate does not react with the normal stereospecific enzyme test for lactate; chemical methods measure both forms. D-lactate is slowly metabolized by mammals. Arterial levels are lower than venous.

Mammals lack D-lactate dehydrogenase (189). In hyperlactacidemia excessive lactate production due to increased anaerobic metabolism of carbohydrate or failure of clearance mech-

anisms alters the normal lactate to pyruvate ratio of 10:1 in favor of lactate (116). Lactate is metabolized slower by the liver and kidney in the dog in shock (112). Alkalosis, especially respiratory, enhances lactate production. Lactate is converted to glucose by the liver and kidney, is oxidized by the kidney and skeletal and cardiac muscle to carbon dioxide, or removed by the kidney in the urine. Its renal threshold is high. Lactacidemias are usually normochloremic. Fatal levels in man are 7 to 8 mEq/l (190).

Primary hyperparathyroidism: Parathormone causes bicarbonate loss by direct reduction of its renal tubular resorption. Moderate metabolic acidosis is produced (103).

Filtration failure: Acids, the products of metabolism, are retained when renal filtration mechanisms fail (213). Many acids including hippuric, indole-3-acetic, 3-(3-hydroxyphenol)-3-hydroxypropanoic acid, 4-hydroxyphenylacetic acid, and 3-carboxy-4-methyl-5-propyl-2-furanproprionic acid accumulate. These acids inhibit binding of both endogenous metabolites and acidic drugs. Consequently the efficacy of toxicity of acidic drugs is altered in uremia (254). Bicarbonate is depleted as it buffers these retained acids. The tubular capacity to resorb bicarbonate decreases as the filtration rate drops and the ability to excrete acids is compromised; therefore bicarbonate consumption exceeds production. An increased anion gap appears in uremic acidosis only when the creatinine is markedly elevated. Acidosis is hyperchloremic up to this point.

Renal tubular acidosis: In proximal tubular acidosis there is an inability to resorb bicarbonate, whereas in distal tubular acidosis acid secretion in the distal tubule is decreased (74,103,213).

Ketoacidosis: Ketosis is due to both overproduction and underuse of beta-hydroxybutyric and acetoacetic acids and acetone (136, 157). Commonly, ketoacidosis is associated with diabetes mellitus (4,116), but it is seen in a wide variety of conditions such as starvation, hyperchloremic acidosis, hyperthyroidism, fever, trauma, high-fat/low-carbohydrate diets, and sepsis.

The plasma may be lipemic in hypoinsulinemic diabetes because lipoprotein lipase is activated by insulin.

In hypoinsulinemic diabetes, insulin deficiency deranges several steps in fatty acid metabolism and at the same time probably activates hepatic ketogenic pathways. The activity of carnitine acyltransferase, the rate-limiting enzyme responsible for transport of fatty acids across membranes, is increased. Specifically, in hypoinsulinemic diabetes, pyruvate that is normally converted to acetyl CoA by pyruvic dehydrogenase and then oxidized to CO_2 and H_2O need insulin for the activation step involving pyruvic dehydrogenase. Insulin deficiency mobilizes stored alanine, which in turn is transaminated, providing more pyruvate to enhance the lactacidosis (179). Excess ketone bodies are produced; normal use by peripheral tissues is impaired (136).

Overproduction and underuse of ketones is also a feature of starvation ketosis.

Ketone acids, beta-hydroxybutyric and acetoacetic, are strong acids that donate protons readily and use up body buffers. They are also interconvertible; more beta-hydroxybutyric and less acetoacetate is formed as oxygen tension of mitochondria falls.

Ketone bodies are produced in the rat, cow, and sheep by identical processes (24).

Interpretation of tests for ketones is often misleading if certain information is ignored. Beta-hydroxybutyrate does not react with nitroprusside reagent; acetoacetic acid does. The colorimetric assay for creatinine is falsely elevated by increased acetoacetate levels. Caution should also be exercised in interpetation of the plasma potassium levels—diabetic acidosis produces serious body deficits. Plasma potassium, however, represents the combined effects of volume contraction and metabolic alkalosis.

Ethylene glycol intoxication: Glycolic acid, a catabolic product of ethylene glycol, is a strong acid which consumes bicarbonate and produces hypobicarbonatemia. Renal failure from tubular crystal accumulation complicates the later stages of intoxication as acids are retained by the kidney and buffers (bicarbonate and ammonia) are lost.

Methanol: Hypobicarbonatemia in methanol intoxication is due to formic acid, the metabolic product of methanol.

Acid intake: (1) Hypobicarbonatemia with hyperchloremia is produced by administration of chloride-containing acids (ammonium chloride, arginine hydrochloride, hydrochloric acid, and lysine hydrochloride). The titrated bicarbonate is replace by chloride. (2)

Hypobicarbonatemia with hyperchloremia results when sulfuric, phosphoric, and sulfur-containing amino acids are given. Bicarbonate is titrated by the acid, while the anion replaces bicarbonate. At the time of this replacement the plasma chloride is normal and the anion gap increased. It does not remain so. Rapid excretion of sodium salts of the retained anion and water increases plasma chloride and contracts extracellular fluid. The condition progresses because hypovolemia stimulates sodium chloride retention.

Salicylic acid: Salicylates cause metabolic acidosis, metabolic alkalosis, and respiratory alkalosis. Salicylic acid is a strong acid and directly consumes bicarbonate. Also, salicylates alter intermediary metabolism. Lactic acid, ketoacids, and a number of other organic acids are produced in excess. Metabolic alkalosis is secondary to gastric irritation and loss of gastric acid. Respiratory alkalosis is caused by the effect of salicylate on the brainstem respiratory center.

Benzoic acid: N-benzoyl-L-tyrosyl-p-aminobenzoic acid may produce metabolic acidosis (benzoic acid acidosis) when it is used as a test of pancreatic function in animals with immature livers. Normal conjugation of benzoic acid and its derivatives with glycine and subsequent excretion as hippuric acid derivatives does not occur (237).

Hyperventilation: Moderate degrees of hypobicarbonatemia are due to acute hyperventilation; more pronounced hypobicarbonatemia is seen when the condition is chronic.

In the acute condition hydrogen ions are released from tissue buffers and these combine with bicarbonate.

In chronic hyperventilation renal bicarbonate resorption is reduced by the decreased PCO_2. This mechanism establishes a lower bicarbonate concentration.

If alkalosis occurs, pH-sensitive phosphofructokinase increases glycolytic acitivity so that greater amounts of lactic and pyruvic acid are produced. These acids lower bicarbonate further.

Ptyalism: Loss of bicarbonate in saliva, especially in herbivorous animals, produces hypobicarbonatemia (161).

Diarrhea: Bicarbonate is lost in the feces in diarrhea, caused by infectious agents, osmotic effects, and malabsorption.

Starvation: Ketones are produced by starving

animals as body fat is used for energy. However skeletal muscle, heart, and kidney become unable to use ketone bodies during starvation (11,181). Ketone acids reduce bicarbonate. Ruminants are especially prone to ketosis, however it is less likely in dogs and cats.

Expansion of extracellular fluid volume: Expansion of the extracellular fluid volume reduces proximal sodium resorption and promotes bicarbonate diuresis.

Dilution acidosis: Dilution of the extracellular fluid by isotonic sodium chloride causes a small increase in hydrogen ion concentration.

Physiologic: *Pregnancy.* In women, plasma bicarbonate is reduced in the third trimester of pregnancy (145). There are no reports of this effect in animals.

Hypophosphatemia. In severe chronic hypophosphatemia due to hyperparathyroidism and other causes, hyperchloremic acidosis develops. The acidosis is most likely due to PTH, because PTH is able to reduce bicarbonate resorption and increase bicarbonaturia (229).

Loss of renal ammoniagenesis. Glutaminase is inhibited by phosphate depletion and the reaction it catalyzes, hydrolysis of glutamine to glutamate with the release of free ammonia, is blocked (255).

Laboratory error

See section under Hyperbicarbonatemia for Laboratory Error.

Temperature effect: When the measuring temperature is higher than the storage temperature, more plasma is sampled by the electrode and the pH will be spuriously high (33). A change in temperature does not affect hydrogen ion distribution between cells and plasma.

Lactate: Delay in sample deproteinization, separation and measurement, or freezing will spuriously elevate lactate concentration (116).

Accompanying changes

Analytes: *Hypoglycemia.* Blood glucose is decreased by starvation (ketones), diarrhea (bicarbonate loss), and salicylate intoxication (salicylic acid). Glucose is decreased in many other conditions that cause hypobicarbonatemia.

Hyperglycemia. Extreme stress, seen in diseases (causing hypobicarbonatemia), elevates blood glucose. Hyperglycemia is also seen in hypercorticism and diabetes mellitus.

Hyperchloremia. Simultaneous increases in chloride and decreases in bicarbonate occur in the following conditions: diarrhea, proximal and distal renal tubular acidosis, early uremic acidosis, acidosis that follows respiratory alkalosis, intestinal loss of bicarbonate or organic acid anions, dilutional acidosis, administration of chloride- and nonchloride-containing acid, sulfur-containing amino acids, and some ketoacids.

Hypertriglyceridemia. Lipoprotein lipase is dependent on insulin for activation. Lipemia is often a feature of ketoacidosis because of the failure of activation of this enzyme (116).

Creatine kinase. In both man and animals there is a causal relationship between ketoacidosis and elevated creatine kinase values (136).

Urinary ketones. Ketones are usually elevated in lactic acidosis when they are measured using an enzymatic method able to detect 3-hydroxybutyrate (the nitroprusside reagent reacts with acetoacetate) (152).

Potassium. Potassium concentration is low in diarrhea and renal tubular acidosis because it is lost. Potassium is elevated in obstructive uropathy and ketoacidosis because it is retained. Acutely decreasing bicarbonate by infusing mineral acids (NH_4Cl and HCl) increases potassium in the dog (193). Nonmineral acids (lactic, beta-hydroxybutyric, and methyl malonic) mostly decrease potassium (193). In acute conditions the plasma potassium depends on the chemical nature of the acidifying agent and the severity of the acidosis (193).

Hyperuricemia. Organic acid anions block secretion of urate by actively competing with it for secretion in humans (179).

Anion gap. Organic acids (citric, lactic, formic, and others) increase the anion gap by adding an unmeasured anion. The plasma chloride remains normal.

Leukemoid reaction. In man severe acidosis causes a leukemoid reaction (90,000 WBC) due to catecholamine release and subsequent release of marginated cells (116).

Physiologic: *Oxygen dissociation.* Acidosis shifts the oxygen dissociation curve to the right.

Bilirubin binding. Acidosis and benzoate, salicylate, sulfisoxizole, free fatty acids, and probably gentamicin inhibit binding of bilirubin to albumin (1).

Enzymes. Acidosis is inhibitory on some key enzymes (phosphofructokinase). Such inhibition slows energy production from the glycolytic pathway.

Severe acidosis inhibits hepatic gluconeogenesis from lactate, causing lactic acidosis in addition to the already preexisting acidosis.

Cardiac contractility. Acidosis is inhibitory on cardiac contraction; however, cardiac output and blood pressure rise (116).

Hydrogen Ion

Hydrogen ions are generated by oxidative metabolism (158) in the form of fixed acids produced by metabolism of phosphate- and sulfur-containing amino acids (for example, sulfuric acid is formed from cysteine, cystine, and methionine, and phosphoric acid from oxidation of nucleoproteins and phospholipids) and are excreted in the urine. Carbonic acid is produced by the reaction of CO_2 and water, is volatile, and is excreted by the lungs.

Free hydrogen ion concentration is expressed as pH (107,262). As this is a logarithmic value, conventional statistics are not applicable to this quantity. Although hydrogen ions are hydrated (hydroxonium ion), they are regarded as protons bound to water. A change in their concentration is always accompanied by a change in other electrolytes.

Most species have a normal arterial blood pH close to 7.4. In the dog, mean arterial blood pH is 7.427 (285). Blood pH is lower than plasma pH because of a bias introduced by the erythrocytes. Venous pH is lower than arterial pH and in the dog the difference is 0.038 units (285). Women have higher pH values than men and pH decreases in old age; other species may be similar to man in this respect. Newborn animals, and humans have respiratory acidosis at birth. Poikilotherms, both vertebrates and nonvertebrates, increase the hydrogen ion concentration as body temperature is increased (207).

Enzymes and structural proteins are directly affected by hydrogen ion concentration (215). The systemic pH influences both neural and humoral mediators of intestinal transport (59).

Hydrogen ions are secreted by the stomach and excreted by the kidney. Excretion is influenced by the concentration of aldosterone, PTH, carbonic anhydrase, glutaminase, and potassium. A transport maximum in the kidney limits urine acidity in humans and dogs (and probably other laboratory species) to a pH of around 4.5. Hydrogen ions are excreted by the tubule combined with a base, resorbable in the case of bicarbonate and nonresorbable in the case of ammonia.

Ammonia is generated by the renal tubules mostly from glutamine, diffuses into the filtrate, and takes on a proton that prevents its back-diffusion (255). This mechanism, enhancing hydrogen ion excretion, is adaptive, but it takes several days to equilibrate.

Plasma hydrogen ion concentration is a function of titratable hydrogen ion concentration and PCO_2, independently variable. Strong electrolytes (completely dissociated) affect hydrogen ion concentration by the strong ion difference. A change in one variable induces a compensatory change in the other to offset a pH change. Hydrogen ion concentration is also a function of the titratable hydrogen ion concentration and PCO_2. Titratable hydrogen ion concentration in venous blood is less than it is in arterial blood because of hydrogen ion binding to deoxyhemoglobin.

Rigid control is maintained over chemical buffers, pulmonary regulation of carbonic acid, and excretion of acid or base by the kidney. Ultimate control of hydrogen ions is vested in those processes that control intake, distribution, metabolism, and excretion (107).

Whole blood pH is ideally measured on an anaerobically collected sample of arterial blood from an undisturbed, unanesthetized animal. The animal is unfortunately always disturbed by arteriopuncture, but every effort should be made to limit the degree of disturbance. Values from anesthetized animals are unacceptable except when used to monitor the anesthetic effect. Blood pH decreases as the body temperature rises ($\Delta pH/\Delta T = -0.0147$ per degree celcius (-0.016 to -0.0120) (220).

Increased Hydrogen Ions

Levels of biologic significance

The limits of life for most homeotherms are in the pH range of 6.8 to 7.8. Acute disturbances only are tolerated in the extremes of pH. A pH below 7.2 is considered life-threatening in man (179).

Mechanisms

The concentration of free hydrogen ions or the pH of arterial plasma is affected by metabolic (addition of titratable acid) and respiratory (increases in PCO_2) disturbances and by increased temperature. The respiratory disturbances are discussed under Carbon Dioxide.

Titratable hydrogen ion/base excess: See section under Decreased Hydrogen Ion.

Disease states

Lactic acidosis: See section under Hypobicarbonatemia.

Ketosis: See section under Hypobicarbonatemia.

Temperature: Plasma-free hydrogen ion concentration is increased by increased temperature; titratable hydrogen ion concentration is not affected (155). The relationship between arterial pH and body temperature is: $\Delta pH/\Delta T = +0.03K^{-1}$ (58) for homeotherms, $\Delta pH/\Delta T = 0.015K^{-1}$ (206,261) for poikilotherms, and $\Delta pH/\Delta T = -0.010K^{-1}$ (156) for hibernating animals (all seasons). These constants are affected by changes in PCO_2, plasma protein concentration, and hemoglobin concentration (54).

Renal failure and urinary obstruction: Hydrogen ions, the products of metabolism, accumulate in blood when clearance by renal excretion is blocked.

Tubular dysfunction: Buffers are lost and hydrogen ion accumulates when renal tubular function fails. Hydrogen ion accumulates because the sodium-hydrogen ion exchange, the normal removal mechanism, fails, In tubular failure, ammonia generation, mostly from glutamine by glutaminase, ceases (255). A valuable pairing base for hydrogen ions is lost. Malfunctioning tubular cells no longer reclaim bicarbonate; a hydrogen ion buffer fails to replenish itself.

Renal tubular acidosis: The tubular hydrogen ion excretion mechanism fails in distal tubular acidosis. Failure of the tubules to resorb bicarbonate occurs in proximal tubular acidosis. Hyperchloremic metabolic acidosis with normal glomerular filtration is present (103,213).

Increased intake: Increased intake of acids, because of the great ability of the kidney to compensate, causes only a slight increase in the concentration of titratable hydrogen ion.

Secondary or compensatory increase: Hydrogen ions are retained by the kidney in response to primary respiratory alkalosis.

Bicarbonate loss: Hydrogen ions are normally buffered by bicarbonate. Processes that cause its loss or failure of its reclamation mechanism produce increases in titratable hydrogen ions. Bicarbonate loss can occur through the saliva, feces, or urine (87). Tubular defects interfere with resorption of bicarbonate.

Dilution acidosis: Dilution of the plasma causes a small rise in the concentration of titratable hydrogen ion (243).

Hyperventilation: An acute fall in carbon dioxide redistributes hydrogen ions. They leave the cell and move into the plasma, replacing the volatile lost acid.

Laboratory error

See section under Hyperbicarbonatemia.

Heparin: Acidic heparin used as an anticoagulant produces a small error in pH (112). Too large a volume of heparin also affects the PCO_2 and PO_2 because they are both soluble in this diluent (33).

Storage: Glycolysis increases the titratable hydrogen ion concentration by 0.5 mmol/l per hour at room temperature and 0.1 mmol/l per hour at 0 to 4°C. The increase is greater when leukocytosis is present (243).

Insufficient arterialization: If blood is not sufficiently arterialized, the pH is erroneously low.

Accompanying changes

Biochemical: *Aciduria.* The urine hydrogen ion concentration is dependent on both glomerular filtration and tubular secretion of titratable hydrogen ion. Excretion of hydrogen ion is maximal when the compensatory fall in filtration, caused by increased titratable hydrogen ion, balances increased tubular secretion, caused by increased concentration of plasma-free hydrogen ion. The maximal urine acid pH for man is 4.3, whereas the most alkaline is 8.0 (198). Acid excretion is limited by the cation exchange mechanism and not by renal ammoniogenesis (231).

pH. Hydrogen ions diffuse slowly into other

water compartments and the pH is thus slow to change. Carbon dioxide diffuses rapidly.

Buffer bases. Increased titratable hydrogen ion concentration is reflected by decreased buffer concentration (HCO_3^-, phosphate, and net protein anion).

Leukocytosis. Severe metabolic acidosis decreases the margination of leukocytes caused by the action of catecholamines released in response to the acidosis.

Anions. Accumulated organic acids (not carbonic) are accompanied by their accumulated bases (chloride, lactate, sulfate, and beta-hydroxybutyrate). In man, these bases compete with uric acid for renal removal and are responsible for causing hyperuricemia (92).

Cations. Hydrogen ions are mainly exchanged for sodium and potassium by the kidney. When excess hydrogen ion is excreted, sodium or potassium excretion is limited. Plasma potassium concentration is related to pH (hydrogen ion) in acute respiratory disturbances ($\Delta cK^+/\Delta pH = -1$ to -3 mmol/l). As one ion enters a cell, the other ion leaves (243).

Ion binding. Increased free hydrogen ion concentration releases calcium from its albumin bonding. (Δ log concentration of free Ca^{++} ΔpH -0.24) (243). Free bilirubin increases as the concentration of free hydrogen rises.

Drug binding. The literature correlating drug binding by albumin with the concentration of free hydrogen ion is limited (215).

Physiologic: Respiration. Increased titratable hydrogen ion concentration causes increased plasma-free hydrogen ion concentration. The increased free hydrogen ions stimulate peripheral chemoreceptors rapidly, and central chemoreceptors after hydrogen ions have time to diffuse across the blood-brain barrier.

Oxygen dissociation (P50). The oxygen dissociation curve is shifted to the right by increased free hydrogen ion concentration and to the left by decreased 2,3-diphosphoglycerate. (An overall decrease in organic phosphates is caused by an increased free hydrogen ion concentration.)

Cardiovascular effect. Increases in free hydrogen ion concentration cause vasodilation, increased sympathetic activity (increased epinephrine and norepinephrine), and decreased tissue responsiveness to catecholamines. Cardiac output, peripheral resistance, and blood pressure increase.

Intermediary metabolism. Glycolysis is decreased by the effect of increased free hydrogen ion concentration on phosphofructokinase (215).

Decreased Hydrogen Ion

Levels of biologic significance

See section on Increased Hydrogen Ion.

Mechanisms

Free hydrogen ion concentration in arterial plasma is reduced by (1) metabolic disturbances (loss of titratable acid), (2) respiratory disturbances (decreases in PCO_2), and (3) decreased temperature. The respiratory disturbances are discussed in the section on Hypocarbia.

The titratable hydrogen ion concentration (of plasma or blood) is called the base excess. Base excess is a measure of metabolic disturbance. Net loss and redistribution of hydrogen ion alter base excess. Positive values for *base excess* indicate a deficiency of hydrogen ions. The two quantities, free hydrogen ion concentration and concentration of titratable hydrogen ions will be discussed.

Disease states

Increased oral intake: Bicarbonate, citrate, lactate, and other weak bases increase total plasma base and cause secondary decreases in hydrogen ion concentration. Titratable hydrogen ion concentration may decrease up to 3 mmol/l because of added bases (243).

Infused sodium bicarbonate initially distributes itself in a volume equal to that of the extracellular fluid, but after 3 to 4 hours the volume distribution is double and therefore the change in hydrogen ion is halved. After several days bone starts to buffer the change.

Postprandial alkali tide: There is postprandial hydrogen ion loss into gastric juice.

Dehydration (contraction alkalosis): Water loss is represented by a loss of titratable hydrogen ion. Hydrogen ion loss may be offset by other changes such as decreased glomerular filtration and reduced tissue perfusion.

Potassium depletion: Both free hydrogen and titratable hydrogen ion concentrations are decreased by potassium depletion and intracellular pH decreases. For acute changes in pH, $\Delta K/\Delta pH = -1$ to -3 mmol/l (3). Extracellular loss of potassium causes a loss of intracellular potassium. Potassium is exchanged for hydrogen ion; intracellular pH decreases and extracellular pH rises.

Haldane effect: Decreased oxygen saturation decreases the concentration of titratable hydrogen ion.

Vomiting: Hydrogen ion is lost in gastric and abomasal contents. The plasma bicarbonate rises in response to the loss of hydrogen ion. The increased plasma bicarbonate causes an alkali diuresis and a small amount of sodium and chloride are lost together with potassium in the urine (233). The water loss causes contraction of the extracellular fluid and subsequent reduction of the glomerular filtration rate. The renal bicarbonate threshold is elevated by an increase in the rate of the sodium-hydrogen exchange (loss of hydrochloric acid in both man and dog influences tubular transport processes) (180). Hypochloremia limits the amount of sodium able to be resorbed with an anion. The kidney resorbs sodium without chloride by increasing its cation exchange mechanism instead of losing filtered sodium without anion and bicarbonate into the urine (128). The body maintains fluid volume at the expense of acid base equilibrium.

Temperature: Decreased free (not titratable) hydrogen ion concentration in plasma occurs with lowered temperature. See section on Hypobicarbonatemia for details on temperature effects.

Renal elimination: The secondary or compensatory response to increased arterial PCO_2 is a decrease in hydrogen ion caused by increased renal excretion.

Increased acid excretion: Sodium and chloride depletion with the resultant secondary aldosteronism cause increased renal acid secretion as sodium is retained under the influence of aldosterone while hydrogen ion is excreted.

Low sodium diet and dehydration: Giving a neutral salt with a nonresorbable anion to a dehydrated animal on a low sodium diet increases the sodium-hydrogen exchange mechanism. The increase results from increased avidity for sodium; it results in increased loss of hydrogen ion. Enhanced hydrogen ion secretion increases urine potassium loss (233).

Potassium depletion: Enhanced renal secretion of hydrogen ion is caused by hypokalemia.

Cushing's syndrome: See foregoing section on Increased Acid Excretion.

Laboratory error

Hemolysis: Hemolysis causes an erroneously low pH (243).

Insufficient arterialization: If the arterialized site is insufficiently prepared, an erroneously low pH will be obtained.

Body temperature: Analyzer sample chamber temperature must be adjusted to body temperature. The results can be corrected mathematically when the body temperature is different form the analyzer setting. This is not a good method because the value is not as accurate as is a directly measured one.

Storage: One hour at 2 to 4°C is probably the maximum storage time allowable as pH falls 0.003 unit per hour (normal leukocyte counts) and may reach 0.01 unit per hour when leukocytosis is present (243).

Syringes and tubes are best stored on their sides, preventing sedimentation of erythrocytes. Blood should be mixed well prior to analysis (244). Inadequate mixing produces pH errors as a result of different pH-temperature coefficients for plasma and blood and because of the effect erythrocytes have on the liquid junction potential (33).

Protein: Malfunctioning glass electrodes may be caused by protein coating resulting from inadequate cleaning (19).

Temperature: Both the liquid junction and glass electrode must be maintained accurately at the same temperature (19). Temperature errors are detected by checking several buffers of different composition: they should all read the same. For this reason and others it is safest to use calibration buffers from two sources (80).

Liquid junction potential: The potassium chloride solution is vulnerable to contamination and dilution. Frequent checks and regular replacement of potassium chloride are important (33).

Accompanying changes

Biochemistry: *Cations and anions.* Lost hydrogen ion is replaced by an equivalent amount of another cation such as sodium or potassium.

If cations do not replace the lost hydrogen ion, there is an equivalent loss of an anion such as chloride.

Ion binding. The percentage of albumin-bound calcium, magnesium, bilirubin, and others is decreased as hydrogen ion increases (123,254). Total blood calcium is unchanged; ionized calcium is decreased (Δ log concentration of free $Ca^{++}/\Delta pH \sim -0.24$) (243).

Physiologic: *Respiration.* Oxygen dissociation, intermediary metabolism and cardiovascular effects have all been previously discussed.

BLOOD GASES

Oxygen

Oxygen is carried in two forms by the blood: physically dissolved in blood (about 3 per cent) and attached to hemoglobin. Dissolved oxygen does not become a significant part of the oxygen transported until the PO_2 rises to several atmospheres. Dissolved oxygen concentration is identical in plasma and whole blood.

Free physically dissolved oxygen concentration is proportional to PO_2 (0.003 ml/dl of blood/mmHg PO_2) (243). The PO_2 is extrapolated from the measured dissolved oxygen.

The solubility coefficient of oxygen at 37°C in plasma is 0.00126 mmol/l^{-1}/mmHg^{-1} and for whole blood 0.00140 mmol/l^{-1}/mmHg^{-1} (243). Oxygen solubility is decreased by increased ionic strength and increased protein concentration and is increased by increased lipid content.

Hemoglobin carries oxygen bound reversibly to ferrous iron. Hemoglobin saturation is increased as the PO_2 is increased. Saturation is about 97 per cent in arterial blood and 70 per cent in venous blood. Calculated oxygen saturation is not a satisfactory substitute for measurement because of the variability of P50 (67,196). The P50 is shifted when hemoglobin species change, such as A to C in sheep, fetal to adult (45,132,210,214,216,230).

Tissue delivery of oxygen is regulated by the lung, vascular system, oxygen-carrying capacity of the blood, and intrinsic qualities of the blood including hemoglobin characteristics and hematocrit. Hematocrits that are too low or too high are deleterious to oxygen exchange. Low hematocrits cause hypoxia because of insufficient hemoglobin and high hematocrits hinder oxygen transport by slowing up flow.

Release and uptake of oxygen by hemoglobin are handled in a carefully controlled manner (132,216,230). The sigmoid shape of the oxyhemoglobin dissociation curve reflects the changes in hemoglobin affintiy for oxygen (53,245,253). Its position is defined by the P50 which indicates the available oxygen supply to the tissues. Displacement to the right indicates decreased oxygen affinity and easier unloading of oxygen. The following list of conditions (216) shifts the curve to the right:

1. Increased hydrogen ion concentration (Bohr effect) (Δlog $PO_2/\Delta pH = 0.040$ to 0.050 for most mammals) (5,18,120,141,214).
2. Increased CO_2 (120)
3. Increased temperature (17,34,141,214).
4. Increased 2,3-diphosphoglycerate except in ruminants and some other species (18,31,34,68,81,210,223).
5. Hemoglobins with low oxygen affinity (human Hb Seattle and Kansas).
6. Increased ATP.
7. Inorganic phosphate and other anions.
8. Anemia, the effect due mainly to increased ATP.
9. Hyperthyroidism.
10. Aged erythrocytes.
11. Aldosterone and cortisol.

It is shifted to the left when the foregoing conditions are reversed and by the presence of fetal hemoglobin and abnormal hemoglobins (human Hb Yakima, Malmo, Rainier) and hexokinase deficiency (33,281). Both carbon monoxide and methemoglobin increase oxygen affinity of the unused heme groups and shift the curve to the left (119,186)

In chronic hypoxia, erythrocytic 2,3-diphosphoglyerate (DPG) is increased. It is also increased in chronic acidosis and is responsible for shifting the curve back to its normal position after being displaced by acidosis. Not all species use this compound and in those species in which DPG is low or absent, separate nomograms must be calculated (99,221). Measured oxygen saturation is preferred to a calculated value. The dog, mouse, rat, rabbit, and monkey have high levels of DPG, whereas pig, sheep, cattle, and the horse have low levels (45). The level of DPG is decreased by hypophosphatemia, metabolic acidosis, and hyperglycemia. Hyperglycemia increases the activity of the sorbitol pathway and the intracellular redox (259). It is probable that other organic phosphates replace DPG in those species in which the compound is low or absent.

The dog, cat, and pig do not have fetal hemoglobin.

For most species PO_2 values increase from birth and reach adult values by several months of age. A slight aging-related decrease in PO_2 occurs in humans and may be present in animals. There are no sex differences in oxygen levels.

The arterial PO_2 is influenced by atmospheric pressure, composition of alveolar air, rate and depth of breathing, cardiac function, and blood flow and distribution. Central and peripheral receptors control and modulate lung, heart, and vascular activity. The PO_2 is under both voluntary and involuntary control.

Many reasons exist for measuring arterial and venous oxygen. Arterial PO_2 at rest indicates whether blood is carrying the desired amount of oxygen, and venous oxygen gives an indication of the degree of oxygen unloading and is a measure of tissue activity.

The P50 indicates if hemoglobin-bound oxygen is meeting tissue needs. It may be altered by many conditions.

Satisfactory blood gas samples may be obtained with relative ease from most laboratory species, except rats and mice. Marsupialization of the carotid artery in the rat may provide an adequate site for obtaining arterial samples in this species.

Hyperoxemia

Levels of biologic significance

Hyperoxemia produced by pressures greater than 3 atmospheres and for periods of time longer than 5 hours is mostly associated with toxicity in man (280).

Mechanisms

Hyperoxemia, increased dissolved oxygen, is produced by the administration of hyperbaric oxygen.

Toxicity is probably due to the effect of increased superoxides (60) and inhibition of sulfhydryl groups. In the rat hyperbaric oxygen decreases brain gamma aminobutyric acid and brain, liver, and kidney ATP content. Oxygen toxicity causes blindnesss, chest pain, cough, tinnitis, decreased pulmonary function, muscle twitching, dizziness, vasoconstriction of cerebral vessels, convulsions, coma, and death.

Hypoxemia

Levels of biologic significance

In man oxygen values compatible with life range from 4.0 to 400 kPa in arterial blood. For long-term survival the PO_2 must be maintained above 40 mmHg. Arterial PO_2 decreases at sea level from 95 to 75 mmHg in man between the ages of 20 and 70 years (243). In chronic hypoxia the ventilatory response becomes blunted, and hypoxic pulmonary edema develops along with muscularization of small pulmonary arteries (227,228).

Mechanisms

Hypoxia is caused by (1) decreased partial pressure of oxygen in inspired air, (2) obstruction to the flow of air in and out of the lungs, (3) decreased exchange of oxygen between the alveoli and blood, (4) changes in the cellular or matrix components of blood, (5) structural alterations in the membrane and intracellular components of the erythrocyte, (6) alterations in the rheogenic properties of the lung and vascular system, and (7) changes in the nervous sensory and regulatory mechanisms.

Disease states

Decreased alveolar ventilation: Decreased alveolar ventilation occurs when the diaphragm and intercostal muscle action is defective. Other variables that produce decreased ventilation originate at three levels: central (respiratory center), intermediate (conduction of impulses), and local (compliance, pneumothorax, airway resistance, positional, structural, muscular, and tissue viability). In turn, tissue viability is affected by local nervous influences, sepsis, structural changes, vascular supply, and secretory products.

Decreased partial pressure of inspired air: The arterial PO_2 is essentially equivalent to that of both the alveolar and inspired air. Thus, the arterial PO_2 is reduced 11 per cent for every kilometer of altitude above sea level. Motionless air, as in mines and wells, has a decreased oxygen content.

Increased consumption: The PO_2 falls by about 4 per cent when consumption is increased by 50 per cent.

Pulmonary edema: Both interstitial and

alveolar edema interfere with gaseous diffusion. Oxygen diffuses less readily than does carbon dioxide.

Decreased ventilation: Parts of the lungs may be less ventilated than others because of the presence of mechanical obstruction, decreased compliance, paralysis of respiratory muscles, skeletal abnormalities, and postural effects. Mechanical obstruction of the airways results from tumors, secretions, exudates, and broncho-constriction. Decreased compliance may be due to emphysema, fibrosis, and atelectasis.

Vascular shunting: Blood passing through the lungs may bypass functioning alveoli or, in congenital heart disease, may bypass the lungs and move directly from the venous to the arterial system. In both cases the blood is prevented normal access to the alveolar air and is improperly oxygenated.

Temperature: The PO_2 is increased by increased temperature because its plasma solubility is decreased (243).

Other solutes: Increased plasma solute concentrations reduce the solubility of oxygen.

Laboratory error

Insufficient arterialization: Inadequate preparation of the collection site causes an erroneously low PO_2 because the venular and arteriolar blood becomes admixed. This error is especially pronounced when the arteriolar PO_2 is high because of the inherent characteristics of hemoglobin-oxygen dissociation.

See the section on Analysis, Precision, and Accuracy for details of laboratory errors due to equipment and refer to Clinical Arterial Blood Gas Analysis (140,238).

Exposure to air: Samples with high true PO_2 levels, exposed to air, have an erroneously low PO_2. Low true PO_2 values are erroneously increased by air exposure. Significant errors are produced in the sample by air bubbles occupying 0.5 to 1.0 per cent of the sample volume (166,167).

Storage: Glycolysis in stored blood increases PO_2 as it is liberated from oxyhemoglobin, and cellular respiration consumes oxygen. The overall change caused by two opposing effects is a decrease of 0.4 kPa/h at 37°C for normal arterial PO_2 and 0.3 kPa/h when the PO_2 is greater than 50 kPa (243). Erythrocytes oxidize glucose by the pentose

pathway, whereas other cells use the tricarboxylic acid cycle.

Improper mixing: Insufficient mixing before sample measurement produces erroneous results because of the effect pH has on the oxygen dissociation curve (244).

Halothane and nitrous oxide: Halothane anesthetic is reduced at the cathode and a falsely high oxygen value is produced (185, 199,236). Both halothane and nitrous oxide produce spurious oxygen values.

Heparin: Heparin may produce two analytic errors: a small change in PO_2 (112) (heparin is in equilibrium with air) and a change in pH if heparin is in an acidic form.

Aspiration rate: For some analyzers the rate of sample aspiration is highly critical to the value obtained and a difference of 2 seconds was found to cause errors (101,112,217).

Microbial contamination: Falsely low values are caused by microbial contamination of the PO_2 membrane (33).

Temperature: Both the oxygen solubility and the equilibrium between oxyhemoglobin and dissolved oxygen are affected by the temperature (118,224,266). Measurement at temperatures other than body temperature can partially be corrected by the equation (53):

$$\Delta \log PO_2 / \Delta T = 0.031.$$

Because the PO_2 of blood changes by 2 to 7 per cent for each centigrade degree, it is necessary to operate PO_2 electrodes within ± 0.2°C (243).

Plastic syringes: False PO_2 reading can be caused by using plastic syringes (33).

Correction factors: Instruments that are calibrated with gases need to have a correction factor applied to measured values (166).

Accompanying changes

Biochemical: *Hemoglobin saturation.* Oxygen saturation decreases as PO_2 falls.

Lactic acidosis. If the decrease in PO_2 is sufficiently rapid, aerobic metabolism is replaced by anaerobic metabolism and lactic acid concentration rises (190). Hypoxemia causes increased inorganic phosphate, urate, and hypoxanthine concentrations. Lactic acidosis arises in chronic hypoxia when the PO_2 is below 35 mmHg in man.

Erythrocytosis. Chronic hypoxia stimulates

erythropoietin production which in turn results in erythrocytosis.

Cerebrospinal fluid pH. The cerebrospinal fluid is more alkaline in man, dog, and horse during chronic hypoxia (47,75,97,274).

Physiologic: *Chemoreceptors.* The peripheral chemoreceptors, aortic and carotid bodies, respond immediately to a fall in PO_2 and are also important in stimulating respiration in chronic hypoxia (35). Hyperventilation is not marked until the PO_2 falls to about 60 mmHg. The carotid receptors are most sensitive to decreased pH and increased PCO_2. Aortic receptors are depressed by a decrease in arterial pH. A progressive increase in activity occurs as the PO_2 falls from 500 to 100 mmHg (36). At 100 mmHg, activity increases markedly, but below 30 mmHg in man and 18.6 mmHg in the dog, chemoreceptor activity is depressed (36,164). Hypoxia and hypercapnia potentiate each other.

In humans, dogs, and cats, central chemoreceptors respond to changes in cerebrospinal fluid hydrogen ion concentration.

Erythropoietin. Low PO_2 stimulates production of erythropoietin with resultant polycythemia.

Cerebral hypoxia. Severe reduction in PO_2 causes cerebral hypoxia. Anaerobic metabolism replaces aerobic. Coma and death result if the oxygen supply to the brain is interrupted in mature humans for longer than 3 minutes. Longer periods are tolerated at lower body temperatures and by neonatal animals.

Cyanosis. Severe hypoxia is accompanied by a bluish color of the skin and mucous membranes. The severity of hypoxia should not be judged by the degree of coloration. Hematocrit, methemoglobin, sulfhemoglobin, blood flow, oxygen consumption, and pigmentation of the skin all affect skin colour. Arteriovenous anastomoses hypertrophy in hypoxia.

Carbon Dioxide

The total carbon dioxide content of human arterial blood is approximately 49 ml/dl. Carbon dioxide exists in arterial blood in a number of different forms: as bicarbonate (25 mmol/l), in carbamino compounds (2.4 mmol/l), as physically dissolved CO_2 (1.2 mmol/l), and as carbonic acid (0.2 μmol/l) (33). The PCO_2 refers to an imaginary gas phase in the blood. The PCO_2 is identical in plasma and erythrocytes. Arteriolar PCO_2 is slightly higher than that of alveolar air because some blood is always shunted in the lungs bypassing functioning alveoli

Free dissolved carbon dioxide concentration is proportional to the PCO_2. Carbon dioxide solubility increases with increased plasma lipid content and decreases with increased protein content. In plasma the solubility coefficient is 0.0306 ± 0.003 mmol/l^{-1}/mmHg^{-1} at 37°C, about 20 times more soluble than oxygen (53).

Values for PCO_2 are slightly lower in human females than in males. They fall further in the last trimester of gestation. Sex differences in animals have not been documented. Cats have similar PCO_2 values to those of man, whereas those in dogs are lower. The PCO_2 is higher when the animal is recumbent. High altitudes result in a reduction of PCO_2 of 5 mmHg per mile. Anxiety decreases PCO_2 (243). Arterial PCO_2 values are fairly constant, whereas venous values are higher than arterial and vary considerably depending on the site, temperature, and muscular activity.

Carbonic anhydrase catalyzes the hydration of CO_2 in erythrocytes and renal tubular cells. In erythrocytes the resultant H_2CO_3 dissociates and HCO_3^- diffuses into the plasma, whereas H^+ is buffered primarily by hemoglobin. Deoxyhemoglobin is a better buffer than oxyhemoglobin.

Carbon dioxide forms carbamino compounds with amino groups of proteins. Deoxyhemoglobin forms carbamino compounds more readily than does oxyhemoglobin. About 20 per cent of the carbon dioxide is carried in systemic capillaries by proteins.

Ventilatory adjustments to changes in metabolism are linear because of their regulation by carbon dioxide (153). Both central and peripheral receptors respond to changes in carbon dioxide concentration (35). Receptor response to carbon dioxide is rapid compared to that elicited by hydrogen ion. Carbon dioxide diffuses rapidly across the blood-brain barrier; hydrogen ion diffuses slowly.

Carbon dioxide partial pressure is measured when there is clinical indication of a respiratory disturbance. It is evaluated along with the pH and PO_2. Appropriate arterial samples are readily obtained from all species of laboratory animal with the exception of the rat, mouse, and guinea pig. In the rat and guinea pig, marsupialization of the carotid artery may provide a site where samples can be collected.

Hypercarbia

Levels of biologic significance

In man hypercarbia rarely produces a pH below 7.0 and the sensitivity to carbon dioxide decreases with age (280).

Mechanisms

In respiratory acidosis the blood pH falls and the plasma bicarbonate increases. The rise in bicarbonate in dogs is curvilinear, whereas the decrease in pH is linear (64,232). The principal mechanisms increasing the PCO_2 are increased metabolic rate, decreased elimination by the lungs, decreased diffusion across the alveolar wall, and increased inspired carbon dioxide.

Disease states

Increased inspired carbon dioxide: Increased inspired carbon dioxide produces a relatively small change in PCO_2 because of the strong opposing ventilatory response (270).

Increased metabolism: A twofold increase in metabolism causes a 10 per cent increase in PCO_2. The metabolic effect is offset by ventilation.

Decreased alveolar ventilation: Decreased alveolar ventilation causes hypercarbia, which may occur under a variety of conditions. When the diaphragmatic and intercostal muscle contraction is defective due to paralysis, muscle degeneration, or pain, alveolar ventilation is compromised. If there is reduced thoracic or lung compliance, as occurs in kyphoscoliosis, hyaline membrane disease, fibrosis, and atelectasis, alveolar ventilation is reduced. Trauma, producing loss of thoracic integrity (pneumothorax), or loss of lung tissue (edema, atelectasis, fibrosis, and bronchiectasis) decreases alveolar ventilation by a variety of mechanisms. Increased resistance to air movement, as seen with obstruction, edema, exudate, bronchiolar constriction, and loss of surfactant, reduces minute volume and causes hypercarbia. Hypercarbia resulting from pulmonary edema and pneumonia is not usually seen in the dog and

cat unless the condition is very severe (LMC, unpublished data).

Temperature: The PCO_2 changes with temperature (54). In plasma the change is expressed as $(\Delta \log PCO2 / \Delta T = +0.019 \text{ K}^{-1})$ and in blood the coefficient is $+0.021 \text{ K}^{-1}$. Varying protein and hemoglobin concentrations and the PCO_2 change these coefficients (54).

In homeothermic animals ventilation increases relatively more than does the production of carbon dioxide as temperature rises (58), and in hibernating animals carbon dioxide production falls relatively more than does ventilation as temperature falls (156). The PCO_2 of arterial blood is related to body temperature by $\log CO_2/T = +0.03 \text{ K}^{-1}$ in homeotherms, $\log PCO_2/T - 0.008 \text{ K}^{-1}$ in hibernating animals, and $\log PCO_2/T = 0.021 \text{ K}^{-1}$ in poikilotherms (58,156,206).

Carbonic anhydrase activity: Slight hypercarbia occurs when carbonic anhydrase activity is deficient. The dehydration of carbonic acid to CO_2 and water is delayed.

Decreased diffusion: Conditions increasing thickness of the alveolar membrane have to be very severe before CO_2 diffusion is slowed. Similarly, shunting of blood from right to left, because of the small arteriolar-venous PCO_2 difference, causes only a slight increase in arteriolar PCO_2.

Laboratory error

Insufficient arterialization of collection site: Improper arterialization of the collection site produces a falsely increased PCO_2. Contamination by a small amount of venous blood causes only a small error because the arteriovenous difference for PCO_2 is small.

Temperature: The PCO_2 of blood decreases by about 5 per cent per degree centigrade increase in temperature because the plasma solubility of CO_2 is decreased (33). Also, protein buffer dissociation affects the temperature response of PCO_2 (33).

Exposure to air: Carbon dioxide is lost from blood when it is exposed to air. Carbon dioxide equilibrates with heparin in the collection syringe. Errors of 17 per cent in measurement of CO_2 were recorded when excess heparin was used improperly in samples (114).

Storage: Glycolysis in normal blood causes an increase in PCO_2 of about 5 mmHg per hour at 37°C. The rate is reduced by a factor of 10 if the sample is cooled to 2 to 4°C. Maximum storage time before analysis should be less than 1 hour (257).

Analyzer: In some analyzers (Corning 175®) a difference of 5 to 9 per cent in values occurs if aspiration time is prolonged by 2 seconds over that recommended (101,217).

Calculated PCO_2: Significant errors arise when PCO_2 is calculated from the Henderson-Hasselbalch equation because samples with abnormal protein, lipid, and ionic composition alter the pK of carbonic acid and the solubility coefficient of CO_2.

Interpolation of pH on the CO_2 equilibrium curve is prone to cause errors when the PCO_2 is at either extreme and when the degree of desaturation is not taken into account.

Inaccurate calibration: Improperly humidified gases, slow electrode responses, dirty or ruptured membranes, incorrect calibrating gas mixtures, incorrect electrode temperature, and other factors affect the validity of PCO_2 measurements (35). The electrode should be thermostated so that a temperature of $\pm 0.2°C$ is maintained by the analyzer (243). Gas-calibrated electrodes do not measure the PCO_2 of blood accurately and the error is greatest at high PCO_2 levels (30).

Temperature: The PCO_2 measurement is dependent on temperature. If the blood sample is not measured at body temperature (preferable), a correction factor needs to be applied.

Accompanying changes

Biochemical: *Bicarbonate ion.* Increased PCO_2 increases both H_2CO_3 and bicarbonate (111). Bicarbonate is increased as CO_2 becomes hydrated (slowly in plasma and rapidly by carbonic anhydrase in the red cell). Following hydration and dissociation, bicarbonate is extruded from the erythrocyte into the plasma. This increase in bicarbonate is not a compensating mechanism.

In acute hypercarbia the increase in bicarbonate is small (3 to 4 mEq/l) and there is no acceleration of renal excretion (49,64).

In severe chronic hypercarbia, that is, hypercarbia of several days' duration, bicarbonate can be increased to around 40 mEq/l, whereas the plasma pH is slightly decreased (243). This response is due to an increase in hydrogen ion excretion and generation by the kidney.

Carbamates. Carbamates increase in hypercarbia. Preferential binding of CO_2 to deoxyhemoglobin decreases the hemoglobin oxygen affintiy in hypercarbia.

Hydrogen ion. Acute hypercarbia increases the concentration of total hydrogen ion in erythrocytes and whole blood and decreases hydrogen ion in plasma and interstitial fluid. Acute hypocarbia produces the opposite effect (143).

Hamburger shift. Increases in PCO_2 drive the chemical reaction $CO_2 + H_2O \rightarrow H_2CO_3 \rightarrow H^+ + HCO_3^-$ to the right. Hydrogen ions from the reaction are buffered in erythrocytes by hemoglobin. Because of the buffering action of hemoglobin, HCO_3^- rises more in the erythrocyte than in plasma. Bicarbonate leaves the erythrocyte as hydrogen, and chloride ions move into the cell from the plasma.

Secondary effects. These effects are the result of changes in free hydrogen ion concentration.

Chloride. Plasma chloride is normal or slightly decreased in hypercapnia. It moves into erythrocytes during hypercarbia. In chronic hypercarbia chloriuresis leads to chloride depletion, an increase in renal acid excretion, and an elevation of plasma bicarbonate (202,203,233).

Urine. Urine acidity and ammonia, phosphate, potassium, and chloride content are increased by hypercarbia (202,203). This results in hypochloremia, hyperbicarbonatemia, and possibly hypokalemia.

Physiologic: *Decreased hemoglobin oxygen affinity.* Carbon dioxide binding to deoxyhemoglobin in moderate hypercarbia abolishes the Bohr effect; it is reversed at very high PCO_2 values (120).

Hyperventilation. Both central and peripheral chemoreceptors respond to hypercapnia. Peripheral receptors are the more rapid in their response; however, CO_2 diffuses readily across the blood-brain barrier (35).

Renal response. The renal response to hypercarbia is identical to that seen in hyperprotonemia (excess hydrogen ion loss). It consists of an increased $Na^+ - H^+$ exchange, increased ammonia formation, and increased resorption of bicarbonate.

Central nervous system depression. Accumulation of carbon dioxide depresses the central nervous system and eventually leads to coma, respiratory depression, and death.

Intestinal electrolyte transport. Hypercapnia in rats and rabbits increases sodium and chloride absorption in the ileum and colon, respectively (59).

Chronic metabolic acid base disorders. Chronic metabolic acid base disorders influence the response to acute hypercapnia (254). As the chronic level of bicarbonate increases, the organism (dog) finds it easier to defend plasma hydrogen ion concentration.

Hypocarbia

Levels of biologic significance

Carbon dioxide diffuses rapidly along its concentration gradient and may fall to values in the range of 15 mmHg.

Mechanisms

Hypocarbia is caused by conditions that produce hyperventilation (increase the rate and/or depth of breathing), decrease body temperature, change the plasma composition, and decrease inspired CO_2. The lowered PCO_2 produces an increase in pH and a decrease in bicarbonate concentration.

Disease states

Hyperventilation: Hypocarbia is produced by an increase in the rate and/or depth of respiration. Carbon dioxide is able to diffuse rapidly across the alveolar membrane to lower the arteriolar PCO_2. Hyperventilation is caused by some drugs, lesions of the central nervous system, hyperthyroidism, Gram-negative bacteremia, and interstitial pulmonary disease.

Periodic breathing: Periodic breathing is associated with hypocarbia because of heightened sensitivity to CO_2. Hyperventilation, a consequence of the supersensitivity, is seen in conditions such as heart failure and uremia and in animals with organic brain disease.

Periodic breathing in cardiac insufficiency is due to oscillatory behavior of the respiratory system. Oscillation occurs because the time lag between removal of CO_2 at the lungs and return of the blood to the brain is not synchronous with the inherent respiratory timer.

Excitement: Hypocarbia caused by excitement is due to an increase in the rate and/or depth of respiration. Carbon dioxide is removed rapidly by the lungs.

Fever: Hyperventilation arising from increased body temperature causes hypocarbia.

Drugs: Certain drugs, by their action on the respiratory center, produce hyperventilation and hypocarbia.

Reduced inspired carbon dioxide: Reduced CO_2 in inspired air increases the concentration gradient for CO_2 between air and blood. Increased removal of CO_2 from the blood follows.

Temperature: See under Hypercarbia for temperature effects.

Laboratory error

Insufficient arterialization of collection site: Improper arterialization of capillary blood causes an increase in PCO_2. Contamination by a small amount of venous blood causes only a small error because the arteriovenous difference for PCO_2 is small (53).

Air exposure: Carbon dioxide is rapidly lost from blood when it is exposed to air.

Storage: Glycolysis in normal blood causes a rise in PCO_2 of about 5 mmHg per hour at 37°C. The rate is reduced by a factor of 10 if the sample is cooled to 2 to 4°C. Blood samples should not be stored longer than 1 hour.

Calculated PCO_2: Significant errors arise if PCO_2 is calculated from the Henderson-Hasselbalch equation (243). Abnormalities affecting the protein, lipid, and ionic composition alter the pK of carbonic acid and the solubility coefficient of CO_2.

Interpolation of pH on the CO_2 equilibrium curve (another method of calculation) is prone to errors when the PCO_2 is at either extreme and when the degree of desaturation is not taken into account.

Inaccurate calibration: Improperly humidified gases, slow electrode responses, dirty or ruptured membranes, incorrect calibrating gas mixture, incorrect electrode temperature, and other factors affect the validity of the PCO_2 measurement (33,148).

Temperature: PCO_2 is dependent on temperature. If the blood sample is not measured at body temperature, the values must be corrected for the temperature difference (33).

Accompanying changes

Biochemical: *Bicarbonate.* Hypocarbia lowers the plasma bicarbonate directly because the reaction $CO_2 + H_2O \rightleftharpoons H_2CO_3 \rightleftharpoons H^+ + HCO_3^-$ is shifted to the left. Indirectly hypocarbia decreases renal bicarbonate resorption because low PCO_2 inhibits renal acid secretion (231). The latter effect is a compensatory change brought about by alteration in the tubular chloride transport and is independent of the plasma pH (231). In the dog with chronic hypocarbia the plasma bicarbonate is decreased 0.50 mEq/l for every millimeter of mercury decrease in PCO_2 (231).

Secondary effects. These effects of hypocarbia are the result of changes in free hydrogen ion concentration.

Calcium. Ionized plasma calcium is decreased by alkalosis.

Ketones. Prolonged hypocarbia (alkalosis) increases ketone bodies because carbohydrate utilization is decreased.

Phosphate. Plasma phosphate is decreased in hypocarbia (193).

Lactate. Plasma lactate is increased in hypocarbia. Reduced hepatic perfusion probably accounts for most of the lactate increase. Alkalosis stimulates glycolysis by enzymatic activation of phosphofructokinase.

Hydrogen ion. Acute hypocarbia reduces whole blood titratable hydrogen ion concentration and causes a rise in the plasma concentration of titratable hydrogen ion; therefore, the plasma pH rises. Chronic hypercarbia has the opposite effect.

Urine. Urine acidity and ammonia content are decreased by hypocarbia.

Physiologic: *Respiration.* Periodic breathing occurs during hypocarbia because respiration is being driven by hypoxia.

During apnea PO_2 falls and PCO_2 rises. The PO_2 reaches a threshold level before PCO_2 and triggers the respiratory receptors.

Central nervous effects. Dizziness and parathesia are caused by hypocarbia.

Tetany. Decreased ionized calcium causes tetany. This secondary efect is due to the alkalosis that hypocarbia produces.

Cardiac output. Cardiac output is increased and there is constriction of cerebral and some other vessels in hypocarbia (71,286).

Vasomotor center. The vasomotor center is depressed by hypocarbia.

Oxygen dissociation. When the PCO_2 falls, the oxygen dissociation curve is shifted to the left.

ANION GAP

The anion gap (AG) is generally taken as the difference between the summed values of the measured cations, sodium and potassium, and the summed values of the measured anions, bicarbonate and chloride. Under normal circumstances in man these account for all except 8 to 16 mEq/l (mean 12) of the total anions (85). Animal data of comparable nature are not available, except for the dog in which the AG has been reported to be 1.03 mmol/l (285) and to range form 16.7 to 20 mEq/l (64) and 14 to 23 mEq/l (2,142). In the dog the contribution of sulfate and organic acids to the gap is smaller than that in man (285):

$$\text{anion gap} = (Na + K) - (Cl + HCO_3).$$

Under most circumstances the value of unaccounted for cations (proteins, magnesium, calcium, and others) is small, and their contribution to a disturbance is usually not significant (calcium and phosphate concentrations can be converted to milliequivalents per liter by dividing by 4 and 3, respectively). However, the anions proteinate, sulfate, phosphate, lactate, and others individually, may change the gap significantly (69). Normally proteins contribute two thirds of the unmeasured anions, and others such as lactate (2.4 mmol/l) and pyruvate (0.4 mmol/l) contribute minimally in the dog and other species (2,64).

The principle of electrical neutrality dictates that the sum of positive and negative charges is zero. The gap exists because routine clinical pathology measurements omit measurements of certain ions. The omitted anions provide vital information needed for basic interpretation of laboratory data by medically qualified persons.

Anion gaps are used in data interpretation to disclose those situations in which acidosis is not accompanied by decreased pH or an increase in free hydrogen (222). The hidden anions are those of organic and inorganic acids and proteans, such as lactate, sulfate, beta-hydroxybutyrate, acetate, formate, oxalate, and proteinate. They are "hidden" because the efficient tissue buffers and PCO_2 adjustments are able to keep the pH or free hydrogen ion concentration within the normal range. However, although the facade appears undisturbed due to buffer action, lurking below this veneer is excess accumulated acid.

Systems controlling acid base and blood gas balance are exquisitely sensitive and highly responsive. Precision and accuracy are of prime concern in the collection and measurement of these analytes (176). Most often overlooked in this regard are bicarbonate measurements because they are not strictly monitored or controlled. A calculated bicarbonate value, calculated from CO_2 and pH with due regard to temperature and other effects, is preferable to a poorly measured value for bicarbonate.

Laboratory computers simplify the calculations necessary for derived values used in data interpretation. Anion gap computations are now readily accessible. Calculated values are important. Calculation of the gap discloses serious and potentially fatal disturbance that may otherwise go unnoticed except for unexplained death.

Increased Anion Gap

Increased anion gaps arise from conditions that cause acidosis, but not all acidoses increase the anion gap. It is increased by decreased unmeasured cations and/or increased unmeasured anions, dehydration, and laboratory error.

Organic and inorganic acids donate hydrogen ions and convert bicarbonate to carbonic acid. Dehydration of carbonic acid produces water and volatile CO_2 (given off at the lungs). Bicarbonate is consumed by its acid interactions, and sodium and/or other cation is freed from its attachment to bicarbonate. The freed sodium pairs with the conjugate base of the offending acid, the conjugate base replacing bicarbonate. Hypobicarbonatemia signals the presence of an existing acidosis.

If acidosis arises simultaneously with a condition causing hyperbicarbonatemia, the telltale bicarbonate deficit just described is absent. Anions gaps provide a convenient means of identifying these hidden disorders (69,271).

Disease states

Metabolic acidosis: Metabolic acidoses are the most common and largest group of disturbances that increase the anion gap (85,98).

Uremia: Uremia causes a moderate increase in the anion gap (178). A number of factors operate to produce uremic acidosis. As glomerular filtration fails, the normal acid load from metabolism is not removed in a timely fashion. Retained hydrogen ions deplete bicarbonate as the retained conjugate base of the acid replaces the lost bicarbonate. By this replacement an increased gap is generated. Plasma chloride is elevated acutely but normalizes as the acidosis becomes chronic.

The tubular secretion of hydrogen ion, ammonia formation, and retrieval of bicarbonate fail in uremia. Anions, particularly phosphate and sulfate, are retained in uremic states and may contribute several milliequivalents to the anion gap.

Ketoacidosis: Ketone bodies are produced when the normal, largely oxidative metabolism of fatty acids is replaced by a predominantly ketogenic path. Both ketoacids, acetoacetic and beta-hydroxybutyrate, are strong acids, consume bicarbonate, and replace it with acid anions. The acid anions produce the gap. (*Note:* Acetone in high concentrations causes positive nitroprusside test results. Acetone is slowly metabolized and excreted. Acetoacetate spuriously elevates the colorimetric test for creatinine [85,113].)

Lactic acidosis: Increased lactate formation and impaired lactate usage result from failure of oxidative metabolism. Lactic acidosis is frequently fulminating, whereas other acidoses develop slowly (189). Bicarbonate is replaced mole for mole by lactate (179).

Conditions particularly prone to produce lactic acidemia in laboratory animals are shock, severe anemia, hypoxia, and malignancies. Other causes of lactic acidosis are alkalosis, seizures (192), severe exercises (215), catecholamines (215), carbohydrate infusion, and diabetic ketosis.

Toxicities: Anions commonly seen in toxicities are salicylate, formate, oxalate, and acetate. Salicylate intoxication produces respiratory alkalosis and increases in organic acids (178,247).

Alkalosis: Metabolic and respiratory alkalosis increases serum lactate. Lactic acidosis is the result of stimulation of the rate-limiting enzyme phosphofructokinase. Acidosis inhibits phosphofructokinase (8,202,215,284). Clinical assessment of the degree of hyperventilation necessary to produce lactic acidosis in animals is unavailable. In man, hyperventilation produces a 2 to 3 mEq/l increase in lactate (85).

Dehydration: Acutely decreased plasma water increases the anion gap, that is, it increases the proteinate.

Iatrogenic: Sodium acetate, sodium citrate, and sodium lactate, and drug anions including bromide, nitrate, and carbenicillin increase the anion gap only until such time as the anions are metabolized to bicarbonate, as in the case of the organic ions, or excreted, as in the case of the inorganic. Antibiotics containing sodium and associated unmeasured anion increase the anion gap but do not cause acidosis (152).

Protein: The anion gap is increased by elevated IgA concentrations as in multiple myeloma (2,194), polyclonal gammopathy seen with septic glomerulonephritis in the cow (JHR, unpublished data), and titration of nonbicarbonate buffers.

During periods of acidosis the non-bicarbonate buffers, especially proteins, are titrated with acids, gain hydrogen ions, and thus decrease their net negative charge. Their contribution to the total anions is decreased and the anion gap decreased (152).

Rhabdomyolysis: Muscle necrosis releases proteins, phosphates, uric acid, and sulfates. Hydrogen ions from intracellular components lower bicarbonate concentration and the anions increase the anion gap ("unmeasured" anions) (149).

Metabolic alkalosis: Alkalemia induces an increase in the net negative charge of plasma proteins. By doing so the contribution of protein to unmeasured anions is increased and the anion gap increased. About 15 per cent (2) of the increased gap is due to titration of proteins, whereas an alkalosis-induced increase in lactic acid accounts for 13 per cent. The remainder is accounted for by elevation of plasma protein (volume contraction). The nonbicarbonate buffers, especially protein, are titrated against the negatively charged plasma. Experimental models validating alkalosis induced increases in the anion gap are gastric alkalosis in man and diuretic-induced alkalosis in the dog.

Laboratory error

Laboratory errors must be considered as part of the anion gap interpretation.

Cations

Individual decreases in calcium, magnesium, and potassium rarely increase the anion gap, but simultaneous decreases in all, as seen in hypomagnesemia, do.

Decreased Anion Gap

Decreased anion gaps arise from increases in the unmeasured cations and/or decreases in the unmeasured anions and laboratory errors.

Disease states

Hemodilution

Acute dilution of plasma decreases the concentration of plasma electrolytes and decreases the anion gap (194).

Acute dilution of plasma bicarbonate produces acidosis. The acidosis is corrected by increased renal excretion of acid and increased renal chloride excretion, facilitating the regeneration of bicarbonate.

Proteins

Increased plasma cationic paraproteins decrease the anion gap. This condition is seen with multiple myeloma and is due to the cationic paraprotein IgG (2,130).

Hypoalbuminemia

Decreased plasma albumin concentration, the largest protein anion moiety in plasma, produces a decrease in the unmeasured anions and thus decreases the anion gap (189).

Hyperlipemia or hyperproteinemia

Hyperlipemia and hyperproteinemia (hyperviscosity) exert a number of effects on blood electrolyte composition. The cations sodium and potassium and anions chloride and bicarbonate, used to estimate anion gap, are affected by hyperlipemia and hyperproteinemia. Plasma sodium and chloride concentrations may be underestimated in hyperproteinemia and hyperlipemia. The error is due to the method used in measurement. Ion-specific measurement tends to be free of this error. Carbon dioxide's solubility is increased by increased lipid concentration and decreased by increased protein concentration. The overall change depends on the outcome of the two opposing effects. Proteins alter the bicarbonate concentration indirectly via their effect on pH and PCO_2. Lithium, calcium, and magnesium, when present in sufficiently large enough concentrations, lower the anion gap (84).

Hydrochloric acid acidosis

Chronic hydrochloric acid acidosis decreases the anion gap. The decrease (40 per cent) is mainly caused by titration of plasma nonbicarbonate buffers, especially protein, with acid (2). Net negative charge of the plasma proteins is decreased. Slight decreases in plasma organic anions probably accounts for the remainder of the decreased gap.

Laboratory error

Careful monitoring of quality control is essential to valid interpretation of the anion gap (130,176). Two very common and significant errors cause false decreases in anion gap. Plasma sodium measured by flame photometry does not obey Beer's law when true hypernatremia is present. Underestimation of an elevated sodium causes a spurious decrease in the anion gap (194). Increased plasma viscosity results in less sample aspirated into the measuring instrument (130). The values for sodium and potassium are decreased; a falsely decreased anion gap is produced (194).

Interfering halides

Halides, other than chloride, in plasma often react preferentially, especially in methods in which intensity of color or electrode selectivity are used (194). They falsely elevate plasma chloride concentration. Frequently high values are obtained which appear to be impossible. The renal tubular epithelium preferentially retains bromide over chloride.

OSMOLALITY

Osmolality is an expression of the total number of particles in solution. Plasma (urine) osmolality is a colligative property dependent only on the total number of particles irrespective of their species (246). Osmolality is a measure of the activity of water in solution.

The molal concentration of solute is a measure of the osmolality. Osmolality (solute concentration per kilogram of solvent) is used instead of osmolarity because it accurately describes the quality (solute per liter of solvent). Osmolarity depends on temperature and is cumbersome to use in physiology (249).

Electrolytes in dilute solution completely dissociate. Plasma is not a dilute solution: sodium chloride produces only 1.86 moles of particles (ie, 93 per cent dissociation) (102,177). Fortunately plasma is only about 93 per cent water (7 per cent solids). Plasma sodium can therefore be looked upon as contributing 2 moles of particles because its incomplete dissociation is made up for by overestimation of the plasma water volume.

Very little of the total plasma osmolality is contributed by analytes other than sodium and its anions, chloride and bicarbonate. The extracellular solutes are confined by their molecular size, electrical charge, and active pumps.

A number of receptors regulate osmolality. Central osmoreceptors, sensitive to alterations in impermeable solutes, act on the kidney through their mediator, antidiuretic hormone (ADH), producing either retention or excretion of water. Peripheral volume receptors cause ADH release when plasma volume decreases. Stimuli from the aortic and carotid baroreceptors respond to blood pressure variations and are the most potent in causing ADH release. When an emergency arises, volume stimuli take precedence over osmotic regulation of ADH secretion. Nervous impulses from the pharyngeal mucosa stimulate thirst. Cholinergic and beta-adrenergic as well as numerous psychic influences and drugs alter ADH output. In the dog an increase in epinephrine inhibits ADH release and an increase in ACTH increases water clearance. The osmoreceptors are very sensitive: a 1 percentile increase in osmolality alters ADH secretion.

Changes in the calculated osmolality necessitate measurement of plasma osmolality. Suspicion of altered hydration or of low molecular weight substances in the blood dictate that osmolality be measured (57). Instruments that measure osmolality must be accurate, that is, able to measure within ± 1.0 mOsm/l (2), because slight changes in tonicity in the order of 1 to 2 per cent cause major responses in ADH secretion, renal water metabolism, and thirst (117).

Osmolality is measured to determine if the plasma water content is altered. Additional use in detection of foreign low molecular weight substances in the plasma is equally as important (272). Interpretation of osmolality requires both measured and calculated osmolality be known. Recently Evans (90) proposed that urine osmolal gaps be used to identify unassayed solutes.

Tonicity

Tonicity and osmolality are different and changes in one do not have the same connotation as changes in the other. Analytes that alter tonicity, for example, protein, sodium, and mannitol, also change the osmolality. Urea and ammonia affect only the osmolality because their diffusion across cell membranes does not move water. Tonicity determines hydration or effective osmolality. Impermeable solutes alter tonicity by moving water across cell borders.

Generally an increase in tonicity indicates relative dehydration and a decrease indicates relative overhydration (102).

Calculations

Calculated osmolality (plasma) $= 2Na + (Glucose/18) + (Urea\ nitrogen/2.8)$

$$= mOsm/kg\ H_2O$$

where Na is in mEq/l and all other substances are in mg/dl (76,93). Calculated Effective Osmolality (Tonicity) $= 2Na + (Glucose/18) + (mannitol/18) + (sorbitol/18) + (glycerol/9) = mOsm/kg\ H_2O$ (93).

Calculated Osmolality $= (Na + K + Cl + urea + 24) \times 1.044$ (urine) where all values are in mmol/l.

Hyperosmolality

Levels of Biologic Significance

In man, when the serum osmolality is outside of 285 ± 5 mOsm/Kg of water, it is clinically recognized as hypo- or hyperosmolality (39, 102). Severe neurologic and circulatory signs are seen at 300 mOsm/kg of water and death at

355 mOsm/kg of water (39). Severe neurologic signs occur in dogs at >375 mOsm/kg of water (LMC, unpublished data).

Sensitive central osmoreceptors secrete ADH when the plasma osmolality reaches 280 mOsm/kg of water in man, rats, monkeys, dogs (12). Individual variation must be considered in interpretation of osmolality values (12). In dogs the threshold may be as high as 290 mOsm/kg of water.

Mechanisms

Plasma osmolality is increased by addition of soluble particulate matter or the net loss of water. Electrolytes cause greater increases than undissociated substances; the magnitude of the increase depends on the degree of dissociation of the substance and the number of ions dissociating. In general, it is the nature of the analyte responsible for the increase and not the magnitude of the increase that is important. Urea and alcohol increase plasma osmolality, cross cell membranes readily, and cause no movement of water: there is no alteration in the state of hydration. Interpretation of what an increase in one of these substances means depends entirely on the nature of the substance. Elevation of urea, a waste product of protein metabolism, indicates either an increase in production or a failure in clearance. Elevated plasma alcohol means either abnormal fermentative processes have occurred in the gut leading to its production or alcohol has been administered.

Increased plasma osmolality due to increased sodium concentration raises the plasma tonicity, causes water movement, and produces cellular dehydration.

Disease States

Reduced fluid intake

Animals in altered states of mentation, with neuromuscular disease, or with other debilitating conditions often do not drink enough to maintain their fluid balance. Small animals especially become dehydrated if water is withheld for prolonged periods before sampling procedures. The fasting period for laboratory animals must be dictated by their metabolic rate and not by limits set for man.

Water loss: Water is lost in sweat during fever or thyrotoxicosis, from the lungs, and in diarrhea and salivary secretions (117,177).

Failure of renal concentration: Failure to concentrate urine results from a number of conditions. Nephrogenic and neurogenic diabetes insipidus produce hyperosmolality because water losses exceed water intake. In the former there is an inability of the tubules to respond to ADH and in the latter there is a lack of ADH (165,177).

Hyperglycemia

Excesses of osmotically active compounds cause osmotic diuresis and a water deficit. These substances are not absorbed by the tubules when the threshold is exceeded; rather, they remain in the lumen of the tubule and take water away with them (177). Glucose diuresis occurs when the filtered load exceeds the transport maximum and it remains in the tubule. Solutes that are filtered but poorly resorbed, such as mannitol and related polysaccharides, simply remain in the tubule. Head injuries and tumors interfere with the osmoreceptors or ADH secretion and cause excessive water loss (133). Lack of urea, due to malnutrition, impairs concentration. Urea is needed to drive the counter-current mechanism (134). Lack of urea in the papillary area causes the concentrating defect of chronic renal failure. Collecting tubules fail to respond to ADH when hypokalemia and/or hypercalcemia are present (134).

In sickle cell anemia in man the medullary circulation is probably disturbed. This causes a counter-current disturbance and results in a concentrating defect (134). Animal counterparts to this disease have not been recognized.

Solute accumulation

Accumulations of glucose (diabetes), urea (renal failure), sodium (aldosteronism), and some absorbed topical applications lead to a decrease in plasma water content and hyperosmolality (149).

Laboratory Error

Lipemia

Dewpoint methods overestimate serum sodium in lipemic samples (159,177).

Accompanying Changes

Biochemical

Electrolytes: Hyperosmolality due to fluid loss is usually accompanied by increases in all electrolytes and most other analytes, including hemoglobin, hematocrit, erythrocytes, leukocytes, and protein.

Urea nitrogen: Hyperosmolality due to water loss is usually accompanied by azotemia due to reduced urea nitrogen clearance.

Hyponatremia: Hyperglycemia sufficient to produce hyperosmolality reduces plasma sodium. Sodium falls 1.3 to 1.6 mEq/l per 100 mg/dl increase in plasma glucose (177).

Urine osmolality: Changes in urine osmolality usually reflect plasma osmolality. Maximal concentrating and diluting ability varies widely among the species (139). Maximal urine concentration for man is 1,200, dog 2,500, laboratory rat 3,200, and desert rodents 5,000 mOsm/kg of water. The minimal urine concentration for man is 50 mOsm/kg of water.

Physiologic

Cardiac function: Hyperosmolality decreases ventricular performance (201).

Fatty acids: Release of fatty acids is inhibited by hyperosmolality (222).

Hyperglycemia: Hyperosmolality inhibits insulin release and thus causes hyperglycemia (222).

Thirst: The conscious animal's first sign of hyperosmolality is a desire for water. In man thirst is stimulated when osmolality reaches 295 mOsm/kg of water (93).

Neurologic signs: Increased effective osmolality dehydrates brain cells and others, causing a variety of signs including hyperpnea, confusion, coma, and death (93).

Skin turgor: Hyperosmolality due to salt and water losses reduces skin turgor. Dry mucous membranes characterize water deficits.

Cardiovascular: Tachycardia, hypotension, and hyperthermia occur with hyperosmolality.

Idiogenic osmoles: Erythrocytes and neurones synthesize intracellular solute as an adaptive response to hyperosmolality (93,146).

Hypoosmolality

Levels of Biologic Significance

In man, dog, and cat no signs arise until the serum sodium is less than 120 mEq/l. At 100 mEq/l the condition is extremely severe and likely to result in death (93).

Mechanisms

Osmolality is decreased by decreased particles in solution. Dilution-induced decreases follow failure to excrete endogenous or exogenous water, excessive water intake, and decreases in solute. Sodium and its anions are the dominant osmotic forces in plasma; true hypoosmolality is always associated with hyponatremia. Most hypoosmolar problems stem from failure to dilute urine and deliver adequate volumes of glomerular filtrate to the diluting sites.

Disease States

Excessive water intake

Excessive intake of fluid, low in solute, dilutes plasma electrolytes. The condition is rare in animals because water diuresis due to inhibition of ADH usually prevents its occurrence. It does occur when vomiting is severe and water is drunk to replace fluid and electrolyte loss.

Impaired renal dilution

Two mechanisms impair renal dilution. Free water (water free of electrolytes) generation is reduced by a decrease in glomerular filtration. Excessive free water is resorbed because of enhanced proximal tubular water and sodium resorption, that is, a decrease in the tubular flow of water increases the amount of sodium resorbed (159).

Limited renal medullary perfusion affects the counter-current mechanism and results in an abnormally diltue fluid leaving the ascending loop after processing. Proximal tubular resorption is enhanced in hypervolemic and edematous diseases. The recently discovered atrial hormone may be a factor involved in failure of the dilution mechanism.

Glucocorticoids

Glucocorticoid deficiencies slow glomerular filtration, impair medullary perfusion, and decrease permeability of the distal tubules. Cortisol deficiency increases sodium loss; hypercortisolism has the opposite effect.

Hypoaldosteronism enhances the effect of deficiencies of the glucocorticoids.

Inappropriate ADH secretion

Acute and chronic diseases are frequently associated with increases in ADH. Inappropriate ADH secretion caues hyponatremic hypoosmolality (177).

Sick cell syndrome

Severe trauma such as surgery and excoriation may cause renal sodium conservation and hyponatremia. This process occurs in an animal that is initially not saving water and has a normal sodium concentration. Alternative mechanisms, one or more of which may induce this effect, include elevated intracellular sodium resulting from impairment of the sodium pump by hypoxia, water overload, impaired renal dilution, increased permeability in areas sensitive to ADH (ADH normal), and inappropriate ADH secretion (177).

Spurious hyponatremia

Increases in the protein or lipid portion of plasma, normally about 5 to 7 per cent, reduce the volume of water containing sodium proportionately. Calculated osmolality will be abnormally low, whereas measured osmolality will be normal when osmolality is measured using a freezing point method. Dewpoint methods overestimate osmolality in lipemic samples (159,177).

Addison's disease

See Glucocorticoids. Sodium moves from the extracellular compartment into urine and into cells.

Accompanying Changes

Biochemical

Electrolytes: Accumulated water decreases the plasma levels of electrolytes and most other analytes. When there are solute deficits, the situation is variable. Hypoosmolarity releases potassium chloride into the plasma from brain cells. In most animals potassium is released into plasma from erythrocytes when hyponatremic (hypoosmolar) conditions prevail. The dog has high intracellular sodium and low potassium erthrocytes and loses sodium from its erythrocytes when plasma osmolality is decreased.

Physiologic

Central nervous system: Osmotic swelling of the brain causes anorexia, vomiting, and restlessness when hypoosmolality is mild. Irritability, uncooperativeness, muscle weakness, stupor, convulsions, and death occur in severe hypoosmolality as cells overhydrate.

Osmolal Gap

Osmolal gaps are determined because, like anion gaps, they are used to reveal hidden disease. Determinations are performed on serum or urine. The urine osmolar gap is complex. A detailed description of calculations and limitations is given by Evans (89,90).

To estimate the serum osmolal gap the calculated osmolality is subtracted from measured osmolality:

Measured Serum Osmolality $-$ (2Na $+$ glucose/18 $+$ urea nitrogen/2.8) $=$ Osmolal gap (147).

where 2Na $+$ glucose/18 $+$ urea nitrogen/2.8 is the calculated osmolality. In man, if the difference is greater than 10, then the following interpretations should be considered: (1) decreased plasma water, (2) low molecular weight substances in the plasma, and (3) laboratory error (176).

Substances that decrease serum water are usually protein or lipid. Lipidemia severe enough to cause decreases in plasma water is usually visible. A maximum serum osmolar gap comparable to the value of 10 for man has not been determined for other species.

BUFFERS

A buffer is a mixture of a weak acid and its corresponding salt or a weak base and its corresponding salt. Buffers resist changes in pH and are most effective when their pH is equal to their pK. The bicarbonate-carbonic acid system has a pK of approximately 6.1, and as such it is not an effective blood buffer! The buffer does possess unique qualities; its effectiveness in the animal stems from its ability to rapidly exchange CO_2 at the lungs and to be regenerated as bicarbonate by the kidney.

All body buffers (intravascular, interstitial, and cellular) are in equilibrium (51). Hemoglobin, plasma protein, and erythrocyte DPG make up 25 per cent of the total blood buffers (33). The ratio of the effectiveness of these buffers is 6:1:1 (33). Buffers work best when the concentration of acid is equal to the concentration of the corresponding base. Buffer action is limited to certain pH ranges; phosphate buffer works best close to pH 7.38, that is, close to blood pH. Buffer pH changes with temperature (235). The pH of acid and neutral buffers changes relatively less with temperature than do alkaline buffers (235). Buffers become more sensitive to changes induced by acids and bases when they are diluted with water. Alkaline buffers absorb atmospheric CO_2 and change their pH.

Blood Buffer Functions

Buffers perform two functions in the plasma. They resist hydrogen ion change associated with CO_2 transport and minimize changes occurring when acids or bases are added to plasma from metabolic processes.

The bicarbonate buffer system, the main blood buffer, is used when an acid other than carbonic is added to the blood. Protein (hemoglobin) buffers guard against changes associated with CO_2 transport. Bone is an important replacement source of bicarbonate. The skeleton acts as a buffer reservoir during chronic metabolic acidosis (159). Experimental evidence in the dog and cat shows that after 5 hours of acidosis most of the tissue buffering is performed by bone (38). Flat bones are the most effective buffer reservoirs. Because bone contains no salts of acids weaker than carbonic acid, it buffers very little of the change in respiratory acidosis. Nonbicarbonate buffers include imidazole rings from histidine residues of protein, terminal amino groups of protein, and inorganic and organic phosphates. Extracellular fluid contains larger amounts of bicarbonate buffer than does intracellular fluid. Both dissolved CO_2 and carbonic acid are considered weak acids in the body. Carbon dioxide can be hydrated rapidly to the acid.

Buffer Action

Carbonic acid is formed by hydration of CO_2 in the plasma and erythrocytes. Hydration, assisted by carbonic anhydrase, is rapid in erythrocytes.

Addition of CO_2 to blood is buffered by hemoglobin: the exchange of oxygen with hemoglobin is associated with a simultaneous exchange of hemoglobin and hydrogen ion. Hemoglobin, a zwitterion, combines with oxygen giving off a hydrogen ion, whereas oxygen is released as a hydrogen ion is accepted. The arterial-venous pH difference is about 0.01 to 0.02 pH units as a result of this process (243).

Hemoglobin-hydrogen ion exchange produces bicarbonate. Inside erythrocytes, hydrated carbon dioxide (carbonic acid) donates a proton to hemoglobin and the residual bicarbonate diffuses into the plasma. The departing bicarbonate is replaced by chloride from the plasma.

The mechanism just described in which hemoglobin acts as a buffer is confined to erythrocytes. In the plasma, proteins buffer CO_2.

The addition of acids, other than carbonic, is buffered by the carbonic acid buffer system. This system protects the body from sudden pH changes induced when acids and bases other than bicarbonate are added. The interactions of this system are described by the Henderson-Hasselbalch equation.

The Henderson-Hasselbalch formula expresses the relationship between PCO_2, pH, and bicarbonate:

$$pH = pK' + log\,(HCO_3^-)/H_2CO_3$$

pK' is the dissociation constant used when molar concentrations are used (ie, 6.1) and it varies with temperature and ionic strength (96). (HCO_3^- is the bicarbonate concentration expressed in millimoles per liter. H_2CO_3 consists of (1) physically dissolved carbon dioxide -99 per cent ($aPCO_2$), and (2) hydrated carbon dioxide -1 per cent (H_2CO_3). Alpha, the solubility coefficient for CO_2, is 0.03 for human plasma at 38°C (51).

When an acid (HCl) is added to the blood the following reaction takes place:

$$HCl + NaHCO_3(salt) \rightarrow NaCl + H_2CO_3 \text{ and}$$
$$H_2CO_3 \rightarrow H_2O + CO_2.$$

Bicarbonate is lowered.

Addition of a base (NaOH) produces:

$$NaOH + H_2CO_3 \ (acid) \rightarrow NaHCO_3 + H_2O.$$

Bicarbonate rises.

There is a continual supply of CO_2 from metabolism to react with added bases. No similar mechanism exists to take care of acid additions. Added acid results in the formation of carbonic acid, which is normally readily removed by the lungs.

ACID BASE DISTURBANCES

Acid base disturbances, characterized by changes in hydrogen ion concentration affect the ionization of molecules and reactive groups (13,254). Proteins and other substances become more or less charged as pH is altered; consequently, reaction rates, membrane activity, molecular binding, and the action and distribution of drugs are affected (215,254). Acid base disturbances are interpreted from arterial blood measurements because it reflects both respiratory and metabolic disturbances (42,171, 191,239,242,279).

Classification of Acid Base Disturbances

Acid base disturbances are interpreted with the knowledge of what is a normal or expected response for a given time (14,15,32,86,91,127, 241,277). They are classified in several ways:

1. *Depending on the cause*—They are called respiratory when the primary change is an alteration in the partial pressure of CO_2 and metabolic when the primary change is an alteration in bicarbonate concentration. Carbonic acid is produced endogenously and its concentration is regulated by respiration. Metabolic conditions are due to alterations in the nonvolatile or fixed acids. Respiratory and metabolic disturbances may be present concurrently as a mixed disturbance.
2. *Depending on the time*—They may be acute or longer than a few hours' duration in which case they are termed chronic.
3. *Depending on the severity and the body's response to the acid base disturbance*—They are uncompensated, partially compensated, and compensated.

Compensation for a metabolic disturbance is mainly respiratory, whereas compensation for a respiratory disturbance is mainly due to renal mechanisms.

Metabolic acidoses are further divided into:

1. *High anion gap acidoses* in which bicarbonate is replaced by other anions (keto-anions, lactate, and salicylate), and chloride is normal.

2. Normal anion gap acidoses are further divided into:

(A) *Hyperkalemic acidoses* due to acidifying agents, RTA, dilution of the plasma, chloride-containing acids, mineralocorticoid deficiency, systemic lupus erythematosus nephritis, acidosis following respiratory alkalosis, intestinal bicarbonate loss, organic anions, amyloidosis, hydronephrosis, sickle cell nephropathy, non-chloride-containing acids, nonspecific renal failure, and some katoacidoses (125).

(B) *Hypokalemic forms* including diarrhea and renal tubular acidosis (3).

(C) *Hyperchloremic acidoses* including those due to diarrhea, small bowel drainage, carbonic anhydrase inhibitors, and proximal and distal tubular acidosis (103,177).

Metabolic alkaloses are defined as:

1. *Volume contracted*, retaining sodium including gastric alkalosis (125).

2. *Volume expanded*, excreting large amounts of sodium chloride with bicarbonate production predominating over bicarbonate excretion (3).

3. *Chloride wasting* due to impaired chloride resorption possibly seen with hypercalcemia and severe hypokalemia (177).

Each condition is identified by the primary cause, duration, and degree of compensation. A primary change in PCO_2 is a respiratory disturbance. Mechanisms that react to the altered PCO_2, by changing bicarbonate, are secondary or compensatory mechanisms. A primary change in bicarbonate is a metabolic disturbance and the mechanisms that operate to change the PCO_2 as a result of the bicarbonate change are secondary or compensatory mechanisms. Compensation for changes in the pH of blood are affected by respiratory and renal systems. Respiratory compensation is rapid, whereas renal compensation may take several days. To interpret acid base balance requires correlation of the clinical finding with the appropriate laboratory data.

Acidosis

Respiratory Acidosis

Definition

Respiratory acidosis is defined as an increase in PCO_2 and subsequent to this a proportionate increase in the carbonic acid concentration of blood. (125,150). The pH may be unchanged, that is, acidemia may be absent, but the hydrogen ion concentration is increased.

Increased PCO_2 due to greater tissue output or as a consequence of inadequate alveolar ventilation produces an immediate increase in bicarbonate concentration. Moderate elevations in PCO_2 usually do not alter pH. In acute hypercapnia in dog and man there is no elevation in metabolic acids (49).

Intracellular acidosis occurs rapidly in respiratory acidosis because dissolved CO_2 crosses cell membranes readily.

Compensation

A compensated respiratory acidosis is one in which the pH has been restored to normal while the PCO_2 remains elevated. Renal compensation of respiratory acidosis is of paramount importance (49). Steady state chronic respiratory acidosis is reached in dogs in 3 to 5 days, in man in 2 to 4 days, and rapidly in the rat (56).

The pH changes less in chronic respiratory acidosis than in acute respiratory acidosis. Acute respiratory acidosis superimposed on chronic metabolic acidosis produces progressively smaller changes in pH as the chronic level of bicarbonate increases (154). Moderate degrees of respiratory acidosis usually do not change pH. When the PCO_2 is greater than 80 mmHg, acidosis is always seen in man (49,150). The apparent lack of response in chronic respiratory acidosis is explained by increased renal acid secretion and generation of bicarbonate. Plasma bicarbonate is elevated (113). The tubular exchange of hydrogen is stimulated by hypercarbia and bicarbonate is increased (231). Because sodium exchanged for hydrogen ion is not resorbed with chloride, chloriuresis occurs (231). Also chloride absorption from the gut is reduced and possibly some chloride is shifted into erythrocytes (221).

Ammonia formation from glutamine in both acute and chronic acidosis in man, rat, and dog is increased (94). In chronic respiratory acidosis the amount of urinary ammonia excreted may increase 10-fold. There is no glutaminase adaptation in the dog (204). In acidotic dogs in addition to glutamine, the glycine, citrulline, tryptophane, asparagine, and proline concentration of renal arterial blood is decreased, thereby facilitating acid excretion as ammonium ion (94,198,255). These amino acids are increased in alkalosis. The concentration of glutaminase, 1-amino acid oxidase, and glycine oxidase in renal tissue of the rat is increased by acidosis and decreased by alkalosis (72,73,255).

The compensatory renal response of sodium, potassium, and chloride to hypercapnia returns to normal in 24 hours and the elevated CO_2 is taken care of by an increase in respiratory exchange.

In most animals potassium and sodium are released from the cells into the plasma by acute hypercapnia, and serum chloride is decreased (56,105,143,205). The shift is probably due to intracellular buffering of hydrogen ion, sodium and potassium moving between cells, and the extracellular fluid to maintain ionic balance. Rats excrete both potassium and chloride, but osseous sodium and calcium are not decreased by acute respiratory acidosis because bone contains no salts of acids weaker than carbonic (143).

Accompanying changes

At high levels CO_2 has a depressant effect on the central nervous system. Comas occur when the PCO_2 reaches the 70 to 80 mmHg in acute situations and 70 to 100 mmHg in chronic conditions.

The cerebrospinal fluid pressure is increased by increased blood flow, the result of hypercarbia. Cardiac output rises in hypercarbia and cardiac contractility decreases.

Autonomic reactions are altered by hypercarbia. Gastric acid secretion increases and hepatic blood flow decreases. Bromsulfophthalein clearance is reduced. Hypercarbia causes vasoconstriction of the pulmonary circulation and splanchnic vessels and vasodilation of most other regions. The effect of carbon dioxide on the bronchi varies with the species.

Hypercarbia affects enzymatic activity indirectly via pH, and the mass effect on CO_2 inhibits its decarboxylation. Acute acidosis in rats causes a rise in plasma corticosterone (276). Intestinal absorption of chloride and sodium in the rat and rabbit is increased by systemic acidemia and hypercapnia (59).

Laboratory assessment

To determine the exact nature of an alteration in CO_2 it is useful to calculate, using the Henderson-Hasselbalch equation, the anticipated change in pH and bicarbonate. In this way the condition may be defined as a pure or mixed acid base disturbance and the degree of compensation may be assessed. Mixed disturbances are indicated when observations fall outside the significance band for the disturbance.

1. In acute respiratory acidosis for each millimeter of mercury increase in PCO_2 the hydrogen ion concentration in arterial blood increases linearly by 0.8 nmol/l in man and by 0.77 nmol/l in the dog (49,64,225,230). There is no renal compensation in acute respiratory acidosis. The acidotic changes are buffered by non-bicarbonate buffers. One third of the acute increase in hydrogen ions is buffered by hemoglobin and two thirds by tissue buffers (32). The response is minimally altered by hemoglobin levels (7 to 20 Hb = ± 1.0 mEq/l H^+) (10).

2. In chronic respiratory acidosis the anticipated change in hydrogen ion concentration is 0.24 nmol/l for each millimeter of mercury increase in CO_2 for man (32) and 0.32 nmol/l for each millimeter of mercury increase for the dog (230).

Metabolic Acidosis

Metabolic acidosis results from conditions that cause a primary decrease in bicarbonate concentration (32,78,116,125,175). Bicarbonate concentration is reduced by: increased endogenous production of acids (other than carbonic, eg, lactic or sulfuric) producing an increased anion gap, loss of bicarbonate in ptyalism or diarrhea, or failure to excrete the normal acid load as in renal tubular acidosis. The latter two mechanisms result in a normal anion gap.

An increase in hydrogen ions causes a rapid weak respiratory response, lowering PCO_2 and returning pH toward the norm. The response is weak in both man and animals because as PCO_2

falls the cerebrospinal fluid pH rises and inhibits ventilatory drive. Other buffers, including bicarbonate, oxyhemoglobin, hemoglobin, phosphate, and protein buffers, act in defense of pH when a strong acid is added to the blood. The main buffer, bicarbonate, is able to buffer twice as much acid as is the hemoglobin system.

In the dog, cat, rat, goat, and man the cerebrospinal fluid is about 4 mV positive to the blood. The potential is linearly related to pH by a slope of -45 mV per pH unit for metabolic acidosis and alkalosis and -30 mV per pH unit for respiratory acidosis and alkalosis in the dog (36).

Laboratory assessment

In acute metabolic acidosis for each milliequivalent decrease in bicarbonate a 1.1 mmHg fall in PCO_2 occurs (32,225). In chronic metabolic acidosis the degree of renal compensation is dependent on the acid anion and the state of hydration. The PCO_2 response is hard to predict (243). For example, animals with lactic acidosis have the lowest PCO_2. Renal compensation is by increased hydrogen ion excretion and increased ammonia formation (142). In steady state acidosis a 1 to 1.3 mmHg decrease in PCO_2 occurs for each milliequivalent fall in HCO_3^- (243).

Compensation

Kussmaul respiration is a characteristic response to metabolic acidosis as the acidified extracellular fluid stimulates the respiratory center (116). Maximal respiratory compensation occurs in man in 24 to 36 hours. Slower renal compensation, increased ammonia formation, and bicarbonate synthesis facilitate both buffering and excretion of excess acid (142). The increase in ammonia formation takes several days to reach its maximum. The rate-limiting factor in acid excretion is $Na^+ - H^+$ exchange. In the dog and rat, bone accounts for most of the tissue buffering of hydrogen ion after 5 hours of acidosis (38).

The ventilatory response to acute metabolic acidosis is both rapid and effective; CO_2 is quickly removed. No similar effective mechanism exists for compensation of respiratory acidosis. Respiratory compensation guards pH by lowering PCO_2, but it simultaneously produces an unfavorable decrease in bicarbonate.

In chronic metabolic acidosis the persistent ventilatory response is stronger than the acute response because bicarbonate has decreased and the cerebrospinal fluid pH is decreased toward its normal value. With the central chemoreceptor drive restored the PCO_2 is lowered further. In chronic steady state metabolic acidosis the cerebrospinal fluid is essentially normal. In severe metabolic acidosis the plasma bicarbonate reaches 5.0 mEq/l when PCO_2 is 15 mmHg in man and this is the limit of the respiratory response. The serious side effect of chronic compensatory hyperventilation is depression of renal acid excretion (231).

Accompanying changes

Organic acidoses increase the anion gap because of the accumulation of organic ions that replace bicarbonate. In diabetic acidosis there is an accompanying hyperglycemia and in uremic acidosis an accompanying azotemia. Dehydration accompanies the acidosis of severe diarrhea.

The alterations in plasma sodium in metabolic acidosis are unpredictable (187). Acidosis caused by mineral acids produces increased plasma potassium, whereas nonmineral acids decrease plasma potassium. Phosphate is increased by lactic and beta-hydroxybutyric acids, unchanged by hydrochloric acid, and decreased by methylmalonic acid in dogs (193).

Leukocytosis is caused by severe metabolic acidemia because catecholamines decrease margination (179). Organic anions compete with urate in the kidney, and in man acidosis may be accompanied by hyperuricemia.

Alkalosis

Respiratory Alkalosis

Respiratory alkalosis is a reduction in physically dissolved CO_2 in the blood (82,125,142). Alkalemia may or may not be present. Respiratory alkalosis results from any process that reduces PCO_2. Hyperventilation in response to heat, cold, fear, exercise, hyperthyroidism, central nervous system disease, chronic liver disease, and administration of progesteronal compounds lowers PCO_2. A steady state of hypocapnia, in which all physiologic adjustments have been made, occurs in about 10 minutes. Anesthesia has little effect on the response (10).

Laboratory assessment

In acute respiratory alkalosis for each millimeter decrease in PCO_2 there is a decrease in hydrogen ion concentration of 0.8 nmol/l (142). The significance band for CO_2 tensions of 15 to 45 mmHg is 6 nmol/l of hydrogen ion and 5 mEq/l for bicarbonate (10). There is no renal loss of bicarbonate in respiratory alkalosis. Bicarbonate is reduced by its titration with hydrogen ions that are released from the acid component of noncarbonic acid buffers; hemoglobin accounts for one third, tissue buffers for two thirds of these.

In compensated chronic respiratory alkalosis for each millimeter decrease in PCO_2 there is a decrease of 0.17 nmol/l in hydrogen ion concentration in the dog (32,104). The regulation of pH in man is not as effective as it is in dogs (104).

Compensation

In acute respiratory alkalosis there are declines in pH and extracellular bicarbonate that coincide with the decrease in PCO_2, but there is no actual loss of bicarbonate (278). Renal bicarbonate loss does not occur in respiratory alkalosis. Bicarbonate reduction takes place by release of hydrogen ions from hemoglobin and tissue buffers and by a small increase in lactic acid (104). Hemoglobin accounts for approximately one third of this effect, tissue buffers two thirds.

Chronic respiratory alkalosis is compensated when pH has been returned to normal while CO_2 remains lowered. Renal compensation is achieved by retention of hydrogen ions and excretion of sodium (104,231). Actual bicarbonate loss occurs in chronic respiratory alkalosis while chloride remains unchanged (232). There is no loss of bicarbonate in acute respiratory alkalosis. In chronic hypocapnia chloride is increased (104). Compensation for chronic hypocapnia is excellent; the bicarbonate decrease usually parallels the fall in CO_2 (9,104). In man about 5 per cent of the bicarbonate deficit is due to renal bicarbonate loss with the largest reduction in bicarbonate accounted for by increased concentrations of lactic and pyruvic acids. Lactic acidosis accompanies all chronic respiratory alkaloses (190).

A paradoxical respiratory alkalosis accompanies rapid recovery from metabolic acidosis. It develops because the bicarbonate concentration is slow to equalize across the blood-brain barrier. The respiratory center remains stimulated by the acidic cerebrospinal fluid even though the plasma hydrogen ion concentration has normalized.

Accompanying changes

Alterations that occur during hypocarbia and respiratory alkalosis are decreases in urine volume, renal phosphate and ammonia excretion, and titratable acidity, and increases in renal sodium and potassium excretion, serum lactic and pyruvic acid production, and urine bicarbonate and pH (204,231,234). Alkalemia and hypocapnia decrease intestinal absorption of sodium and chloride in the rat and rabbit (59). Plasma sodium generally falls in respiratory alkalosis, probably because of intracellular buffering of hydrogen ion. Both sodium and potassium move to maintain ionic balance. Plasma phosphate is usually lowered by respiratory alkalosis (105,187). Ionized calcium and magnesium are decreased by hypocarbia.

Hypocarbia decreases both cardiac output and stroke volume, causing a decrease in blood pressure (286). Cerebral vessels constrict whereas pulmonary blood flow is increased by hypocarbia due to decreased resistance. The electroencephalogram and cardiogram show evidence of hypocarbia.

Metabolic Alkalosis

Metabolic alkalosis is an increase in bicarbonate and a decrease in hydrogen ion (32,125,169) resulting from excessive loss of fixed acids, excessive secretion of hydrogen ion, or excessive intake of base. In the rat uncomplicated potassium and chloride depletion produces metabolic alkalosis (9). Experimentally in dog and man alkalosis cannot be produced by these methods (122). Metabolic alkaloses are conveniently classified on the basis of urine chloride levels. Those with low urine chloride levels are caused by loss of hydrochloric acid and those in which an increased concentration of chloride appears in the urine are associated with mineralocorticoid excess.

Metabolic alkaloses resulting from loss of gastric acid produce a deficiency of chloride, the anion that is normally resorbed with sodium in the proximal tubule. Because sodium is not resorbed in the proximal tubule, an excess of sodium is delivered to the distal tubule and exchanges there with hydrogen ion and potassium. The excessive sodium results in potassium and hydrogen ion secretion while bicarbonate is retained.

Metabolic alkalosis stemming from mineralocorticoid excess (adrenal hyperfunction) is produced by steroidal action on the distal tubule. Excess steroid enhances cation exchange and both sodium and bicarbonate are retained at the expense of hydrogen ions and potassium. Water retention and an expanded plasma volume result from the excess retained sodium. The expanded plasma volume increases the glomerular filtration rate, this in turn results in more sodium chloride filtered, and in this way a vicious cycle is set up.

Laboratory assessment

In metabolic alkalosis an increase in PCO_2 is the exception, taking place only when the bicarbonate is about 45 mEq/l. The PCO_2 compensatory increase ranges from 55 to 60 mmHg in man. All animals have a distinct preference to be well oxygenated and forego acid base adjustments.

Compensation

Both bicarbonate and nonbicarbonate buffers respond to metabolic alkalosis (278). Bicarbonate excretion by the kidney is enhanced and occurs within the first hour of the disturbance. Volume deficits from the alkalosis itself hamper renal removal of bicarbonate. Respiratory compensation is proportional to the degree of arterial hydrogen ion depression (9). The PCO_2 is usually only slightly decreased because lowering the PCO_2 has the undesirable limiting effect of lowering the PO_2. In extreme alkalosis respiration is lowered and PCO_2 raised. In man bicarbonate is rarely greater than 28 mEq/l, the renal threshold for bicarbonate. Bicarbonate is rapidly excreted in the urine (147).

Accompanying changes

Plasma sodium and inorganic phosphate changes are unpredictable in metabolic alkalosis. Lactate is increased because of activation of phosphofructokinase by the alkalosis (215). Metabolic alkalosis depresses renal use of ketone bodies in the rat (6).

In chronic metabolic alkalosis urine pH is usually low. This paradoxical aciduria was once attributed to potassium depletion, but is now best explained by another mechanism. Poorly resorbed bases such as sulfate require pairing with cations, Na^+, K^+, or H^+ before renal excretion. Neither sodium nor potassium is available for this purpose in metabolic alkalosis; therefore hydrogen ions must be chosen. Sodium is unavailable, as it is saved in response to the volume deficit. Potassium is also retained by the kidney as it too is depleted by alkalosis. Therefore, the kidney must excrete the only remaining cation, hydrogen, in the urine. An increase in sodium conservation is in essence an increase in the cation exchange, with more hydrogen ion excretion and higher bicarbonate values generated (233). To correct the situation hydrochloric acid is required. Chloride functions as a resorbable base, and pH and bicarbonate are restored to normal. Hydrogen ion given with a nonresorbable base only results in excretion of the added acid (233). In man both nausea and vomiting occur with metabolic alkalosis.

Mixed Disorders

Acid base disorders may be superimposed on each other. It is therefore essential that laboratory data be carefully considered alongside predicted values and clinical correlates (32,40, 125,211).

As a general rule, when a normal pH is seen with abnormal bicarbonate or CO_2, a mixed disorder is expected. When the pH moves in the opposite direction to that predicted for the primary disturbance, a mixed disturbance exists.

To interpret an acid base disturbance correctly, the following information is required: (1) the environment, (2) state of hydration, (3) body temperature, (4) respiratory rate and character, (5) evidence of diarrhea, vomiting, and excoriation, (6) physical appearance, and (7) duration of the condition.

The normal expected compensatory adjustments are calculated in order to categorize a set of acid base values. Clinical input is needed to explain why compensation may not be as expected. For example, pain and decreased compliance hinder respiratory compensation and urine retention limits renal compensation.

The anion gap is calculated to define the presence of a hidden acidosis that may be superimposed on a primary disturbance.

Information provided by urinalysis includes the presence of ketones and glucose and the levels of electrolytes excreted.

REFERENCES

1. Ackerman U (1986) Structure and function of atrial natriuretic peptides. Clin Chem 32: 241–247
2. Adrogue HJ, Brensilver J, Madias NE (1978) Changes in the plasma anion gap during chronic metabolic acid-base disturbances. Am J Physiol 235: F291–F297
3. Adrogue HJ, Madias NE (1981) Changes in plasma potassium concentration during acute acid-base disturbances. Am J Med 71: 456–467
4. Adrogue HJ, Wilson H, Boyd AE, Suki WN, Eknoyan G (1982) Plasma acid-base patterns in diabetic ketoacidosis. N Engl J Med 307: 1603–1610
5. Agostini A, Berfasconi C, Gerli G, Luzzana M, Rossi-Bernardi L (1973) Oxygen affinity and electrolyte distribution of human blood: Changes induced by propanolol. Science 182: 300–301
6. Angielski S, Lukowics J (1978) The role of the kidney in the removal of ketone bodies under different acid-base status of the rat. Am J Clin Nutr 31: 1635–1641
7. Anonymous (1950) Standardization of definitions and symbols in respiratory physiology. Fed Proc 9: 602–605
8. Anrep GV, Cannan RK (1924) The concentration of lactic acid in the blood in experimental alkalaemia and acidaemia. J Physiol 58: 244–258
9. Aquino HC, Luke RG (1973) Respiratory compensation to potassium-depletion and chloride-depletion alkalosis. Am J Physiol 225: 1444–1448
10. Arbus GS, Hebert LA, Levesque PR, Etsten BE, Schwartz WB (1969) Characterization and clinical application of the "significance band" for acute respiratory alkalosis. N Engl J Med 280: 117–123
11. Arieff AI, Felts PW, Frawley TF (1974) Hyperosmolar Coma. Upjohn, Kalamazoo
12. Arieff AI, Guisado R, Lazarowitz VC (1977) Pathophysiology of hyperosmolar states. In Andreoli TE (ed), Disturbances in Body Fluid Osmolality. American Physiological Society, Bethesda
13. Astrup P (1958) Ultra-micro-methods for determining pH, PCO_2 and standard bicarbonate in capillary blood. Technical Publication 29, Radiometer, Copenhagen
14. Astrup P (1961) A new approach to acid-base metabolism. Clin Chem 7: 1–15
15. Astrup P, Jorgensen K, Siggaard Andersen O, Engel K, Classification of disturbances in the acid-base metabolism. Technical Publication 8, Radiometer, Copenhagen
16. Astrup P, Engel K (1965) Acid-base problems in hypothermia. Arch Intern Med 116: 739–742
17. Astrup P, Engel K, Severinghaus JW, Munson E (1965) The influence of temperature and pH on the dissociation curve of oxyhemoglobin of human blood. Scand J Clin Lab Invest 17: 515–523
18. Astrup P, Rorth M, Thorshauge C (1970) Dependency on acid-base status of oxyhemoglobin dissociation and 2,3-diphosphoglycerate level in human erythrocytes. II. In vivo studies. Scand J Clin Lab Invest 26: 47–52
19. Austin WH, Littlefield SC (1966) The difference in apparent pH of blood and buffer caused by raising the liquid junction from room temperature to 37.5 C. J Lab Clin Med 67: 517–519
20. Avioli LV (1979) Management of osteomalacia. Hosp Pract 14: 109–114
21. Bach JR (1963) The Astrup Method. A micromethod for determination of pH and other acid base values in blood. Technical Publication 16, Radiometer, Copenhagen
22. Bach JR (1963) The measurement of blood pH with Radiometer capillary blood electrodes. Technical Publication 17, Radiometer, Copenhagen
23. Baer DM, The clinical use of the Astrup pH, PCO_2 and acid base excess determination. Technical Publication 31, Radiometer, Copenhagen
24. Baird G (1977) Aspects of ruminant intermediary metabolism in relation to ketosis. Biochem Rev 5: 819–827
25. Bakerman S, Khazanie P (1982) Calcium metabolism and hypercalcemia. Lab Man July: 17–25
26. Banerjee CM, Alarie Y, Woolard M (1968) Gas tensions in conscious monkeys. Proc Soc Exp Biol Med 128: 1183–1185
27. Baron DN, Broughton PMG, Cohen M, Lansley TS, Lewis SM, Shinton NK (1974) The use of SI units in reporting results obtained in hospital laboratories. J Clin Pathol 27: 590–597
28. Bartness TJ, Waldbillig RJ (1981) Handling induced changes in plasma volume and osmolality: Adrenal modulation of blood parameters. Physiol Behav 26: 177–182
29. Bartels H, Dejours P, Kellogg RH, Mead J (1973) Glossary on respiration and gas exchange. J Appl Physiol 14: 549–558
30. Bateman NT, Musch TI, Smith CA, Dempsey JA (1980) Problems with the gas calibrated PCO_2 electrode. Resp Physiol 41: 217–226
31. Bauer C (1970) Reduction of the carbon dioxide affinity of human haemoglobin solutions by 2,3-diphosphoglycerate. Resp Physiol 10: 10–19
32. Bean RA, Gribik M (1974) Assessing acid-base imbalances through laboratory parameters. Hosp Pract 9: 157–165
33. Beetham R (1982) A review of pH and blood-gas analysis. Ann Clin Biochem 19: 198–213
34. Benesch R, Benesch RE, Yu CI (1968) Reciprocal binding of oxygen and diphosphoglycerate by human hemoglobin. Proc Nat Acad Sci 59: 526–532
35. Berger AJ, Krassney JA, Dutton RE (1973) Respiratory recovery from CO_2 breathing in intact and chemodenervated awake dogs. J Appl Physiol 35: 35–41

36. Berger AJ, Mitchell RA, Severinghaus JW (1977) Regulation of respiration. N Engl J Med 297: 92–97, 194–201

37. Bergstrom J (1981) Determination of electrolytes. Methodological problems. Acta Med Scand 647: 39–46

38. Bettice JA, Gamble JL (1975) Skeletal buffering of acute metabolic acidosis. Am J Physiol 229: 1618–1624

39. Bevan DR (1978) Osmometry: Clinical applications. Anaesthesia 33: 809–814

40. Bia M, Thier SO (1981) Mixed acid base disturbances: A clinical approach. Med Clin North Am 65: 347–361

41. Biddulph DM, Gallimore LB (1974) Sensitivity of the kidney to parathyroid hormone and its relationship to serum calcium in the hamster. Endocrinology 94: 1241–1246

42. Blackwood WD (1965) Some practical aspects of the measurement of acid-base balance in blood. Arch Intern Med 116: 654–657

43. Blair E (1969) Generalized hypothermia. Fed Proc 28: 1456–1462

44. Bloom SA, Canzanella VJ, Strom JA, Madias NE (1985) Spurious assessment of acid-base status due to dilutional effect of heparin. Am J Med 79: 528–530

45. Blunt MH, Kitchens JL, Mayson SM, Huisman THJ (1971) Red cell 2,3-diphosphoglycerate and oxygen affinity in newborn goats and sheep. Proc Soc Exp Biol Med 138: 800–803

46. Boutilier RG, Randall DJ, Shelton G, Toews DP (1978) Some response characteristics of CO_2 electrodes. Resp Physiol 32: 381–388

47. Bouverot P, Bureau M (1975) Ventilatory acclimatization and csf acid-base balance in carotid chemodenervated dogs at 3550 m. Pfluegers Arch 361: 17–23

48. Bowers GN, Brassard C, Sena SF (1986) Measurement of ionized calcium in serum with ion-selective electrodes: a mature technology that can meet the daily service needs. Clin Chem 32: 1437–1446

49. Brackett NC, Cohen JJ, Schwartz WB (1965) Carbon dioxide titration curve of normal man. N Engl J Med 272: 6–12

50. Brodda K (1975) On the theory of base excess curve in the Siggaard Andersen nomogram. Respiration 32: 378–388

51. Brown EB (1965) Blood and tissue buffers. Arch Intern Med 116: 665–669

52. Brown MJ, Brown DC, Murphy MB (1983) Hypokalemia from beta 2 receptor stimulation by circulating epinephrine. N Engl J Med 309: 1414–1419

53. Burnett RW, Noonan DC (1974) Calculations and correction factors used in determination of pH and blood gases. Clin Chem 20: 1499–1506

54. Burton GW (1965) Effects of the acid-base state upon the temperature coefficient of pH of blood. Br J Anaes 37: 89–102

55. Bush M, Custer R, Smeller J, Bush LM (1977) Physiologic measures of non human primates during physical restraint and chemical immobilization. J Am Vet Med Assoc 171: 866–869

56. Carter NW, Seldin DW, Teng HC (1959) Tissue and renal response to chronic respiratory acidosis. J Clin Invest 38: 949–960

57. Chalmers RA, Bickle S, Watts RWE (1974) A method for the determination of volatile organic acids in aqueous solutions and urine, and the results obtained in propionic acidaemia methylcrotonylglycinuria and methylmalonic aciduria. Clin Chim Acta 52: 31–41

58. Chapot G, Barrault N, Muller M, Dargnat D (1972) Comparative study of $PaCO_2$ in several homeothermic species. Am J Physiol 223: 1354–1357

59. Charney AN, Feldman GM (1984) Systemic acid-base disorders and intestinal electrolyte transport. Am J Physiol 247: G1–G12

60. Clark JM (1974) The toxicity of oxygen. Am Rev Resp Dis 110: 40–50

61. Coe FL (1981) Nephrolithiasis. Causes, classification and management. Hosp Pract 16: 33–45

62. Cogan MG, Huang CL, Liu FY, Madden D, Wong KR (1986) Effect of atrial natriuretic factor on acid-base homeostasis. J Hypertension 4: S31–S34

63. Cohen JJ (1979) Disorders of potassium balance. Hosp Pract 14: 119–128

64. Cohen JJ, Brackett NC, Schwartz WB (1964) The nature of the carbon dioxide titration curve in the normal dog. J Clin Invest 43: 777–786

65. Cohen JJ, Gennari FJ, Harrington JT (1981) In Brenner BM, Rector FC (eds), The Kidney. Saunders, Philadelphia, pp 908–939

66. Cohen RD, Simpson BR (1975) Lactate metabolism. Anaesthesiology 43: 661–673

67. Cole FV, Hawkins LH (1967) The measurement of the oxygen content of whole blood. Biomed Eng 2: 56–63

68. Comline RS, Silver M (1974) A comparative study of blood gas tensions, oxygen affinity and red cell 2,3 DPG concentrations in foetal and maternal blood in the mare, cow and sow. J Physiol 242: 805–826

69. Coude FX, Ogier H, Grimber G, Parvy P, Pham Dinh D, Charpentier C, Saudubray JM (1982) Correlation between blood ammonia concentration and organic acid accumulation in isovaleric and propionic acidemia. Pediatrics 69: 115–117

70. Cox MC, Sterns RH, Singer I (1978) The defense against hyperkalemia: The roles of insulin and aldosterone. N Engl J Med 299: 525–531

71. Cristina M, de Hurtado C, Genda OA, Cingolani HE (1979) Species differences in the chronotropic response to acid-base alterations. Arch Int Physiol Biochim 87: 592–602

72. Davies BMA, Yudkin J (1951) Role of glutaminase in the production of urinary ammonia. Nature 167: 117

73. Davies BMA, Yudkin J (1952) Studies in biochemical adaptation: The origin of urinary ammonia as indicated by the effect of chronic acidosis and alkalosis on some renal enzymes in the rat. Biochem J 52: 407–412

74. Defronzo RA, Their SO (1982) Inherited tubule disorders. Hosp Pract 17: 111–128

75. Dempsey JA, Forster JV, doPico GA (1974) Ventilatory acclimatization to moderate hypoxemia in man: The role of spinal fluid $[H^+]$. J Clin Invest 53: 1091–1100

76. Dharan M (1978) Increase your awareness of clinical osmometry. Lab Man January: 38–42

77. Diengott D, Roza O, Levy N, Muammar S (1964) Hypokalemia in barium poisoning. Lancet II: 343–345

78. Doe RP (1965) Metabolic acidosis nondiabetic. Arch Intern Med 116: 717–728

79. D'Silva JL (1934) The action of adrenaline on serum potassium. J Physiol 82: 393–398

80. Durst RA (1975) Temperature variation detection in a blood pH-gas analyser. Clin Chem 21: 176–177

81. Eaton JW, Brewer GJ (1968) The relationship between red cell 2,3-diphosphoglycerate and levels of hemoglobin in the human. Proc Natl Acad Sci 61: 756–760

82. Eichenholz A (1965) Respiratory alkalosis. Arch Intern Med 116: 699–708

83. Elser RC, Sitler J, Garver C (1982) A flexible and versatile program for blood-gas quality control. Am J Clin Pathol 78: 471–478

84. Emmett M, Goldfarb S, Agus ZS, Narins RG (1977) The pathophysiology of acid base changes in chronically phosphate-depleted rats. Bone-kidney interactions. J Clin Invest 59: 291–298

85. Emmett M, Narins RG (1977) Clinical use of the anion gap. Medicine 56: 38–54

86. Englesson S, Grevsten S, Olin A (1973) Some numerical methods of estimating acid-base variables in human blood with a haemoglobin concentration of 5 gm/100 cm³. Scand J Clin Lab Invest 32: 289–295

87. English PB (1967) A study of water and electrolyte metabolism in sheep. III. Sodium depletion. Brit Vet J 123: 111–121

88. Epstein FH, Rosa RM (1983) Adrenergic control of serum potassium. N Engl J Med 309: 1450–1451

89. Evans JR (1987) Osmolal gaps in urine. Clin Chem 32: 1415

90. Evans JR (1987) More on osmolal gaps in urine. Clin Chem 33: 746

91. Fairley HB (1964) Untitled presentation. Technical Publication 38, Radiometer, Copenhagen

92. Faller J, Fox IH (1982) Ethanol-induced hyperuricemia. N Engl J Med 307: 1598–1602

93. Feig PU, McCurdy DK (1977) The hypertonic state. N Engl J Med 297: 1444–1454

94. Fine A, Bennett FI, Alleyne GAO (1978) Effects of acute acid-base alterations on glutamine metabolism and renal ammoniagenesis in the dog. Clin Sci Mol Med 54: 503–508

95. Fitzgerald F (1978) Clinical hypophosphatemia. Ann Rev Med 29: 177–189

96. Flear CTG (1987) pK′1 and bicarbonate concentration in plasma. Clin Chem 33: 13–20

97. Forster HV, Bisgard GE, Rasmussen B (1976) Ventilatory control in peripheral chemoreceptor-denervated ponies during chronic hypoxemia. J Appl Physiol 41: 878–885

98. Gabow PA, Kaehny WD, Fennessey PV, Goodman SI, Gross PA, Schrier RW (1980) Diagnostic importance of an increased serum anion gap. N Engl J Med 303: 854–858

99. Gattinoni L, Samaja M (1979) Acid-base equilibrium in the blood of sheep. Experientia 9: 1247–1348

100. Gault MH, Dixon ME, Doyle M, Cohen WM (1968) Hypernatremia, azotemia and dehydration due to high-protein tube feeding. Ann Intern Med 68: 778–791

101. Geary TD (1978) A clarification on the Corning 175 Blood Gas Analyser. Clin Chem 24: 1085–1086

102. Gennari FJ (1984) Serum osmolality. N Engl J Med 310: 102–105

103. Gennari FJ, Cohen JJ (1978) Renal tubular acidosis. Ann Rev Med 29: 521–541

104. Gennari JF, Goldstein MB, Schwartz WB (1972) The nature of the renal adaptation to chronic hypocapnia. J Clin Invest 51: 1772–1730

105. Giebisch G, Berger L, Pitts RF (1955) The extrarenal response to acute acid-base disturbances of respiratory origin. J Clin Invest 34: 231–245

106. Girndt J, Henning HV, Delling G (1979) Correlation of calcium and acid-base metabolism. Horm Metab Res 11: 587–588

107. Gleason DF (1965) pH measurements. Arch Intern Med 116: 649–653

108. Goldfarb S, Cox M, Singer I, Goldberg M (1976) Acute hyperkalemia induced by hyperglycemia: Hormonal mechanisms. Ann Intern Med 84: 426–432

109. Gordon EE (1973) Etiology of lactic acidosis. Am J Med Sci 265: 463–465

110. Gullick JD, Schauble MK (1972) SD unit system for standardized reporting and interpretation of laboratory data. Am J Clin Pathol 57: 517–525

111. Guttler F, Pedersen A (1973) Baseosis and hypopotassaemia in chronic hypercapnia: The influence of chloride and potassium intake during administration of diuretics. Scand J Clin Lab Invest 31: 159–164

112. Hamilton RD, Crockett RJ, Alpers JH (1978) Arterial blood gas analysis: Potential errors due to the addition of heparin. Anaesth Intensive Care 6: 251–255

113. Hansen AC, Wamberg S, Engel K, Kildeberg P (1979) Balance of net base in the rat: Adaptation to and recovery from sustained hypercapnia. Scand J Clin Lab Invest 39: 723–730

114. Hansen JE, Simons DH (1977) A systematic error in the determination of blood PCO_2. Am Rev Resp Dis 115: 1061–1063

115. Hansen JE, Stone ME, Ong ST, Van Kessel AL (1982) Evaluation of blood gas quality control and proficiency testing materials by tonometry. Am Rev Resp Dis 125: 480–483

116. Hare JW, Rossini AA (1979) Diabetic comas: The overlap concept. Hosp Pract 14: 95–108

117. Harrington JT (1982) Evaluation of serum and urinary electrolytes. Hosp Pract 17: 28–39

118. Hedley-White J, Laver MB (1964) O_2 solubility in blood and temperature correction factors for PO_2. J Appl Physiol 196: 901–906

119. Hellung-Larsen P, Kjeldsen K, Mellemgaard K, Astrup P (1966) Photometric determination of oxyhemoglobin saturation in the presence of carbon monoxide hemoglobin, especially at low oxygen tensions. Scand J Clin Lab Invest 18: 443–449

120. Hilpert P, Fleischmann RG, Kempe D, Bartels H (1963) The Bohr effect related to blood and erythrocyte pH. Am J Physiol 205: 337–340

121. Humes HD, Narins RG, Brenner BM (1979) Disorders of water balance. Hosp Pract 14: 113–145

122. Johnson JJ (1975) Neonatal hemolytic jaundice. N Engl J Med 292: 194–197

123. Hulter HN, Sigala JF, Sabastian A (1978) K^+ deprivation potentiates the renal alkalosis-producing effect of mineralocorticoid. Am J Physiol 235: F298–F309

124. Karselis TC (1982) Electrolyte instrumentation: Then and now. Am J Med Technol 48: 329–335

125. Kassirer JP (1974) Serious acid-base disorders. N Engl J Med 291: 773–776

126. Kassirer JP, Bleich HL (1965) Rapid estimation of plasma carbon dioxide tension from pH and total carbon dioxide content. N Engl J Med 272: 1067–1068

127. Kassirer JP, Madias N (1980) Respiratory acid-base disorders. Hosp Pract 15: 57–71

128. Kassirer JP, Schwartz WB (1966) The response of normal man to selective depletion of hydrochloric acid. Am J Med 40: 10–18

129. Kazushige L, Isao I, Tosio O, Hiroko H, Junko S, Kunio K, Huichi K (1987) Radioimmunoassay of atrial natriuretic polypeptide in heat treated human plasma. Clin Chem 33(5): 674–676

130. Keshgegian AA (1980) Anion gap and immunoglobin concentration. Am J Clin Pathol 74: 282–286

131. Key A (1974) Non-linearity of in vitro blood PO_2 measurements. Biomeg Eng 9: 154–156

132. Kirschbaum TH, Dehaven JC, Shapiro N, Assali NS (1966) Oxyhemoglobin dissociation characteristics of human and sheep maternal and fetal blood. Am J Obstet Gynecol 96: 741–759

133. Kleeman CR (1979) CNS manifestations of disordered salt and water balance. Hosp Pract 14: 59–73

134. Kokko JP (1979) Renal concentrating and diluting mechanisms. Hosp Pract 14: 110–116

135. Kreisberg RA (1977) Phosphorus deficiency and hypophosphatemia. Hosp Pract 12: 121–128

136. Kreisberg RA (1978) Diabetic ketoacidosis: New concepts and trends in pathogenesis and treatment. Arch Intern Med 88: 681–695

137. Kurtzman NA (1982) Chronic renal failure: metabolic and clinical consequences. Hosp Pract 17: 107–122

138. Kwarecki K, Debiec H, Koter Z (1980) Rhythms of electrolytes and hydroxyproline excretion in urine of rats after three weeks of weightlessness. The Physiologist 23: S34–S37

139. Ladenson JH, Lewis JW, Boyd JC (1978) Failure of total calcium corrected for protein, albumen, and pH to correctly assess free calcium status. J Clin Endocrinol Metab 46: 986–993

140. Lane EE, Walker J (ed) (1987) Clinical Arterial Blood Gas Analysis. Mosby, St Louis

141. Lawson WH (1966) Interrelation of pH, temperature, and oxygen on deoxygenation rate of red cells. J Appl Physiol 21: 905–914

142. Lennon EJ, Lemann J (1966) Defense of hydrogen ion concentration in chronic metabolic acidosis. Ann Intern Med 65: 265–274

143. Levitin H, Amick CJ, Epstein FH (1961) Response of tissue electrolytes to respiratory acidosis. Am J Physiol 200: 1151–1154

144. Levitin H, Epstein FH (1961) Effects of potassium deficiency on renal response to respiratory acidosis. Am J Physiol 200: 1148–1150

145. Lim VS, Katz AI (1976) Acid-base regulation in pregnancy. Am J Physiol 231: 1764–1770

146. Lockwood AH (1980) Adaptation to hyperosmolality in the rat. Brain Research 200: 216–219

147. Loeb JN (1974) The hyperosmolar state. N Engl J Med 290: 1184–1187

148. Lott JA, Bibbey D (1980) Determination of pH, PCO_2, and PO_2 on whole blood: Steps to maximize accuracy. Lab Med 11: 455–461

149. McCarron DA, Elliott WC, Rose JS, Bennett WM (1979) Severe mixed metabolic acidosis secondary to rhabdomyolysis. Am J Med 67: 905–908

150. MacDonald FM (1965) Respiratory alkalosis. Arch Intern Med 116: 689–698

151. McLean FC, Hastings AB (1935) The state of calcium in the fluids of the body. J Biol Chem 108: 285–322

152. Madias NE, Carlos Ayus J, Adrogue HJ (1979) Increased anion gap in metabolic alkalosis. The role of plasma-protein equivalency. N Engl J Med 300: 1421–1423

153. Madias NE, Adrogue HJ, Cohen JJ, Schwartz WB (1979) Effect of natural variations in $PaCO_2$ on plasma $[HCO_3]$ in dogs: A redefinition of normal. Am J Physiol 236: F30–F35

154. Madias NE, Adrogue HJ (1983) Influence of chronic metabolic acid base disorders on the acute CO_2 titration curve. J Appl Physiol 55: 1187–1195

155. Malan A (1977) Blood acid-base state at a variable temperature. A graphical representation. Resp Physiol 31: 259–275

156. Malan A, Arens H, Waechter A (1973) Pulmonary respiration and acid-base state in hibernating marmots and hamsters. Resp Physiol 17: 45–61

157. Marks CE, Goldring RA, Becchione JJ, Gordon EE (1973) Cerebrospinal fluid acid-base relationships in ketoacidosis and lactic acidosis. J Appl Physiol 35: 813–819

158. Masaro EJ (1982) An overview of hydrogen ion regulation. Arch Intern Med 142: 1019–1023

159. Mercier DE, Feld RD, Witte DL (1978) Comparison of dewpoint and freezing point osmometry. Am J Med Technol 44: 1066–1069

160. Metzger G, Kenny M (1987) Temperature dependent results with the ChemPro-1000. Clin Chem 33: 443

161. Michell AR (1970) Protons, pH, and survival. J Am Vet Med Assoc 157: 1540–1548

162. Mitnick P, Greenberg A, Coffman T, Kelepouris E, Wolf CJ, Goldfarb S (1982) Effects of two models of hypercalcemia on renal acid base metabolism. Kidney Int 21: 613–620

163. Moore-Ede MC, Herd JA (1977) Renal electrolyte circadian rhythm: Independence from feeding and activity patterns. Am J Physiol 232: F128–F135

164. Morrill CG, Meyer JR, Weil JV (1975) Hypoxic ventilatory depression in dogs. J Appl Physiol 38: 143–146

165. Moses AM, Miller M (1974) Drug-induced dilutional hyponatremia. N Engl J Med 291: 1234–1238

166. Mueller RG, Lang GE (1982) Blood gas analysis: Effect of air bubbles in syringe and delay in estimation. Brit Med J 285: 1659–1660

167. Mueller RG, Lang GE, Gordon E, Beam JM (1976) Bubbles in samples for blood gas determinations. Am J Clin Path 65: 242–249

168. Mueller RG, Lang GE, Daskam JM, Lewis PJ (1975) Phase equilibria of oxygen in blood-gas control samples. Clin Chem 21: 165–166

169. Mulhausen RO, Blumentals AS (1965) Metabolic alkalosis. Arch Intern Med 116: 729–728

170. Munson ES, Gillespie JR, Wagman IH (1970) Respiratory blood gases and pH in two species of unanesthetized monkeys. J Appl Physiol 28: 108–109

171. Murray JF (1969) Acid-base balance. J Am Vet Med Assoc 154: 528–530

172. Murray JF (1979) Uniform requirements for manuscripts submitted to biomedical journals. Am Rev Resp Dis 119: 3–10

173. Nadiminti Y, Wang JC, Chou SY, Pineles E, Tobin MS (1980) Lactic acidosis associated with Hodgkin's disease. N Engl J Med 303: 15–17

174. Naik DV, Valtin H (1969) Hereditary vasopressin-resistant urinary concentrating defects in mice. Am J Physiol 217: 1183–1190

175. Nandrup E (1958) Metabolic changes in acid-base equilibrium during operation and anesthesia. Scand J Clin Lab Invest 10: 346–347

176. Nanji AA, Blank D (1982) Spurious increases in anion gap due to exposure of serum to air. N Engl J Med 307: 190–191

177. Narins RG, Jones ER, Stom MC, Rudnick MR, Bastil CP (1972) Diagnostic strategies in disorders of fluid, electrolyte and acid-base homeostasis. Am J Med 72: 496–520

178. Narins RG, Rudnick MR, Bastl CP (1980) Lactic acidosis and the elevated anion gap. II. Hosp Pract 15: 91–98

179. Narins RG, Rudnick MR, Bastl CP (1980) Lactic acidosis and the elevated anion gap. I. Hosp Pract 15: 125–136

180. Needle MA, Kalovanides GJ, Schwartz WB (1964) The effects of selective depletion of hydrochloric acid on acid-base and electrolyte equilibrium. J Clin Invest 43: 1836–1846

181. Newsholme EA, Start C (1973) Regulation in Metabolism. John Wiley & Sons, London

182. Ng RH (1987) Temperature dependent results with ChemPro-1000. Clin Chem 33: 444

183. Nixon DE, Moyer TP, Johnson P, McCall JT, Ness AB, Fjerstad WH, Wehde MB (1986) Routine measurement of calcium, magnesium, copper, zinc and iron in urine and serum by inductivity coupled plasma emission spectroscopy. Clin Chem 32: 1660–1664

184. Noonan DC, Burnett RW (1974) Quality-control system for blood pH and gas measurements with use of tonometered bicarbonate-chloride solution and duplicate samples of whole blood. Clin Chem 20: 660–665

185. Norden AGW, Flynn FV (1979) Halothane interference with PO_2 measurements and a method of inhibiting its effects. Clin Chim Acta 99: 229–234

186. Norman JN, Douglas TA, Smith G (1966) Respiratory and metabolic changes during carbon monoxide poisoning. J Appl Physiol 21: 848–852

187. Nuttall FQ (1965) Serum electrolytes and their relation to acid-base balance. Arch Intern Med 116: 670–680

188. Nuttall FQ (1965) Metabolic acidosis-diabetic. Arch Intern Med 116: 709–716

189. Oh MS, Phelps KR, Traube M, Barbosa-Saldivar JL, Boxhill C, Carrill HJ (1979) D-lactic acidosis in a man with the short-bowel syndrome. N Engl J Med 301: 249–251

190. Oliva PB (1970) Lactic acidosis. Am J Med 48: 209–225

191. O'Regan S, Carson S, Chesney RW, Drummond KN (1977) Electrolyte and acid-base disturbances in the management of leukemia. Blood 49: 345–353

192. Orringer CE, Eustace JC, Wunsch CD, Gardner LB (1977) Natural history of lactic acidosis after grandmal seizures. A model for the study of an anion-gap acidosis not associated with hyperkalemia. N Engl J Med 297: 796–799

193. Oster JR, Perez GO, Vaamonde CA (1978) Relationship between blood pH and potassium and phosphorus during acute metabolic acidosis. Am J Physiol 235: F345–F351

194. Paladini G, Sala PG (1979) Anion gap in multiple myeloma. Acta Hematol 62: 148–152

195. Pandian MR (1986) Atrial natriuretic peptide. Clin Chem News 12: 14

196. Parker JT (1967) The O_2 dissociation curve of blood of the rhesus monkey (*Macaca mulatta*). Resp Physiol 2: 168–172

197. Payne RB, Carver ME, Morgan DB (1979) Interpretation of serum total calcium: Effects of adjustment for albumin concentrations on frequency of abnormal values and on detection of change in the individual. J Clin Pathol 32: 56–60

198. Pfohl RA (1965) The kidney in acid-base balance. Arch Intern Med 116: 681–688

199. Piernan S, Roizen MF, Severinghaus JW (1979) Oxygen analyser dangerous-senses nitrous oxide as battery fails. Anaesthesiology 50: 146–149

200. Plant SB, McCarron DA (1952) Effects of sample freezing on ion-selective electrode determinations of serum calcium. Clin Chem 28: 1362–1363

201. Pog'atsa G, Dubecz E (1978) The influence of hyperosmolality on heart function. Experientia 34: 1600–1601

202. Polak A, Haynie GD, Hays RM, Schwartz WB (1961) Effect of chronic hypercapnia on electrolyte and acid-base equilibrium. I. Adaptation. J Clin Invest 40: 1223–1237

203. Polak A, Haynie GD, Hays RM, Schwartz WB (1961) Effects of chronic hypercapnia on electrolyte and acid-base equilibrium. II. Recovery, with special reference to the influence of chloride intake. J Clin Invest 40: 1238–1249

204. Pollak VE, Mattenheimer H, De Bruin H, Weinman KJ (1965) Experimental metabolic acidosis: The

enzymatic basis of ammonia production. J Clin Invest 44: 169–181

205. Poole-Wilson PA, Cameron IA (1975) Intracellular pH and K^+ of cardiac and skeletal muscle in acidosis and alkalosis. Am J Physiol 289: 1305–1310

206. Rahn H (1974) PCO_2, pH and body temperature. In Nahas GG, Schaefer KE (eds), Carbon Dioxide and Metabolic Regulation. Springer-Verlag, New York

207. Rahn H, Garey WF (1973) Arterial CO_2, O_2, pH, and HCO_3 values of ectotherms living in the Amazon. Am J Physiol 225: 735–738

208. Raisz LG, Mundy GR, Dietrich W, Canalis EM (1977) Hormonal regulation of mineral metabolism. Inter Rev Physiol 16: 199–240

209. Ramsey DJ, Ganong WF (1977) CNS regulation of salt and water intake. Hosp Pract 12: 63–69

210. Rand PW, Norton JM, Barker ND, Lovell MD, Austin WII (1973) Responses to graded hypoxia at high and low 2,3-diphosphoglycerate concentrations. J Appl Physiol 34: 827–832

211. Randall IIT (1976) Fluid, electrolyte, and acid-base balance. Surg Clin NA 56: 1019–1057

212. Rasmussen H (1970) Cell communication, calcium ion, and cyclic adenosine monophosphate. Science 170: 404–412

213. Rector FC, Cogan MG (1980) The renal acidoses. Hosp Pract 15: 99–111

214. Reeves RB (1978) Temperature and acid-base balance effects on oxygen transport by human blood. Resp Physiol 33: 99–102

215. Relman AS (1972) Metabolic consequences of acid-base disorders. Kidney Int 1: 347–359

216. Riggs TE, Shafer AW, Guenter CA (1973) Acute changes in oxyhemoglobin affinity: Effects on oxygen transport and utilization. J Clin Invest 52: 2660–2663

217. Rippin SJ, Elston DJ, Fuller BC, Geary TD (1978) Source of error in use of the Corning 175 Blood-Gas Analyser. Clin Chem 24: 722

218. Rodkey WG, Hannon JP, Dramise JG, White RD, Welsh DC, Persky BN (1978) Arterialized capillary blood used to determine the acid-base and blood gas of dogs. Am J Vet Res 39: 459–464

219. Rogers N, Laver M, Pain MC (1968) Oxygen electrode calibration. Med J Aust 2: 585–587

220. Rosenthal TB (1948) The effect of temperature on the pH of blood and plasma in vitro. J Biol Chem 173: 25–30

221. Rossing RG, Cain SM (1966) A nomogram relating PO_2, pH, temperature, and hemoglobin saturation in the dog. J Appl Physiol 21: 195–201

222. Rossini AA, Galway CW (1977) Hyperosmolar nonketotic coma. Compr Ther 3: 29–36

223. Rorth M, Nygaard SF, Parving H-H, Hansen V, Kalsig T (1973) Human red cell metabolism and in vivo oxygen affinity of red cells during 24 hours' exposure to simulated high altitude (4500 m). Scand J Clin Lab Invest 31: 447–452

224. Roughton FJW, Severinghaus JW (1973) Accurate determination of O_2 dissociation curve of human blood above 98.7 per cent saturation with data on O_2 solubility in unmodified human blood from 0 to 37°C J Appl Physiol 31: 865–869

225. Russell CD, Hoeher HD, Deland EC, Maloney JV (1978) Acute response to acid-base stress. Ann Surg 187: 417–422

226. Sachs C (1987) More on determination of ionized calcium in blood with ion selective electrodes. Clin Chem 33: 445

227. Said SI, Yoshida T, Kitamura S, Vreim C (1974) Pulmonary alveolar hypoxia: Release of prostaglandins and other humoral mediators. Science 185: 1181–1182

228. Schade DS, Eaton RP (1975) Modulation of fatty acid metabolism by glucagon in man. I. Effects in normal subjects. Diabetes 24: 502–509

229. Schmidt RW (1978) Effects of phosphate depletion on acid-base status in dogs. Metabolism 27: 943–952

230. Schwartz WB, Brackett NC, Cohen JJ (1965) The response of extracellular hydrogen ion concentration to graded degrees of chronic hypercapnia: The physiologic limits of the defense of pII. J Clin Invest 44: 291–301

231. Schwartz WB, Cohen JJ (1978) The nature of the renal response to chronic disorders of acid-base equilibrium. Am J Med 64: 417–428

232. Schwartz WB, Lemieux G, Falbriard A (1959) The physiological significance of renal bicarbonate reabsorption during acute respiratory alkalosis. J Clin Invest 38: 2197–2202

233. Schwartz WB, Van Ypersele DE, Stihou C, Kassirer JP (1968) Role of anions in metabolic alkalosis and potassium deficiency. N Engl J Med 279: 630–639

234. Sehy JT, Roseman MK, Arruda JAL, Kurtzman NA (1978) Characterization of distal hydrogen ion secretion in acute respiratory alkalosis. Am J Physiol 235: F203–F208

235. Seal US (1965) The chemistry of buffers. Arch Intern Med 116: 658–664

236. Severinghaus JW, Weiskopf RB, Nishimura M, Bradley AF (1971) Oxygen electrode errors due to polarographic reduction of halothane. J Appl Physiol 31: 640–642

237. Sharpe S, Llino L (1986) Two indirect tests of exocrine pancreatic function evaluated. Clin Chem 33: 5–10

238. Shrout JB (1982) Controlling the quality of blood gas results. Am J Med Technol 48: 347–351

239. Siggaard Andersen O (1960) A graphic representation of changes of the acid base status. Scand J Clin Lab Invest 12: 311–314

240. Siggaard Andersen O (1961) Factors affecting the liquid-junction potential in electrometric blood pH measurement. Scand J Clin Lab Invest 13: 205–211

241. Siggaard Andersen O (1961) Acute experimental acid-base disturbances in dogs. Scand J Clin Lab Invest 14: 1–20 (suppl 66)

242. Siggaard Andersen O (1962) The pH-log CO_2 blood acid-base nomogram revised. Scand J Clin Lab Invest 14: 1–7

243. Siggaard Andersen O (1979) Hydrogen ions and blood gases. In Brown SS, Mitchell FL, Young DS (eds), Chemical Diagnosis of Disease. Elsevier/North Holland Biomedical Press, Amsterdam

244. Siggaard Andersen O (1974) The Acid-Base Status of the Blood, 4th ed. Williams & Wilkins, Baltimore

245. Siggaard Andersen O, Jorgensen K, Naera N (1962) Spectrophotometric determination of oxygen saturation in capillary blood. Scand J Clin Lab Invest 14: 298–302

246. Smithline N, Gardner KD (1976) Gaps—anion and osmolal. JAMA 236: 1594–1597

247. Spencer J, Kibachi A (1983) Lethargy and vomiting after insulin thawed. Hosp Pract 18: 100A–100H

248. Spinner MB, Petersen GK (1961) Determining the pH of a phosphate buffer solution for blood measurements. Scand J Clin Lab Invest 13: 1–7

249. Streng WH, Huber HE, Carstensen JT (1978) Relationship between osmolality and osmolarity. J Pharm Sci 67: 384–386

250. Stewart PA (1978) Independent and dependent variables of acid-base control. Resp Physiol 33: 9–26

251. Sussman KE, Alfrey A, Krisch WM, Zweig P, Felig P, Messner F (1970) Chronic lactic acidosis in an adult. A new syndrome associated with an altered redox state of certain NAD/NADH coupled reactions. Am J Med 48: 104–112

252. Tarail R, Elkinton JRK (1949) Potassium deficiency and the role of the kidney in its production. J Clin Invest 28: 99–113

253. Takano N, Lever MJ, Lambertsen CJ (1979) Acid-base curve nomogram for chimpanzee blood and comparison with human blood characteristics. J Appl Physiol 46: 381–386

254. Takedo N, Toshimitsu N, Takematsu A, Suzuki M (1987) Identification and quantification of protein-bound ligand in uremic serum. Clin Chem 33: 682–685

255. Tannen RL (1978) Ammonia metabolism. Am J Physiol 235: F265–F277

256. Tachijian AH, Voelkel EF, Levine L, Goldhaber P (1972) Evidence that the bone resorption stimulating factor produced by mouse fibrosarcoma cells is prostaglandin E2: A new model for the hypercalcemia of cancer. J Exp Med 136:1329–1343

257. Tietz NW (ed) (1976) Fundamentals of Clinical Chemistry, 2nd ed. Saunders, Philadelphia

258. Todd EP, Vick RL (1971) Kalemotropic effect of epinephrine: Analysis with adrenergic agonists and antagonists. Am J Physiol 220: 1964–1969

259. Trippoda NC, Kardon MB, Pegram BL, Cole FE, MacPhee AA (1966) Acute haemodynamic effects of the atrial natriuretic hormone in rats. J Hypertension 4: S35–S40

260. Travis SF, Morrison AD, Clements RS, Winegrad AI, Osk A (1971) Metabolic alterations in the human erythrocyte produced by increases in glucose concentration. J Clin Invest 50: 2104–2112

261. Truchot JP (1973) Temperature and acid-base regulation in the shore crab Carcinus maenas (L). Resp Physiol 17: 11–20

262. Van Kampen EJ (1979) Interparametric quality control in acid-base balance. In Maas AHJ (ed), Blood pH and Gases. University Press, Utrecht

263. Van Kessel AL (1979) The bloodgas laboratory. An update. Lab Med 10: 419–429

264. Van Leeuwen AM (1964) Net cation equivalency ("base binding power") of the plasma proteins. Acta Med Scand 176, (suppl 242)

265. Van Slyke DD, Hastings AB, Hiller A, Sendroy J (1928) Studies of gas and electrolyte equilibria in blood. XIV. The amounts of alkali bound by serum albumin and globulin. J Biol Chem 79: 769–780

266. Van Stekelenburg GJ (1970) The influence of temperature changes on the PO_2 of normal anaerobic blood samples. Resp Physiol 8: 245–259

267. Voelkel EF, Tashijian AH, Franklin R, Wasserman E, Levine L (1975) Hypercalcemia and tumor-prostaglandins: The VX2 carcinoma model in the rabbit. Metabolism 24: 973–986

268. Wamberg S, Engel K, Kildberg P (1983) Corticotropin-induced alkalosis in the weanling rat and its relation to the balance of non-metabolizable base. Scand J Clin Lab Invest 43: 73–83

269. de Wardener HE (1978) The control of sodium excretion. Am J Physiol 235: F163–F173

270. Wasserman K, Whipp BJ, Casaburi R, Huntsman DJ, Castagna J, Lugliani R (1975) Regulation of arterial PCO_2 during intravenous CO_2 loading. J Appl Physiol 38: 651–656

271. Wathen RL, Ward RA, Harding GB, Meyer LC (1982) Acid-base responses to anion infusion in the anesthetized dog. Kidney Int 21: 592–599

272. Weil MH, Michaels S, Klein D (1982) Measurement of whole blood osmolality. Am J Clin Pathol 77: 447–448

273. Weisbrot IM, Vijaykant BK, Gorton L (1974) An evaluation of clinical laboratory performance of pH-blood gas analysis using whole-blood tonometer specimens. Am J Clin Pathol 61: 923–935

274. Weiskopf RB, Gabel RA, Fenci V (1976) Alkaline shift in lumbar and intracranial CSF in man after 5 days at high altitude. J Appl Physiol 41: 93–97

275. Weitzman R, Kleeman CR (1980) Water metabolism and the neurohypophyseal hormones. In Maxwell MH, Kleeman CR (eds), Clinical Disorders of Fluid and Electrolyte Metabolism. McGraw-Hill, New York

276. Welbourne TC (1976) Acidosis activation of the pituitary-adrenal-renal glutaminase I axis. Endocrinology 99: 1071–1079

277. Wilson RF (1978) Get the venous blood too. Am Surg 44: 396–400

278. Winters RW (1967) Studies of acid-base disturbances. Pediatrics 39: 700–712

279. Winters RW, Some comments on the validity of the Astrup technique for the measurement of acid-base status of blood. Technical Publication 36, Radiometer, Copenhagen

280. Wise WC (1973) Normal arterial blood gases and chemical components in the unanesthetized dog. J Appl Physiol 35: 427–429

281. Yawata Y, Craddock P, Hebbel R, Howe R, Silvis S, Jacob H (1973) Hyperalimentation hypophosphatemia: Hematologic-neurologic dysfunction due to ATP depletion. Clin Res 21: 729

282. Young DS (1975) "Normal laboratory values" (Case Records of the Massachusetts General Hospital) in SI units. N Engl J Med 292: 795–802

283. Young DS (1979) Biological variability. In Brown SS, Mitchell FL, Young DS (eds), Chemical Diagnosis of Disease, Elsevier/North Holland Biomedical Press, Amsterdam, pp 1–113

284. Zborowska-Sluis DT, Dossetor JB (1967) Hyperlactemia of hyperventilation. J Appl Physiol 22: 746–755

285. Zweens J, Frankena H, Van Kampen EJ, Rispens P, Zijlstra WG (1977) Ionic composition of arterial and mixed venous plasma in the unanesthetized dog. Am J Physiol 233: F412–F415

286. Zwillich CW, Pierson DJ, Creagh EM, Weil JV (1976) Effects of hypocapnia and hypocapnic alkalosis on cardiovascular function. J Appl Physiol 40: 333–337

Appendix
Reference Values for
Clinical Chemical Analytes

GLUCOSE

SPECIES	SEX/AGE	SAMPLE	NUMBER	METHOD	MEAN	UNITS	S.D.	REF.
<u>Mouse CD-1</u>	M 20-22g		6		278	mg/dl	14	21
CD-1	M 20-22g		6		245	mg/dl	30	21
A/HeJ	M 20-22g		6		235	mg/dl	9	21
A/HeJ	M 20-22g		6		201	mg/dl	17	21
C3H/HeJ	M 20-22g		6		252	mg/dl	18	21
C3H/HeJ	M 20-22g		6		232	mg/dl	7	21
C3H/HeN	M 20-22g		6		202	mg/dl	9	21
C3H/HeN	M 20-22g		6		197	mg/dl	10	21
C57BL/6 x DBA/2 F$_1$	M 45 d	Cardiac	561	o-Toluidine	196	mg/dl	32	42
<u>Rat (CRL: COBS CD (SD) BR)</u>	M 4 mos		42		83	mg/dl	14.1	75
CRL: COBS CD (SD) BR	F 4 mos		40		80	mg/dl	12.7	75
CRL: COBS CD (SD) BR	M 7 mos		45		94	mg/dl	12.5	75
CRL: COBS CD (SD) BR	F 7 mos		45		89	mg/dl	15.4	75
CRL: COBS CD (SD) BR	M 13 mos		40		102	mg/dl	14.9	75
CRL: COBS CD (SD) BR	F 13 mos		40		93	mg/dl	9.7	75
CRL: COBS CD (SD) BR	M 19 mos		40		96	mg/dl	13.2	75
CRL: COBS CD (SD) BR	F 19 mos		40		84	mg/dl	9.7	75
CRL: COBS CD (SD) BR	M 25 mos		62		90	mg/dl	14.9	75
CRL: COBS CD (SD) BR	F 25 mos		66		93	mg/dl	10.2	75
CD (CRL: CD (SD) BR)	M 6-8 wks	Cardiac	20	Glucose Oxidase	245	mu/ml	77	27
CD (CRL: CD (SD) BR)	F 6-8 wks	Cardiac	20	Glucose Oxidase	226	mu/ml	89	27
CD (CRL: CD (SD) BR)	M 19-21 wks	Cardiac	20	Glucose Oxidase	196	mu/ml	96	27
CD (CRL: CD (SD) BR)	F 19-21 wks	Cardiac	20	Glucose Oxidase	225	mu/ml	76	27
CD (CRL: CD (SD) BR)	M 32-34 wks	Cardiac	20	Glucose Oxidase	267	mu/ml	120	27
CD (CRL: CD (SD) BR)	F 32-34 wks	Cardiac	20	Glucose Oxidase	247	mu/ml	150	27
Pooled age and strain	M		66	Hycel	215.7	mgs %	46.7	68
Pooled age and strain	F		60	Hycel	160.5	mgs %	45.2	68
SD	M Cardiac			SMAC	152.4			75
SD	F Cardiac			SMAC	157.6			75
Sprague-Dawley - CD	M 30-91 d	Orbital	30	MCA	148.74	mg/dl	10.56	93
Sprague-Dawley - CD	M 30-91 d	Cardiac	70	MCA	268.20	mg/dl	87.64	93

Glucose (cont.)

SPECIES	AGE/SEX	SAMPLE	NUMBER	METHOD	MEAN	UNITS	S.D.	REF.
Rat (cont.)								
Sprague-Dawley – CD	F 30–91 d	Orbital	30	MCA	143.10	mg/dl	15.30	93
Sprague-Dawley – CD	F 30–91 d	Cardiac	69	MCA	237.89	mg/dl	77.74	93
Sprague-Dawley – CD	M 92–182 d	Orbital	20	MCA	134.27	mg/dl	8.31	93
Sprague-Dawley – CD	M 92–182 d	Cardiac	55	MCA	242.23	mg/dl	87.62	93
Sprague-Dawley – CD	F 92–182 d	Orbital	19	MCA	133.52	mg/dl	11.15	93
Sprague-Dawley – CD	F 92–182 d	Cardiac	55	MCA	247.53	mg/dl	78.45	93
Sprague-Dawley – CD	M 183–273 d	Orbital	10	MCA	128.72	mg/dl	7.39	93
Sprague-Dawley – CD	M 183–273 d	Cardiac	10	MCA	133.40	mg/dl	9.85	93
Sprague-Dawley – CD	F 183–273 d	Orbital	10	MCA	125.55	mg/dl	13.34	93
Sprague-Dawley – CD	F 183–273 d	Cardiac	10	MCA	131.48	mg/dl	11.26	93
Sprague-Dawley – CD	M 274–450 d	Orbital	10	MCA	125.08	mg/dl	10.81	93
Sprague-Dawley – CD	F 274–450 d	Orbital	10	MCA	114.80	mg/dl	12.07	93
Hamster (Golden) Syrian								
Lak: LVG	M 3 mos/100g	Cardiac–fasted	31	Hexokinase	120.9	mg/dl	33.7	81
Lak: LVG	F 3 mos/100g	Cardiac–fasted	32	Hexokinase	134	mg/dl	37.6	81
B$_{10}$F$_1$D Alexander	M 3 mos/100g	Cardiac–fasted	30	Hexokinase	124	mg/dl	31.3	81
B$_{10}$F$_1$D Alexander	F 3 mos/100g	Cardiac–fasted	30	Hexokinase	104	mg/dl	25.0	81
Syrian	M 50g				117	mg/dl	17.9	120
Syrian	F 50g				105	mg/dl	23.1	120
Syrian	M 100g				84	mg/dl	18.5	34
Syrian	F 100g				100	mg/dl	16.6	34
Syrian	F/M 2½–4 mos	24 hr fasted	25		123	mg/dl	62.7	120
Syrian	F/M 2–5 mos		138		73.4	mg/dl	20.3	120
Syrian	M 75–100g		84		73.4	mg/dl	12.6	86
Syrian	F 75–100g		80		65.0	mg/dl	10.5	86
Syrian	M Mature				144.8	mg/dl	7.7	120

Glucose (cont.)

SPECIES	SEX/AGE	SAMPLE	NUMBER	METHOD	MEAN	UNITS	S.D.	REF.
Guinea Pig – Hartley	M 500–800g		110		95.3	mg/dl	11.9	86
Hartley	F 500–800g		85		89.0	mg/dl	9.60	86
Rabbit (Oryctolagus cuniculus)	M		120		120.5	mg/dl	15.5	46
Oryctolagus cuniculus	M				144	mg/dl	11	66
Oryctolagus cuniculus	M				129	mg/dl	15	66
Oryctolagus cuniculus	F		120		120.2	mg/dl	10.3	46
Oryctolagus cuniculus	F				135	mg/dl	15	66
Oryctolagus cuniculus	F				126	mg/dl	13	66
Rabbit (Pooled age & strain)	M		109	Hycel	112.0	mgs %	31.9	68
(Pooled age & strain)	F		113	Hycel	113.4	mgs %	31.6	68
Canine Breed not specified	M 150–350 d	Jugular vein	394	MCA	96.6	mg/dl	15.05	93
Breed not specified	F 150–350 d	Jugular vein	386	MCA	97.4	mg/dl	8.35	93
(Pooled over breed, age, reproductive status)	M	57		Hycel	100.1	mgs %	23.5	68
(Pooled over breed, age, reproductive status)	F	54		Hycel	109.8	mgs %	33.0	68
Non-human primates								
Pan troglodytes			223–224		78	mg/dl	16.3	82
Pongo pygmaeus			89–92		78	mg/dl	17.0	84
Gorilla gorilla			44		79	mg/dl	12.3	83
Papio sp.			12		121	mg/dl	20.8	20
Cercopithecus aethiops			40–102		104	mg/dl	23.6	5
Cercocebus atys			39–71		86	mg/dl	31.6	5
Presbytis entillis			34–60		107	mg/dl	20.4	5
Saimiri sciureus			41–44		80	mg/dl	28.0	9, 77
Aotus trivirgatus			43–75		113	mg/dl	40.0	128
Saguinus fusicollis or nigricollis			49–95		228	mg/dl	59.0	56
Saguinus oedipus			13–40		157	mg/dl	31.5	56

Glucose (cont.)

SPECIES	SEX/AGE	SAMPLE	NUMBER	METHOD	MEAN	UNITS	S.D.	REF.
Non-human primates (cont.)								
Macaca mulatta			20–253		70	mg/dl	17.0	11
Macaca mulatta			867		73.4	mg/dl		75
Macaca mulatta (Pooled age and sex)			20	Hycel	70.1	mg/dl	17.2	68
Macaca fascicularis	M Adult	Venous or arterial-fasted	33	Glucose Oxidase	59	mg/dl	10.3	122
Macaca arctoides	M Adult	Venous or arterial-fasted	7	Glucose Oxidase	51	mg/dl	4.9	122

ALKALINE PHOSPHATASE

SPECIES	SEX/AGE	SAMPLE	NUMBER	METHOD	MEAN	UNITS	S.D.	REF.
Mouse								
CD-1	M 20–22 g		6		207	IU/L	9	21
CD-1	M 20–22 g		6		171	IU/L	3	21
A/HeJ	M 20–22 g		6		171	IU/L	3	21
A/HeJ	M 20–22 g		6		226	IU/L	3	21
C3H/HeJ	M 20–22 g		6		262	IU/L	4	21
C3H/HeJ	M 20–22 g		6		258	IU/L	2	21
C3H/HeN	M 20–22 g		6		177	IU/L	3	21
C3H/HeN	M 20–22 g		6		184	IU/L	10	21
C57BL/6 x DBA/2 F$_1$	M 45 d	Cardiac	574	p–Nitrophenyl phosphate	66	IU/L	19	42
Rat (pooled age and strain)	M		66	Hycel	18.3	U	6.5	68
(pooled age and strain)	F		60	Hycel	14.5	U	6.6	68
(CD (CRL: CD (SD) BR)	M 6–8 wks	Cardiac	20	Modified Bessey–Lowry & Brock	405	IU/L	116	27
CD (CRL: CD (SD) BR)	F 6–8 wks	Cardiac	20	Modified Bessey–Lowry & Brock	252	IU/L	110	27
CD (CRL: CD (SD) BR)	M 19–21 wks	Cardiac	20	Modified Bessey–Lowry & Brock	152	IU/L	106	27
CD (CRL: CD (SD) BR)	F 19–21 wks	Cardiac	20	Modified Bessey–Lowry & Brock	170	IU/L	94	27
CD (CRL: CD (SD) BR)	M 32–34 wks	Cardiac	20	Modified Bessey–Lowry & Brock	133	IU/L	96	27
CD (CRL: CD (SD) BR)	F 32–34 wks	Cardiac	20	Modified Bessey–Lowry & Brock	133	IU/L	134	27

Alkaline Phosphatase (cont.)

Rat (cont.)

SPECIES	SEX/AGE	SAMPLE	NUMBER	METHOD	MEAN	UNITS	S.D.	REF.
(CRL: COBS CD (SD) BR)	M 4 mos		40		151	mu/ml	47	75
(CRL: COBS CD (SD) BR)	F 4 mos		39		103	mu/ml	40	75
(CRL: COBS CD (SD) BR)	M 7 mos		40		127	mu/ml	37	75
(CRL: COBS CD (SD) BR)	F 7 mos		39		69	mu/ml	21	75
(CRL: COBS CD (SD) BR)	M 13 mos		40		106	mu/ml	23	75
(CRL: COBS CD (SD) BR)	F 13 mos		40		49	mu/ml	16	75
(CRL: COBS CD (SD) BR)	M 19 mos		40		124	mu/ml	29	75
(CRL: COBS CD (SD) BR)	F 19 mos		40		66	mu/ml	25	75
(CRL: COBS CD (SD) BR)	M 25 mos		64		101	mu/ml	34	75
(CRL: COBS CD (SD) BR)	F 25 mos		66		55	mu/ml	20	75
SD	M	Cardiac	10	SMAC	204.86			75
SD	F	Cardiac	10	SMAC	136.25			75
Sprague–Dawley – CD	M 30–91 d	Orbital	30	MCA	264.10	U/l	71.62	93
Sprague–Dawley – CD	M 30–91 d	Cardiac	70	MCA	201.34	U/l	70.48	93
Sprague–Dawley – CD	F 30–91 d	Orbital	30	MCA	181.55	U/l	55.73	93
Sprague–Dawley	F 30–91 d	Cardiac	69	MCA	144.48	U/l	54.36	93
Sprague–Dawley	M 92–182 d	Orbital	20	MCA	132.00	U/l	47.76	93
Sprague–Dawley	M 92–182 d	Cardiac	55	MCA	127.61	U/l	42.29	93
Sprague–Dawley	F 92–182 d	Orbital	19	MCA	96.87	U/l	33.15	93
Sprague–Dawley	F 92–182 d	Cardiac	55	MCA	94.74	U/l	36.86	93
Sprague–Dawley	M 183–273 d	Orbital	10	MCA	111.74	U/l	53.60	93
Sprague–Dawley	M 183–273 d	Cardiac	10	MCA	93.45	U/l	22.41	93
Sprague–Dawley	F 183–273 d	Orbital	10	MCA	70.58	U/l	23.50	93
Sprague–Dawley	F 183–273 d	Cardiac	10	MCA	63.47	U/l	25.31	93
Sprague–Dawley	M 274–450 d	Orbital	10	MCA	103.32	U/l	20.11	93
Sprague–Dawley	F 274–450 d	Orbital	10	MCA	74.97	U/l	24.61	93

Alkaline Phosphatase (cont.)

SPECIES	SEX/AGE	SAMPLE	NUMBER	METHOD	MEAN	UNITS	S.D.	REF.
Hamster (Golden) Syrian								
Lak: LVG	M 3 mos or 100g	Cardiac-fasted	18	P-nitro phenylphosphate	121	IU/L	17.2	81
Lak: LVG	F 3 mos or 100g	Cardiac-fasted	25	P-nitro phenylphosphate	143	IU/L	22.2	81
B10F1D Alexander	M 3 mos or 100g	Cardiac-fasted	21	P-nitro phenylphosphate	159	IU/L	16.5	81
B10F1D Alexander	F 3 mos or 100g	Cardiac-fasted	15	P-nitro phenylphosphate	202	IU/L	23.0	81
Syrian	M 3 mos/100g				8.0	IU/L	1.2	115
Syrian	M 3 mos/100g				17.5	IU/L	6.1	86
Syrian	F 3 mos/100g				9.8	IU/L	0.9	115
Syrian	F 3 mos/100g				15.4	IU/L	4.2	86
Guinea Pig – Hartley	M 500–800 g		110		74.2	IU/l	6.92	86
Hartley	F 500–800 g		85		65.8	IU/l	5.46	86
Rabbit (Oryctolagus cuniculus)								
Oryctolagus cuniculus (pooled age and strain)	M		120		13.8	IU	6.2	46
(pooled age and strain)	F		120		13.6	IU	6.1	46
NZW	M		109	Hycel	12.34	U	4.84	68
Dutch belted	F		113	Hycel	10.33	U	4.29	68
					4.90–15.6	K.A.		
					2.10–16.0	K.A.		
Polish					4.30–5.60	K.A.		
Canine Breed not specified	M 150–350 d	Jugular vein	394	MCA	44.3	u/l	16.25	93
Breed not specified	F 150–350 d	Jugular vein	386	MCA	43.4	u/l	17.05	93
Beagle			63		70		26	60
(pooled breed, age, reprod. status)	M		57	Hycel	17.8	U	13.4	68
(pooled breed, age, reprod. status)	F		54	Hycel	21.6	U	17.4	68

Alkaline Phosphatase (cont.)

SPECIES	SEX/AGE	SAMPLE	NUMBER	METHOD	MEAN	UNITS	S.D.	REF.
Non-human primates								
Macaca mulatta			428		149.2	mu/ml		75
Macaca fascicularis	M Adult	venous or arterial fasted	33	P-nitro phenylphosphate hydrolysis	127.0	mIU/ml	38.5	122
Macaca arctoides	M Adult	venous or arterial fasted	7	P-nitro phenylphosphate hydrolysis	205.0	mIU/ml	51.0	122
Macaca mulatta (pooled over age and sex)				Hycel	43.4	U	21.2	68

SERUM GLUTAMIC PYRUVIC TRANSAMINASE
SGPT (ALT)

SPECIES	SEX/AGE	SAMPLE	NUMBER	METHOD	MEAN	UNITS	S.D.	REF.
Mouse – CD-1								
CD-1	M 20–22g		6		100	IU/l	22	21
A/HeJ	M 20–22g		6		98	IU/l	21	21
A/HeJ	M 20–22g		6		131	IU/l	19	21
C3H/HeJ	M 20–22g		6		143	IU/l	40	21
C3H/HeJ	M 20–22g		6		118	IU/l	21	21
C3H/HeJ	M 20–22g		6		102	IU/l	20	21
C3H/HeJ	M 20–22g		6		138.7	IU/l	29	21
C3H/HeJ	M 20–22g		6		84	IU/l	15	21
B6C3F1	M 50 d		8		94.65	mu/ml	53	21
B6C3F1	F 50 d		6		90.50	mu/ml	47.7	21
B6C3F1	M 8 wks		5		189.0	mu/ml	89.9	75
B6C3F1	F 8 wks		5		121.6	mu/ml	121.2	75
B6C3F1	M 9 wks		8		94.6	mu/ml	74.6	75
B6C3F1	F 9 wks		6		39.0	mu/ml	55.7	75
B6C3F1	M 19 wks		8		389.6	mu/ml	380.5	75
B6C3F1	F 19 wks		9		62	mu/ml	23.4	75
C57BL/6 x DBA/2 F1	M 45 d	Cardiac	574	NADH	40	IU/l	14.0	42
Rats								
F344	M 8 wks		5		42.2	mu/ml	2.8	75
F344	F 8 wks		5		39.0	mu/ml	4.4	75
F344	M 9 wks		15		42.8	mu/ml	4.8	75
F344	F 9 wks		13		45.0	mu/ml	7.0	75
F344	M 10 wks		11		50.8	mu/ml	10.2	75
F344	F 10 wks		9		41.8	mu/ml	6.6	75
F344	M 19 wks		30		49.2	mu/ml	13.6	75
F344	F 19 wks		30		47.8	mu/ml	14.2	75
CD (CRL: CD (SD) BR)	M 6–8 wks	Cardiac	20	Kessler, Leon Delea & Cupiola	150	IU/l	74	27
CD (CRL: CD (SD) BR)	F 6–8 wks	Cardiac	20	Kessler, Leon Delea & Cupiola	132	IU/l	70	27
CD (CRL: CD (SD) BR)	M 19–21 wks	Cardiac	20	Kessler, Leon Delea & Cupiola	111	IU/l	72	27

SGPT (ALT) (cont.)

SPECIES	SEX/AGE	SAMPLE	NUMBER	METHOD	MEAN	UNITS	S.D.	REF.
Rats CD (CRL: CD (SD) BR)	F 19–21 wks	Cardiac	20	Kessler, Leon Delea & Cupiola	146	IU/l	116	27
CD (CRL: CD (SD) BR)	M 32–34 wks	Cardiac	20	Kessler, Leon Delea & Cupiola	153	IU/l	52	27
CD (CRL: CD (SD) BR)	F 32–34 wks	Cardiac	20	Kessler, Leon Delea & Cupiola	118	IU/l	66	27
SD	M 30–91 d	Orbital	30	MCA	37.18	U/l	6.57	93
SD	M 30–91 d	Cardiac	70	MCA	26.49	U/l	7.43	93
SD	F 30–91 d	Orbital	30	MCA	34.11	I/l	6.18	93
SD	F 30–91 d	Cardiac	69	MCA	23.69	U/l	7.13	93
SD	M 92–182 d	Orbital	20	MCA	26.67	U/l	3.62	93
SD	M 92–182 d	Cardiac	55	MCA	29.34	U/l	6.42	93
SD	F 92–182 d	Orbital	19	MCA	26.29	U/l	4.59	93
SD	F 92–182 d	Cardiac	55	MCA	30.58	U/l	11.97	93
SD	M 183–273 d	Cardiac	10	MCA	26.52	U/l	4.64	93
SD	F 183–273 d	Cardiac	10	MCA	31.61	U/l	9.28	93
SD	M 274–450 d	Cardiac	10	MCA	35.14	U/l	13.31	93
SD	F 274–450 d	Cardiac	10	MCA	141.38	U/l	280.97	93
CRL: COBS CD (SD) BR	M 4 mos		36		49	mu/ml	13	75
CRL: COBS CD (SD) BR	F 4 mos		35		38	mu/ml	7	75
CRL: COBS CD (SD) BR	M 7 mos		45		37	mu/ml	8	75
CRL: COBS CD (SD) BR	F 7 mos		45		38	mu/ml	14	75
CRL: COBS CD (SD) BR	M 13 mos		40		80	mu/ml	35	75
CRL: COBS CD (SD) BR	F 13 mos		40		73	mu/ml	37	75
CRL: COBS CD (SD) BR	M 19 mos		40		53	mu/ml	18	75
CRL: COBS CD (SD) BR	F 19 mos		40		47	mu/ml	12	75
CRL: COBS CD (SD) BR	M 25 mos		39		46	mu/ml	12	75
CRL: COBS CD (SD) BR	F 25 mos		40		40	mu/ml	10	75
SD	M	Cardiac	10	SMAC	53.14			75
SD	F	Cardiac	10	SMAC	46.88			75

Hamster (Golden)

SPECIES	SEX/AGE	SAMPLE	NUMBER	METHOD	MEAN	UNITS	S.D.	REF.
Lak: LVG	M 3 mos/100g	Cardiac–fasted	19	UV Kinetic	38	IU/l	26.1	81
Lak: LVG	F 3 mos/100g	Cardiac–fasted	21	UV Kinetic	49	IU/l	18.3	81
$B_{10}F_1D$ Alexander	M 3 mos/100g	Cardiac–fasted	21	UV Kinetic	107	IU/l	31.6	81
$B_{10}F_1D$ Alexander	F 3 mos/100g	Cardiac–fasted	16	UV Kinetic	80	IU/l	17.5	81

SGPT (ALT) (cont.)

SPECIES	SEX/AGE	SAMPLE	NUMBER	METHOD	MEAN	UNITS	S.D.	REF.
Hamster (cont.)								
Syrian	M 3 mos/100g				44.7	IU/l	25.9	81
Syrian	M 3 mos/100g				26.9	IU/l	4.6	86
Syrian	M 3 mos/100g				35.0	IU/l	9.0	34
Syrian	F 3 mos/100g				50.3	IU/l	18.3	81
Syrian	F 3 mos/100g				20.6	IU/l	4.0	86
Syrian	F 3 mos/100g				32	IU/l	9.5	34
Guinea Pig – Hartley	M 500–800g		110		44.6	IU/l	6.75	86
Hartley	F 500–800g		85		38.8	IU/l	7.15	86
Rabbit (Oryctolagus cuniculus)	M		109	Hycel	50.8	U	28.8	68
Oryctolagus cuniculus	M			Wroblewski LaDue	35	U	16	66
Oryctolagus cuniculus	M		113	Hycel	22	U	9	66
Oryctolagus cuniculus	F			Wroblewski	47.3	U	11.6	68
Oryctolagus cuniculus	F			LaDue	33	U	10	66
Oryctolagus cuniculus	F				28	U	4	66
Dog (pooled breed, age & reproductive status)	M		57	Hycel	91.2	U	65.5	68
	F		54	Hycel	72.7	U	43.4	68
			32		36		9	60
Beagle	M 150–350 d	Jugular vein	394	MCA	21.7	U/l	8.35	93
	F 150–350 d	Jugular vein	386	MCA	20.1	U/l	6.4	93

SGPT (ALT) (cont.)

SPECIES	SEX/AGE	SAMPLE	NUMBER	METHOD	MEAN	UNITS	S.D.	REF.
Non-human primates								
Pan troglodytes (Chimpanzee)			223-224		5.7	IU	4.3	82
Pongo pygmaeus (Orangutan)			89-92		5.1	IU	2.3	84
Gorilla gorilla (Gorilla)			44		5.3	IU	2.5	83
Papio sp. (Baboon)			12		15.8	IU	3.5	20
Cercopithicus aethiops (African green)			40-102		14.5	IU	8.3	5
Cercocebus atys (Sooty mangabey)			39-71		13.8	IU	6.6	5
Presbytis entillis (Indian langur)			34-60		11.2	IU	4.4	5
Saimiri sciureus (Squirrel monkey)			41-44		83.5	IU	25.4	9, 77
Aotus trivirgatus (Owl monkey)			43-75		22.6	IU	11.0	128
Saguinus oedipus (Cotton-topped marmoset)			13-40		9.6	IU	3.8	56
Macaca mulatta (Rhesus)			20-253		42.1		21.1	11
Macaca mulatta (Rhesus)			286	Hycel	27.2	mu/ml		75
Macaca mulatta (Rhesus) (pooled over age and sex)			20		42.1	U	21.2	68

SERUM GLUTAMIC OXALOACETIC TRANSAMINASE
SGOT (AST)

SPECIES	SEX/AGE	SAMPLE	NUMBER	METHOD	MEAN	UNITS	S.D.	REF.
Mouse								
CD-1	M 20–22 g		6		383	IU/l	81	21
CD-1	M 20–22 g		6		352	IU/l	108	21
A/HeJ	M 20–22 g		6		345	IU/l	24	21
A/HeJ	M 20–22 g		6					21
C3H/HeJ	M 20–22 g		6		260	IU/l	47	21
C3H/HeJ	M 20–22 g		6		290	IU/l	49	21
C3H/HeN	M 20–22 g		6		308.3	IU/l	90	21
C3H/HeN	M 20–22 g		6		305	IU/l	84	21
B6C3F1	M 50 d		8		77.65	mu/ml	20.80	21
B6C3F1	F 50 d		6		87.20	mu/ml	13.70	21
B6C3F1	M 8 wks		5		300.6	mu/ml	59.6	75
B6C3F1	F 8 wks		5		318.8	mu/ml	45.6	75
B6C3F1	M 9 wks		8		77.6	mu/ml	31.8	75
B6C3F1	F 9 wks		6		87.2	mu/ml	12.3	75
B6C3F1	M 19 wks		8		262.9	mu/ml	160.2	75
B6C3F1	F 19 wks		9		226.8	mu/ml	68.7	75
C57BL/6 x DBA/2 F1	M 45 d	Cardiac	592	NADH	153	IU/l	79.0	42
Rat – F344								
F344	M 8 wks		5		116.6	mu/ml	29.7	75
F344	F 8 wks		5		102.0	mu/ml	7.9	75
F344	M 9 wks		15		111.2	mu/ml	21.6	75
F344	F 9 wks		13		159.9	mu/ml	81.0	75
F344	M 10 wks		11		144.4	mu/ml	70.9	75
F344	F 10 wks		9		122.8	mu/ml	45.7	75
F344	M 19 wks		30		104.3	mu/ml	13.4	75
F344	F 19 wks		30		114.0	mu/ml	20.1	75
CD (CRL: CD (SD) BR	M 6–8 wks	Cardiac	20	Kessler, Leon, Delea & Cupiola	262	IU/l	107	27
CD (CRL: CD (SD) BR	F 6–8 wks	Cardiac	20	Kessler, Leon, Delea & Cupiola	203	IU/l	152	27
CD (CRL: CD (SD) BR	M 19–21 wks	Cardiac	20	Kessler, Leon, Delea & Cupiola	192	IU/l	82	27

SGOT (AST) continued

Rat (cont.)

SPECIES	SEX/AGE	SAMPLE	NUMBER	METHOD	MEAN	UNITS	S.D.	REF.
CD (CRL: CD (SD) BR	F 19–21 wks	Cardiac	20	Kessler, Leon, Delea & Cupiola	240	IU/l	123	27
CD (CRL: CD (SD) BR	M 32–34 wks	Cardiac	20	Kessler, Leon, Delea & Cupiola	210	IU/l	140	27
CD (CRL: CD (SD) BR	F 32–34 wks	Cardiac	20	Kessler, Leon, Delea & Cupiola	229	IU/l	109	27
SD	M 30–91 d	Orbital	30	MCA	52.49	U/l	7.08	93
SD	M 30–91 d	Cardiac	70	MCA	55.89	U/l	10.55	93
SD	F 30–91 d	Orbital	30	MCA	52.54	U/l	10.75	93
SD	F 30–91 d	Cardiac	69	MCA	52.90	U/l	8.32	93
SD	M 92–182 d	Orbital	20	MCA	41.91	U/l	6.43	93
SD	M 92–182 d	Cardiac	55	MCA	54.36	U/l	11.97	93
SD	F 92–182 d	Orbital	19	MCA	39.52	U/l	5.52	93
SD	F 92–182 d	Cardiac	55	MCA	58.65	U/l	17.5	93
SD	M 183–273 d	Cardiac	10	MCA	41.00	U/l	4.90	93
SD	F 183–273 d	Cardiac	10	MCA	43.08	U/l	6.81	93
SD	M 274–450 d	Cardiac	10	MCA	42.87	U/l	10.15	93
SD	F 274–450 d	Cardiac	10	MCA	155.52	U/l	223.1	93
CRL: COBS CD (SD) BR	M 4 mos		37		139	mu/ml	36	75
CRL: COBS CD (SD) BR	F 4 mos		38		121	mu/ml	30	75
CRL: COBS CD (SD) BR	M 7 mos		45		114	mu/ml	29	75
CRL: COBS CD (SD) BR	F 7 mos		45		122	mu/ml	61	75
CRL: COBS CD (SD) BR	M 13 mos		37		114	mu/ml	30	75
CRL: COBS CD (SD) BR	F 13 mos		40		129	mu/ml	53	75
CRL: COBS CD (SD) BR	M 19 mos		39		111	mu/ml	32	75
CRL: COBS CD (SD) BR	F 19 mos		40		116	mu/ml	46	75
CRL: COBS CD (SD) BR	M 25 mos		63		114	mu/ml	39	75
CRL: COBS CD (SD) BR	F 25 mos		65		107	mu/ml	33	75
SD	M	Cardiac	10	SMAC	106.57			75
SD	F	Cardiac	10	SMAC	110.38			75

SGOT (AST) continued

SPECIES	SEX/AGE	SAMPLE	NUMBER	METHOD	MEAN	UNITS	S.D.	REF.
Hamster (Golden) Syrian								
Lak: LVG	M 3 mos/100g	Cardiac-fasted	18	UV Kinetic	121	IU/l	17.2	81
Lak: LVG	F 3 mos/100g	Cardiac-fasted	25	UV Kinetic	143	IU/l	22.2	81
B10F1D Alexander	M 3 mos/100g	Cardiac-fasted	21	UV Kinetic	159	IU/l	16.5	81
B10F1D Alexander	F 3 mos/100g	Cardiac-fasted	15	UV Kinetic	202	IU/l	23	81
Syrian	M 3 mos/100g				61.2	IU/l	39.1	81
Syrian	M 3 mos/100g				124.	IU/l	22	86
Syrian	F 3 mos/100g				53.3	IU/l	22.7	81
Syrian	F 3 mos/100g				77.6	IU/l	14.5	86
Guinea pig								
Hartley	M 500–800 g		110		48.2	IU/l	9.50	86
Hartley	F 500–800 g		95		45.5	IU/l	7.00	86
Rabbit (Oryctolagus cuniculus)								
Oryctolagus cuniculus	M				59.5	U	25.3	68
Oryctolagus cuniculus	M			Karmen	42	U	31	66
Oryctolagus cuniculus	M				35	U	14	66
Oryctolagus cuniculus	F				63.0	U	18.9	68
Oryctolagus cuniculus	F			Karmen	44	U	26	66
Oryctolagus cuniculus	F				40	U	22	66
Pooled age and strain	M		109	Hycel	50.8	U	28.8	68
Pooled age and strain	F		113	Hycel	47.3	U	11.6	68
Dog (pooled over breed, age, reproductive status)	M		57	Hycel	75.8	U	30.5	68
	F		54	Hycel	86.6	U	77.4	68
Beagle			32		31		7	60
Breed not specified	M 150–350 d	Jugular vein	394	MCA	20.6	U/l	4.9	93
Breed not specified	F 150–350 d	Jugular vein	386	MCA	19.6	U/l	3.5	93

SGOT (AST) continued

SPECIES	SEX/AGE	SAMPLE	NUMBER	METHOD	MEAN	UNITS	S.D.	REF.
Non-human primates								
Pan troglodytes			223–224		8.7	IU	4.7	82
Pongo pygmaeus			89–92		6.7	IU	3.0	84
Gorilla gorilla			44		10.1	IU	5.1	83
Papio sp.			12		24.5	IU	2.6	20
Cercopithecus aethiops			40–102		26.1	IU	9.4	5
Cercocebus atys			39–71		24.8	IU	7.3	5
Presbytis entillis			34–60		17.3	IU	7.5	5
Saimiri sciureus			41–44		87.0	IU	31.0	9, 77
Aotus trivirgatus			43–75		73.9	IU	34.0	128
Saguinus fusicollis or nigricollis			49–95		47.5	IU	18.0	56
Saguinus oedipus			13–40		54.2	IU	5.3	56
Macaca mulatta			20–253		27.0	IU	6.5	11
Macaca mulatta			262		59.5	mu/ml	45.2	75
Macaca mulatta (pooled age and sex)			20		79.9	U		68
Macaca fascicularis	M Adult	Venous or arterial-fasted	33	Oxaloacetate production	38.4	mIU/ml	18.3	122
Macaca arctoides	M Adult	Venous or arterial-fasted	7	Oxaloacetate production	32.7	mIU/ml	6.58	122

LACTIC DEHYDROGENASE

SPECIES	SEX/AGE	SAMPLE	NUMBER	METHOD	MEAN	UNITS	S.D.	REF.
Rat								
F344	M 9 wks		10		394.6	mu/ml	263.9	75
F344	F 9 wks		7		447.1	mu/ml	278.1	75
Sprague–Dawley	M 30–91 d	Cardiac	65		96.01	IU	53.46	93
Sprague–Dawley	F 30–91 d	Cardiac	64		102.46	IU	63.45	93
Sprague–Dawley	M 92–182 d	Cardiac	55		137.44	IU	135.72	93
Sprague–Dawley	F 92–182 d	Cardiac	55		149.10	IU	176.64	93
Sprague–Dawley	M 274–450 d	Cardiac	10		46.63	IU	22.05	93
Sprague–Dawley	F 274–450 d	Cardiac	10		105.90	IU	77.83	93
Sprague–Dawley	M	Cardiac		SMAC	452.86			75
Sprague–Dawley	F	Cardiac		SMAC	301.75			75
Wistar	M				186	IU/24 hr	12	14
F344/N	M				573	IU/1	94	14
F344/N					99	IU/1	9	14
F344/N	F				63	IU/1	7	14
Hamster (Golden) Syrian								
Lak: LVG	F 3 mos/100g	Cardiac– 12 hr fasted	15	UV Kinetic	217	IU/L	74.4	81
Lak: LVG	M 3 mos/100g	Cardiac– 12 hr fasted	18	UV Kinetic	211	IU/L	52.7	81
$B_{10}F_1D$ Alexander	F 3 mos/100g	Cardiac– 12 hr fasted	15	UV Kinetic	208	IU/L	60.9	81
$B_{10}F_1D$ Alexander	M 3 mos/100g	Cardiac– 12 hr fasted	15	UV Kinetic	204	IU/L	72.4	81
No strain	M 3 mos/100g				222.2	IU/L	69.7	81
No strain	M 3 mos/100g				257	IU/L	63.6	34
No strain	F 3 mos/100g				225.7	IU/L	179.3	81
No strain	F 3 mos/100g				208.0	IU/L	54.7	34
Rabbit (Oryctolagus cuniculus)								
Pooled inbred	F	Venous	120	Hycel	104.8	U	29.9	68
Pooled inbred	M	Venous	119	Hycel	94.3	U	28.8	68

LDH (cont.)

SPECIES	SEX/AGE	SAMPLE	NUMBER	METHOD	MEAN	UNITS	S.D.	REF.
Canine (Pooled over breed, age, reproductive status)	F		54	Hycel	58.3	U	27.8	68
	M		57	Hycel	73.0	U	55.1	68
Canine	M	Jugular vein	394	MCA	68.0	U/l	37.85	93
	F	Jugular vein	386	MCA	48.2	U/l	25.75	93
Non-human primates								
Macaca fascicularis	M Adult	Venous or arterial-fasted 17 hrs.	33	Lactate oxidation	283	mIU/ml	123	122
Macaca arctoides	M Adult	Venous or arterial-fasted 17 hrs.	7	Lactate oxidation	289	mIU/ml	84.8	122
Macaca mulatta		Venous	20	Hycel	186.9	U	68.4	68

SORBITOL DEHYDROGENASE

SDH

SPECIES	SEX/AGE	SAMPLE	NUMBER	METHOD	MEAN	UNITS	S.D.	REF.
Mouse								
B6C3F1	M 8 wks		5		31.0	mu/ml	5.1	75
B6C3F1	F 8 wks		4		26.8	mu/ml	3.4	75
B6C3F1	M 9 wks		8		30.9	mu/ml	4.6	75
B6C3F1	F 9 wks		5		32.0	mu/ml	1.84	75
B6C3F1	M 19 wks		7		29.6	mu/ml	7.4	75
B6C3F1	F 19 wks		9		34.4	mu/ml	3.0	75
B6C3F1	M 50 d		8		30.9	mu/ml	3.5	21
B6C3F1	F 50 d		5		32.0	mu/ml	1.87	21
Rat								
F344	M 8 wks		5		18.2	mu/ml	4.1	75
F344	F 8 wks		5		20.6	mu/ml	3.4	75
F344	M 9 wks		15		19.5	mu/ml	5.7	75
F344	F 9 wks		12		18.6	mu/ml	5.3	75
F344	M 10 wks		11		22.0	mu/ml	4.4	75
F344	F 10 wks		9		30.7	mu/ml	6.1	75
F344	M 19 wks		30		20.3	mu/ml	4.16	75
F344	F 19 wks		30		23.1	mu/ml	3.12	75

CREATINE PHOSPHOKINASE
CPK

SPECIES	AGE/SEX	SAMPLE	NUMBER	METHOD	*MEAN	*UNITS	S.D.	REF.
Mouse (Albino) ICR	M 20–25g		145		3.70	IU/L	1.45	86
(Albino) ICR	F 20–25g		128		2.50	IU/L	1.52	86
Rat								
(CRL: COBS CD (SD) BR)	M 25 mos		27		216	mIU/ml	119	75
(CRL: COBS CD (SD) BR)	F 25 mos		29		309	mIU/ml	655	75
Wistar (Albino)	M 180–250g		160		5.60	IU/L	1.30	86
Wistar (Albino)	F 180–250g		140		6.80	IU/L	2.40	86
Hamster (Golden) Syrian								
Lak: LVG	M 3 mos or 100g	Cardiac–fasted	18	Enzymatic	469	IU/L	174	81
Lak: LVG	F 3 mos or 100g	Cardiac–fasted	15	Enzymatic	520	IU/L	184	81
B$_{10}$F$_1$D Alexander	M 3 mos or 100g	Cardiac–fasted	9	Enzymatic	1218	IU/L	336	81
B$_{10}$F$_1$D Alexander	F 3 mos or 100g	Cardiac–fasted	7	Enzymatic	1553	IU/L	386	81
Syrian Hamster	M 3 mos or 100g				0.56	IU/L	0.08	81
	F 3 mos or 100g				0.59	IU/L	0.15	81
	M 3 mos or 100g				0.45	IU/L	0.13	115
	F 3 mos or 100g				0.39	IU/L	0.04	115
Guinea pig – Hartley								
Hartley	M 500–800g		110		0.95	IU/L	0.15	86
	F 500–800g		95		1.10	IU/L	0.20	86
Rabbit – Oryctolagus cuniculus								
Pooled over age and breed	M		109	Hycel	170.7	U	43.9	68
Pooled over age and breed	F		113	Hycel	176.6	U	54.1	68
Canine – Mongrel								
Mongrel	M 12–16 Kg		18		1.20	IU/L	0.30	86
	F 12–16 Kg		10		0.80	IU/L	1.10	86

Non-human primates

Species	Sex	Age	Specimen	n	Method	Mean	Units		
Macaca mulatta									
Macaca mulatta (pooled over age and strain)				146	Hycel	124.1	mu/ml	69.6	75
				20		172.8	U		68
Macaca fascicularis	M	Adult	venous or arterial	33	Creatinine phosphate ADP reaction	507	mIU/ml	386	122
Macaca arctoides	M	Adult	venous or arterial	7	Creatinine phosphate ADP reaction	301	mIU/ml	118	122

* Editors' Note: In the measurement of enzymes, results are markedly influenced by methodology. Values obtained by diverse methods may not be able to be compared to one another simply. Unitage expressed in International Units (IU) related to moles of end-product produced from substrate per minute per ml or l of specimen. By definition this can be increased or decreased by a factor of 10^3. Inspection of the data in this table suggests that the mean CPK values of 0.39–1.20 may represent 10^{-3} of the mean values of 216–1553, a difference more in calculation than in methodology.

CALCIUM

SPECIES	SEX/AGE	SAMPLE	NUMBER	METHOD	MEAN	UNITS	S.D.	REF.
Mouse								
CD-1	M 20-22g		6		10.5	mg/dl	0.16	21
CD-1	M 20-22g		6		9.6	mg/dl	1.21	21
A/HeJ	M 20-22g		6		10.5	mg/dl	0.1	21
A/HeJ	M 20-22g		6		9.6	mg/dl	0.2	21
C3H/HeJ	M 20-22g		6		9.7	mg/dl	0.25	21
C3H/HeJ	M 20-22g		6		9.3	mg/dl	0.2	21
C3H/HeN	M 20-22g		6		8.4	mg/dl	0.2	21
C3H/HeN	M 20-22g		6		7.9	mg/dl	0.3	21
C57BL/6 x DBA/2 F_1	M 45 days	Heart	585	Sodium Alizarin sulfonate	9.0	mg/dl	1.0	42
Rat								
CD Crl:CD (SD) BR	M 6-8 wks	Cardiac Puncture non-fasting	20	Modified Kessler & Gitelman	10.5	mg/dl	1.4	27
CD Crl:CD (SD) BR	M 19-21 wks	Cardiac Puncture non-fasting	20	Modified Kessler & Gitelman	11.0	mg/dl	1.1	27
CD Crl:CD (SD) BR	M 32-34 wks	Cardiac puncture non-fasting	20	Modified Kessler & Gitelman	11.3	mg/dl	1.3	27
CD Crl:CD (SD) BR	F 6-8 wks	Cardiac puncture non-fasting	20	Modified Kessler & Gitelman	12.9	mg/dl	2.2	27
CD Crl:CD (SD) BR	F 19-21	Cardiac puncture non-fasting	20	Modified Kessler & Gitelman	11.6	mg/dl	1.7	27
CD Crl:CD (SD) BR	F 32-34	Cardiac puncture non-fasting	20	Modified Kessler & Gitelman	12.4	mg/dl	3.4	27

Calcium (cont.)

Species	Sex/Age	Sample	Number	Method	Mean	Units	S.D.	Ref.
Rat (cont.)								
Sprague-Dawley	M 30–91 d	Cardiac	65		12.07	mg/dl	0.56	93
Sprague-Dawley	F 30–91 d	Cardiac	64		11.85	mg/dl	0.48	93
Sprague-Dawley	M 92–182 d	Cardiac	55		11.65	mg/dl	0.83	93
Sprague-Dawley	F 92–182 d	Cardiac	55		11.75	mg/dl	0.89	93
Sprague-Dawley	M 274–450 d	Cardiac	10		11.67	mg/dl	0.62	93
Sprague-Dawley	F 274–450 d	Cardiac	10		11.90	mg/dl	0.46	93
CRL: COBS CD (SD) BR	M 25 Mos		25		10.9	mg/dl	0.5	75
CRL: COBS CD (SD) BR	F 25 Mos		26		11.5	mg/dl	0.5	75
Sprague-Dawley	M 25 Mos	Cardiac	10	SMAC Analyzer	11.4	mg/dl		75
Sprague-Dawley	F 25 Mos	Cardiac	10	SMAC Analyzer	11.6	mg/dl		75
Hamster (Syrian) Golden								
Lak:LVG	F 3 Mos or 100g	Cardiac–fasted	29	CC[1]	11.0	mg/dl	0.61	81
Lak:LVG	M 3 Mos or 100g	Cardiac–fasted	30	CC	11.1	mg/dl	0.75	81
B10F$_1$D Alexander	F 3 Mos or 100g	Cardiac–fasted	28	CC	12.1	mg/dl	1.09	81
B10F$_1$D Alexander	M 3 Mos or 100g	Cardiac–fasted	28	CC	11.3	mg/dl	1.39	81
Syrian	M 3 Mos or 100g				11.1	mg/dl	1.6	115
Syrian	M 3 Mos or 100g				12.4	mg/dl	0.6	34
Syrian	F 3 Mos or 100g				10.4	mg/dl	2.0	5
Syrian	F 3 Mos or 100g				11.4	mg/dl	0.9	34
Guinea pig – Hartley	M 500–800g		110		9.6	mg/dl	0.63	86
Hartley	F 500–800g		95		10.7	mg/dl	0.58	86
Rabbit (Oryctolagus cuniculus)	M				14.4	mg/dl	0.5	104
Canine Breed not specified	M	Jugular vein	394	MCA[2]	10.75	mg/dl	0.43	93
Breed not specified	F	Jugular vein	386	MCA	10.73	mg/dl	0.43	93
Beagle			32		5.3	mg/dl	0.2	60

Calcium (cont.)

Species	Sex/Age	Sample	Number	Method	Mean	Units	S.D.	Ref.
Non-human primates								
Macaca fascicularis	M Adult	Venous or arterial fasted 17 hrs.	33	CC	8.9	mg/dl	0.39	122
Macaca arctoides	M Adult		7	CC	9.2	mg/dl	0.45	122
Pan troglodytes			223–224		9.3	mg/dl	0.9	82
Pongo pygmaeus			89–92		9.3	mg/dl	0.9	84
Gorilla gorilla			44		9.5	mg/dl	0.7	83
Papio sp.			12		8.4	mg/dl	1.5	20
Cercopithicus aethiops			40–102		10.1	mg/dl	0.8	5
Cercocebus atys			39–71		10.4	mg/dl	0.8	5
Presbytis entillis			34–60		11.5	mg/dl	1.1	5
Saimiri sciureus			41–44		9.0	mg/dl	0.7	9, 77
Saguinus fusicollis or nigricollis			49–95		10.4	mg/dl	1.3	56
Saguinus oedipus			13–40		10.0	mg/dl	0.6	56
Macaca mulatta			20–253		9.7	mg/dl	1.6	11
Macaca mulatta			267		10.82	mg/dl		75

1   Cresolphthalein complexone

2   IL MCA Multistat

PHOSPHORUS

SPECIES	SEX/AGE	SAMPLE	NUMBER	METHOD	MEAN	UNITS	S.D.	REF.
Mouse (albino)	M 20–25 g		145		5.60	mg/dl	1.61	86
Albino	F 20–25 g		128		6.55	mg/dl	1.30	86
C57BL/6 x DBA/2 F₁	M 45 d	Cardiac	578	Phosphomolyb–date reaction	9.2	mg/dl	1.9	42
Rat CD (CRL: CD (SD) BR)	M 6–8 wks		20	Modified Hurst & Kreml	13.4	mg/dl	2.6	27
CD (CRL: CD (SD) BR)	F 6–8 wks		20	Modified Hurst & Kreml	13.4	mg/dl	3.0	27
CD (CRL: CD (SD) BR)	M 19–21 wks		20	Modified Hurst & Kreml	9.7	mg/dl	2.2	27
CD (CRL: CD (SD) BR)	F 19–21 wks		20	Modified Hurst & Kreml	15.9	mg/dl	1.5	27
CD (CRL: CD (SD) BR)	M 32–34 wks		20	Modified Hurst & Kreml	12.3	mg/dl	3.2	27
CD (CRL: CD (SD) BR)	F 32–34 wks		20	Modified Hurst & Kreml	11.2	mg/dl	4.2	27
CRL: COBS CD (SD) BR	M 25 mos		24		5.5	mg/dl	0.54	75
CRL: COBS CD (SD) BR	F 25 mos		26		5.3	mg/dl	0.61	75
SD	M	Cardiac	10	SMAC	7.26			75
SD	F	Cardiac	10	SMAC	6.89			75
Pooled over age and strain	M		66	Hycel	4.93	mgs %	1.73	68
Pooled over age and strain	F		60	Hycel	5.75	mgs %	2.58	68
Sprague-Dawley – CD	M 30–91 d		50	MCA	10.09	mg/dl	1.51	93
Sprague-Dawley	F 30–91 d		50	MCA	9.07	mg/dl	1.32	93
Sprague-Dawley	M 92–182 d		45	MCA	7.92	mg/dl	1.47	93
Sprague-Dawley	F 92–182 d		45	MCA	6.87	mg/dl	1.36	93
Sprague-Dawley	M 274–450 d		10	MCA	7.08	mg/dl	1.19	93
Sprague-Dawley	F 274–450 d		10	MCA	7.24	mg/dl	0.76	93

Phosphorus (cont.)

SPECIES	SEX/AGE	SAMPLE	NUMBER	METHOD	MEAN	UNITS	S.D.	REF.
Hamster (Golden) Syrian								
Lak: LVG	M 3 mos or 100g	Cardiac-fasted	31	Phosphomolybdate complex	8.2	mg/dl	1.07	81
Lak: LVG	F 3 mos or 100g	Cardiac-fasted	32	Phosphomolybdate complex	6.3	mg/dl	1.23	81
$B_{10}F_1D$ Alexander	M 3 mos or 100g	Cardiac-fasted	29	Phosphomolybdate complex	7.5	mg/dl	0.93	81
$B_{10}F_1D$ Alexander	F 3 mos or 100g	Cardiac-fasted	28	Phosphomolybdate complex	7.0	mg/dl	0.98	81
Hamster-Syrian								
Syrian	M 3 mos/100g				6.6	mg/dl	0.8	115
Syrian	M 3 mos/100g				5.3	mg/dl	1.0	86
Syrian	M 3 mos/100g				6.3	mg/dl	1.0	34
Syrian	F 3 mos/100g				6.5	mg/dl	1.6	115
Syrian	F 3 mos/100g				6.0	mg/dl	1.1	86
Syrian	F 3 mos/100g				6.4	mg/dl	0.6	34
Guinea pig (Albino)								
Hartley	M 500–800g		110		5.33	mg/dl	1.15	86
Hartley	F 500–800g		95		5.30	mg/dl	1.10	86
Rabbit								
Pooled over age and strain	M		109	Hycel	4.08	mgs %	0.86	68
Pooled over age and strain	F		113	Hycel	3.89	mgs %	0.80	68
Oryctolagus cuniculus	M				4.16	mg/dl	0.46	46
Oryctolagus cuniculus	M				7.89	mg/dl	0.22	104
Oryctolagus cuniculus	F				4.12	mg/dl	0.70	46
Dutch belted					3.10–8.15	mg/dl		86
Polish					4.00–5.10	mg/dl		86
Canine Breed not specified	M 150–350 d	Jugular vein	394	MCA	5.50	mg/dl	0.77	93
Breed not specified	F 150–350 d	Jugular vein	386	MCA	5.35	mg/dl	0.87	93
(Pooled over age, breed and reproductive status)	M		57	Hycel	4.68	mgs %	1.87	68
	F		54	Hycel	4.41	mgs %	1.79	68

Phosphorus (cont.)

SPECIES	SEX/AGE	SAMPLE	NUMBER	METHOD	MEAN	UNITS	S.D.	REF.
Non-human primates								
Pan troglodytes			223–224		4.8	mg/dl	1.2	82
Pongo pygmaeus			89–92		4.4	mg/dl	1.0	84
Gorilla gorilla			44		5.2	mg/dl	0.7	83
Papio sp.			12		7.0	mg/dl	1.5	20
Cercopithicus aethiops			40–102		5.1	mg/dl	1.4	5
Cercocebus atys			39–71		5.5	mg/dl	1.4	5
Presbytis entillis			34–60		5.2	mg/dl	1.4	5
Saimiri sciureus			41–44		4.5	mg/dl	2.2	9, 77
Saguinus fusicollis or nigricollis			49–95		5.5		2.0	56
Saguinus oedipus			13–40		4.7	mg/dl	1.6	56
Macaca mulatta			20–253		5.0	mg/dl	0.9	11
Macaca mulatta			223		4.78	mg/dl		75
Macaca mulatta (pooled over age and sex)			20	Hycel	4.37	mgs %	1.52	68
Macaca fascicularis	M Adult	Venous or arterial–fasted	33	Phosphomolyb-date reaction	5.2	mg/dl	2.09	122
Macaca arctoides	M Adult	Venous or arterial	7	Phosphomolyb-date reaction	4.3	mg/dl	0.83	122

SODIUM

SPECIES	AGE/SEX	SAMPLE	NUMBER	METHOD	MEAN	UNITS	S.D.	REF.
Mouse – Albino (ICR)	M 20–25 g		145		138	mEq/l	2.9	86
Albino (ICR)	F 20–25 g		138		134	mEq/l	2.6	86
C57BL/6 x DBA/2 F_1	M 45 d	Cardiac	542	flame photo-meter	147	mEq/l	15	42
C57BL/6	M 8–10 mos	Cardiac–fasted	41	flame photo-meter	186	mEq/l	29.4	43
C57BL/6	M 25–28 mos	Cardiac–fasted	45	flame photo-meter	181	mEq/l	29.3	43
Rat								
CRL: COBS CD (SD) BR	M 25 mos		24		150	mEq/l	4.4	75
CRL: COBS CD (SD) BR	F 25 mos		25		149	mEq/l	3.5	75
CD (CRL: CD (SD) BR)	M 6–8 wks	Cardiac	20	IL–ISE 502	143	mg/l	5.0	27
CD (CRL: CD (SD) BR)	F 6–8 wks	Cardiac	20	IL–ISE 502	144	mg/l	5.0	27
CD (CRL: CD (SD) BR)	M 19–21 wks	Cardiac	20	IL–ISE 502	147	mg/l	3.0	27
CD (CRL: CD (SD) BR)	F 19–21 wks	Cardiac	20	IL–ISE 502	143	mg/l	4.0	27
CD (CRL: CD (SD) BR)	M 32–34 wks	Cardiac	20	IL–ISE 502	145	mg/l	6.0	27
CD (CRL: CD (SD) BR)	F 32–34 wks	Cardiac	20	IL–ISE 502	143	mg/l	7.0	27
SD	M	Cardiac	10	SMAC	147.4			75
SD	F	Cardiac	10	SMAC	148.4			75
Sprague–Dawley – CD	M 30–91 d	Cardiac	64	IL 443 flame photometer	146.96	mEq/l	1.66	93
Sprague–Dawley – CD	F 30–91 d	Cardiac	62	IL 443 flame photometer	145.89	mEq/l	3.04	93
Sprague–Dawley – CD	M 92–182 d	Cardiac	45	IL 443 flame photometer	146.76	mEq/l	2.0	93
Sprague–Dawley – CD	F 92–182 d	Cardiac	44	IL 443 flame photometer	145.84	mEq/l	2.16	93
Sprague–Dawley – CD	M 274–450 d	Cardiac	10	IL 443 flame photometer	146.84	mEq/l	0.93	93
Sprague–Dawley – CD	F 274–450 d	Cardiac	10	IL 443 flame photometer	145.19	mEq/l	1.33	93

Sodium (cont.)

SPECIES	SEX/AGE	SAMPLE	NUMBER	METHOD	MEAN	UNITS	S.D.	REF.
Hamsters – Syrian								
Syrian	M 3 mos/100g				144.0	mEq/1	3.1	34
Syrian	M 3 mos/100g				128.0	mEq/1	1.9	86
Syrian	F 3 mos/100g				145.0	mEq/1	3.4	34
Syrian	F 3 mos/100g				134.0	mEq/1	2.3	86
Guinea pig – Hartley	M 500–800 g		110		122	mEq/1	0.98	86
Hartley	F 500–800 g		95		125	mEq/1	0.96	86
Rabbit								
Oryctolagus cuniculus	M				141.0	mEq/1	4.5	66
Oryctolagus cuniculus	M				147.3	mEq/1	4.6	66
Oryctolagus cuniculus	F				139.0	mEq/1	3.5	66
Oryctolagus cuniculus	F				147.7	mEq/1	3.4	66
Dutch belted					138–156	mEq/1		86
Polish					114–146	mEq/1		86
Canine Breed not specified	M 150–350 d	jugular vein	394	IL 443 flame photometer	146.8	mEq/1	2.0	93
Breed not specified	F 150–350 d	jugular vein	386	IL 443 flame photometer	147.2	mEq/1	2.1	93
Beagle			32		144		3.0	60
Non-human Primates								
Pan troglodytes			223–224		139.0	mEq/1	3.6	82
Pongo pygmaeus			89–92		138.0	mEq/1	3.8	84
Gorilla gorilla			44		135	mEq/1	3.9	83
Papio sp.			12		142	mEq/1	3.5	20
Cercopithecus aethiops			40–102		154	mEq/1	4.6	5
Cercocebus atys			39–71		151	mEq/1	4.4	5
Presbytis entillis			34–60		154	mEq/1	4.6	5
Saimiri scuireus			41–44		149	mEq/1	6.0	9, 77
Saguinus fusicicollis or nigricollis			49–95		169	mEq/1	9.0	56
Saguinus oedipus			13–40		161	mEq/1	5.5	56

Sodium (cont.)

SPECIES	SEX/AGE	SAMPLE	NUMBER	METHOD	MEAN	UNITS	S.D.	REF.
Non-human primates (cont.)								
Macaca mulatta			20–253		158	mEq/1	13.0	11
Macaca mulatta			382		154.1	mEq/1		75
Macaca fascicularis	M Adult	venous or arterial fasted	33	flame emission spectrophotometry	146	mEq/1	3.60	122
Macaca arctoides	M Adult	venous or arterial fasted	7	flame emission spectrophotometry	147	mEq/1	1.89	122

POTASSIUM

SPECIES	SEX/AGE	SAMPLE	NUMBER	METHOD	MEAN	UNITS	S.D.	REF.
Mice – Albino ICR	M 20–25 gr		145		5.25	mEq/l	0.13	86
Albino ICR	F 20–25 gr		128		5.40	mEq/l	0.15	86
C57BL/6 x DBA/2 F$_1$	M 45 days		552	flame photo-meter	6.28	mEq/l	1.28	42
Rat								
CRL: COBS CD (SD) BR	M 25 mos		25		5.78	mEq/l	0.80	75
CRL: COBS CD (SD) BR	F 25 mos		26		5.17	mEq/l	0.82	75
CD (CRL: CD (SD) BR)	M 6–8 wks	Cardiac	20	IL–ISE 502	6.6	mEq/l	2.6	27
CD (CRL: CD (SD) BR)	F 6–8 wks	Cardiac	20	IL–ISE 502	6.8	mEq/l	2.6	27
CD (CRL: CD (SD) BR)	M 19–21 wks	Cardiac	20	IL–ISE 502	6.2	mEq/l	2.2	27
CD (CRL: CD (SD) BR)	F 19–21 wks	Cardiac	20	IL–ISE 502	5.8	mEq/l	2.2	27
CD (CRL: CD (SD) BR)	M 32–34 wks	Cardiac	20	IL–ISE 502	7.4	mEq/l	1.8	27
CD (CRL: CD (SD) BR)	F 32–34 wks	Cardiac	20	IL–ISE 502	5.9	mEq/l	3.6	27
SD	M	Cardiac	10	SMAC	6.27			75
SD	F	Cardiac	10	SMAC	5.26			75
Sprague–Dawley – CD	M 30–91 d		64	IL 443 flame photometer	7.26	mEq/l	1.27	93
Sprague–Dawley – CD	F 30–91 d	Cardiac	62	IL 443 flame photometer	7.37	mEq/l	0.88	93
Sprague–Dawley – CD	M 92–182 d	Cardiac	45	IL 443 flame photometer	7.47	mEq/l	1.30	93
Sprague–Dawley – CD	F 92–182 d	Cardiac	44	IL 443 flame photometer	7.29	mEq/l	1.44	93
Sprague–Dawley – CD	M 274–450 d	Cardiac	10	IL 443 flame photometer	6.50	mEq/l	1.33	93
Sprague–Dawley – CD	F 274–450 d	Cardiac	10	IL 443 flame photometer	6.46	mEq/l	1.06	93
Hamsters – Syrian	M 3 Mos or 100g				4.7	mEq/l	0.5	86
Syrian	F 3 Mos or 100g				5.3	mEq/l	0.5	86
Guinea pig – Hartley	M 500–800 g		110		4.87	mEq/l	0.84	86
Guinea pig – Hartley	F 500–800 g		85		5.06	mEq/l	0.93	86

Potassium (cont.)

SPECIES	SEX/AGE	SAMPLE	NUMBER	METHOD	MEAN	UNITS	S.D.	REF.
Rabbit								
Oryctolagus cuniculus	M				5.1	mEq/l	0.6	66
Oryctolagus cuniculus	M				5.9	mEq/l	0.5	66
Oryctolagus cuniculus	F				5.3	mEq/l	0.5	66
Dutch belted					4.40–7.40	mEq/l		86
Polish					5.00–5.70	mEq/l		86
Canine Breed not specified	M 150–350 d	jugular vein	394	IL 443 flame photometer	4.79	mEq/l	0.37	93
Breed not specified	F 150–350 d	jugular vein	386	IL 443 flame photometer	4.77	mEq/l	0.38	93
Beagle				32	4.5	mEq/l	0.3	60
Non-human Primates								
Pan troglodytes			223–224		3.7	mEq/l	0.5	82
Pongo pygmaeus			89–92		4.4	mEq/l	1.0	84
Gorilla gorilla			44		4.1	mEq/l	0.4	83
Papio Sp.			12		3.8	mEq/l	0.5	20
Cercopithicus aethiops			40–102		4.8	mEq/l	0.7	5
Cercocebus atys			39–71		5.3	mEq/l	0.8	5
Presbytis entillis			34–60		5.7	mEq/l	0.7	5
Saimiri scuireus			41–44		4.4	mEq/l	0.9	9, 77
Saguinus fusicollis or nigricollis			49–95		5.7	mEq/l	0.9	56
Saguinus oedipus			13–40		6.0	mEq/l	1.3	56
Macaca mulatta			20–253		4.7	mEq/l	0.8	11
Macaca mulatta			368		4.62	mEq/l		75
Macaca fascicularis	M Adult	venous or arterial	33	flame emission spectro-photometry	3.6	mEq/l	0.32	122
Macaca arctoides	M Adult	venous or arterial	7	flame emission spectro-photometry	3.6	mEq/l	0.10	122

CHLORIDE

SPECIES	SEX/AGE	SAMPLE	NUMBER	METHOD	MEAN	UNITS	S.D.	REF.
Mouse C57BL/6 x DBA/2 F_1	M 45 d	Cardiac	184	Mercuric thiocyanate	99	mEq/l	7.0	42
Albino (ICR)	M 20-25g		145		108	mEq/l	0.60	86
Albino (IRC)	F 20-25g		128		107	mEq/l	0.55	86
Rat – CD (CRL: CD (SD) BR)	M 6-8 wks	Cardiac	20	Zall, Fisher & Garner	99	mEq/l	5.0	27
CD (CRL: CD (SD) BR)	F 6-8 wks	Cardiac	20	Zall, Fisher & Garner	102	mEq/l	7.0	27
CD (CRL: CD (SD) BR)	M 19-21 wks	Cardiac	20	Zall, Fisher & Garner	96	mEq/l	3.0	27
CD (CRL: CD (SD) BR)	F 19-21 wks	Cardiac	20	Zall, Fisher & Garner	89	mEq/l	5.0	27
CD (CRL: CD (SD) BR)	M 32-34 wks	Cardiac	20	Zall, Fisher & Garner	100	mEq/l	5.0	27
CD (CRL: CD (SD) BR)	F 32-34 wks	Cardiac	20	Zall, Fisher & Garner	85	mEq/l	19.0	27
(CRL: COBS CD (SD) BR)	M 25 mos		25		103	mEq/l	4.0	75
(CRL: COBS CD (SD) BR)	F 25 mos		25		101	mEq/l	4.0	75
SD	M	Cardiac	10	SMAC	101.4			75
SD	F	Cardiac	10	SMAC	101.1			75
Sprague–Dawley – CD	M 30-91 d	Cardiac	45	MCA	98.84	mmol/l	2.71	93
Sprague–Dawley – CD	F 30-91 d	Cardiac	41	MCA	100.61	mmol/l	2.79	93
Sprague–Dawley – CD	M 92-182 d	Cardiac	35	MCA	99.57	mmol/l	1.98	93
Sprague–Dawley – CD	F 92-182 d	Cardiac	34	MCA	100.82	mmol/l	2.48	93
Sprague–Dawley – CD	M 274-450 d	Cardiac	10	MCA	97.60	mmol/l	2.72	93
Sprague–Dawley – CD	F 274-450 d	Cardiac	10	MCA	96.50	mmol/l	2.80	93
Hamster – Syrian	M 3 mos				99.0	mEq/l	2.1	34
Syrian	M 3 mos				96.7	mEq/l	1.2	86
Syrian	F 3 mos				99.0	mEq/l	2.2	34
Syrian	F 3 mos				93.8	mEq/l	1.2	86

Chloride (cont.)

SPECIES	SEX/AGE	SAMPLE	NUMBER	METHOD	MEAN	UNITS	S.D.	REF.
Guinea pig (Albino)								
Hartley	M	500-800g	110		92.3	mEq/l	1.04	86
Hartley	F	500-800g	95		96.5	mEq/l	1.19	86
Rabbit (Oryctolagus cuniculus)	M				108.7	mEq/l	4.0	66
Oryctolagus cuniculus	F				109.1	mEq/l	5.7	66
NZW					98.0–116	mEq/l		86
Dutch belted					102–120	mEq/l		86
Polish					89.0–112	mEq/l		86
Dog								
Breed not specified	M	Jugular vein	394	MCA	110.9	mmol/l	2.45	93
Breed not specified	F	Jugular vein	386	MCA	111.5	mmol/l	2.30	93
Beagle			32		108	mmol/l	3.0	60
Non-human Primates								
Pan troglodytes			223–224		100	mEq/l	4.1	82
Pongo pygmaeus			89–92		101	mEq/l	3.6	84
Gorilla gorilla			44		98	mEq/l	4.5	83
Papio sp.			12		107	mEq/l	3.7	20
Cercopithicus aethiops			40–102		107.5	mEq/l	4.0	5
Cercocebus atys			39–71		105	mEq/l	3.8	5
Presbytis entillis			34–60		106	mEq/l	4.2	5
Saimiri sciureus			41–44		114	mEq/l	6.0	9, 77
Saguinus fusicollis or nigricollis			49–95		114	mEq/l	6.0	56
Saguinus oedipus			13–40		108	mEq/l	5.0	56
Macaca mulatta			20–253		114	mEq/l	9.0	11
Macaca mulatta			145		109.6	mEq/l		75

MAGNESIUM

SPECIES	SEX/AGE	SAMPLE	NUMBER	METHOD	MEAN (RANGE)	UNITS	S.D.	REF.
Mouse								
Albino – ICR Strain	M	20–25 g	145		3.11	mg/dl	0.37	86
Albino – ICR strain	F	20–25 g	128		1.38	mg/dl	0.28	86
Rat								
Albino – Wistar	M	180–250 g	160		3.12	mg/dl	0.41	86
Albino – Wistar	F	180–250 g	140		2.60	mg/dl	0.21	86
Fisher 344/cr					1.60–4.35	mg/dl		86
Osborne – Mendel					1.50–4.10	mg/dl		86
Long–Evans BLU: (LE)					2.10–4.20	mg/dl		86
Germ-free (axenic)					1.80–2.30	mg/dl		86
Hamsters								
Syrian	M	3 mos/100g			2.5	mg/dl	0.2	86
Syrian	F	3 mos/100g			2.2	mg/dl	0.1	86
Golden Syrian	M	75–100g	84		2.54	mg/dl	0.22	86
Golden Syrian	F	75–100g	80		2.20	mg/dl	0.14	86
Guinea pig – Hartley	M	500–800 g	110		2.35	mg/dl	0.25	86
Hartley	F	500–800 g	95		2.46	mg/dl	0.27	86
Rabbit								
Oryctolagus cuniculus	M				2.25	mg/dl	0.16	104
New Zealand White	M	3–5 Kg	120		2.52	mg/dl	0.24	86
New Zealand White	F	3–5 Kg	80		3.20	mg/dl	0.22	86
Dutch belted					1.98–41.0	mg/dl		86
Polish					2.00–4.50	mg/dl		86

Magnesium (cont.)

SPECIES	SEX/AGE	SAMPLE	NUMBER	METHOD	MEAN	UNITS	S.D.	REF.
Canine								
Mongrel	M 12–16 Kg		18		2.10	mg/dl	0.30	86
Mongrel	F 12–16 Kg		10		2.20	mg/dl	0.28	86
Non-human primates								
Macaca mulatta	M 2–5 Kg		38		1.65	mg/dl	0.32	86
Macaca mulatta	F 2–5 Kg		30		1.82	mg/dl	0.41	86

SERUM IRON

SPECIES	SEX/AGE	SAMPLE	NUMBER	METHOD	MEAN	UNITS	S.D.	REF.
Mice – CD-1	M 20–22g		6		473	ug/dl	16	21
CD-1	M 20–22g		6		474	ug/dl	44	21
A/HeJ	M 20–22g		6		336	ug/dl	12	21
A/HeJ	M 20–22g		6		236	ug/dl	4	21
C3H/HeJ	M 20–22g		6		256	ug/dl	7	21
C3H/HeJ	M 20–22g		6		210	ug/dl	5.7	21
C3H/HeN	M 20–22g		6		230	ug/dl	9.5	21
C3H/HeN	M 20–22g		6		259	ug/dl	19	21
Rats CD (CRL: CD (SD) BR)	M 6–8 wks	Cardiac	20	Giouoniellow automated	202	ug/dl	49	27
CD (CRL: CD (SD) BR)	F 6–8 wks	Cardiac	20	Giouoniellow automated	314	ug/dl	230	27
CD (CRL: CD (SD) BR)	M 19–21 wks	Cardiac	20	Giouoniellow automated	152	ug/dl	70	27
CD (CRL: CD (SD) BR)	F 19–21 wks	Cardiac	20	Giouoniellow automated	220	ug/dl	130	27
CD (CRL: CD (SD) BR)	F 32–34 wks	Cardiac	20	Giouoniellow automated	220	ug/dl	124	27
Rabbit – (Oryctolagus cuniculus)	M		120		204.2	ug/dl	19.2	47
Oryctolagus cuniculus	F		120		209.7	ug/dl	20.5	47

URIC ACID

SPECIES	AGE/SEX	SAMPLE	NUMBER	METHOD	MEAN	UNITS	S.D.	REF.
Rat								
(CRL: COBS CD (SD) BR)	M		25		1.52	mg/dl	0.30	75
(CRL: COBS CD (SD) BR)	F		26		1.25	mg/dl	0.36	75
SD	M	Cardiac	10	SMAC	2.44			75
SD	F	Cardiac	10	SMAC	2.44			75
Pooled over age and strain	M		66	Hycel	2.07	mgs %	1.17	68
Pooled over age and strain	F		60	Hycel	2.80	mgs %	1.87	68
Hamster (Golden Syrian)								
Lak. LVG	M 3 mos/100g	Cardiac–fasted	30	Uricase	2.8	mg/dl	0.83	81
Lak. LVG	F 3 mos/100g	Cardiac–fasted	31	Uricase	5.1	mg/dl	0.89	81
B10F1D Alexander	M 3 mos/100g	Cardiac–fasted	27	Uricase	1.3	mg/dl	0.81	81
B10F1D Alexander	F 3 mos/100g	Cardiac–fasted	30	Uricase	2.5	mg/dl	0.94	81
Hamster – Syrian	M 3 mos/100g				4.6	mg/dl	0.5	86
Syrian	F 3 mos/100g				4.4	mg/dl	0.5	86
Rabbit Oryctolagus cuniculus								
pooled over age and strain	M		109	Hycel	1.18	mgs %	0.28	68
pooled over age and strain	F		113	Hycel	1.15	mgs %	0.30	68
Canine Pooled over breed, age and reproduction status	M		57	Hycel	1.15	mgs %	1.43	68
Pooled over breed, age and reproduction status	F		54	Hycel	1.06	mgs %	1.45	68

Uric Acid (cont.)

SPECIES	SEX/AGE	SAMPLE	NUMBER	METHOD	MEAN	UNITS	S.D.	REF.
Non-humans primates								
Macaca mulatta (pooled over age and sex)			191		0.26	mg/dl	0.11	75
Macaca mulatta			20	Hycel	0.66	mgs %		68
Macaca fascicularis	M Adult	venous or arterial fasted	33	Phosphotung-state reaction	0.14	mg/dl	0.13	122
Macaca arctoides	M Adult	venous or arterial fasted	7	Phosphotung-state reaction	1.2	mg/dl	0.28	122

CHOLESTEROL

SPECIES	SEX/AGE	SAMPLE	NUMBER	METHOD	MEAN	UNITS	S.D.	REF.
Rat CD (CRL: CD (SD) BR)	M 6-8 wks	Cardiac	20	Allain & Roeschlau	55	mg/dl	18	27
CD (CRL: CD (SD) BR)	F 6-8 wks	Cardiac	20	Allain & Roeschlau	38	mg/dl	24	27
CD (CRL: CD (SD) BR)	M 19-21 wks	Cardiac	20	Allain & Roeschlau	39	mg/dl	19	27
CD (CRL: CD (SD) BR)	F 19-21 wks	Cardiac	20	Allain & Roeschlau	52	mg/dl	22	27
CD (CRL: CD (SD) BR)	M 32-34 wks	Cardiac	20	Allain & Roeschlau	36	mg/dl	12	27
CD (CRL: CD (SD) BR)	F 32-34 wks	Cardiac	20	Allain & Roeschlau	60	mg/dl	42	27
Sprague-Dawley - CD	M 30-91 d	Cardiac	70	MCA	54.99	mg/dl	12.72	93
Sprague-Dawley - CD	F 30-91 d	Cardiac	69	MCA	58.72	mg/dl	15.61	93
Sprague-Dawley - CD	M 92-182 d	Cardiac	45	MCA	67.73	mg/dl	15.52	93
Sprague-Dawley - CD	F 92-182 d	Cardiac	45	MCA	73.19	mg/dl	17.35	93
Sprague-Dawley - CD	M 274-450 d	Cardiac	10	MCA	82.57	mg/dl	23.03	93
Sprague-Dawley - CD	F 274-450 d	Cardiac	10	MCA	100.52	mg/dl	24.04	93
(CRL: COBS (CD) SD BR)	M 25 mos		25		73	mg/dl	22	75
(CRL: COBS (CD) SD BR)	F 25 mos		26		67	mg/dl	26	75
Pooled over age and strain	M		66	Hycel	49.9	mgs %	11.7	68
Pooled over age and strain	F		60	Hycel	49.5	mgs %	17.9	68
F344	M 9 wks		10		56.8	mg/dl	7.1	75
F344	F 9 wks		10		53.2	mg/dl	7.3	75

Cholesterol (cont.)

SPECIES	SEX/AGE	SAMPLE	NUMBER	METHOD	MEAN	UNITS	S.D.	REF.
Hamster (Golden) Syrian								
Lak: LVG	M 3 mos/100g	Cardiac-fasted	31	Enzymatic	94	mg/dl	23.0	81
Lak: LVG	F 3 mos/100g	Cardiac-fasted	32	Enzymatic	136	mg/dl	20.4	81
B10F1D Alexander	M 3 mos/100g	Cardiac-fasted	28	Enzymatic	99	mg/dl	11.8	81
B10F1D Alexander	F 3 mos/100g	Cardiac-fasted	30	Enzymatic	95	mg/dl	14.9	81
Hamster								
Syrian	M 3 mos/100g				237	mg/dl	28.7	34
Syrian	F 3 mos/100g				182	mg/dl	48.7	34
Rabbit (Oryctolagus cuniculus)								
Sex mixed or not specified					69	mg/dl	15	129
Sex mixed or not specified					45	mg/dl	18	16
	M				21.5	mg/dl	5.4	69
	F				38.7	mg/dl	11.2	69
Pooled over age and strain	M		109	Hycel	19.35	mgs %	5.60	68
Pooled over age and strain	F		113	Hycel	35.1	mgs %	15.21	68
Dog	M 150–350 d	Jugular vein	394	MCA	151.9	mg/dl	29.35	93
	F 150–350 d	Jugular vein	386	MCA	146.7	mg/dl	31.1	93
Pooled over breed, age and	M		57	Hycel	195.3	mgs %	71.6	68
reproductive status	F		54	Hycel	206.1	mgs %	66.6	68
Non-human primates								
Pan troglodytes			223–224		209	mg/dl	48	82
Pongo pygmaeus			89–92		216	mg/dl	52	84
Gorilla gorilla			44		337	mg/dl	49	83
Cercopithicus aethiops			40–102		141	mg/dl	28.2	5
Cercocebus atys			39–71		155	mg/dl	32.3	5
Presbytis entillis			34–60		173	mg/dl	30.3	5

Cholesterol (cont.)

458

SPECIES	SEX/AGE	SAMPLE	NUMBER	METHOD	MEAN	UNITS	S.D.	REF.
Non-human primates (cont.)								
Saimiri sciureus			41–44		167	mg/dl	40.0	9, 77
Macaca mulatta					128	mg/dl	34	11
Macaca mulatta			61		171.4	mg/dl		75
Macaca mulatta (pooled over age and sex)			20	Hycel	169.8	mgs %	36.4	68
Macaca fascicularis	M Adult	Venous or arterial-fasted	33	Liebermann–Burchard	127	mg/dl	20.9	122
Macaca arctoides	M Adult	Venous or arterial-fasted	7	Liebermann–Burchard	130	mg/dl	18.0	122

TRIGLYCERIDES

SPECIES	SEX/AGE	SAMPLE	NUMBER	METHOD	MEAN	UNITS	S.D.	REF.
Rats								
Sprague-Dawley – CD	M 30–91 d	Cardiac	5		205.58	mg/dl	112.0	93
Sprague-Dawley – CD	F 30–91 d	Cardiac	5		99.48	mg/dl	40.13	93
Sprague-Dawley – CD	M 92–182 d	Cardiac	5		173.28	mg/dl	25.89	93
Sprague-Dawley – CD	F 92–182 d	Cardiac	5		97.46	mg/dl	46.24	93
SD	M	Cardiac	10	SMAC	168.86			75
SD	F	Cardiac	10	SMAC	183.33			75
Hamster (Golden) Syrian								
Lak: LVG	M 3 mos/100g	Cardiac-fasted	30	Enzymatic	126.3	mg/dl	42.7	81
Lak: LVG	F 3 mos/100g	Cardiac-fasted	32	Enzymatic	129.8	mg/dl	27.0	81
B10F1D Alexander	M 3 mos/100g	Cardiac-fasted	29	Enzymatic	123	mg/dl	34.3	81
B10F1D Alexander	F 3 Mos/100g	Cardiac-fasted	30	Enzymatic	100	mg/dl	14.6	81
Non-human primates								
Macaca fascicularis	M Adult	venous or arterial fasted	32	Enzymatic	60.2	mg/dl	16.2	122
Macaca arctoides	M Adult	venous or arterial fasted	7	Enzymatic	44.3	mg/dl	8.86	122

BLOOD UREA NITROGEN
BUN

SPECIES	SEX/AGE	SAMPLE	NUMBER	METHOD	MEAN	UNITS	S.D.	REF.
Mouse – CD-1								
CD-1	M 20–22 g		6		25	mg/dl	1.6	21
A/HeJ	M 20–22 g		6		21.3	mg/dl	2.47	21
A/HeJ	M 20–22 g		6		25	mg/dl	1.0	21
C3H/HeJ	M 20–22 g		6		26	mg/dl	1.7	21
C3H/HeJ	M 20–22 g		6		23	mg/dl	1.3	21
C3H/HeN	M 20–22 g		6		23	mg/dl	1.7	21
C3H/HeN	M 20–22 g		6		22.5	mg/dl	1.7	21
C3H/HeN	M 20–22 g		6		22.5	mg/dl	1.1	21
C57BL/6 x DBA/2 F$_1$	M 45 d	Cardiac	587	Diacetyl monoxime	20.7	mg/dl	5.1	42
Rat – F344								
F344	M 9 wks		12		33.1	mg/dl	8.67	75
F344	F 9 wks		8		36.7	mg/dl	15.01	75
F344	M 19 wks		20		20.8	mg/dl	1.66	75
F344	F 19 wks		20		21.45	mg/dl	2.78	75
CD (CRL: CD (SD) BR)	M 6–8 wks	Cardiac	20	Nod Marsh	13	mg/dl	4	27
CD (CRL: CD (SD) BR)	F 6–8 wks	Cardiac	20	Nod Marsh	19	mg/dl	12	27
CD (CRL: CD (SD) BR)	M 19–21 wks	Cardiac	20	Nod Marsh	18	mg/dl	5	27
CD (CRL: CD (SD) BR)	F 19–21 wks	Cardiac	20	Nod Marsh	23	mg/dl	8	27
CD (CRL: CD (SD) BR)	M 32–34 wks	Cardiac	20	Nod Marsh	16	mg/dl	3	27
CD (CRL: CD (SD) BR)	F 32–34 wks	Cardiac	20	Nod Marsh	25	mg/dl	17	27
Pooled over age and strain	M		66		19.17	mgs %	3.73	68
Pooled over age and strain	F		60		21.54	mgs %	9.45	68
SD	M 30–91 d	Orbital	30	MCA	15.77	mg/dl	1.75	93
SD	M 30–91 d	Cardiac	70	MCA	16.31	mg/dl	2.98	93
SD	F 30–91 d	Orbital	30	MCA	17.48	mg/dl	2.52	93
SD	F 30–91 d	Cardiac	69	MCA	17.54	mg/dl	4.14	93
SD	M 92–182 d	Orbital	20	MCA	17.34	mg/dl	2.22	93
SD	M 92–182 d	Cardiac	55	MCA	19.00	mg/dl	2.78	93
SD	F 92–182 d	Orbital	19	MCA	18.33	mg/dl	2.78	93
SD	F 92–182 d	Cardiac	55	MCA	19.93	mg/dl	3.41	93
SD	M 183–273 d	Orbital	10	MCA	15.75	mg/dl	0.81	93
SD	M 183–273 d	Cardiac	10	MCA	17.36	mg/dl	1.17	93

BUN (cont.)

SPECIES	SEX/AGE	SAMPLE	NUMBER	METHOD	MEAN	UNITS	S.D.	REF.
Rat (cont.)								
SD	F 183–273 d	Orbital	10	MCA	17.38	mg/dl	2.53	93
SD	F 183–273 d	Cardiac	10	MCA	16.47	mg/dl	3.74	93
SD	M 274–450 d	Orbital	10	MCA	16.87	mg/dl	2.13	93
SD	F 274–450 d	Orbital	10	MCA	19.06	mg/dl	5.48	93
CRL: COBS CD (SD) BR	M 4 mos		41		13.7	mg/dl	1.9	75
CRL: COBS CD (SD) BR	F 4 mos		39		16.5	mg/dl	2.7	75
CRL: COBS CD (SD) BR	M 7 mos		45		13.3	mg/dl	1.4	75
CRL: COBS CD (SD) BR	F 7 mos		45		14.6	mg/dl	2.4	75
CRL: COBS CD (SD) BR	M 13 mos		40		13.4	mg/dl	1.9	75
CRL: COBS CD (SD) BR	F 13 mos		40		14.2	mg/dl	2.1	75
CRL: COBS CD (SD) BR	M 19 mos		40		12.3	mg/dl	1.7	75
CRL: COBS CD (SD) BR	F 19 mos		40		13.6	mg/dl	2.1	75
CRL: COBS CD (SD) BR	M 25 mos		64		13.3	mg/dl	5.8	75
CRL: COBS CD (SD) BR	F 25 mos		66		12.0	mg/dl	2.7	75
SD	M	Cardiac	10	SMAC	15.86			75
SD	F	Cardiac	10	SMAC	13.75			75
Hamster – (Golden) Syrian								
Lak: LVG	M 3 mos/100g	Cardiac-fasted	30	Urease	19	mg/dl	4.2	81
Lak: LVG	F 3 mos/100g	Cardiac-fasted	32	Urease	19	mg/dl	2.3	81
B$_{10}$F$_1$D Alexander	M 3 mos/100g	Cardiac-fasted	28	Urease	14	mg/dl	1.9	81
B$_{10}$F$_1$D Alexander	F 3 mos	Cardiac-fasted	29	Urease	16	mg/dl	2.4	81
Strain not specified	F/M $2\frac{1}{2}$–4 mos	Fasted	33		20.5	mg/dl	3.9	120
Strain not specified	M 50 g				24.9	mg/dl	3.4	120
Strain not specified	F 50 g				21.9	mg/dl	3.1	120
Strain not specified	M 100 g				23.2	mg/dl	4.1	120
Strain not specified	F 100 g				27.5	mg/dl	4.6	120
Syrian	M 75–100 g		84		23.4	mg/dl	6.7	86

BUN (cont.)

SPECIES	SEX/AGE	SAMPLE	NUMBER	METHOD	MEAN	UNITS	S.D.	REF.
Hamster (cont.)								
Syrian	F 75-100 g		80		20.8	mg/dl	5.6	86
Syrian	M 3 mos/100g		10		30.1	mg/dl	3.9	115
Syrian	F 3 mos/100g		9		28.4	mg/dl	2.6	115
Guinea pig								
Hartley	M 500-800g		110		25.2	mg/dl	6.37	86
Hartley	F 500-800g		95		21.5	mg/dl	5.84	86
Rabbit (Oryctolagus cuniculus)	M				14.3	mg/dl	3.0	46
Oryctolagus cuniculus	M				17.0	mg/dl	4.4	66
Oryctolagus cuniculus	M				22.1	mg/dl	7	66
Oryctolagus cuniculus	M				23.3	mg/dl	5.2	66
Oryctolagus cuniculus	F				17.0	mg/dl	4.6	46
Oryctolagus cuniculus	F				20.0	mg/dl	3.5	66
Sex not specified or combined					19.23	mg/dl	5.0	66
Sex not specified or combined					38.0	mg/dl	10.0	66
Pooled over age and breed	M		109	Hycel	20.93	mgs %	4.5	68
Pooled over age and breed	F		113	Hycel	21.92	mgs %	5.9	68
Dog - breed not specified	M 150-350 d	Jugular vein	394	MCA	13.1	mg/dl	2.65	93
breed not specified	F 150-350 d	Jugular vein	386	MCA	13.2	mg/dl	3.25	93
Beagle			32		13		2	60
Pooled over breed, age, reproductive status	M		57	Hycel	16.4	mgs %	7.4	68
	F		54	Hycel	16.7	mgs %	10.4	68

BUN (cont.)

SPECIES	SEX/AGE	SAMPLE	NUMBER	METHOD	MEAN	UNITS	S.D.	REF.
Non-human primates								
Pan troglodytes			223–224		14.2	mg/dl	4.8	82
Pongo pygmaeus			89–92		14.5	mg/dl	5.3	84
Gorilla gorilla			44		13.8	mg/dl	4.2	83
Papio sp.			12		8.6	mg/dl	4.6	20
Cercopithicus aethiops			40–102		21.0	mg/dl	5.6	5
Cercocebus atys			39–71		18.0	mg/dl	3.7	5
Presbytis entillis			34–60		25.0	mg/dl	4.9	5
Saimiri sciureus			41–44		31.0	mg/dl	8.0	9, 77
Aotus trivirgatus			43–75		14.0	mg/dl	3.0	128
Saguinus fusicollis or nigricollis			49–95		10.0	mg/dl	4.0	56
Saguinus oedipus			13–40		9.0	mg/dl	3.0	56
Macaca mulatta			20–253		16.9	mg/dl	2.7	11
Macaca mulatta			479		20.8	mg/dl		75
Macaca mulatta (pooled over age and sex)			20	Hycel	16.9	mgs %	2.7	68
Macaca fascicularis	M Adult	Venous or arterial-fasted	33	Diacetyl-monoxime	18	mg/dl	2.8	122
Macaca arctoides	M Adult	Venous or arterial-fasted	7	Diacetyl-monoxime	19	mg/dl	2.3	122

CREATININE

SPECIES	SEX/AGE	SAMPLE	NUMBER	METHOD	MEAN	UNITS	S.D.	REF.
Mouse								
C57BL/6 x DBA/2 F_1	M 45 d	Cardiac	544	Alkaline Picrate	0.5	mg/dl	0.56	42
Rats								
CD (CRL: CD (SD) BR)	M 6–8 wks	Cardiac	20	Chasson	0.6	mg/dl	0.2	27
CD (CRL: CD (SD) BR)	F 6–8 wks	Cardiac	20	Grady & Stanley	0.8	mg.dl	0.3	27
CD (CRL: CD (SD) BR)	M 19–21 wks	Cardiac	20	Chasson	1.0	mg/dl	0.4	27
CD (CRL: CD (SD) BR)	F 19–21 wks	Cardiac	20	Grady & Stanley	0.7	mg/dl	0.4	27
CD (CRL: CD (SD) BR)	M 32–34 wks	Cardiac	20	Chasson	0.9	mg/dl	0.3	27
CD (CRL: CD (SD) BR)	F 32–34 wks	Cardiac	20	Grady & Stanley	0.8	mg/dl	0.2	27
(CRL: COBS CD (SD) BR)	M 4 mos		41		.65	mg/dl	.11	75
(CRL: COBS CD (SD) BR)	F 4 mos		39		.75	mg/dl	.10	75
(CRL: COBS CD (SD) BR)	M 7 mos		40		.65	mg/dl	.11	75
(CRL: COBS CD (SD) BR)	F 7 mos		40		.75	mg/dl	.13	75
(CRL: COBS CD (SD) BR)	M 13 mos		40		.67	mg/dl	.16	75
(CRL: COBS CD (SD) BR)	F 13 mos		40		.71	mg/dl	.15	75
(CRL: COBS CD (SD) BR)	M 19 mos		40		.70	mg/dl	.11	75
(CRL: COBS CD (SD) BR)	F 19 mos		40		.72	mg/dl	.07	75
(CRL: COBS CD (SD) BR)	M 25 mos		64		.80	mg/dl	.32	75
(CRL: COBS CD (SD) BR)	F 25 mos		66		.70	mg/dl	.09	75
SD	M	Cardiac	10	SMAC	.51			75
SD	F	Cardiac	10	SMAC	.60			75
Rat (Continued)								
F344	M 9 wks		8		1.39	mg/dl	0.46	75
F344	F 9 wks		3		0.90	mg/dl	0.87	75
F344	M 19 wks		10		0.61	mg/dl	0.06	75
F344	F 19 wks		10		0.50	mg/dl	0.07	75

Creatinine (cont.)

SPECIES	SEX/AGE	SAMPLE	NUMBER	METHOD	MEAN	UNITS	S.D.	REF.
Hamster (Golden) Syrian								
Lak: LVG	M 3 mos or 100g	Cardiac-fasted	30	Alkaline picrate	0.6	mg/dl	0.08	81
Lak: LVG	F 3 mos or 100g	Cardiac-fasted	32	Alkaline picrate	0.6	mg/dl	0.15	81
B₁₀F₁D Alexander	M 3 mos or 100g	Cardiac-fasted	29	Alkaline picrate	0.5	mg/dl	0.10	81
B₁₀F₁D Alexander	F 3 mos or 100g	Cardiac-fasted	28	Alkaline picrate	0.5	mg/dl	0.11	81
Guinea pig (Albino)								
Hartley	M 500–800g		110		1.38	mg/dl	0.39	86
Hartley	F 500–800g		95		1.40	mg/dl	0.35	86
Rabbit								
Oryctolagus cuniculus	M				1.52	mg/dl	0.19	104
	M				1.4	mg/dl	0.22	66
	M				1.22	mg/dl	0.15	66
	F				1.2	mg/dl	0.10	66
	F				1.25	mg/dl	0.22	66
	Sexes Pooled or Not Stated				1.59	mg/dl	0.34	66
	Sexes Pooled or Not Stated				1.78	mg/dl	0.62	66
NZW					0.80–2.57	mg/dl		86
Dutch belted					0.80–1.70	mg/dl		86
Polish					1.30–2.90	mg/dl		86
Dog								
Beagle			32		0.9		0.2	58
Mongrel	M 12–16 Kg		18		1.35	mg/dl	0.35	82
Mongrel	F 12–16 Kg		10		1.08	mg/dl	0.15	82
Non-human primates								
Macaca mulatta	M				1.50	mg/dl	0.9	82
Macaca mulatta	F				1.28	mg/dl	0.6	82
Papio sp.	M				4.90	mg/dl	0.5	82
Papio sp.	F				4.60	mg/dl	0.6	82

TOTAL PROTEIN

SPECIES	SEX/AGE	SAMPLE	NUMBER	METHOD	MEAN	UNITS	S.D.	REF.
Mouse								
CD-1	M 20–22 g		6		6.2	g/dl	0.2	21
CD-1	M 20–22 g		6		5.3	g/dl	0.6	21
A/HeJ	M 20–22 g		6		6.5	g/dl	0.2	21
A/HeJ	M 20–22 g		6		6.6	g/dl	0.4	21
C3H/HeJ	M 20–22 g		6		6.2	g/dl	0.25	21
C3H/HeJ	M 20–22 g		6		5.0	g/dl	0.0	21
C3H/HeN	M 20–22 g		6		5.9	g/dl	0.3	21
C3H/HeN	M 20–22 g		6		5.2	g/dl	0.2	21
C57BL/6 x DBA/2 F$_1$	M 45 d	Cardiac	591	Biuret	4.96	g/dl	0.39	42
C57BL/6	M 8–10 mo	Cardiac-fasted	41	Lowry	6.4	g/dl	1.11	42
C56BL/6	M 8–10 mo	Cardiac-fasted	44	Lowry	6.3	g/dl	1.13	42
Rat								
CD (CRL:CD (SD) BR)	M 6–8 wks	Cardiac	20	Biuret	6.3	gms/dl	0.5	27
CD (CRL: CD (SD) BR)	F 6–8 wks	Cardiac	20	Biuret	7.5	gms/dl	1.3	27
CD (CRL: CD (SD) BR)	M 19–21 wks	Cardiac	20	Biuret	7.3	gms/dl	0.6	27
CD (CRL: CD (SD) BR)	F 19–21 wks	Cardiac	20	Biuret	6.7	gms/dl	0.8	27
CD (CRL: CD (SD) BR)	M 32–34 wks	Cardiac	20	Biuret	7.3	gms/dl	0.7	27
CD (CRL: CD (SD) BR)	F 32–34 wks	Cardiac	20	Biuret	7.2	gms/dl	2.4	27
(CRL: COBS CD (SD) BR)	M 4 mos		41		7.18	g/dl	.29	75
(CRL: COBS CD (SD) BR)	F 4 mos		39		7.52	g/dl	.40	75
(CRL: COBS CD (SD) BR)	M 7 mos		40		7.29	g/dl	.36	75
(CRL: COBS CD (SD) BR)	F 7 mos		40		7.74	g/dl	.67	75
(CRL: COBS CD (SD) BR)	M 13 mos		40		7.32	g/dl	.44	75
(CRL: COBS CD (SD) BR)	F 13 mos		40		7.97	g/dl	.44	75
(CRL: COBS CD (SD) BR)	M 19 mos		40		7.41	g/dl	.38	75
(CRL: COBS CD (SD) BR)	F 19 mos		40		7.95	g/dl	.61	75
(CRL: COBS CD (SD) BR)	M 25 mos		62		6.89	g/dl	.42	75
(CRL: COBS CD (SD) BR)	F 25 mos		68		7.48	g/dl	.49	75
SD	M	Cardiac	10	SMAC	7.19			75
SD	F	Cardiac	10	SMAC	7.54			75
Pooled over age and strain	M		66	Hycel	5.34	gms %	0.43	68
Pooled over age and strain	F		60	Hycel	5.41	gms %	0.75	75

Total Protein (cont.)

Rat (cont.)

SPECIES	SEX/AGE	SAMPLE	NUMBER	METHOD	MEAN	UNITS	S.D.	REF.
CD–Sprague-Dawley	M 30–91 d	Orbital	30	MCA	6.37	g/dl	0.73	93
CD–Sprague-Dawley	M 30–91 d	Cardiac	70	MCA	6.30	g/dl	0.43	93
CD–Sprague-Dawley	F 30–91 d	Orbital	30	MCA	6.68	g/dl	0.60	93
CD–Sprague-Dawley	F 30–91 d	Cardiac	69	MCA	6.37	g/dl	0.51	93
CD–Sprague-Dawley	M 92–182 d	Orbital	20	MCA	7.41	g/dl	0.56	93
CD–Sprague-Dawley	M 92–182 d	Cardiac	55	MCA	6.84	g/dl	0.45	93
CD–Sprague-Dawley	F 92–182 d	Orbital	19	MCA	7.61	g/dl	0.50	93
CD–Sprague-Dawley	F 92–182 d	Cardiac	55	MCA	7.25	g/dl	0.63	93
CD–Sprague-Dawley	M 183–273 d	Orbital	10	MCA	7.33	g/dl	0.52	93
CD–Sprague-Dawley	M 183–273 d	Cardiac	10	MCA	7.64	g/dl	0.54	93
CD–Sprague-Dawley	F 183–273 d	Orbital	10	MCA	8.06	g/dl	0.76	93
CD–Sprague-Dawley	F 183–273 d	Cardiac	10	MCA	8.32	g/dl	0.59	93
CD–Sprague-Dawley	M 274–450 d	Orbital	10	MCA	7.52	g/dl	0.27	93
CD–Sprague-Dawley	M 274–450 d	Cardiac	10	MCA	7.48	g/dl	0.31	93
CD–Sprague-Dawley	F 274–450 d	Orbital	10	MCA	8.45	g/dl	0.72	93
CD–Sprague-Dawley	F 274–450 d	Cardiac	10	MCA	8.26	g/dl	0.79	93
F344	M 9 wks		10	MCA	6.06	g/dl	0.48	75
F344	F 9 wks		10	MCA	5.74	g/dl	0.89	75
Hamster (Golden) Syrian								
Lak: LVG	M 3 mos/100g	Cardiac-fasted	31	Biuret	6.3	g/dl	0.32	81
Lak: LVG	F 3 mos/100g	Cardiac-fasted	32	Biuret	5.9	g/dl	0.34	81
B10F1D Alexander	M 3 mos/100g	Cardiac-fasted	28	Biuret	5.4	g/dl	0.64	81
B10F1D Alexander	F 3 mos/100g	Cardiac-fasted	27	Biuret	5.3	g/dl	0.67	81
Hamster								
Syrian	M 3 mos/100g				6.9	g/dl	0.3	86
Syrian	M 3 mos/100g				6.3	g/dl	0.3	34
Syrian	F 3 mos/100g				7.3	g/dl	0.5	86
Syrian	F 3 mos/100g				6.4	g/dl	0.3	34

Total protein (cont.)

SPECIES	SEX/AGE	SAMPLE	NUMBER	METHOD	MEAN	UNITS	S.D.	REF.
Guinea pig								
Hartley	M 500–800 g		110		5.60	g/dl	0.28	86
Hartley	F 500–800 g		95		4.80	g/dl	0.34	86
Rabbit (Oryctolagus cuniculus)								
Oryctolagus cuniculus	M				6.45	g/dl	.31	46
Oryctolagus cuniculus	M				6.02	g/dl	.52	104
Oryctolagus cuniculus	M				5.25	g/dl	.38	104
Oryctolagus cuniculus	M				6.3	g/dl	.50	66
Oryctolagus cuniculus	M				7.2	g/dl	1.0	66
Oryctolagus cuniculus	F				6.36	g/dl	.32	46
Oryctolagus cuniculus	F				7.1	g/dl	0.4	66
Oryctolagus cuniculus	F				8.5	g/dl	1.0	66
Pooled over age and breed	M		109	Hycel	6.11	gms %	0.44	68
Pooled over age and breed	F		113	Hycel	6.14	gms %	0.54	68
Dog Breed not specified	M 150–350 d	jugular vein	394	MCA	5.83	g/dl	0.39	93
Breed not specified	F 150–350 d	jugular vein	386	MCA	5.70	g/dl	0.37	93
Beagle			32		5.9		0.3	60
Pooled over breed, age and reproductive status	M		57	Hycel	6.11	gms %	1.2	68
	F		54	Hycel	5.8	gms %	0.73	68
Non-human primates								
Pan troglodytes			223–224		7.4	g/dl	0.7	82
Pongo pygmaeus			89–92		7.5	g/dl	0.7	84
Gorilla gorilla			44		6.8	g/dl	0.6	83
Papio sp.			12		6.3	g/dl	0.6	20
Cercopithecus aethiops			40–102		7.6	g/dl	0.8	5
Cercocebus atys			39–71		8.5	g/dl	0.7	5
Presbytis entillis			34–60		7.7	g/dl	0.7	5
Saimiri sciureus			41–44		7.5	g/dl	0.6	9, 77
Aotus trivirgatus			43–75		7.0	g/dl	1.2	128

Total Protein (cont.)

SPECIES	SEX/AGE	SAMPLE	NUMBER	METHOD	MEAN	UNITS	S.D.	REF.
Non-human primates (cont.)								
Saguinus fusicollis or nigricollis			49–95		7.2	g/dl	1.5	56
Saguinus oedipus			13–40		7.4	g/dl	1.2	56
Macaca mulatta			20–253		6.6	g/dl	0.5	11
Macaca mulatta			124		8.0	g/dl		75
Macaca mulatta – pooled over age and sex			20	Hycel	6.61	gms %	0.46	68
Macaca fascicularis	M Adult	venous or arterial fasted	33	Biuret	7.6	g/dl	0.39	122
Macaca arctoides	M Adult	venous or arterial fasted	7	Biuret	7.5	g/dl	0.63	122

ALBUMIN

SPECIES	SEX/AGE	SAMPLE	NUMBER	METHOD	MEAN	UNITS	S.D.	REF.
Mouse – CD-1	M 20-22g		6		3.4	g/dl	0.1	21
CD-1	M 20-22g		6		3.0	g/dl	0.5	21
A/HeJ	M 20-22g		6		3.0	g/dl	0.5	21
A/HeJ	M 20-22g		6		4.0	g/dl	0.3	21
C3H/HeJ	M 20-22g		6		3.9	g/dl	0.2	21
C3H/HeJ	M 20-22g		6		3.5	g/dl	0.0	21
C3H/HeN	M 20-22g		6		3.58	g/dl	0.2	21
C3H/HeN	M 20-22g		6		3.5	g/dl	0.0	21
C57BL/6 x DBA/2 F$_1$	M 45 d	Cardiac	590	Bromcresol Green	3.09	g/dl	0.25	42
C57BL/6	M 8-10 mos	Cardiac fasted	41	Electrophoresis	3.68	g/dl	0.58	43
C57BL/6	M 25-28 mos	Cardiac fasted	43	Electrophoresis	3.56	g/dl	0.68	43
Rat (CD (CRL: CD (SD) BR)	M 6-8 wks	Cardiac	20	Bromcresol Green	3.8	g/dl	0.5	27
(CD (CRL: CD (SD) BR)	F 6-8 wks	Cardiac	20	Bromcresol Green	4.2	g/dl	0.6	27
(CD (CRL: CD (SD) BR)	M 19-21 wks	Cardiac	20	Bromcresol Green	3.8	g/dl	0.2	27
(CD (CRL: CD (SD) BR)	F 19-21 wks	Cardiac	20	Bromcresol Green	3.8	g/dl	0.6	27
(CD (CRL: CD (SD) BR)	M 32-34 wks	Cardiac	20	Bromcresol Green	3.5	g/dl	0.5	27
(CD (CRL: CD (SD) BR)	F 32-34 wks	Cardiac	20	Bromcresol Green	4.0	g/dl	0.7	27
(CRL: COBS CD (SD) BR)	M 25 mos		25		3.27	g/dl	.35	75
(CRL: COBS CD (SD) BR)	F 25 mos		26		3.85	g/dl	.31	75
SD	M	Cardiac	10	SMAC	3.86			75
SD	F	Cardiac	10	SMAC	4.33			75
F344	M 9 wks		10		3.84	g/dl	.25	75
F344	F 9 wks		9		3.84	g/dl	.27	75
CD Sprague-Dawley	M 30-91 d	Orbital	30	MCA	4.14	g/dl	0.30	93
CD Sprague-Dawley	M 30-91 d	Cardiac	70	MCA	4.32	g/dl	0.27	93
CD Sprague-Dawley	F 30-91 d	Orbital	30	MCA	4.32	g/dl	0.29	93
CD Sprague-Dawley	F 30-91 d	Cardiac	69	MCA	4.41	g/dl	0.25	93

Albumin (cont.)

SPECIES	SEX/AGE	SAMPLE	NUMBER	METHOD	MEAN	UNITS	S.D.	REF.
Rat (cont.)								
CD Sprague-Dawley	M 92–182 d	Orbital	20	MCA	4.53	g/dl	0.365	93
CD Sprague-Dawley	M 92–182 d	Cardiac	55	MCA	4.36	g/dl	0.32	93
CD Sprague-Dawley	F 92–182 d	Orbital	19	MCA	4.85	g/dl	0.42	93
CD Sprague-Dawley	F 92–182 d	Cardiac	55	MCA	4.86	g/dl	0.49	93
CD Sprague-Dawley	M 183–273 d	Orbital	10	MCA	4.29	g/dl	0.38	93
CD Sprague-Dawley	M 183–273 d	Cardiac	10	MCA	4.43	g/dl	0.30	93
CD Sprague-Dawley	F 183–273 d	Orbital	10	MCA	5.39	g/dl	0.58	93
CD Sprague-Dawley	F 183–273 d	Cardiac	10	MCA	5.35	g/dl	0.61	93
Sprague-Dawley – CD	M 274–450 d	Orbital	10	MCA	4.17	g/dl	0.21	93
Sprague-Dawley – CD	M 274–450 d	Cardiac	10	MCA	4.33	g/dl	0.27	93
Sprague-Dawley – CD	F 274–450 d	Orbital	10	MCA	5.30	g/dl	0.53	93
Sprague-Dawley – CD	F 274–450 d	Cardiac	10	MCA	5.27	g/dl	0.73	93
Hamster (Golden) Syrian								
Lak: LVG	M 3 mos/100g	Cardiac-fasted	31	Bromcresol Green	4.3	g/dl	0.22	81
Lak: LVG	F 3 mos/100g	Cardiac-fasted	31	Bromcresol Green	4.1	g/dl	0.28	81
B10F1D Alexander	M 3 mos/100g	Cardiac-fasted	30	Bromcresol Green	4.0	g/dl	0.22	81
B10F1D Alexander	F 3 mos/100g	Cardiac-fasted	30	Bromcresol Green	4.2	g/dl	0.28	81
Syrian	M 3 mos/100g				3.2	g/dl	0.4	86
Syrian	M 3 mos/100g				3.7	g/dl	0.3	34
Syrian	F 3 mos/100g				3.5	g/dl	0.3	86
Syrian	F 3 mos/100g				3.6	g/dl	0.2	34

Albumin (cont.)

SPECIES	SEX/AGE	SAMPLE	NUMBER	METHOD	MEAN	UNITS	S.D.	REF.
Guinea pig								
Hartley	M 500–800 g		110		2.73	g/dl	0.30	86
Hartley	F 500–800 g		85		2.42	g/dl	0.14	86
Rabbit								
NZW M	3–5 Kg		120		3.39	g/dl	0.29	86
NZW F	3–5 Kg		80		3.04	g/dl	0.26	86
Canine Breed not specified	M 150–350 d	Jugular	394	MCA	3.31	g/dl	0.28	93
Breed not specified	F 150–350 d	Jugular	386	MCA	3.34	g/dl	0.27	93
Mongrel	M 12–16 Kg		18		3.68	g/dl	0.22	86
Mongrel	F 12–16 Kg		10		3.10	g/dl	0.27	86
Non-human primates								
Pan troglodytes			223–224		3.7	g/dl	0.4	82
Pongo pygmaeus			89–92		4.7	g/dl	0.5	84
Gorilla gorilla			44		4.6	g/dl	0.5	83
Papio sp.			12		3.7	g/dl	0.4	20
Cercopithecus aethiops			40–102		3.7	g/dl	1.0	5
Cercocebus atys			39–71		4.2	g/dl	1.0	5
Presbytis entillis			34–60		4.1	g/dl	0.8	5
Saimiri sciureus			41–44		4.1	g/dl	0.6	9, 77
Aotus trivirgatus			43–75		2.7	g/dl	0.7	128
Saguinus fusicollis or nigricollis			49–95		3.6	g/dl	0.8	56
Saguinus oedipus			13–40		3.5	g/dl	0.6	54
Macaca mulatta			20–253		4.4	g/dl	0.9	11
Macaca mulatta			113		4.29	g/dl		75
Macaca fascicularis	M Adult	Venous or arterial	33	Bromcresol green	4.0	g/dl	0.21	122
Macaca arctoides	M Adult	Venous or arterial	7	Bromcresol green	4.4	g/dl	0.34	122

LIVER FUNCTION TESTS

IN LABORATORY AND DOMESTIC ANIMALS

Sulfobromophthalein (BSP) clearances in various laboratory animals.

Species	Dose Level (mg/kg) (1V)	Half-Life (minutes)	Disappearance Rate (%/min)	Plasma Concentration (mg/dl)	% Retention 30-minutes (unless otherwise stated)	Ref.
Cat	5	2.2	34.7	-	0.6	25
Cattle	2	3.3–4.2	-	-	-	99
Chickens	5	1	-	-	-	99
Dog	5	-	-	-	1.81	121
Dog	5	-	-	-	5	53
Dog	5	-	-	-	3.4	113
Dog	5	4.2	17.0	-	1.9	24
Dog	5	-	-	-	0	54
Dog	5	-	-	1 mg at 32 min.	0.8/45 min.	70
Dog	7.5	-	-	-	-	63
Dog	10	-	-	-	2–5	52
Dog	15	-	-	2 mg at 32 min.	-	63
Dog	30	-	-	8 mg at 32 min.	-	63
Dog	60	-	-	30 mg at 32 min.	-	63
Horse	2–5	2.3	-	-	-	99
Macaca mulatta newborn	5	18	-	-	-	71
5 day old	5	10	-	-	-	71
Alouatta	5	2.6	-	-	5%/45 min.	61
Alouatta	20	6.1	-	-	5%/45 min.	61
Mice	50	-	-	0.46 mg at 30 min.	6.5	130
Mice	50 IP	-	-	-	-	22
Rabbit	30	-	-	1 mg at 32 min.	-	63
Rabbit	60	-	-	2 mg at 32 min.	-	63
Rabbit	120	-	-	20 mg at 32 min.	-	63

(continued)

Sulfobromophthalein (BSP) clearances in various laboratory animals.

Species	Dose Level (mg/kg) (IV)	Half-Life (minutes)	Disappearance Rate (%/min)	Plasma Concentration (mg/dl)	% Retention 30-minutes (unless otherwise stated)	Ref.
Rat Gunn	5	–	–	–	0.0%/30 min.	103
Rat	30	–	–	3 mg at 32 min.	–	63
Rat M	50	–	–	–	3.7%/10 min.	17
Rat F	50	–	–	–	4.79%/10 min.	17
Rat	50	–	–	–	1.1%/10 min.	74
Rat Wistar M	–	–	–	–	–	30
Rat	60	–	–	4 mg at 32 min.	–	63
Rat	120	–	–	30 mg at 32 min.	–	63
Sheep & Goat	2	3.3–4.2	–	–	–	99
Sheep	2–6	–	–	–	5.9%/10 min.	28

LIVER FUNCTION TESTS IN

LABORATORY AND DOMESTIC ANIMALS

Indocyanine green clearances in various laboratory animals.

Species	Dose Level (mg/kg)	Half-Life (minutes)	Disappearance Rate (%/min)	Clearance (ml/min/kg)	30-minute % Retention	Ref.
Cat	1.5	3.8	19.2	3.6	7.3	25
Dog	1	-	7.6	-	-	57
Dog	0.5	8.9	8.77	-	-	121
Dog Beagle	0.5	5.5	13.1	-	-	123
Dog Mongrel	0.5	8.3	9.7	-	-	123
Dog Beagle M	0.5	5.64	-	-	-	67
Dog Beagle F	0.5	7.03	-	-	-	67
Dog	0.5	8.4	8.9	5.2	-	13
Dog	0.4-0.6	10.8	6.9	3.2	-	62
Dog	1	9.1	7.6	-	-	57
Dog	1	9.0	8.1	3.7	14.7	24
Dog	1	7	10	-	-	64
Dog	1.5	8.4	8.7	3.9	11.4	24
Dog	2	17	4	-	-	64
Dog	4	30	2.3	-	-	64
Dog	9	-	3.8	-	-	57
M mulatta F	0.5	1.9	36.5	-	1.13	124
M mulatta M	0.5	1.3	52.9	-	2.03	124
M mulatta anesthetized	0.5	3.5	25.5	-	-	124
Mice	10	6.0	-	-	-	99
Rat Gunn	4	-	43.1	-	-	57
Rat	4	2.5	28	-	-	64
Rat	8	4	17	-	-	64

(continued)
Indocyanine green clearances in various laboratory animals.

Species	Dose Level (mg/kg)	Half-Life (minutes)	Disappearance Rate (%/min)	Clearance (ml/min/kg)	30-minute % Retention	Ref.
Rat	16	6.5	11	-	-	64
Rat	32	8.5	8	-	-	64
Rat	64	18	4	-	-	64
Rabbit	3.5	-	36.5	-	-	57
Rabbit	8	1.5	46	-	-	64
Rabbit	16	3.5	20	-	-	64
Rabbit	32	7	10	-	-	64

LIVER FUNCTION TESTS IN

LABORATORY AND DOMESTIC ANIMALS

Total serum bilirubin and conjugated bilirubin levels in various non-human primates.

Species	Total bilirubin (mg/dl)			Conjugated bilirubin (direct reacting, mg/dl)			Ref.
	Mean	SD	Range	Mean	SD	Range	
Gorilla	0.40	–	0.2–0.8	–	–	–	80
Gorilla	0.23	0.15	–	–	–	–	83
Orangutan	0.90	–	0.6–1.4	–	–	–	80
Orangutan	0.55	0.63	–	–	–	–	84
Chimpanzee	0.50	–	0.2–0.8	–	–	–	80
Chimpanzee	–	–	0.0–0.4	–	–	0.0–0.1	32
Chimpanzee	0.17	0.05	–	–	–	–	131
Chimpanzee	0.17	0.11	–	–	–	–	82
Papio							
African	–	–	–	0.30	–	–	31
Domestic	–	–	–	0.23	–	–	31
Cross	–	–	–	0.23	–	–	31
Nairobi	–	–	–	0.34	–	–	31
Male	–	–	–	0.24	–	–	31
Female	–	–	–	0.24	–	–	31
Species	0.30	0.16	0.10–0.90	–	–	–	31
Cercopithecus aethiops	0.27	0.13	0.04–0.80	–	–	–	5
Cercocebus atys	0.37	0.10	0.08–0.70	–	–	–	5
Presbytis entellus	0.28	0.15	0.04–0.71	–	–	–	5

(continued)

Total serum bilirubin and conjugated bilirubin levels in various non-human primates.

Species	Total bilirubin (mg/dl)			Conjugated bilirubin (direct reacting, mg/dl)			Ref.
	Mean	SD	Range	Mean	SD	Range	
Macaca							
mulatta newborn	4.10	–	–	–	–	–	71
mulatta 5 days	1.00	–	–	–	–	–	71
mulatta	0.36	0.21	–	–	–	–	95
mulatta M	0.38	0.18	0.05–1.32	–	–	–	86
mulatta F	0.57	0.20	0.05–1.32	–	–	–	86
mulatta	0.35	–	–	–	–	–	1
mulatta	0.38	0.28	–	0.80	0.28	–	6
mulatta	0.10	–	0.08–0.18	–	–	–	41
mulatta	0.15	0.15	–	–	–	–	18
mulatta	–	–	–	–	–	0–0.2	125
mulatta	0.21	–	–	–	–	–	49
mulatta	0.38	0.28	–	–	–	–	11
mulatta	0.07	0.21	–	–	–	–	68
mulatta	0.33	–	–	–	–	–	75
arctoides M	0.46	0.39	0.03–2.79	–	–	–	91
arctoides F	0.44	0.36	0.03–2.20	–	–	–	91
arctoides M	0.26	0.09	0.13–0.59	0.03	0.03	0.00–0.10	4
arctoides F	0.29	0.09	0.10–0.47	0.08	0.02	0.00–0.92	4
arctoides M	0.14	0.08	–	–	–	–	122
fascicularis M	0.25	0.05	0.19–0.40	0.05	0.09	0.00–0.32	4
fascicularis F	0.25	0.12	0.04–0.88	0.07	0.05	0.00–0.63	4
fascicularis M	0.06	0.06	–	–	–	–	122
radiata	0.25	0.09	0.10–0.45	0.03	0.02	0.00–0.08	4
radiata	0.22	0.11	0.04–0.60	0.00	0.01	0.00–0.02	4
Saimiri							
sciureus	0.20	0.30	0.00–1.90	–	–	–	87
sciureus	0.50	–	–	0.20	–	–	85
sciureus	0.30	0.23	–	–	–	–	9, 77
Alouatta	0.75	0.06	–	0.17	0.03	–	61

(continued)

Total serum bilirubin and conjugated bilirubin levels in various non-human primates.

Species	Total bilirubin (mg/dl)			Conjugated bilirubin (direct reacting, mg/dl)			Ref.
	Mean	SD	Range	Mean	SD	Range	
Marmoset	0.20	–	–	0.10	–	0–0.3	33
Marmoset, adult M	0.48	0.54	0.02–4.41	–	–	–	132
Marmoset, adult F	0.25	0.22	0.00–0.95	–	–	–	132
Marmoset, juvenile M	0.51	0.45	0.00–1.45	–	–	–	132
Marmoset, juvenile F	0.55	0.50	0.00–1.36	–	–	–	132
Tamarins	0.21	–	–	0.10	–	0–2.11	56
Cotton top	0.20	–	–	0.11	–	0–2.07	56

LIVER FUNCTION TESTS IN

LABORATORY AND DOMESTIC ANIMALS

Total and conjugated serum bilirubin levels in various laboratory animals.

Species	Total bilirubin (mg/dl)			Conjugated bilirubin (direct reacting, mg/dl)			Ref.
	Mean	SD	Range	Mean	SD	Range	
Armadillo	0.10	–	0.00–0.19	–	–	–	111
Cat M	0.18	0.05	0.10–1.89	–	–	–	86
Cat F	0.15	0.04	0.10–1.89	–	–	–	86
Cat	–	–	0.15–0.30	–	–	–	36
Cattle	–	–	0.01–1.00	–	–	–	36
Chinchilla	–	–	0.00–0.23	–	–	–	86
Dog	–	–	0.07–0.61	–	–	0.06–0.12	110
Dog	0.22	–	0.05–0.55	–	–	–	121
Dog	–	–	0.10–0.60	–	–	–	36
Dog M	0.25	0.11	0.00–0.50	–	–	–	86
Dog F	0.21	0.10	0.00–0.05	–	–	–	86
Canine M 150–350d	0.16	0.30	–	–	–	–	93
Canine F 150–350d	0.19	0.30	–	–	–	–	93
Canine M pooled (bred, age, repro. status)	0.82	1.60	–	–	–	–	68
Canine F pooled (bred, age, repro. status)	0.37	0.68	–	–	–	–	68
Gerbil	–	–	0.20–0.60	–	–	–	86

(continued)

Total and conjugated serum bilirubin levels in various laboratory animals.

Species	Total bilirubin (mg/dl)			Conjugated bilirubin (direct reacting, mg/dl)			Ref.
	Mean	SD	Range	Mean	SD	Range	
Guinea Pig	1.00	–	–	–	–	–	48
Guinea Pig							
Male	0.30	0.08	0.00–0.90	–	–	–	86
Female	0.32	0.07	0.00–0.09	–	–	–	86
Horse	–	–	0.01–1.00	–	–	–	36
Mice	0.54	–	–	–	–	–	58
Mice	0.40	0.50	–	0.15	0.10	–	130
Mice	1.00	–	–	–	–	–	42
Mice M	0.75	0.05	–	–	–	–	86
Mice F	0.70	0.04	–	–	–	–	86
Mice	0.43	–	–	–	–	–	130
Opposum	–	–	0.30–0.80	–	–	–	86
Opposum	0.48	0.16	0.30–0.80	–	–	–	118
Rabbit M	0.32	0.04	0.00–0.74	–	–	–	86
Rabbit F	0.30	0.04	0.00–0.74	–	–	–	86
Rabbit M	0.28	0.12	–	–	–	–	47
Rabbit F	0.21	0.11	–	–	–	–	47
Rabbit pooled age & strain	0.28	0.33	–	–	–	–	68
Rabbit pooled age & strain	0.21	0.26	–	–	–	–	68
Rat 9 wks	0.41	–	–	–	–	–	30
Rat 24 wks	0.40	–	–	–	–	–	30
Rat M	0.35	0.02	0.05–0.55	–	–	–	86
Rat F	0.24	0.07	0.05–0.55	–	–	–	86

(continued)

Total and conjugated serum bilirubin levels in various laboratory animals.

Species	Total bilirubin (mg/dl)			Conjugated bilirubin (direct reacting, mg/dl)			Ref.
	Mean	SD	Range	Mean	SD	Range	
Rat (cont.)							
Fisher	–	–	0.15–0.36	–	–	–	86
Osborne–Mendel	–	–	0.10–0.52	–	–	–	86
Long–Evans	–	–	0.00–0.55	–	–	–	86
Germ–Free	–	–	0.24–0.64	–	–	–	86
Sprague–Dawley M	0.30	0.20	–	–	–	–	89
Sprague–Dawley F	0.20	0.10	–	–	–	–	89
Sprague–Dawley M	0.10	–	–	–	–	–	75
Sprague–Dawley F	0.10	–	–	–	–	–	75
Sprague–Dawley M 30–91d	0.15	0.24	–	–	–	–	93
Sprague–Dawley F 30–91d	0.13	0.21	–	–	–	–	93
Sprague–Dawley M 92–182d	0.17	0.20	–	–	–	–	93
Sprague–Dawley F 92–182d	0.17	0.20	–	–	–	–	93
Sprague–Dawley M 274–450d	0.30	0.14	–	–	–	–	93
Sprague–Dawley 274–450d	0.39	0.28	–	–	–	–	93
Wistar M	0.10	–	–	0.01	–	–	103
Wistar Gunn	8.09	2.85	–	0.21	0.05	–	103
Rat							
pooled age & strain M	0.24	0.34	–	–	–	–	68
pooled age & strain F	0.07	0.15	–	–	–	–	68

(continued)
Total and conjugated serum bilirubin levels in various laboratory animals.

Species	Total bilirubin (mg/dl)			Conjugated bilirubin (direct reacting, mg/dl)			Ref.
	Mean	SD	Range	Mean	SD	Range	
Rat (cont.)							
CD (CRL:CD(SD)BR)							
M 6-8 wks	0.30	0.2	-	-	-	-	27
F 6-8 wks	0.40	0.3	-	-	-	-	27
M 19-21 wks	0.40	0.3	-	-	-	-	27
F 19-21 wks	0.90	0.4	-	-	-	-	27
M 32-34 wks	0.40	0.4	-	-	-	-	27
F 32-34 wks	0.30	0.3	-	-	-	-	27
CRL: COBS CD(SD)BR							
M 25 mos.	0.16	0.09	-	-	-	-	75
F 25 mos.	0.14	0.05	-	-	-	-	75
F344 M 9 wks	0.11	0.30	-	-	-	-	75
F344 F 9 wks	0.34	0.23	-	-	-	-	75
Hamster							
LAK: LVG M 3 mos.	0.4	0.18	-	-	-	-	81
LAK: LVG F 3 mos.	0.3	0.16	-	-	-	-	81
$B_{10}F_1D$ Alexander							
M 3 mos.	0.5	0.26	-	-	-	-	81
F 3 mos.	0.2	0.10	-	-	-	-	81
M 3 mos.	0.52	0.16	-	-	-	-	115
M 3 mos.	0.42	0.12	-	-	-	-	86
F 3 mos.	0.54	0.11	-	-	-	-	115
F 3 mos.	0.36	0.11	-	-	-	-	86

ACID-BASE PARAMETERS
ARTERIAL BLOOD
ALBINO RAT (UNANESTHETIZED)

REFERENCE	NUMBER	pH	PaCO$_2$ mm Hg	HCO$_3$ mM/1	BE mEq/1
2	9	7.40 $\pm$ 0.05	38.0 $\pm$ 1.0	23.1 $\pm$ 0.	-0.8
19	6	7.416 $\pm$ 0.027	40.7 $\pm$ 1.0	25.2 $\pm$ 2.0	
59	8	7.40 $\pm$ 0.03	39.9 $\pm$ 1.8		
72	128	7.43 $\pm$ 0.45	40.9 $\pm$ 4.5	27.5 $\pm$ 2.3	+4.2 $\pm$ 2.3
73	10	7.44 $\pm$ 0.03	32.7 $\pm$ 7.6	21.8 $\pm$ 4.4	-1.6 $\pm$ 3.8
76	8	7.476 $\pm$ 0.03	37.4 $\pm$ 2.3	26.6 $\pm$ 1.7	
94	120	7.466 $\pm$ 0.020	41.2 $\pm$ 1.87	29.5	
106	52	7.48 (7.34–7.56)	27.1 (20.5–34.5)		-1.1 (1.15 – – 3.31)
78	26	7.433 $\pm$ 0.020	35.7 $\pm$ 3.5	24.0 $\pm$ 2.2	
8	10	7.450 $\pm$ 0.020	35.5 $\pm$ 2.6	24.7 $\pm$ 1.9	+1.5 $\pm$ 2.1

Values are mean $\pm$ S.D.

ACID-BASE PARAMETERS
ARTERIAL BLOOD
GUINEA PIGS (UNANESTHETIZED)

	TEST	NUMBER	MEAN	UNITS	S.D.	REF.
1.	pH	69	7.444		0.032	102
2.	$PaCO_2$	69	35.7	mmHg	4.4	102
3.	PaO_2	25	91.9	mmHg	7.3	102
4.	HCO_3	69	24.4	mM/l	2.8	102
5.	BE	69	+0.4	mEq/l	2.1	102
6.	HCO_3STD	69	24.7	mM/l	1.8	102
7.	Cl	30	99.3	mEq/l	3.6	102
8.	T_B	69	39.5	°C	0.6	102
1.	pH	6	7.452		0.012	8
2.	$PaCO_2$	6	32.0	mmHg	2.4	8
3.	PaO_2	6	93.6	mmHg	5.9	8
4.	HCO_3	6	22.0	mM/l	1.3	8
5.	BE	6	+0.6	mEq/l	0.5	8
6.	HCO_3STD	6	24.4	mM/l	0.3	8
7.	T_B	6	39.8	°C	0.5	8

SYRIAN HAMSTERS

	TEST	MEAN	UNITS	S.D.	REF.
1.	pH	7.48		0.03	88
2.	$PaCO_2$	41.1	mm Hg	2.4	88
3.	PaO_2	71.8	mm Hg	4.9	88
4.	HCO_3	29.9	mEq/l	2.9	88

REPORTED URINE VALUES

Species	Strain	Variable	Value	Units	Reference
Rat	Wistar (male)	Volume	5–23	ml/24 hr	126
	Wistar (male)		18.2 ± 5.6	ml/24 hr	127
	F–344/N		4–5	ml/16 hr	65
	F–344/N		11.3 ± 2.9	ml/24 hr	98
	F–344/N		8.1 ± 1.1	ml/24 hr	79
	NS (not specified)		4.3 – 24.0	ml/24 hr	3
	Sprague–Dawley		9.3–12.3	ml/24 hr	98
	Wistar		6.2 ± 3.0	ml/100g/24 hr	109
	Wistar	Specific Gravity	1.030–1.078		10
	F–344/N		1.054 ± 0.008		98
	F–344/N		1.046–1.057		79
	Sprague–Dawley		1.050–1.062		98
	F–344/N	pH	6–6.5		65
	F–344/N		7.9 ± 0.7		98
	Wistar (male)		6.6 ± 0.4		127
	Sprague–Dawley		7.7–8.1		98
	F–344/N	Osmolality	1905–2498	mOsm/kg	79
	F–344/N		1300–1900	mOsm/kg	98
	Sprague–Dawley		2686 ± 19	mOsm/kg (U max)	50
	Sprague–Dawley	Chloride	2.7 ± 0.4	mEq/24 hr	116
	NS		0.4–1.9	mEq/24 hr	3
	F–344/N		165.9 ± 30.8	mEq/L	98
	NS		96	mEq/L	3
	NS		0.9–8.2	mEq/kg/24 hr	3
	Sprague–Dawley		142–220	mEq/L	98

REPORTED URINE VALUES

Species	Strain	Variable	Value	Units	Reference
Rat (cont.)	Wistar (male)	Sodium	191.6 + 57.2	µEq/100g/d	112
	NS		0.2-1.9	mEq/24 hr	3
	Sprague-Dawley		2.4-0.4	mEq/24 hr	116
	Wistar (male)		22.8 + 8.8	mM/L	127
	F-344/N		143.0 + 27.6	mEq/L	98
	NS		90.4	mEq/L	3
	Sprague-Dawley		94-124	mEq/L	98
	Wistar		62 + 52	mEq/L	109
	Wistar (male)	Potassium	794.4 + 161.4	µEq/100g/d	112
	Sprague-Dawley		3.8 + 0.5	mEq/24 hr	116
	NS		0.4-1.9	mEq/24 hr	3
	Wistar (male)		165.0 + 94.8	mM/L	127
	F-344/N		357.0 + 65.1	mEq/L	98
	NS		190-260	mEq/L	3
	Sprague-Dawley		367-477	mEq/L	98
	Wistar		246.6 + 70.2	mEq/L	109
	F-344/N	Phosphorus	104.5 + 41.7	mg/dl	98
	NS		0.27-0.55	mEq/24 hr	3
	NS		0.8-3.6	mEq/kg/24 hr	3
	F-344/N (male)	Creatinine	3.1 + 0.12	mg/100g/24 hr	98
	F-344/N (female)		2.8 + 0.31	mg/100g/24 hr	98
	F-344/N	Glucose	10-30	mg/dl	65
	Wistar		negative		10
	F-344/N (male)		0.5 + 0.05	mg/100g/24 hr	98
	F-344/N (female)		0.6 + 0.06	mg/100g/24 hr	98

REPORTED URINE VALUES

Species	Strain	Variable	Value	Units	Reference
Rat (cont.)	Wistar (male)	Protein	5–20	mg/24 hr	126
	F-344/N		30–100	mg/dl	65
	F-344/N		100–400	mg/dl	65
	Wistar		30 ± 15	mg/dl	37
	F-344/N (males)		1.8 ± 0.68	mg/100g/24 hr	98
	F-344/N (females)		0.2 ± 0.07	mg/100g/24 hr	98
	Wistar (male)	Alkaline Phosphatase	59.0 ± 5.4	IU/24 hr	126
	Wistar		211 ± 25	mU/dl	97
	F-344/N		176 ± 23	U/hr	100
	F-344/N		263 ± 26	IU/L	65
	F-344/N (male)		358 ± 108	IU/L	35
	F-344/N (female)		171 ± 43	IU/L	35
	Wistar (male)	Lactic Dehydrogenase	186 ± 12	IU/24 hr	126
	F-344/N		573 ± 94	IU/L	65
	F-344/N (male)		99 ± 9	IU/L	35
	F-344/N (female)		63 ± 7	IU/L	35
	Wistar (male)	Leucine Amino-peptidase	1483 ± 153	IU/24 hr	126
	Wistar	Isocitric Dehydrogenase	51 ± 20	mU/24 hr	97
	Wistar		6.3 ± 1.4	mU/ml	97
	F-344/N	N-Actyl-Glucosaminase	125 ± 7	u/hr	100
	Wistar (male)	Acid Phosphatase	598 ± 49	IU/24 hr	126
	Wistar		15.5 ± 7.5	IU/hr	119

REPORTED URINE VALUES

Species	Strain	Variable	Value	Units	Reference
Rat (cont.)	Wistar (male)	Glutamic Oxaloacetic Transaminase	148 + 11	IU/24 hr	126
	Wistar		16-48	IU/ml	118
	F-344/N (male)		59 + 9	IU/L	35
	F-344/N (female)		62 + 20	IU/L	35
	F-344/N	Glutamic Pyruvic Transaminase	32 + 22	IU/L	65
	Wistar (male)	Gamma Glutamyl Transpeptidase	11490 + 630	IU/24 hr	126
	F-344/N (male)		4964 + 780	IU/L	35
	F-344/N (female)		1873 + 215	IU/L	35
	Wistar	Cholinesterase	132 + 17	mU/ml	97
	Wistar	Creatinine Clearance	7.2	ml/min/kg	37
	Wistar (male)	Inulin Clearance	857 + 263	ul/min/100g	117
	NS (female)		0.673 + 0.019	ml/min/100g	105
	Sprague-Dawley (male)		857 + 178	ul/min/100g	117
	Wistar (male)	PAH Clearance	1.341 + 0.129	ml/min/100g	51
	NS (female)		2.90 + 0.091	ml/min/100g	105
	Sprague-Dawley	Glomerular Filtration Rate	1236 + 27	ul/min/100g	50
	Sprague-Dawley		275 + 33	ul/min	38
	Wistar (male)	PSP Clearance	27 + 5	%	37
	Wistar (female)		37 + 7	%	37
	Wistar (male)	Urine Flow	4.8 + 0.6	ul/min/100g	117
	Sprague-Dawley (male)		5.2 + 2.0	ul/min/100g	117

REPORTED URINE VALUES

Species	Variable	Value	Units	Reference
Mouse	Volume	0.5-2.5	ml/24 hr	42
		0.5-2.5	ml/24 hr	55
		0.5-2.5	ml/24 hr	108
		3.7 + 1.70	ml/24 hr	98
	Specific Gravity	1.034 + 0.005		98
	pH	5.011		26
	Osmolality	1.06-2.63	Osm	42
		2300-3100	mOsm/kg	98
	Creatinine	0.57-0.67	mg/24 hr	42
		2.6 + 0.91	mg/100g/24 hr	98
	Glucose	1.98-3.09	mg/24 hr	42
		0.53 + 0.19	mg/24 hr	98
	Protein	6.8-25.8	mg/24 hr	42
		0.6-3.1	mg/24 hr	45
		3.21+1.05 (male)	mg/24 hr	98
		0.7+0.33 (female)	mg/24 hr	98
	Albumin	11.9 + 0.2	mg/ml	55
Dog	Volume	600 + 125	ml/24 hr	39,40
		596 + 34	ml/24 hr	101
		223 + 142	ml/24 hr	98
		20-167	ml/kg/24 hr	86

REPORTED URINE VALUES

Species	Variable	Value	Units	Reference
Dog (cont.)	Specific Gravity	1.026 + 0.003		39,40
		1.001 + 1.060		29
		1.036 + 0.014		98
		1.015-1.050		86
	pH	7.5 + 0.14		98
		6.0-7.0		86
	Osmolality	176-1292	mOsm/kg	14
		1550-1700	mOsm/kg	98
		2006 + 74	mOsm/kg (Umax)	101
		1322 + 544	mOsm/kg	98
	Chloride	0-222	mEq/24 hr	3
		0-10.2	mEq/kg/24 hr	3
		0-289	mEq/L	3
		28.5 + 12.0	mEq/24 hr	98
		5.0-15.0	mg/kg/24 hr	86
	Sodium	80-620	uM/kg/hr	14
		1-209	mEq/24 hr	3
		0.04-13	mEq/kg/24 hr	3
		2-189	mEq/L	3
		25.8 + 9.3	mEq/24 hr	98
		2-189	mg/kg/24 hr	86
	Potassium	30-630	uM/kg/hr	14
		3-128	mEq/24 hr	3
		0.1-2.4	mEq/kg/24 hr	3
		18-234	mEq/L	3
		25.5 + 9.0	mEq/24 hr	98
		40-100	mg/kg/24 hr	86

REPORTED URINE VALUES

Species	Variable	Value	Units	Reference
Dog (cont.)	Phosphorus	0–38	mEq/24 hr	3
		0–1.04	mEq/kg/24 hr	3
		0–120	mEq/L	3
		20–50	mg/kg/24 hr	86
	Creatinine	233 ± 68	mg/24 hr	98
		15–80	mg/kg/24 hr	86
	Glucose	negative		29
		18.7 ± 14.2	mg/24 hr	98
	Protein	117 ± 15	mg/24 hr	39,40
		200	mg/24 hr	29
		42.1 ± 29.1	mg/24 hr	98
		1.6–5.0	mg/kg/24 hr	86
	Alkaline Phosphatase	201 ± 31	uM/h/24 hr	39,40
		16.2 ± 13.0	IU/24 hr	98
	Lactic Dehydrogenase	12.6 ± 2.0	IU/24 hr	39,40
		19 ± 3	mU/ml	114
		5.7 ± 1.0	IU/hr	119
	β-Glucuronidase	5.0 ± 0.6	uM/h/24 hr	39,40
	N-Acetyl- β- Glucosaminase	33.8 ± 6.8	uM/h/24 hr	39,40
	β-D-Galactosidase	4.9 ± 0.3	uM/h/24 hr	39,40
	Acid Phosphatase	9.7 ± 1.8	uM/h/24 hr	39,40
		1.02 ± 0.56	IU/24 hr	98

REPORTED URINE VALUES

Species	Variable	Value	Units	Reference
Dog (cont.)	Glutamic Oxaloacetic Transaminase	2.2 + 0.4 0.5 + 0.2	mU/ml IU/24 hr	114 98
	Glutamic Pyruvic Transaminase	1.23 + 1.21	IU/24 hr	98
	Creatinine Clearance	3.26 + 0.39 2.8-3.7 66 + 5 2.98 + 0.96 3.7 + 0.77	ml/min/kg ml/min/kg ml/min ml/min/kg ml/min/kg	39,40 29 101 44 15
	Inulin Clearance	3.89 + 0.42 41.8 + 13.9	ml/min/kg ml/min/m^2	39,40 15
	PAH Clearance	8.8 + 1.0 6.6 14-173	ml/min/kg ml/min/kg ml/min	39,40 12 90
	Glomerular Filtration Rate	234 + 16.4 60.2 + 7.8	ml/kg/hr ml/min/m^2	107 15
	Urine Flow Rate	0.4 + 0.1 3.5-9.9	ml/min ml/kg/hr	114 14
	PSP Clearance	43.8 + 11.1	%	44

REPORTED URINE VALUES

Species	Variable	Value	Units	Reference
Cat	Volume	10–30	ml/kg/24 hr	86
	Specific Gravity	1.062 + 1.019		92
		1.001–1.080		29
		1.018–1.040		23
		1.020–1.045		86
	pH	5.5–8.0		29
		5–7		23
		6.0–7.0		86
	Chloride	89–130	mg/kg/24 hr	86
	Potassium	55–120	mg/kg/24 hr	86
	Phosphorus	39–62	mg/kg/24 hr	86
	Creatinine	12–30	mg/kg/24 hr	86
	Glucose	less than 0.1	%	23
	Protein	30–300	mg/dl	92
		3.1–6.8	mg/kg/24 hr	86
	Albumin	less than 10	mg/dl	23
Rabbit	Volume	20–350	ml/kg/24 hr	86
	Specific Gravity	1.003–1.036		86
	pH	7.6–8.8		86

REPORTED URINE VALUES

Species	Variable	Value	Units	Reference
Rabbit (cont.)	Chloride	3.4–94	mEq/L	3
		0.1–1.4	mEq/kg/24 hr	3
		190–300	mg/kg/24 hr	86
	Sodium	60	mEq/L	3
		50–70	mg/kg/24 hr	86
	Potassium	40–55	mg/kg/24 hr	86
	Phosphorus	1.5–6.9	mEq/24 hr	3
		0.3–1.3	mEq/kg/24 hr	3
		10–60	mg/kg/24 hr	86
	Creatinine	20–80	mg/kg/24 hr	86
	Protein	0.7–1.9	mg/kg/24 hr	86
	β-2 Microglobulins	19–221	ug/100g creatinine	96

References

1.   Allen JR, Carstens LA (1968) Veno-occlusive disease in rhesus monkeys. Am J Vet Res 29: 1681-1694

2.   Altland PD, Brubach HF, Parker MG, Highman B (1967) Blood gases and acid-base values of unanesthetized rats exposed to hypoxia. Am J Physiol 212: 142-148

3.   Altman PL, Dittmer DS (1968) Biological handbook of metabolism. Fed Am Soc Exp Biol Med, Bethesda, p 523

4.   Altshuler HL, Stowell RE, Lowe RT (1971) Normal serum biochemical values of Macaca arctoides, Macaca fascicularis and Macaca radiata. Lab An Sci 21: 916-926

5.   Altshuler HL, Stowell RE (1972) Normal serum biochemical values of Cercopithecus aethiops, Cercocebus atys and Presbytis entellus. Lab An Sci 22: 692-704

6.   Anderson DR (1966) Normal values for clinical blood chemistry tests of the Macaca mulatta monkey. Am J Vet Res 27: 1484-1489

7.   Astrup P (1961) A new approach to acid-base metabolism. Clin Chem 7: 1-15

8.   Bar-Ilan A, Marder J (1980) Acid base status in unanesthetized, unrestrained guinea pigs. Pflugers Arch 384: 93-97

9.   Beland MF, Sehgal PK, Peacock WC (1979) Baseline blood chemistry determinations in the squirrel monkey (Saimiri sciureus). Lab An Sci 29: 195

10. Belazs T, Hatch A, Zawidzka Z, Grice HC (1963) Renal tests in toxicity studies on rats. Toxicol Appl Pharmacol 5: 661-674

11. Benjamin MM, McKelvie DH (1978) Clinical biochemistry. In Benirschke, K, Garney FM, Jones TC (eds). Pathology of Laboratory Animals. New York, Springer Verlag, pp 1750-1815

12. Binnion PF, Cumming JK (1967) A study of ^{131} I-Hippuran excretion in dogs as a measure of renal plasma flow. Clin Sci 33: 313-318

13. Bonasch H, Cornelius CE (1964) Indocyanine green clearance — A liver function test for the dog. Am J Vet Res 25: 254-259

14. Borrensen HC, Rorvik S, Guldvog I, Aakvaag A (1982) Angiotensin II and renal excretion of sodium and potassium in unanesthetized dogs. Scand J Clin Lab Invest 42: 87-92

15. Bovee BC, Joyce T (1979) Clinical evaluation of glomerular function: 24-hour creatinine clearance in dogs. JAVMA 174: 488-491

16. Boyd EM (1942) Species variation in normal plasma lipids estimated by oxidative micromethods. J Biol Chem 143: 131-132

17. Brauer RW, Pessotti RL (1949) The removal of bromosulphthalein from blood plasma by the liver of the rat. J Pharmacol Exp Ther 97: 358-370

18. Brooks FP, Deneau GA, Potter HP Jr, Reinhold JG, Norris RG (1963) Liver function tests in morphine-addicted and in non-addicted rhesus monkeys. Gastroenterology 44: 287-290

19. Burlington RF, Maher JT, Sidel CM (1969) Effect of hypoxia on blood gases, acid-base balance and in vitro myocardial function in a hibernator and a non-hibernator. Fed Proc 28: 1042-1046

20. Burns KF, Ferguson FG, Hampton SH (1967) Compendium of normal blood values for baboons, chimpanzees and marmosets. Am J Clin Pathol 48: 484

21.   Carlson EC Personal communication

22.   Casals J, Olitsky PK (1946) Tests for hepatic dysfunction of mice.
      Proc Soc Exp Biol Med 63: 383-390

23.   Catcott EJ (1964) Feline Medicine and Surgery. American Veterinary
      Publications, Santa Barbara

24.   Center SA, Bunch SE, Baldwin BH, Hornbuckle WE, Tennant BC (1983)
      Comparison of sulfobromophthalein and indocyanine green
      clearances in the dog. Am J Vet Res 44: 722-726

25.   Center SA, Bunch SE, Baldwin BH, Hornbuckle WE, Tennant BC (1983)
      Comparison of sulfobromophthalein and indocyanine green
      clearance in the cat. Am J Vet Res 44: 727-730

26.   Charles River Digest (1971) Some physiological parameters of small
      animals, vol 10, pp 1-4

27.   Charles River Technical Bulletin (1984) vol 3, No 2

28.   Cornelius CE, Holm LW, Jasper DE (1958) Bromsulphalein clearance in
      normal sheep and in pregnancy toxemia. Cornell Vet 48: 305-312

29.   Cowgill LD (1983) Diseases of the kidney. In Ettinger SJ (ed), Textbook
      of Veterinary Internal Medicine. W B Saunders, Philadelphia

30.   Cutler MG (1974) The sensitivity of function tests in detecting liver
      damage in the rat. Toxicol Appl Pharmacol 28: 349-357

31.   de la Pena A, Goldzieher JW (1967) Clinical parameters of the normal
      baboon. Baboon Med Res 2: 379-389

32.   Deinhardt F, Courtois G, Dherte P, Osterrieth P, Ninane G, Henle G,
      Henle W (1962) Studies of liver function tests in chimpanzees
      after inoculation with human infectious hepatitis virus. Am J Hyg
      75: 311-321

33. Deinhardt F, Holmes AW, Capps RB, Popper H (1967) Studies on the transmission of human viral hepatitis to marmoset monkeys. I. Transmission of disease serial passages, and description of liver lesions. J Exp Med 125: 673-688

34. Dent NJ (1977) In Duncan WA, Leonard BJ (eds). Clinical Toxicology, Exerpta Medica XVIII, Amsterdam

35. Dieter MP, Powers MB, Riley JH, Thorstenson JH, Uriah LC (1984) Utilization of urinary enzyme assays to monitor renal toxicity in Fischer 344 rats after prolonged mercuric chloride treatment. Toxicologist 4: 119

36. Duncan JR, Prasse KW (1977) Veterinary Laboratory Medicine, Clinical Pathology, Iowa State University Press, Ames, Iowa

37. Edwards KDG, Curtis EA, Stoker LM (1971) One-day renal function testing in normal rats and in cases of experimentally-induced analgesic nephropathy, nephrocalcinosis and nephrotic syndrome. Nephron 8: 235-245

38. Eknoyan G, Bulger RE, Dobyan DC (1982) Mercuric chloride-induced acute renal failure in the rat. Lab Invest 46: 613-620

39. Ellis BG, Price RG, Topham JC (1973) The effect of tubular damage by mercuric chloride on kidney function and some urinary enzymes in the dog. Chem Biol Interactions 7: 101-113

40. Ellis BG, Price RG, Topham JC (1973) The effect of papillary damage by ethyleneimine on kidney function and some urinary enzymes in the dog. Chem Biol Interactions 7: 131-142

41. Evans AS, Evans BK, Sturtz V (1953) Standards for hepatic and hematologic tests in monkeys. Observations during experiments with hepatitis and mononucleosis. Proc Soc Exp Biol NY 82: 437–440

42. Everett RM, Harrison SD Jr (1983) Clinical biochemistry. In Foster HL, Small JD, Fox JG (eds), The Mouse in Biomedical Research, vol III. Academic Press, New York, pp 313–325,

43. Finch CE, Foster JR (1973) Hematologic and serum electrolyte values of the $C_{57}BL/6J$ male mouse in maturity and senescence. Lab An Sci 23: 339–349

44. Finco DR (1980) Kidney function. In Kaneko JJ (ed), Clinical Biochemistry of Domestic Animals, Academic Press, New York, p 367

45. Finlayson JS, Baumann CA (1958) Mouse proteinuria. Am J Physiol 192: 69–72

46. Fox RR, Laird CW, Blau EM, Schultz HS, Mitchel BP (1970) Biochemical Parameters of Clinical Significance in Rabbits. I. Strain Variations. J Hered 61: 261–265

47. Fox RR, Laird CW, Kirshenbaum J (1974) Effects of strain, sex and circadian rhythm on rabbit serum bilirubin and iron levels. Proc Soc Exp Biol Med 145: 421–427

48. Gartner LM, Arias IM (1969) The transfer of bilirubin from blood to bile in the neonatal guinea pig. Pediat Res 3: 171–180

49 Gartner LM, Lane DL, Cornelius CE (1971) Bilirubin transport by liver in adult Macaca mulatta. Am J Physiol 220: 1528–1535

50. Gobe GC, Axalson RA (1983) Effects of indomethacin on renal concentrating capacity of lithium-treated rats. Res Comm Chem Pathol Pharmacol 39: 11-28

51. Grosman ME, Elias MM, Comin EJ, Garay EAR (1983) Alterations in renal function induced by aflatoxin B in the rat. Toxicol Appl Pharmacol 69: 319-325

52. Hallesy D, Benitz KF (1963) Sulfobromophthalein sodium retention and morphological liver damage in dogs. Toxicol Appl Pharmacol 5: 650-660

53. Hoe C (1969) Liver function tests. In Medway W, Prier JE, Wilkinson JS, (eds), Textbook of Veterinary Clinical Pathology, Chpt 3. Williams & Wilkins, Baltimore

54. Hoerlein BF, Green JE (1950) The bromsulfalein liver function test as an aid in the diagnosis of canine hepatosis. N Am Vet 31: 662-665

55. Hoffsten PE, Hill CL, Klahr S (1975) Studies of albuminuria and proteinuria in normal mice and mice with immune complex glomerulonephritis. J Lab Clin Med 86: 920-930

56. Holmes AW, Passovoy M, Capps RB (1967) Marmosets as laboratory animals. III. Blood chemistry of laboratory-kept marmosets with particular attention to liver function and structure. Lab An Care 17:41-47

57. Hunton DB, Bollman JL, Hoffman HN, II (1960) Hepatic removal of indocyanine green. Proc Staff Meet Mayo Clin 35: 752-755

58. Joe M, Teasdale JM, Miller JR (1962) A new mutation (sph) causing neonatal jaundice in the house mouse. Can J Genet Cytol 4: 219-225

59. Kaczmarczyk G, Reinhardt HW (1975) Arterial blood gas tensions and
     acid-base status of wistar rats during thiopental and halothane
     anesthesia. Lab An Sci 25: 184-190

60. Kastello M Personal communication

61. Katz S, Gilardoni A, Genovese N, Wikinski RW, Cornelius CE, Malinow
     MR (1968) Liver function studies in free ranging howler monkeys
     with hepatic pigmentation. Lab An Care 18: 626-630

62. Ketterer SG, Weigand BD, Rapoport E (1960) Hepatic uptake and biliary
     excretion of indocyanine green and its use in estimation of
     hepatic blood flow in dogs. Am J Physiol 199: 481-484

63. Klaassen CD, Plaa GL (1967) Species variation in metabolism, storage
     and excretion of sulfobromophthalein. Am J Physiol 213:
     1322-1326

64. Klaassen CD, Plaa GL (1969) Plasma disappearance and biliary
     excretion of indocyanine green in rats, rabbits and dogs.
     Toxicol Appl Pharmacol 15: 374-384

65. Kluwe WM (1981) Renal function tests as indicators of kidney injury in
     subacute toxicity studies. Toxicol Appl Pharmacol 57: 414-424

66. Kozma C, Macklin W, Cummins LM, Mauer R (1974) In: Weisbroth
     SH, Flatt RE, Kraus AL (eds).   The Biology of the Laboratory
     Rabbit. Academic Press, New York

67. Krasavage WJ, Michaelson SM (1965) Indocyanine green-plasma half
     time clearance (T1/2) in normal beagles. Soc Exp Biol Med Proc
     119: 215-218

68. Laird CW (1972) Representative values for animal and veterinary
     populations and their clinical significances. Hycel, Inc., Houston.

69. Laird CW, Fox RR, Schultz HS, Mitchell BP, Blau EM (1970) Strain variation in rabbits: Biochemical indicators of thyroid function. Life Sci 9: 203-214

70. Larson EJ, Morrill CC (1960) Evaluation of the bromsulfophthalein liver function test in the dog. Am J Vet Res 21: 949

71. Levi AJ, Gatmaitan Z, Arias IM (1970) Deficiency of hepatic organic anion-binding protein impaired organic anion uptake by the liver and "physiologic" jaundice in newborn monkeys. N Engl J Med 283: 1136-1139

72. Lewis LD, Ponten U, Seisjo BK (1973) Arterial acid-base change in unanesthetized rat in acute hypoxia. Resp Physiol 19: 311-321

73. Libermann IM, Capano A, Gonzalez F, Brazzuna H, Garcia H, DeGelabert AG (1973) Blood acid-base status in normal albino rats. Lab An Sci 23: 862-865

74. Linder GC, Parker RFG, Selzer G (1953) Bromosulphthalein retention in young rats on diets producing liver necrosis. Br J Exp Pathol 34: 656-660

75. Loeb W Personal communication

76. Mani KV, Weinstein SA (1966) Effect of carbonic anhydrase inhibition on blood gas and acid-base balance during hypoxia. Bull Johns Hopkins Hosp 119: 331-343

77. Manning PJ, Lehner NDM, Feldner MA, Bullock BC (1969) Selected hematologic serum chemical and arterial blood gas characteristics of squirrel monkeys (Saimiri sciureus). Lab An Care 19:381

78. Marder J, Bar-Ilan A (1975) Acid-base metabolism in the albino rat during hypercapnia. Physiol Zool 48: 282-289

79. Maronpot RR Personal communication

80. Maschgan ER (1980) Clinical data for gorillas, orangutans and
    chimpanzees at the Lincoln Park Zoological Gardens. Lincoln Park
    Zoological Gardens, Chicago, IL

81. Maxwell KO, Wish C, Murphy JC, Fox JG (1985) Serum chemistry
    reference values in two strains of syrian hamsters.
    Lab An Sci 35:67–70

82. McClure HM, Keeling ME, Guilloud NB (1972) Hematologic and blood
    chemistry data for the chimpanzee (Pan troglodytes). Folia
    Primatol 18:444

83. McClure HM, Keeling ME, Guilloud NB (1972) Hematologic and blood
    chemistry data for the gorilla (Gorilla gorilla). Folia Primatol
    18: 300

84. McClure HM, Keeling ME, Guillard NB (1972) Hematologic and blood
    chemistry data for the orangutan (Pongo pygmaeus). Folia
    Primatal 18:284

85. Minette HP, Shaffer MF (1968) Experimental leptospirosis in monkeys.
    Am Soc Trop Med Hyg 17: 202–212

86. Mitruka BM, Rawnsley HM (1977) Clinical biochemical and
    hematological reference values in normal experimental
    animals. Masson Publishing USA, Inc., New York

87. New AE (1968) The Squirrel Monkey. Academic Press, New York,
    pp 418–419

88. O'Brien JJ Jr, Lucey EC, Snider GL (1979) Arterial blood gases
    in normal hamsters at rest and during exercise. J Appl Physiol 46:
    806–810

89. Odell GB, Natzschka JC, Storey B (1966) Bilirubin in the liver and kidney in jaundiced rats. Am J Dis Child 112: 351-358

90. Oester A, Wolf H, Madsen PO (1969) Measurement of glomerular filtration rate using ^{131}I-diatriazoate. Lancet 1: 397-399

91. Oser FO, Lang RE, Vogin EE (1970) Blood values in stumptailed macaques (M. arctoides) under laboratory conditions. Lab An Care 20: 462-466

92. Palmore WP, Gaskin IM, Nielson JT (1978) Effects of diet on feline urine. Lab An Sci 28: 551-555

93. Parker P Personal communication

94. Pepelko WE, Dixon GA (1975) Arterial blood gases in conscious rats exposed to hypoxia, hypercapnia or both. J Appl Physiol 38: 581-587

95. Petery JJ (1967) Ultramicroanalysis of selected blood components of normal Macaca mulatta. Lab An Care 17: 342-344

96. Piscator M, Bjorek L, Nordberg M (1981) β_2-Microglobulin levels in serum and urine of cadmium exposed rabbits. Acta Pharmacol Toxicol 49: 1-7

97. Raab WP (1972) Diagnostic value of urinary enzyme determinations. Clin Chem 18: 5-25

98. Ragan HA, Apley GA, Sweeney JK, Debban KH Unpublished data

99. Rossoff IS (1974) Handbook of Veterinary Drugs. Soringer Publishing Co, New York

100. Rush GF, Smith JH, Newton JF, Hook JB (1984) Chemically induced nephrotoxicity: Role of metabolic activation. CRC Crit Rev Toxicol 13: 99-160

101. Rutecki GW, Cox JW, Robertson GW, Francisco LL, Ferris TF (1982) Urinary concentrating ability and diuretic hormone responsiveness in the potassium depleted dog. J Lab Clin Med 100: 53-60

102. Schaefer RE, Messier AA, Morgan C, Baker GT (1975) Effect of chronic hypercapnia on body temperature regulation. J Appl Physiol 38: 900-905

103. Schmid R, Axelrod J, Hammaker L, Swarm RL (1958) Congenital jaundice in rats due to a defect in glucuronide formation. J Clin Invest 37:1123-1130

104. Schtacher G (1969) Selective renal involvement in the early development of hypercalcemia and hypophosphatemia in vx-2 carcinoma bearing rabbits: studies on serum and tissue alkaline phosphatase and renal handling of phosphorus. Cancer Res 29: 1512-1528

105. Sharratt M, Frazer AC (1963) The sensitivity of function tests in detecting renal damage in the rat. Toxicol Appl Pharmacol 5: 36-48

106. Simmons DH, Kahn FH, Guze LB (1966) Blood gases of rats at altitude and sea level. Fed Proc 25: 1247-1252

107. Singhvi SM, Heald AF, Murphy BF, DiFazio LT, Schreiber EC, Poutsiaka JW (1978) Disposition of [14]Nadolol in dogs with reversible renal impairment induced by uranyl nitrate. Toxicol Appl Pharmacol 43: 99-109

108. Smith CR, Felton JS, Taylor RT (1981) Description of a disposable individual-mouse urine collection apparatus. Lab An Sci 31: 80-82

109. Sophansan S, Sorrasuchart S (1984) Factors inducing post-obstructive diuresis in rats. Nephron 38: 125-133

110. Strombeck DR, Qualls C (1978) Hepatic sulfobromophthalein uptake and storage defect in a dog. J Am Vet Med Assoc 172:1423-1426

111. Strozier LM, Blair CB, Evans BH (1971) Armadillos I. Serum chemistry values. Lab An Sci 21: 399-400

112. Suketa Y, Kawahara M, Sahashi K, Suzuki N, Akiyama Y (1983) A role of renal k-stimulated phosphatase activity on elevation of urinary sodium excretion in fluoride-treated rats. Toxicol Appl Pharmacol 69: 225-233

113. Svirbely JL, Monaco AA, Alford WC (1946) The comparative efficiency of various liver function tests in detecting hepatic damage produced in dogs by xylidine. J Lab Clin Med 31: 1133

114. Talner LB, Rushmer HN, Coel MN (1972) The effect of renal artery injection of contrast material on urinary enzyme excretion. Invest Radiol 7: 311-322

115. Thomas RG, London JE, Drake GA, Jackson DE, Wilson JS, Smith DM (1979) The Golden Hamster — Quantitative Anatomy with Age. Los Almos Scientific Laboratory, University of California.

116. Thompson JH, Lee YH, Campbell LB (1966) Urinary electrolyte excretion in the young rat. Am J Vet Res 27: 1093-1098

117. Thomsen K, Olesen OV (1981) Effect of anesthesia and surgery on urine flow and electrolyte excretion in different rat strains. Renal Physiol 4: 165-172

118. Timmons EH, Marques PA (1969) Blood chemical and hematological studies in laboratory confined unanesthetized opossum (Didelphis virginiana). Lab An Care 19: 342-344

119. Tsuzuki Y (1981) Urinary enzymes as indicators of kidney damage by
        methylmercury exposure. Bull Environ Contam Toxicol 27: 55-58

120. Van Hoosier GL Personal communication

121. Van Vleet JF, Albert JO (1968) Evaluation of liver function test and
        liver biopsy in experimental carbon tetrachloride intoxication and
        extrahepatic bile duct obstruction in the dog. Am J Vet Res
        29: 2119-2131

122. Verlangieri AJ, De Priest JC, Kapeghian JC (1985) Normal serum
        biochemical, hematological and EKG parameters in anesthetized
        adult male Macaca fascicularis and Macaca arctoides.
        Lab An Sci 35: 63-66

123. Vogin EE, Scott W, Mattis PA (1965) Hepatic clearance of indocyanine
        green in the beagle. Proc Soc Exp Biol Med 119: 570-573

124. Vogin EE, Moreno OM, Brodie DA, Mattis PA (1966) Indocyanine green
        clearances in the rhesus monkey (Macaca mulatta).
        J Appl Physiol 21: 1880-1882

125. Wakeman AM, Morrell CA (1932) Chemistry and metabolism in
        experimental yellow fever in Macaca rhesus monkeys.
        Arch Intern Med 50: 826-833

126. Watanabe M, Nomura G, Hirata H, Imai K, Koizumi H (1980) Studies on
        the validity of urine enzyme assay in the diagnosis of
        drug-induced renal lesions in rats. Toxicol Pathol 8: 22-33

127. Weiner RN, Reinacher M (1982) Lower nephron toxicity of a highly
        purified cytotoxin from Pseudomonas aeruginosa in rats.
        Exp Mol Pathol 37: 249-271

128. Wellde BT, Johnson AJ, Williams JS, Langhehn HR, Sadun EH
(1971) Hemotologic, biochemical parasitologic parameters of the
night monkey (Aotus trivirgatus). Lab An Sci 21: 575

129. Westerman MP, Wiggins RG III, Mao R (1970) Anemia and
hypercholesterolemia in cholesterol-fed rabbits. J Lab Clin Med
75: 893-902

130. Williams JS, Meroney FC, Hutt G, Sadun EH (1966) Serum chemical
components in mice determined by the use of ultra micro
techniques. J Appl Physiol 21: 1026-1030

131. Wisecup WG, Hodson HH, Hanly WC, Felts PE (1969) Baseline blood
levels of the chimpanzee (Pan troglodytes). Liver function tests.
Am J Vet Res 30: 955-962

132. Yarborough LW, Tollett JL, Montrey RD, Beattie RJ (1984) Serum
biochemical, hematological and body measurement data for
common marmosets (Callithrix jacchus jacchus). Lab An Sci
34: 276-280

133. Yu H, Yanagisawa Y, Forbes MA, Cooper EH, Crockson RA,
MacLennan ICM (1983) Alpha-1-Microglobulin: An indicator
protein for renal tubular function. J Clin Pathol 36: 253-259

Index